Lung Cancer
Volume 1

METHODS IN MOLECULAR MEDICINE™

John M. Walker, Series Editor

METHODS IN MOLECULAR MEDICINE

Lung Cancer

Volume 1:
Molecular Pathology
Methods and Reviews

Edited by

Barbara Driscoll, PhD

Children's Hospital,
Los Angeles, CA

Springer Science+Business Media, LLC

www.humanapress.com

All papers, comments, opinions, conclusions, or recommendations are those of the author(s), and do not necessarily reflect the views of the publisher.

This publication is printed on acid-free paper. ∞
ANSI Z39.48-1984 (American Standards Institute) Permanence of Paper for Printed Library Materials.

Cover design by Patricia F. Cleary.

Cover illustration: Figure 1B from Volume 1, Chapter 2/Clinical and Biological Relevance of Recently Defined Categories of Pulmonary Neoplasia by E. Gabrielson.

Production Editor: Mark J. Breaugh.

For additional copies, pricing for bulk purchases, and/or information about other Humana titles, contact Humana at the above address or at any of the following numbers: Tel.: 973-256-1699; Fax: 973-256-8341; E-mail: humana@humanapr.com; Website: http://humanapress.com

Photocopy Authorization Policy:

Library of Congress Cataloging in Publication Data

Main entry under title: Methods in molecular medicine™.

Lung cancer / edited by Barbara Driscoll.
    p. ; cm. -- (Methods in molecular medicine ; 74-75)
  Includes bibliographical references and index.
  Contents: v. 1. Molecular pathology methods and reviews -- v. 2. Diagnostic and therapeutic methods and reviews.
  ISBN 978-1-4899-3912-8   ISBN 978-1-59259-323-1 (eBook)
  DOI 10.1007/978-1-59259-323-1
  1. Lungs--Cancer--Molecular aspects--Laboratory manuals. 2. Lungs--Cancer--Gene therapy--Laboratory manuals. 3. Molecular diagnosis--Laboratory manuals. 4. Tumor markers--Laboratory manuals. I. Driscoll, Barbara. II. Series.
  [DNLM: 1. Lung neoplasms--physiopathology. 2. Lung Neoplasms--diagnosis. 3. Lung Neoplasms--therapy. 4. Molecular Biology--methods. WF 658 L96062 2002]
  RC280.L8 L76532 2002
  616.99'424--dc21
                                                                    2002024050

Preface

The *Methods in Molecular Medicine* series is intended as a resource for both novice and experienced investigators attempting to diversify their technological base in research. *Lung Cancer: Volume 1: Molecular Pathology Methods and Reviews* presents an overview of the current status of assays employed to detect and characterize the multitude of pathologies that contribute to the development of this deadly disease.

As with all volumes in the *Methods in Molecular Medicine* series, the reader should find that each methods-based chapter provides clear instructions for the performance of various protocols, supplemented by additional technical notes that provide valuable insight. These notes are designed to enable the reader to acquire the techniques described with a proficiency not easily achieved by reading standard method formats.

No volume can exhaustively cover every aspect of biological research and there will be gaps in this endeavor that one or another research group will identify. Each section herein could readily be expanded into a book in its own right. However, I have sought to include a spectrum of techniques that should allow for the acquisition of key skills in each area covered.

It is my hope that the reviews and methods in *Lung Cancer, vol. 1*, describing investigation into the etiology and classification of lung cancers based on molecular analysis of abnormalities, will provide an overview of the complex disease faced daily by those who diagnose and treat patients suffering from this cancer. In addition, the section on model systems for analysis of both development of lung tumors and the testing of novel methods for their treatment, should prove particularly useful to those determined to translate basic research from the laboratory to the clinic.

I would like to express my gratitude to all those who have contributed to this volume and who have been patient over the period required to collate such a work. I am grateful to Professor John Walker for his encouragement and guidance as series editor.

This volume is dedicated with gratitude to my parents, Charles W. Driscoll and Barbara A. Driscoll, for their unflagging love and support.

Barbara Driscoll, PhD

Contents

Lung Cancer

Volume II: Diagnostic and Therapeutic Methods and Reviews

Contributors

BRUCE C. BAGULEY • *Faculty of Medicine and Health Science, Auckland Cancer Society Research Centre, University of Auckland, New Zealand*

SIPRA BANERJEE • *Department of Cancer Biology, Lerner Research Institute, The Cleveland Clinic Foundation, Cleveland, OH*

DAVID G. BEER • *Section of General Thoracic Surgery, Department of Surgery, University of Michigan Medical School, Ann Arbor, MI*

NANDAN BHATTACHARYYA • *Department of Cancer Biology, Lerner Research Institute, The Cleveland Clinic Foundation, Cleveland, OH*

DAVID L. CHEO • *Life Technologies Division, Invitrogen Corporation, Rockville, MD*

TIMOTHY I. CHRISTMAS • *Respiratory Unit, Green Lane Hospital, Auckland, New Zealand*

J. JOHN COHEN • *Department of Immunology, University of Colorado Medical School, Denver, CO*

CARRIE M. COLEMAN • *Division of Endocrinology and Diabetes, The Children's Hospital of Philadelphia, Philadelphia, PA*

JUDY M. COULSON • *Departments of Physiology and Human Anatomy, University of Liverpool, Liverpool, UK*

LLOYD A. CULP • *Department of Molecular Biology and Microbiology, School of Medicine, Case Western Reserve University, Cleveland, OH*

DAVID DINSDALE • *MRC Toxicology Unit, Leicester, UK*

LORI D. DWYER-NIELD • *Department of Pharmaceutical Sciences, School of Pharmacy, University of Colorado Health Sciences Center, Denver, CO*

ARMANDO E. FRAIRE • *Department of Pathology, University of Massachusetts Memorial Medical Center, Worcester, MA*

ERROL C. FRIEDBERG • *Laboratory of Molecular Pathology, Department of Pathology, University of Texas Southwestern Medical Center, Dallas, TX*

EDWARD GABRIELSON • *Departments of Pathology and Oncology, The Johns Hopkins University School of Medicine; Department of Environmental Health Sciences, The Johns Hopkins University School of Public Health, Baltimore, MD*

ADI F. GAZDAR • *Department of Pathology, The Hamon Center for Therapeutic Oncology Research, University of Texas Southwestern Medical Center, Dallas, TX*

JOSEPH GERADTS • *Department of Pathology and Laboratory Medicine, Roswell Park Cancer Institute, Buffalo, NY*

ALEXANDRA GIATROMANOLAKI • *Department of Radiotherapy & Oncology, Laboratory of Pathology, Democritus University of Thrace, Alexandroupolis, Greece*

JONATHAN GODDARD • *University Department of Oncology, Leicester Royal Infirmary, Leicester, UK*

ADDA GRIMBERG • *The Joseph Stokes, Jr. Research Institute of the Children's Hospital of Philadelphia, The University of Pennsylvania School of Medicine, Philadelphia, PA*

LESLIE-ANN M. HALL • *Incyte Genomics, Newark, DE*

ROY S. HERBST • *Department of Thoracic/Head and Neck Medical Oncology, M. D. Anderson Cancer Center, Houston, TX*

EISO HIYAMA • *Department of General Medicine, School of Medicine, Hiroshima University, Hiroshima, Japan*

KEIKO HIYAMA • *The Second Department of Internal Medicine, School of Medicine, Hiroshima University, Hiroshima, Japan*

ROBERT M. HOFFMAN • *AntiCancer Inc., San Diego, CA*

JULIANNE L. HOLLERAN • *Department of Molecular Biology and Microbiology, Case Western Reserve University, School of Medicine, Cleveland, OH*

DAVID M. JABLONS • *Thoracic Oncology Program, University of California San Francisco/Mount Zion Medical Center, San Francisco, CA*

SONIA B. JAKOWLEW • *Cell and Cancer Biology Branch, National Cancer Institute, Rockville, MD*

KRISTIINA JÄRVINEN • *Finnish Institute of Occupational Health, Helsinki, Finland*

SHU-FANG JIA • *Division of Pediatrics, The University of Texas M. D. Anderson Cancer Center, Houston, TX*

ZHONG JIANG • *Department of Pathology, University of Massachusetts Memorial Medical Center, Worcester, MA*

KUSHAGRA KATARIYA • *Division of Cardiothoracic Surgery, University of Miami School of Medicine, Miami, FL*

JANET S. KERR • *Bristol-Myers Squibb Company, Experimental Station, Wilmington, DE*

MICHAEL KERSTING • *GATC Biotech AG, Konstanz, Germany*

TAKASHI KIJIMA • *Department of Adult Oncology, Dana-Farber Cancer Institute, and Department of Medicine, Brigham and Women's Hospital and Harvard Medical School, Boston, MA*

VUOKKO L. KINNULA • *Department of Internal Medicine, University of Oulu, Oulu, Finland*

EUGENIE S. KLEINERMAN • *Division of Pediatrics, The University of Texas M. D. Anderson Cancer Center, Houston, TX*

NANETTE KLEINMAN • *Animal Resource Center, Case Western Reserve University, School of Medicine, Cleveland, OH*

REET KOOMÄGI • *Department of Oncological Diagnostics and Therapy, German Cancer Research Center, Heidelberg, Germany*

PATRICK P. KOTY • *Department of Environmental and Occupational Health, Graduate School of Public Health, University of Pittsburgh, Pittsburgh, PA*

MICHAEL I. KOUKOURAKIS • *Department of Radiotherapy & Oncology, Laboratory of Pathology, Democritus University of Thrace, Alexandroupolis, Greece*

CANDICE M. KRAUTHAUSER • *Bristol-Myers Squibb Company, Wilmington, DE*

TERESA A. LEHMAN • *BioServe Biotechnologies Ltd., Laurel, MD*

WENDONG LEI • *Cancer Institute and Hospital, Chinese Academy of Medical Sciences and Peking Union Medical College, Beijing, China*

MARK L. LEVITT • *Department of Environmental and Occupational Health, Graduate School of Public Health, University of Pittsburgh, Pittsburgh, PA; Sheba Medical Center, Institute of Oncology, Tel Hashomer, Israel*

MELISSA LIM • *Thoracic Oncology Program, University of California San Francisco/Mount Zion Medical Center, San Francisco, CA*

WEN-CHANG LIN • *Institute of Biomedical Sciences, Academia Sinica, Taipei, Taiwan*

ALISON MACKINNON • *Rayne Laboratory, Centre for Inflammation Research, Respiratory Medicine Unit, University of Edinburgh Medical School, Edinburgh, UK*

ALVIN M. MALKINSON • *Department of Pharmaceutical Sciences, School of Pharmacy, University of Colorado Health Sciences Center, Denver, CO*

THOMAS H. MARCH • *Lovelace Respiratory Research Institute, Albuquerque, NM*

JENNIFER MARIANO • *Cell and Cancer Biology Branch, National Cancer Institute, Rockville, MD*

ELAINE S. MARSHALL • *Auckland Cancer Society Research Centre, Faculty of Medicine and Health Science, University of Auckland, Auckland, New Zealand*

ALFREDO MARTÍNEZ • *Intervention Section, Department of Cell and Cancer Biology, National Cancer Institute, National Institutes of Health, Bethesda, MD*

GAUTAM MAULIK • *Department of Adult Oncology, Dana-Farber Cancer Institute; Department of Medicine, Brigham and Women's Hospital and Harvard Medical School, Boston, MA*

CIRO MENDOZA • *INERAM (National Institute of Pulmonary and Enviromental Diseases), Venezuela y Sol, Asuncion, Paraguay*

CARSON J. MILLER • *Department of Molecular Biology and Microbiology, School of Medicine, Case Western Reserve University, Cleveland, OH*

RAMA MODALI • *BioServe Biotechnologies Ltd., Laurel, MD*

MARSHA A. MOSES • *Laboratory of Surgical Research, Department of Surgery, The Children's Hospital and Harvard Medical School, Boston, MA*

JAMES L. MULSHINE • *Department of Cell and Cancer Biology, Intervention Section, National Cancer Institute, National Institutes of Health, Bethesda, MD*

YOSHIHIRO NAMBU • *Department of Internal Medicine, Division of Respiratory Diseases, Kanazawa Medical University, Ishikawa, Japan*

BARRY D. NELKIN • *The Oncology Center, The Johns Hopkins University School of Medicine, Baltimore, MD*

KENNETH J. O'BYRNE • *University Department of Oncology, Leicester Royal Infirmary, Leicester, UK*

MARTA OCEJO-GARCIA • *Academic Unit of Clinical Oncology, University of Nottingham; Nottingham City Hospital, Nottingham, UK*

AMIR ONN • *Department of Thoracic/Head and Neck Medical Oncology, The University of Texas M. D. Anderson Cancer Center, Houston, TX*

MICHAEL S. O'REILLY • *Departments of Radiation Oncology and Cancer Biology, M. D. Anderson Cancer Center, Houston, TX*

RAJANI K. RAVI • *The Oncology Center, The Johns Hopkins University School of Medicine, Baltimore, MD*

WILLIAM N. ROM • *Bellevue Chest Service, NYU Medical Center and Division of Pulmonary and Critical Care Medicine, Department of Medicine, NYU School of Medicine, New York, NY*

RAVI SALGIA • *Department of Medicine, Division of Adult Oncology and Thoracic Oncology Program, Dana-Farber Cancer Institute, Brigham and Women's Hospital and Harvard Medical School, Boston, MA*

LOUIS SAVAS • *Department of Pathology, University of Massachusetts Memorial Medical Center, Worcester, MA*

MARCUS SCHUERMANN • *Department of Hematology, Oncology, and Immunology, Philipps-University of Marburg, Marburg, Germany*

TARIQ SETHI • *Rayne Laboratory, Centre for Inflammation Research, Respiratory Medicine Unit, University of Edinburgh Medical School, Edinburgh, UK*

ANDREW M. SLEE • *Enanta Pharmaceuticals Inc., Watertown, MA*

YLERMI SOINI • *Department of Internal Medicine, University of Oulu, Oulu, Finland*

SABURO SONE • *Third Department of Internal Medicine, The University of Tokushima School of Medicine, Tokushima, Japan*

MARGARET K. T. SQUIER • *Department of Immunology, University of Colorado Medical School, Denver, CO*

EVA SZABO • *Lung and Upper Aerodigestive Cancer Research Group, Division of Cancer Prevention, National Cancer Institute, Bethesda, MD*

KAM-MENG TCHOU-WONG • *Department of Medicine, Division of Pulmonary and Critical Care Medicine, NYU School of Medicine, New York, NY*

RICHARD J. THURER • *Division of Cardiothoracic Surgery, University of Miami School of Medicine, Miami, FL*

KIRSI VÄHÄKANGAS • *Department of Pharmacology and Toxicology, University of Kuopio, Finland*

MANFRED VOLM • *Department of Oncological Diagnostics and Therapy, German Cancer Research Center, Heidelberg, Germany*

SARAH A. WARDLAW • *Department of Thoracic/Head and Neck Medical Oncology, The University of Texas M. D. Anderson Cancer Center, Houston, TX*

ROSEANNE S. WEXLER • *Bristol-Myers Squibb Company, Experimental Station, Wilmington, DE*

IGNACIO I. WISTUBA • *Department of Pathology, Pontificia Universidad Catolica de Chile, Santiago, Chile*

HANSPETER WITSCHI • *CHE and Department of Molecular Biosciences, School of Veterinary Medicine, University of California, Davis, CA*

BRUCE A. WODA • *University of Massachusetts Memorial Medical Center, Department of Pathology, Worcester, MA*

PENELLA J. WOLL • *Department of Clinical Oncology, University of Nottingham, Nottingham City Hospital, Nottingham, UK*

SEIJI YANO • *Third Department of Internal Medicine, The University of Tokushima School of Medicine, Tokushima, Japan*

HAIFAN ZHANG • *Department of Molecular and Cellular Biology, Imclone Systems Inc., New York, NY*

RONG-RONG ZHOU • *Division of Pediatrics, The University of Texas M. D. Anderson Cancer Center, Houston, TX*

I

INTRODUCTION

1

Characteristic Genetic Alterations in Lung Cancer

Ignacio I. Wistuba and Adi F. Gazdar

1. Introduction

Lung cancer is the most frequent cause of cancer deaths in both men and women in the U.S. *(1)*. Although tobacco smoking is accepted as the number one cause of this devastating disease, our understanding of the acquired genetic changes leading to lung cancer is still rudimentary. Lung cancer is classified into two major clinic-pathological groups, small cell lung carcinoma (SCLC) and non-small cell lung carcinoma (NSCLC) *(2)*. Squamous cell carcinoma, adenocarcinoma, and large cell carcinoma are the major histologic types of NSCLC. As with other epithelial malignancies, lung cancers are believed to arise after a series of progressive pathological changes (preneoplastic lesions) *(3)*. Many of these preneoplastic changes are frequently detected accompanying lung cancers and in the respiratory mucosa of smokers *(3)*. Although many molecular abnormalities have been described in clinically evident lung cancers *(4)*, relatively little is known about the molecular events preceding the development of lung carcinomas and the underlying genetic basis of tobacco-related lung carcinogenesis.

To investigate the molecular abnormalities involved in the multistep pathogenesis of lung carcinomas, we have developed a five-step analysis scheme that included the study of: 1) lung cancer cell lines; 2) microdissected primary lung tumors of the three major histologic types (SCLC, squamous cell carcinoma, and adenocarcinoma); and normal and abnormal respiratory epithelium from 3) lung cancer patients; 4) from smoker subjects without lung cancer; and from 5) never smoker subjects (*see* **Fig. 1**). Under this strategy we systematically search for mutations in tumor cell-lines specimens, and in archival tumor tissues, preneoplastic lesions, and normal epithelium, using paraffin-embedded

From: *Methods in Molecular Medicine, vol. 74: Lung Cancer, Vol. 1: Molecular Pathology Methods and Reviews*
Edited by: B. Driscoll © Humana Press Inc., Totowa, NJ

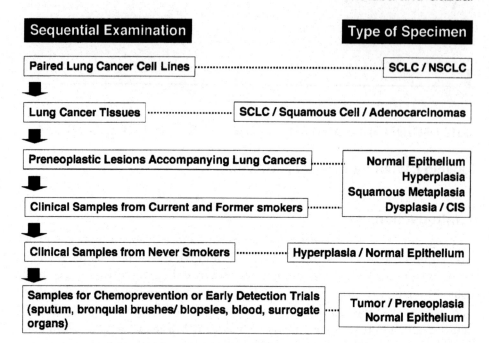

Fig. 1. Schema showing the strategy developed to study the molecular abnormalities involved in the pathogenesis of lung cancer.

materials. Recently, we have also analyzed genetic changes present in cytologic specimens bronchial brushes from smokers *(5)*. In tissues samples, using a precise microdissection technique, under direct microscopic observation a variable number of cells from those areas are precisely isolated along with invasive primary tumor and stromal lymphocytes (as a source of normal constitutional DNA). Using polymerase chain reaction (PCR)-based techniques, these different specimens are examined for molecular abnormalities (mainly gene mutations and allele losses) at chromosomal regions frequently mutated or deleted in clinically evident lung carcinomas.

The risk population for targeting lung cancer early detection efforts has been defined (current and heavy smokers, and patients who have survived one cancer of the upper aerodigestive tract). However, conventional morphologic methods for the identification of premalignant cell populations in the airways have limitations. This has led to a search for other biological properties (including genetic changes) of respiratory mucosa that may provide new methods for assessing the risk of developing invasive lung cancer in smokers, for early detection, and for monitoring their response to chemopreventive regimens.

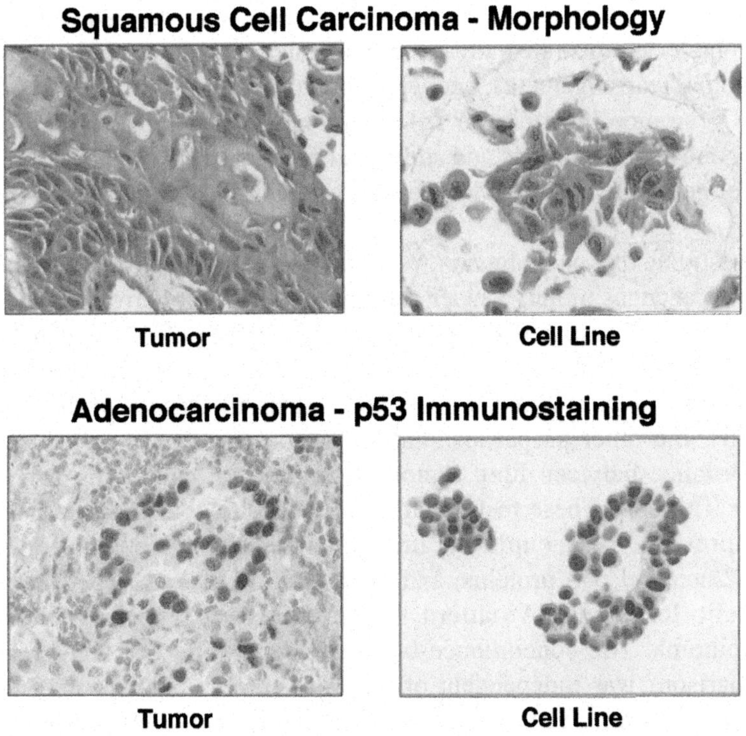

Squamous Cell Carcinoma - Morphology

| Tumor | Cell Line |

Adenocarcinoma - p53 Immunostaining

| Tumor | Cell Line |

Fig. 2. Comparison of phenotypic properties between primary lung cancer tissues and their corresponding cancer cell lines. Upper panels, tumor tissue and corresponding cell line showing squamous cell differentiation with keratinization features. Lower panel, tumor tissue and corresponding cell line showing adenocarcinoma features with gland-like structures formation and p53 nuclear immunostaining.

2. Tumor-Cell and Tissue-Specimens Methodologies Used in the Analysis of Lung Cancer Molecular Abnormalities

To investigate the molecular abnormalities involved in the pathogenesis of lung cancers, we have utilized a panel of paired lung tumor cell lines and corresponding normal lymphoblastoid cells (6), as well as microdissection technique of archival paraffin-embedded tumor and nonmalignant epithelial tissues (7–9) (*see* **Fig. 2**). Both methodologies have played a pivotal role in the study of the molecular abnormalities of the pathogenesis of lung cancer.

2.1. Paired Lung Tumor and Normal Lymphoblastoid Cell Lines

Despite the pivotal role played by human lung cancer cell lines in biomedical research, there is a widespread belief in the scientific community that they are not representative of the tumors from which they were derived. Lung cancer cell lines have demonstrated advanced molecular changes, including extensive chromosomal rearrangements, oncogene mutations, and multiple sites of allelic loss and gene amplification *(10,11)*. Thus, many investigators presume that loss of phenotypic properties and additional molecular changes develop during the prolonged time required for cell-culture establishment and subsequent passage.

To investigate this phenomenon we compared the morphologic, phenotypic, and genetic changes in lung cancer cell lines and in their corresponding tumor tissues *(12)*. We compared the properties of a series of 12 human NSCLC cell lines (cultured for a median period of 39 mo, range 12–69) and their corresponding archival tumor tissues. Other than differences in the degree of aneuploidy, the other properties studied demonstrated a remarkable degree of concordance between lung tumors and their corresponding cancer cell lines (*see* **Table 1**). These features included morphologic characteristics (*see* **Fig. 2**), presence of aneuploidy, immunohistochemical expression profile for HER2/neu and p53 proteins, and a similar *K-RAS* and *TP53* gene mutations allelic loss and MA pattern for multiple loci frequently deleted in lung carcinoma. The concordance between tumors and cell lines for all of the comparisons was independent of the time on culture, indicating that the properties of cell lines usually closely resemble those of their parental tumors for culture periods up to 69 mo.

While p53 immunohistochemical protein expression was detected in all of the lung tumor cell lines and their corresponding tumor tissues (100% correlation). *TP53* gene mutations in exons 5–8 were detected in 10 (83%) of 12 lung tumor cell lines, and six of those corresponding tumor tissues exhibited the identical *TP53* gene mutation. *K-RAS* gene mutations at codon 12 were detected in two adenocarcinomas cell lines (17% of the NSCLCs and 33% of adenocarcinoma cases), and identical *K-RAS* mutations were identified in their corresponding tumors. We also determined chromosomal deletions expressed by loss of heterozygosity (LOH) at 13 chromosomal regions frequently deleted in lung cancers. Nearly identical high LOH frequencies at all chromosomal regions analyzed were detected between tumors and theirs corresponding cell lines (*see* **Table 1**). For all of the individual markers there was an excellent correlation between tumors and cell lines (mean concordance of 89%). In all of the 115 (100%) comparisons, when allelic loss of a particular microsatellite was present in both the tumor and corresponding cell line, the identical parental allele was lost in both, confirming that the allelic loss originated in the original tumor tissue. In addition, tumor cell did not develop greater frequency of genomic instability phenomenon in culture and they retain some of the unstable properties of their parental tumors after lengthy culture periods (up to 69 mo).

Table 1
Comparison of Properties Between 12 Lung Cancer Tumor Tissues and Their Corresponding Cancer Cell Lines

	Frequency	
Feature	Tumor tissue	Cell lines
Aneuploidy	100%	100%
Protein immunohistochemical expression		
HER2/neu	25%	25%
p53 protein	100%	100%
Chromosomal region with LOH		
3p25	38%	38%
3p22–24	55%	55%
3p21	58%	58%
3p14–21	22%	22%
3p14.2 (*FHIT* gene)	50%	50%
3p12	25%	25%
Any 3p	67%	67%
5q22 (*APC-MCC* region)	44%	44%
8p23	91%	91%
8p22	91%	91%
8p21	58%	75%
Any 8p	100%	100%
9p21	78%	89%
13q (*RB* gene)	33%	33%
17p (*TP53* gene)	78%	89%
Microsatellite Alteration (MA)	54%	58%
Gene Mutations		
TP53 gene (Exons 5–8)	58%	83%
K-RAS gene (Codons 12–13)	17%	17%

Our findings also indicated that successfully cultured NSCLCs represent the general population of tumors and their cell lines are useful models for studying this important type of lung neoplasm.

2.2. Tissue Microdissection Technique

The molecular examination of pathologically altered cells and tissues at the DNA, RNA, and protein level has revolutionized research and diagnostics in tumor pathogenesis. However, the inherent heterogeneity of primary tissues with an admixture of various reactive cell populations can affect the outcome and interpretation of molecular studies. Recently, microdissection of tissue sections and cytological preparations has been used increasingly for the

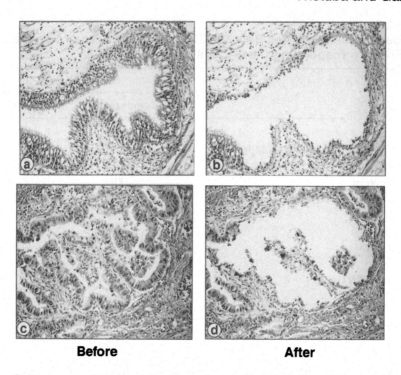

Before   **After**

Fig. 3. Representative example of precise tissue microdissection technique of bronchial epithelium (**a** and **b**) and adenocarcinoma of the lung (**c** and **d**) (*before* and *after* microdissection). Note that only tumor and epithelial cells were microdissected without contamination with stromal cells.

isolation of homogeneous, morphologically identified cell populations, thus overcoming the obstacle of tissue complexity. In conjunction with sensitive analytical techniques, such as the PCR, microdissection allows precise in vitro examination of cell populations, such as normal epithelial or dysplastic cells, which are otherwise inaccessible for conventional molecular studies (*see* **Fig. 3**). However, most of manual microdissection techniques are time-consuming and require a high degree of manual dexterity, which limits their practical use. Microdissection under microscopic visualization using micromanipulator is very precise, but very time-consuming. Laser capture microdissection (LCM), a novel technique developed at the National Cancer Institute, is an important advance in terms of speed, ease of use, and versatility of microdissection *(13)*. LCM is based on the adherence of visually selected cells to a thermoplastic membrane, which overlies the dehydrated tissue section and is focally melted by triggering of a low-energy infrared laser pulse. The melted membrane forms a composite with the selected tissue area, which can be removed by simple lifting of the membrane. LCM can be applied to a wide range of cell and tissue preparations including paraffin wax-embedded material. The use of immunohistochemical stains allows the selection of cells according to phenotypic and functional characteristics. Depending on the starting material, DNA, good-quality mRNA, and proteins can be extracted successfully from captured tissue fragments, down to the single-cell level. In combination with techniques like expression library construction, cDNA array hybridization, and differential display *(14–16)*, the use of this microdissection technique has allowed to us to analyze minute amount of lung tissues and perform most of our studies on the genetic changes involved in lung cancer pathogenesis *(7–9,12,17–25)*.

3. Overview of Molecular Abnormalities in Lung Cancer

Several cytogenetic, allelotyping, and comparative genomic hybridization (CGH) studies have revealed that multiple genetic changes (estimated to be between 10 and 20) are found in clinically evident lung cancers, and involve known and putative recessive oncogenes as well as several dominant oncogenes *(4)*. The major molecular changes detected in lung cancers are summarized in **Table 1**.

3.1. Growth Stimulation and Oncogenes

Many growth factors or regulatory peptides and their receptors are expressed by cancer cells or adjacent normal cells in the lung, and thus provide a series of autocrine and paracrine growth stimulatory loops in this neoplasm *(26)*. Several but not all components of these stimulatory pathways are proto-oncogene products.

3.2. Gastrin-Releasing Peptide (GRP)/Bombesin (BN) Autocrine Loop

There is good evidence that the GRP/BN and GRP receptor autocrine loop is involved in the growth of lung cancer, particularly SCLC *(26)*. Immuno-histochemical studies demonstrate that most SCLCs express the ligand portion of the autocrine loop GRP/BN, whereas NSCLC express GRP/BN less frequently *(27)*.

3.3. Tyrosine Kinases

Neuregulins and their receptors, the ERBB family of transmembrane receptor tyrosine kinases (ERBB1 and ERBB2), constitute a potential growth stimulatory loops in lung cancer *(27)*. However, NSCLCs but not SCLCs often demonstrate abnormalities of *ERBB* gene family. The *KIT* proto-oncogene, which encodes yet another tyrosine kinase receptor, CD117, and its ligand, stem cell factor (SCF), are co-expressed in many SCLC *(28)*. Other putative loops involve insulin-like growth factor 1 (IGF-1), insulin-like growth factor 2 (IGF-2), and the type I insulin-like growth factor receptor (IGF-1R), which are frequently co-expressed in SCLC, as well as platelet-derived growth factor (PDGF) and its receptor *(4)*.

3.4. MYC *Family*

MYC family genes are frequently altered in SCLC and include *MYC*, *MYCN*, and *MYCL*, all of which can be involved in SCLC pathogenesis. Of the well-characterized *MYC* genes, *MYC* is most frequently activated in both SCLC and NSCLC, whereas abnormalities of *MYCN* and *MYCL* usually only affect SCLC. In nearly all cases, only one *MYC* family member is activated in each individual tumor. Activation of the *MYC* genes may occur via gene amplification (20–115 copies per cell) or via transcriptional dysregulation, both of which lead to protein overexpression *(29)*. Amplification or overexpression of *MYC* family members has been reported more frequently in SCLCs (18–31%) than NSCLCs (8–20%) *(27)*.

3.5. BCL-2, BAX, and Apoptosis

There is accumulating evidence that tumor cells acquire the ability to escape pathways leading cells to undergo programmed cell death (apoptosis) when exposed to conditions such as growth factor deprivation or DNA damage. Key members of the normal apoptotic pathways are the *BCL-2* proto-oncogene product and the *TP53* TSG product. BCL-2 protects cells from the apoptotic process and thus probably plays a role in determining the chemotherapy response of cancer cells. Whereas BCL-2 protein immunohistochemical expression (and thus upregulation) is present in most SCLCs (75–95%), BCL-2 immunostaining is far less frequent in NSCLC (10–35%) *(4)*. BAX, which is a BCL-2 related protein that promotes apoptosis, is a downstream transcriptional target of p53. BAX and BCL-2 immunostaining are inversely related in neuroendocrine lung cancers, with most SCLCs having high BCL-2 and low BAX expression *(30)*.

Recent CGH studies have shown that lung cancer cell lines and tumor tissues demonstrate increased copy number consistent with amplification of underlying dominant oncogenes at several chromosomal regions, including 1p, 1q, 2p, 3q, 5q, 11q, 16p, 17q, 19q, and Xq *(31)*. Some of these regions, such as 1p32 (*L-MYC*), 2p25 (*N-MYC*), and 8q24 (*C-MYC*) contain known dominant oncogenes, while in others the genes need to be identified.

3.6. Recessive Oncogenes

The list of recessive oncogenes that are involved in lung cancer is likely to include as many 10–15 known and putative genes *(4)*. These include changes in *TP53* (17p13), *RB* (13q14), *p16^{6ink4}* (9p21), and new candidate recessive oncogenes in the short arms of chromosome 3 (3p) at 3p12 (*DUTT1* gene), 3p14.2 (*FHIT* gene), 3p21 (*RASFF1* gene), 3p22-24 (*BAP-1* gene), and 3p25 regions *(4)*. Recessive oncogenes are believed to be inactivated via a two-step process involving both alleles. Knudson has proposed that the first "hit" frequently is a point mutation, while the second allele is subsequently inactivated via a chromosomal deletion, translocation, or other event such as methylation *(32)*.

3.6.1. TP53 Gene

Loss of p53 function allows inappropriate survival of genetically damaged cells, setting the stage for the accumulation of multiple mutations and the subsequent evolution of a cancer cell *(33)*. Missense *TP53* mutations prolong the protein's half-life, leading to accumulation of high levels of mutant p53 protein readily detected by immunohistochemistry. Multiple studies have shown abnormal p53 protein expression by immunohistochemistry in 40–70% of lung cancer *(4)*. *TP53* abnormalities play a critical role in lung cancer pathogenesis *(4)*. Chromosome 17p13 sequences, the site of the *TP53* locus, are frequently hemizygously lost in SCLC (90%) and NSCLC (65%) *(9)*, and mutational inactivation of the remaining allele occurs in 50–75% of these neoplasms *(34)*. *TP53* mutations in lung tumors correlate with cigarette smoking and are mostly the G-T transversions expected of tobacco-smoke carcinogens *(33)*. Furthermore, in lung cancers a relationship has been described between mutational hot-spots at the *TP53* gene and adduct hot-spots caused by benzo[α]pyrene metabolites of cigarette smoke *(35)*.

3.6.2. The p16-Cyclin D1-CDK4-Retinoblastoma Pathway

In SCLC, this pathway is usually disrupted by retinoblastoma gene (*RB*) inactivation, while cyclin D1, CDK4, and p16 abnormalities are rare in SCLC but common (particularly p16) in NSCLC *(4)*. The major growth-suppressing function of RB protein is to block G1-S progression. Inactivation of both *RB* alleles at chromosomal region 13q14 is common in SCLC *(36)*, with protein abnormalities reported at frequencies of over 90% *(37)*. There is frequent loss of one the *RB* 13q14 alleles. Functional loss of the remaining *RB* allele can include deletion, nonsense mutations, or splicing abnormalities, leading to a truncated *RB* protein encoded by the remaining allele.

3.6.3. PTEN/MMAC1

A new TSG, *PTEN* (Phosphatase and Tensin homolog deleted on chromosome 10), also called *MMAC1* (Mutated in Multiple Advanced Cancers), has been identified and localized to chromosome region 10q23.3 *(38)*. Allelotyping analysis utilizing microsatellite markers in close proximity to the *PTEN/MMAC1* gene have demonstrated high incidence of LOH in lung cancers, especially SCLCs (91% LOH in SCLC, and 41% in NSCLC) *(39)*. Homozygous deletions interrupting the *PTEN/MMAC1* gene have been detected in 8% of SCLC cell lines examined and in a few uncultured primary SCLCs *(40)*. However *PTEN/MMAC1* mutations were detected in only 11% of lung cancers, including both SCLC and NSCLC tumors *(40)*.

3.6.4. Other Candidate TSGs

TSG101 is a recently discovered candidate TSG that maps to 11p15 *(41)*. It has been reported that the mutant *TSG101* transcript was expressed simultaneously with wild-type *TSG101* transcript in almost all SCLC cell lines. In contrast, normal lung tissue, as well primary NSCLC specimens, express only a wild-type transcript. *DMBT1* is a candidate TSG located at 10q25.3-26.1 *(42)*. Recent data demonstrate that *DMBT1* gene expression is frequently lost in both SCLC and NSCLC *(43)*, suggesting that inactivation of *DMBT1* may play an important role in lung tumorigenesis.

3.6.5. Candidate TSGs at Chromosome Region 3p

The very frequent loss of alleles on chromosome 3p in both SCLC (>90%) and NSCLC (>80%) *(24)* provides strong evidence for the existence of one or more TSGs on this chromosomal arm. Several distinct 3p regions have been identified by high-density allelotyping including 3p25-26, 3p24, 3p21.3-22 (several sites), 3p14.2 (*FHIT*), and 3p12 (U2020 deletion site) suggesting that there are several different TSGs located on 3p. The 3p21.3 region has been extensively examined for putative TSGs, although the identity of such gene(s) remains elusive *(44)*. Currently, two distinct 3p21.3 regions are under study because of the existence of multiple homozygous deletion in lung cancer cell lines. Although several genes identified so far in both homozygous deletions none of them have been shown to have frequent mutations in lung cancer *(44)*. Recently, one of the splicing isoforms of the *RASSF1* gene (*RASSF1A*) located in the 370 kb deletion region has been shown to undergo tumor promoter hypermethylation as a mechanism of inactivation (>90% of SCLCs and 60% of NSCLC) *(45)*. This gene when re-expressed in lung cancer cells suppresses the malignant phenotype *(45,46)*.

The *FHIT* gene maps to 3p14.2 and encompasses approx 1 Mb of genomic DNA, which includes the human common fragile site (FRA3B). *FHIT* is a candidate TSG for lung cancer on the basis of frequent 3p14.2 allele loss in lung cancer (100% of SCLCs and 88% of NSCLCs) and homozygous deletion in several lung cancer cell lines *(47,48)*. Lung cancer cells (40–80%) express abnormal mRNA transcripts of *FHIT* but nearly always also express very low levels of wild-type *FHIT* transcripts *(47,48)*. However, unlike classic TSG inactivation, *FHIT* point mutations are rare *(47,48)*, and a few abnormal transcripts can be found in normal lung tissue. Of importance, most lung cancers, expressed undetectable or very low levels of *FHIT* mRNA, and exhibited loss of Fhit protein expression by immunohistochemistry. Recently, it has been demonstrated that hypermethylation of the promoter region of the *FHIT* gene is a frequent event in lung cancer cell lines (SCLC 64% and NSCLC 64%) and noncultured NSCLC primary tumors (37%) *(5)*.

There are other candidate TSGs of lung cancer on chromosome 3p. The Von Hippel-Lindau *(VHL)* TSG at 3p25 and the BRCA1-associated protein, *BAP-1*, at 3p21. However, these genes have been infrequently mutated in lung cancer, including SCLC *(4)*. Recently, a new candidate TSG, *DUTT1*, has been cloned residing in the U2020 3p12 deletion region and crossing a small (>100 KB) lung cancer homozygous deletion at 3p12 *(49)*. However, *DUTT1* tumor-suppressing activity and protein expression patterns in tumors are unknown.

3.6.6. Other Candidate Lung Cancer Tumor Suppressor Genes Loci

Besides the candidate and known TSGs mentioned earlier, cytogenetic and allelotyping studies have shown allelic loss of many other chromosomal regions, in both SCLC and NSCLC, suggesting the involvement of other tumor-suppressor genes in its pathogenesis. The chromosomal regions include 1q, 2q, 5q, 6p, 6q, 8p, 8q, 10q, 11p, 14q, 17q, 18q, and 22q *(11,39)*. These novel sites will direct the search for new candidate TSGs. Future investigations with an even higher resolution of microsatellite markers will be crucial to narrow down the sites of frequent allelic loss. In addition, the presence of homozygously deleted chromosomal regions 2q33, 5p13-q14, 8, and X/Y in lung cancer provide further evidence that these regions harbor as yet unidentified TSGs *(4)*.

3.7. Genetic Instability in Lung Cancer

In addition to the specific genetic changes discussed earlier, other evidence indicates that genomic instability occurs in lung cancer. This evidence includes changes in the number of short-tandem DNA repeats (also known as microsatellite markers), frequently present in a wide variety of cancer types, including SCLC. Microsatellite instability, was initially reported in hereditary nonpolyposis colorectal cancer, resulting from inherited defects in DNA mismatch-repair enzymes, which induce large-scale genetic instability with the formation of a ladder-like pattern replacing the normal allele pattern. This type has not been seen in lung cancer. Another form of microsatellite change, where only a single band of altered size is found, has been described in many forms of sporadic cancers, including SCLC and NSCLC, referred to as microsatellite alteration (MA). While the relationship of MAs to the DNA repair mechanism has not been established, the former probably represents evidence of some form of genomic instability *(50)*. Multiple studies have reported MAs in lung cancers. Overall, 35% (range 0–76%) of SCLCs and 22% (range 2–49%) of NSCLCs have shown some evidence of MA at individual loci *(4)*. Although the mechanisms are unknown, a significantly higher frequency of MAs have been detected in lung tumors arising in HIV-positive individuals *(20)* and in patients with secondary lung tumors after treatment for Hodgkin's disease *(25)*, compared to lung cancers in the general population.

3.8. Aberrant Methylation in Lung Cancer

TSGs need to inactivate both alleles to exert their tumor-promoting effects. One method of gene silencing is via the epigenetic phenomenon of aberrant methylation of gene promoters. DNA methylation only occurs at CpG sites (known as "CpG islands"). In the human genome CpG sites are usually concentrated in the promoter regions of about half of all human genes, and normally these islands are completely unmethylated *(51)*. During carcinogenesis, the promoter regions of several genes are methylated, resulting in gene silencing. It is estimated that the average number of CpG islands methylated in individual human tumors may be as high as 600 (range 0–4500) *(52)*.

As predicted, several genes are methylated in lung cancers, and the list is increasing rapidly. Esteller et al. *(53)*, detected promoter hypermethylation of at least one of four genes examined (*p16^{6ink4}$, *DAP kinase*, *GSTP1*, and *MGMT*) in 15 of 22 (68%) NSCLC tumors but not in any paired normal lung tissue. Interestingly, 11 of 15 (73%) matched serum samples obtained from primary tumors with aberrant methylation also had abnormal methylated DNA. None of the sera from patients with tumors not demonstrating methylation was positive. These findings suggest that detection of aberrant promoter hypermethylation of cancer-related genes in serum may be useful for cancer diagnosis or the detection of recurrence. Recently, Tang et al. *(54)* reported that patients with pathologic stage I NSCLC whose tumors exhibited *DAP kinase* gene promoter hypermethylation (44%) had a statistically significantly poorer probability of overall 5-yr survival after surgery than those without such hypermethylation. These finding suggest that abnormal promoter-gene methylation may be useful as prognostic marker in lung cancer patients.

In lung cancer, regional hypermethylation has been found at chromosome 3p, but the precise gene target(s) until recently have been uncertain. Recently, three reports have shown in lung cancer frequent methylation of promoter sequences of three genes located at chromosome 3p regions, which are frequently deleted in this neoplasm *(46,55)*. Dammann et al. *(46)* and Burbee et al. *(45)* described a human *RAS* effector homologue *(RASSF1)* gene located in a small 120-kb region of minimal homozygous deletion in 3p21.3, with frequent (>90% of SCLC and ~40% of NSCLCs) methylation of its CpG-island promoter sequence, which correlates with loss of gene expression. Virmani et al. *(55)* reported a high frequency of methylation of the *RARβ* gene in lung cancers, particularly SCLC (72%) compared to NSCLC (41%). In addition, high frequencies of methylation of lung cancers has been recently detected in *FHIT* gene (3p14.2), in both SCLC and NSCLC cell lines (64%) and NSCLC primary tumors (37%) *(5)*.

Recently, it has been shown a relatively high frequency of other genes methylation (*TIMP-3* 26%, *p16^{ink4}* 25%, *MGMT* 21%, *DAPK* 19%, *ECAD* 18%, *p14^{ARF}* 8%, and *GSTP1* 7%) in a panel of 107 NSCLC primary tumors *(56)*. Frequent abnormal methylaton of the *CDH13* (H-Cadherin) gene (16q24.2-3) has been also demonstrated in lung cancer, particularly in NSCLC cell lines (50%) and primary tumors (43%) *(57)*. The number of genes showing a high incidence of abnormal methylation in lung cancer is rapidly increasing. All these recent findings suggest that aberrant methylation of genes is a frequent abnormality in lung cancers and may have applications for risk assessment, diagnosis, and for development of novel therapeutic approaches.

4. Tumor Type-Specific Genetic Changes in Lung Cancers

Studies of large numbers of lung cancers have demonstrated different patterns of involvement between the two major groups of lung carcinomas (SCLC and NSCLC) *(39)* and between the three major histologic types of lung carcinomas (SCLC, squamous cell carcinomas, and adenocarcinomas) *(9,22,24,58)*. The major differences found between SCLC and NSCLC are summarized in **Table 1**. Our results *(9,22,24,39,58)* of allelotyping lung cancer cell lines and microdissected invasive primary tumors indicate that SCLC demonstrate more frequent losses at 4p, 4q, 5q21 (*APC-MCC* region), 10q, and 13q14 (*RB*), while losses at 9p21 and 8p21-23 are more frequent in NSCLCs. Recently, Girard et al. *(11)* performed a high-resolution genome-wide allelotyping analysis of a similar panel of lung cancer (SCLC and NSCLC) and detected 22 different "hot spots" for LOH, 13 with a preference for SCLC, 7 for NSCLC, and 2 affecting both. This provides clear evidence on a genome-wide scale that SCLC and NSCLC different significantly in the TSGs that are inactivated during their pathogenesis. Similarly, the recent findings on the methylation pattern of a number of genes in lung cancer indicate that there are differences in between SCLCs and NSCLCs *(55)*.

In addition, we have found different patterns of allelic loss involving the two major types of NSCLC (squamous cell and adenocarcinoma), with higher incidences of deletions at 17p13 (*TP53*), 13q14 (*RB*), 9p21 (*p16^{6ink4}*), 8p21-23, and several 3p regions in squamous cell carcinomas. These results suggest that more genetic changes accumulate during tumorigenesis in squamous cell carcinomas than in adenocarcinomas. Several of those studies have identified different allele loss patterns between SCLC and NSCLC.

5. Preneoplasia and the Development of Lung Cancer

Lung cancers are believed to arise after a series of progressive pathological changes (preneoplastic or precursor lesions) in the respiratory mucosa. While the sequential preneoplastic changes have been defined for centrally arising squamous carcinomas, they have been poorly documented for large-cell carcinomas, adenocarcinomas, and SCLCs *(3)* (*see* **Table 2**). Mucosal changes in the large airways that may precede or accompany invasive squamous cell carcinoma include hyperplasia (basal cell hyperplasia and goblet cell hyperplasia), squamous metaplasia, squamous dysplasia, and carcinoma *in situ (3)*. While hyperplasia and squamous metaplasia are considered reactive and reversible changes, dysplasia and carcinoma *in situ* are the changes most frequently associated with the development of squamous cell lung carcinomas. Adenocarcinomas may be accompanied by changes including atypical adenomatous hyperplasia (AAH) *(3)* in peripheral airway cells, although the malignant potential of these lesions has not been demonstrated. For SCLC, no specific preneoplastic changes have been described in the respiratory epithelium.

Currently available information suggests that lung preneoplastic lesions frequently are extensive and multifocal throughout the lung, indicating a field effect ("field cancerization") by which much of the respiratory epithelium has been mutagenized, presumably from exposure to carcinogens.

6. Genetic Abnormalities in the Sequential Development of Lung Cancer

Although our knowledge of the molecular events in invasive lung cancer is relatively extensive, until recently we knew little about the sequence of events in preneoplastic lesions. A few studies have provided suggestions that molecular lesions can be identified at early stages of the pathogenesis of lung cancer. Myc upregulation, cyclin D1 expression, p53 immunostaining, and DNA aneuploidy have been detected in dysplastic epithelium adjacent to invasive lung carcinomas *(59–61)*. *K-RAS* mutations have been also detected in atypical adenomatous hyperplasia *(62)*, which may be a potential precursor lesion of adenocarcinoma. *TP53* gene abnormalities (including mutations, deletions, and overexpression) have been demonstrated in nonmalignant epithelium of lung specimens resected for lung cancer *(63)*. They also occur in

Table 2
Major Differences in the Pathogenesis of SCLC and NSCLC

	SCLC	NSCLC
Frequency	20%–25%	80%–85%
Neuroendocrine cells	Yes	No
Putative autocrine loop	GRP/GRP receptor	HGM/MET
SCF/KIT	NDF/ERBB	
RAS mutations	<1%	15%–20%
MYC amplification	18%–31%	8%–20%
BCL-2 IHC	75%–95%	10%–35%
TP53 abnormalities		
LOH	90%	65%
Mutation	75%	~50%
p53 IHQ	40%–70%	40%–60%
RB abnormalities		
LOH	67%	31%
rb abnormalities (IHC)	90%	15%–30%
p16^{6ink4} abnormalities		
LOH	53%	66%
Mutation	<1%	10%–40%
p16 IHC	0%–10%	30%–70%
PTEN/MMAC1 loci LOH	91%	41%
TSG101 abnormal transcripts	~100%	0%
DMBT1 abnormal expression	100%	43%
3p LOH various regions	>90%	>80%
4p LOH various regions	50%	~20%
4q LOH various regions	80%	30%
8p21-23 LOH	80%–90%	80%–100%
Other specific LOH regions	1q23, 9q22-32, 10p15, 13q34	13q11, Xq22.1
Microsatellite alterations	35%	22%
Promoter hypermethylation		
RASSF1 gene	>90%	~40%
RARβ gene	72%	41%
Other genes	Not studied	10–40% various genes[*]
Preneoplastic changes		
Histopathology	Unknown	Relatively known
LOH multiple loci	90%	31%
MA frequency	68%	11%

GRP, Gastrin-releasing peptide; HFG, hepatocyte growth factor; MET, MET proto-oncogene; SCF, stem cell factor; KIT, KIT proto-oncogene; NDF, neu differentiation factor; ERBB, neuregulin receptor; LOH, loss of heterozygosity; IHC, immunohistochemistry; BCL-2, BCL-2 anti-apoptotic proto-oncogene. [*]p16, death-associated protein (DAP) kinase, glutathione S transferase P1 (GSTP1), and O6-methylguanine-DNA methyltransferase (MGMT).

the histologically normal and abnormal epithelium of smokers *(7,64)*. Recently, Franklin et al. described an identical *TP53* gene mutation widely dispersed in normal and preneoplastic epithelium of a smoker without lung cancer *(65)*. Our recent studies allowed us to identify some of the genetic changes involved in the pathogenesis of lung cancer (summarized in **Table 2**). Because the preneoplastic changes have been well established only for squamous cell carcinoma of the lung, most of our findings are referred to this histologic type of lung cancer.

6.1. Mutations Follow a Sequence

Our data have demonstrated that in lung cancer the developmental sequence of molecular changes is not random, with LOH at one or more 3p regions (especially telomeric regions 3p21, 3p22-24, and 3p25) and 9p21, and to a lesser extent at 8p21-23, 13q14 *(RB)*, and 17p13 *(TP53)*, being detected frequently very early in pathogenesis (histologically normal epithelium) *(8,22,24)* *(see* **Fig. 4**). In contrast, LOH at 5q21 *(APC-MCC* region) and *K-RAS* mutations were only detected at the carcinoma *in situ* stage, and *TP53* mutations appear at variable times. Detailed examination of all our material suggests that the order of events (allelic losses) is usually either 3p→9p→8p or 3p→8p→9p deletions followed by *TP53* deletions. In early lesions (normal epithelium-metaplasia), the 3p losses are small and multifocal, commencing at the central (3p21) and telomeric end of the chromosomal arm *(24)*. In later lesions (carcinoma *in situ* and invasive cancers), all or almost the entire chromosome is lost. Similar findings were detected on chromosome 8p analysis *(22)*.

6.2. Accumulation of Genetic Changes in the Development of Lung Cancer

The development of epithelial cancers requires multiple mutations stepwise accumulation of which may represent a mutator phenotype. Thus, it is possible that those preneoplastic lesions that have accumulated multiple mutations are at higher risk for progression to invasive cancer. Of interest, using a panel of microsatellite markers targeting chromosomal regions frequently deleted in invasive lung carcinomas, we have detected similar incidences of LOH between histologically normal epithelium and slightly abnormal epithelial changes (hyperplasia and squamous metaplasia) accompanying lung carcinomas *(8)*. These findings may indicate the latter foci may represent reactive foci, and are not at higher risk for progression to invasive carcinomas. However, high-grade dysplasias and carcinoma *in situ* accompanying invasive squamous cell lung carcinomas demonstrated a significant increase of total number of allelic losses *(8)*, suggesting that the accumulation of mutations correlates with the

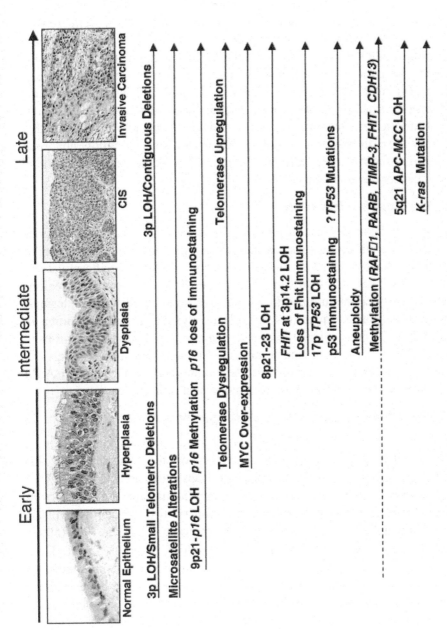

Fig. 4. Sequential histologic and molecular changes during the multistage pathogenesis of lung cancer. Adapted from **ref. 71**.

morphologic changes and may lead to development of invasive carcinomas (sequential theory of lung cancer development).

In our recent study *(9)*, comparing MA frequency in lung cancer types and their accompanying bronchial epithelia, SCLCs (50%) demonstrated a significantly higher incidence of MAs than NSCLC tumor types (24–32%), suggesting that more widespread and more extensive genetic damage is present in bronchial epithelium in patients with SCLC. The finding of some specimens of normal or mildly abnormal epithelia accompanying SCLCs have demonstrated a very high incidence of genetic changes *(9)*, suggests that SCLC may arise directly from histologically normal or from mildly abnormal epithelium, without passing through the entire histologic sequence (parallel theory of cancer development).

6.3. Allele-Specific Mutations

We have noted that the specific parental allelic lost in chromosomal deletions present in preneoplastic lesions and their accompanying cancers are similar *(8,18,19)*. We have referred to this phenomenon as allele-specific mutations (ASM). We have detected ASMs in preneoplastic lesions located in all regions of the respiratory epithelium and in a wide spectrum of preneoplastic lesions, including hyperplasia, squamous metaplasia, dysplasia, and carcinoma *in situ (8,18,19)*. Of great interest, we have detected ASMs in smoking-related damaged epithelium, even in biopsy samples obtained from different lungs *(7)*. Although the mechanism by which this phenomenon occurs is unknown, ASM is likely to be a phenomenon of major biological significance.

6.4. Aberrant Methylation in the Pathogenesis of Lung Cancer

The finding of $p16^{6ink4}$ methylation in the early stages of progression of squamous cell lung carcinoma of the lung support the critical role for this molecular change *(66)*. $p16^{6ink4}$ methylation has been detected in 75% of carcinoma *in situ* adjacent to squamous cell carcinomas and the frequency of this event increased during disease progression from basal cell hyperplasia (17%) to squamous metaplasia (24%) to carcinoma *in situ* lesions (50%). Recently, aberrant methylation of the $p16^{6ink4}$ and/or O^6-methyl-guanine-DNA methyltransferase promoters have been detected in DNA from sputum in 100% of patients with squamous cell lung carcinoma up to 3 yr before clinical diagnosis *(67)*. Preliminary results on methylation analysis of several genes (*RARβ H-cadherin, APC, $p16^{6ink4}$*, and *RASFF1*) indicate that abnormal gene methylation is a relatively frequent (at least one gene, 35%) in oropharyngeal and bronchial epithelial cells in heavy smokers with evidence of sputum atypia (Zöxhbauer-Muller et al., in preparation). Although more studies need to be performed in lung cancer preneoplastic lesions, the recent findings suggest

Table 3
Summary of the Histopathological and Molecular Abnormalities in the Major Three Types of Lung Cancer

Abnormality	SCLC	Squamous cell carcinoma	Adenocarcinoma
Histopathology			
Precursor lesion	Unknown Normal epithelium and hyperplasia?	Known Squamous dysplasia and CIS	Probable Adenomatous atypical hyperplasia (AAH)?
Theory of development	Parallel	Sequential	Probably Sequential
Molecular			
Gene Abnormalities	*MYC* overexpression *TP53* LOH and mutation	*TP53* LOH and mutation	*K-RAS* mutation
LOH			
Frequency	High 10%	Intermediate 54%	Low 90%
Chromosomal regions	9p21, 17p/*TP53*1	8p21-23, 9p21, 17p/*TP53*	5q21, 8p21–23, 9p21, 17p/*TP53*
Genetic instability	High	Intermediate	Low
Frequency	13%	10%	68%

that aberrant gene methylation can be an early event in lung cancer and may constitute in this neoplasm new marker for risk assessment, early detection, and monitoring of chemoprevention trials.

7. Smoking-Damaged Bronchial Epithelium

It has been established that advanced lung preneoplastic changes occur far more frequently in smokers than in nonsmokers and increase in frequency with amount of smoking, adjusted by age. Although morphologic recovery occurs after smoking cessation, elevated lung cancer risk persists. Changes in bronchial epithelium, including metaplasia and dysplasia, have been utilized as surrogate end points for chemoprevention studies. Risk factors that identify normal and premalignant bronchial tissue at risk for malignant progression need to be better defined. However, only scant information is available about molecular changes in the respiratory epithelium of smokers without cancer.

Two independent studies showed that the genetic changes (LOH and MA) found in invasive cancers and preneoplasia can also be identified in morphologically normal-appearing bronchial epithelium from current or former smokers and may persist for many years after smoking cessation *(7,64)*. In general, such genetic changes are not found in the bronchial epithelium from true, lifetime, never-smokers. In our study *(7)* 86% of the individuals who smoked demonstrated LOH in one or more biopsies and 24% showed LOH in all biopsies. Somewhat surprising, about half of the histologically normal epithelium showed LOH; however, the frequency of LOH and the severity of histologic changes did not correspond until the carcinoma *in situ* stage. As it has been observed in epithelial foci accompanying invasive lung carcinoma *(8)*, allelic losses on chromosome 3p and 9p were more frequent than deletions in chromosomes 5q21, 17p13 *(TP53* gene), and 13q14 *(RB* gene). All these findings suggest the hypothesis that identifying biopsies with extensive or certain patterns of allelic loss may provide new methods for assessing the risk in smokers of developing invasive lung cancer and for monitoring response to chemoprevention.

8. Molecular Markers for Early Detection of Lung Cancer

Mutant *K-RAS* and *TP53* genes have been detected in the sputum some months prior to diagnosis of cancer *(68)* and *K-RAS* mutations have been detected in bronchoalveolar lavage fluids from patients with adenocarcinoma (56%), but not in patients with squamous cell carcinoma or with other diagnosis *(69)*. Recently, Ahrendt et al. *(70)* have reported that molecular assays could identify cancer cells in bronchoalveolar lavage fluid from patients with early-stage lung cancers. Using PCR-based assays for *K-RAS* and *TP53* gene mutations, CpG-island methylation of the $p16^{6ink4}$ gene and for microsatellite instability, they were able to detect identical molecular abnormalities in the bronchoalveolar fluid and corresponding tumors in 23 of 43 (53%) of the cases. These findings suggest that molecular strategies may detect the presence of neoplastic cells in the central and peripheral airways in patients with early-stage lung carcinomas.

As we stated earlier, several genes are methylated in lung cancers, and the list is increasing rapidly. Aberrant methylation commences during the multistage pathogenesis, in bronchial epithelium with mildly abnormal changes (hyperplasia/squamous metaplasia) *(66)*. Because methylated DNA sequences can be found even when they represent a small fraction within total normal DNA, they are very attractive candidates for early molecular detection tools and for following chemoprevention studies. The potential of using assays for aberrant $p16^{6ink4}$ methylation to identify disease and/or risk was validated by detection of this change in sputum from a small series of patients with cancer and smoker individual without lung cancer *(66)*. Recently, abnormal methylation of the *FHIT* gene has been shown in bronchial brushes from heavy smokers (17%) subjects *(5)*. Thus, aberrant methylation may be useful for early detection, risk assessment, and for monitoring the efficacy of chemoprevention trials.

9. Summary

Our understanding of the molecular pathology of lung cancer is advancing rapidly with several specific genes and chromosomal regions being identified. Lung cancer appears to require many mutations in both dominant and recessive oncogenes before they become invasive. Several genetic and epigenetic changes are common to all lung cancer histologic types, while others appear to be tumor-type specific. The identification of those specific genes undergoing such mutations and the sequence of cumulative changes that lead the neoplastic changes for each lung tumor histologic type remain to be fully elucidated. Recent findings in normal and preneoplastic bronchial epithelium from lung cancer patients and smoker subjects suggest that genetic changes may provide in this neoplasm new methods for early diagnosis, risk assessment, and for monitoring response to chemoprevention.

References

1. Greenlee, R. T., Hill-Harmon, M. B., Murray, T., and Thun, M. (2001) Cancer statistics, 2001. *CA Cancer J. Clin.* **51,** 15–36.
2. Colby, T. V., Koss, M. N., and Travis, W. D. (1995) Tumors of the lower respiratory tract, 3rd. series, Fascicle 13, Armed Forces Institute of Pathology, Washington, DC, pp. 1–554.

3. Colby, T. V., Wistuba, I. I, and Gazdar, A. (1998) Precursors to pulmonary neoplasia. *Adv. Anat. Pathol.* **5,** 205–215.

4. Sekido, Y., Fong, K. M., and Minna, J. D. (1998) Progress in understanding the molecular pathogenesis of human lung cancer. *Biochim. Biophys. Acta.* **1378,** F21–F59.

5. Zochbauer-Muller, S., Fong, K. M., Maitra, A., Lam, S., Geradts, J., Ashfaq, R., et al. 5′ CpG island methylation of the FHIT gene is correlated with loss of gene expression in lung and breast cancer. *Cancer Res.* In press.

6. Gazdar, A. F. and Minna, J. D. (1996) NCI series of cell lines: an historical perspective. *J. Cell Biochem. Suppl.* **24,** 1–11.

7. Wistuba, I. I., Lam, S., Behrens, C., Virmani, A. K., Fong, K. M., LeRiche, J., et al. (1997) Molecular damage in the bronchial epithelium of current and former smokers. *J. Natl. Cancer Inst.* **89,** 1366–1373.

8. Wistuba, I. I., Behrens, C., Milchgrub, S., Bryant, D., Hung, J., Minna, J. D., and Gazdar, A. F. (1999) Sequential molecular abnormalities are involved in the multistage development of squamous cell lung carcinoma. *Oncogene* **18,** 643–650.

9. Wistuba, I. I., Berry, J., Behrens, C., Maitra, A., Shivapurkar, N., Milchgrub, S., et al. (2000) Molecular changes in the bronchial epithelium of patients with small cell lung cancer. *Clin. Cancer Res.* **6,** 2604–2610.

10. Phelps, R. M., Johnson, B. E., Ihde, D. C., Gazdar, A. F., Linnoila, R. I., Matthews, M. J., et al. (1996) NCI-Navy Medical Oncology Branch cell line data base. *J. Cell. Biochem.* **(Suppl. 24),** 32–91.

11. Girard, L., Zöchbauer-Müller, S., Virmani, A. K., Gazdar, A. F., and Minna, J. D. (2000) Genome-wide allelotyping of lung cancer identifies new regions of allelic loss, differences between small cell and non-small cell lung cancer, and loci clustering. *Cancer Res.* **60,** 4894–4906.

12. Wistuba, II, Bryant, D., Behrens, C., Milchgrub, S., Virmani, A. K., Ashfaq, R., et al. (1999) Comparison of features of human lung cancer cell lines and their corresponding tumors. *Clin. Cancer Res.* **5,** 991–1000.

13. Emmert-Buck, M. R., Bonner, R. F., Smith, P. D., Chuaqui, R. F., Zhuang, Z., Goldstein, S. R., et al. (1996) Laser capture microdissection. *Science* **274,** 998–1001.

14. Maitra, A., Wistuba, II, Virmani, A. K., Sakaguchi, M., Park, I., Stucky, A., et al. (1999) Enrichment of epithelial cells for molecular studies. *Nat. Med.* **5,** 459–463.

15. Fend, F., Emmert-Buck, M. R., Chuaqui, R., Cole, K., Lee, J., Liotta, L. A., and Raffeld, M. (1999) Immuno-LCM: laser capture microdissection of immunostained frozen sections for mRNA analysis. *Am. J. Pathol.* **154,** 61–66.

16. Simone, N. L., Remaley, A. T., Charboneau, L., Petricoin, E. F., Glickman, J. W., Emmert-Buck, M. R., et al. (2000) Sensitive immunoassay of tissue cell proteins procured by laser capture microdissection. *Am. J. Pathol.* **156,** 445–452.

17. Sugio, K., Kishimoto, Y., Virmani, A., Hung, J. Y., and Gazdar, A. F. (1994) K-*ras* mutations are a relatively late event in the pathogenesis of lung carcinomas. *Cancer Res.* **54,** 5811–5815.

18. Hung, J., Kishimoto, Y., Sugio, K., Virmani, A., McIntire, D. D., Minna, J. D., and Gazdar, A. F. (1995) Allele-specific chromosome 3p deletions occur at an early stage in the pathogenesis of lung carcinoma. *JAMA* **273**, 558–563.
19. Kishimoto, Y., Sugio, K., Mitsudomi, T., Oyama, T., Virmani, A., McIntire, D. D., and Gazdar, A. F. (1995) Allele specific loss of chromosome 9p in preneoplastic lesions accompanying non-small cell lung cancers. *J. Natl. Cancer Inst.* **87**, 1224–1229.
20. Wistuba, II, Behrens, C., Milchgrub, S., Virmani, A. K., Jagirdar, J., Thomas, B., et al. (1998) Comparison of molecular changes in lung cancers in HIV-positive and HIV- indeterminate subjects. *JAMA* **279**, 1554–1559.
21. Onuki, N., Wistuba, II, Travis, W. D., Virmani, A. K., Yashima, K., Brambilla, E., et al. (1999) Genetic changes in the spectrum of neuroendocrine lung tumors. *Cancer* **85**, 600–607.
22. Wistuba, II, Behrens, C., Virmani, A. K., Milchgrub, S., Syed, S., Lam, S., et al. (1999) Allelic losses at chromosome 8p21-23 are early and frequent events in the pathogenesis of lung cancer. *Cancer Res.* **59**, 1973–1979.
23. Park, I. W., Wistuba, II, Maitra, A., Milchgrub, S., Virmani, A. K., Minna, J. D., and Gazdar, A. F. (1999) Multiple clonal abnormalities in the bronchial epithelium of patients with lung cancer. *J. Natl. Cancer Inst.* **91**, 1863–1868.
24. Wistuba, II, Behrens, C., Virmani, A. K., Mele, G., Milchgrub, S., Girard, L., et al. (2000) High resolution chromosome 3p allelotyping of human lung cancer and preneoplastic/preinvasive bronchial epithelium reveals multiple, discontinuous sites of 3p allele loss and three regions of frequent breakpoints. *Cancer Res.* **60**, 1949–1960.
25. Behrens, C., Travis, L. B., Wistuba, II, Davis, S., Maitra, A., Clarke, E. A., et al. (2000) Molecular changes in second primary lung and breast cancers after therapy for Hodgkin's disease. *Cancer Epidemiol. Biomarkers Prev.* **9**, 1027–1035.
26. Viallet, J. and Sausville, E. A. (1996) Involvement of signal transduction pathways in lung cancer biology. *J. Cell Biochem.* (**Suppl. 24**), 228–236.
27. Richardson, G. E. and Johnson, B. E. (1993) The biology of lung cancer. *Semin. Oncol.* **20**, 105–127.
28. Krystal, G. W., Hines, S. J., and Organ, C. P. (1996) Autocrine growth of small cell lung cancer mediated by coexpression of c-kit and stem cell factor. *Cancer Res.* **56**, 370–376.
29. Krystal, G., Birrer, M., Way, J., Nau, M., Sausville, E., Thompson, C., et al. (1988) Multiple mechanisms for transcriptional regulation of the myc gene family in small-cell lung cancer. *Mol. Cell. Biol.* **8**, 3373–3381.
30. Brambilla, E., Negoescu, A., Gazzeri, S., Lantuejoul, S., Moro, D., Brambilla, C., and Coll, J. L. (1996) Apoptosis-related factors p53, Bcl2, and Bax in neuroendocrine lung tumors. *Am. J. Pathol.* **149**, 1941–1952.
31. Levin, N. A., Brzoska, P. M., Warnock, M. L., Gray, J. W., and Christman, M. F. (1995) Identification of novel regions of altered DNA copy number in small cell lung tumors. *Genes Chromosomes Cancer* **13**, 175–185.
32. Knudson, A. G. (1989) Hereditary cancers: clues to mechanisms of carcinogenesis. *Br. J. Cancer* **59**, 661–666.

33. Harris, C. C. (1996) p53 Tumor suppressor gene: from the basic research laboratory to the clinic—an abridged historical perspective. *Carcinogenesis* **17,** 1187–1198.
34. Takahashi, T., Nau, M. M., Chiba, I., Birrer, M. J., Rosenberg, R. K., Vinocour, M., et al. (1989) p53: A frequent target for genetic abnormalities in lung cancer. *Science* **246,** 491–494.
35. Denissenko, M. F., Pao, A., Tang, M.-S., and Pfeifer, G. P. (1996) Preferential formation of benz[a]pyrene adducts in lung cancer mutational hotspots in p53. *Science* **274,** 430–433.
36. Harbour, J. W., Sali, S. L., Whang-Peng, J., Gazdar, A. F., Minna, J. D., and Kaye, F. J. (1988) Abnormalities in structure and expression of the human retinoblastoma gene in SCLC. *Science* **241,** 353–357.
37. Cagle, P. T., el-Naggar, A. K., Xu, H. J., Hu, S. X., and Benedict, W. F. (1997) Differential retinoblastoma protein expression in neuroendocrine tumors of the lung. Potential diagnostic implications. *Am. J. Pathol.* **150,** 393–400.
38. Li, J., Yen, C., Liaw, D., Podyspanina, K., Bose, S., Wang, S. I., et al. (1997) PTEN, a putative protein tyrosine phosphatase gene mutated in human brain, breast and prostate cancer. *Science* **275,** 1943–1947.
39. Virmani, A. K., Fong, K. M., Kodagoda, D., McIntire, D., Hung, J., Tonk, V., et al. (1998) Allelotyping demonstrates common and distinct patterns of chromosomal loss in human lung cancer types. *Genes Chromosomes Cancer* **21,** 308–319.
40. Forgacs, E., Biesterveld, E. J., Sekido, Y., Fong, K., Muneer, S., Wistuba, II, et al. (1998) Mutation analysis of the PTEN/MMAC1 gene in lung cancer. *Oncogene* **17,** 1557–1565.
41. Ponting, C. P., Cai, Y. D., and Bork, P. (1997) The breast cancer gene product TSG101: a regulator of ubiquitination? *J. Mol. Med.* **75,** 467–469.
42. Mollenhauer, J., Wiemann, S., Scheurlen, W., Korn, B., Hayashi, Y., Wilgenbus, K. K., et al. (1997) DMBT1, a new member of the SRCR superfamily, on chromosome 10q25.3-26.1 is deleted in malignant brain tumours. *Nat Genet.* **17,** 32–39.
43. Wu, W., Kemp, B. L., Proctor, M. L., Gazdar, A. F., Minna, J. D., Hong, W. K., and Mao, L. (1999) Expression of DMBT1, a candidate tumor suppressor gene, is frequently lost in lung cancer. *Cancer Res.* **59,** 1846–1851.
44. Lerman, M. I. and Minna, J. D. (2000) The 630-kb lung cancer homozygous deletion region on human chromosome 3p21.3: identification and evaluation of the resident candidate tumor suppressor genes. The International Lung Cancer Chromosome 3p21.3 Tumor Suppressor Gene Consortium. *Cancer Res.* **60,** 6116–6133.
45. Burbee, D., Forgacs, E., Zöchbauer-Müller, S., Shivakuma, L., Fong, K., Gao, B., et al. RASFF1A in the 3p21.3 homozygous deletion region: epigenetic inactivation in lung an breast cancer and suppression of the malignant phenotype. *J. Natl. Cancer Inst.* In press.
46. Dammann, R., Li, C., Yoon, J. H., Chin, P. L., Bates, S., and Pfeifer, G. P. (2000) Epigenetic inactivation of a RAS association domain family protein from the lung tumour suppressor locus 3p21.3. *Nat. Genet.* **25,** 315–319.

47. Sozzi, G., Veronese, M. L., Negrini, M., Baffa, R., Corticelli, M. G., Inoue, H., et al. (1996) The FHIT gene at 3p14.2 is abnormal in lung cancer. *Cell* **85**, 17–26.

48. Fong, K. M., Biesterveld, E. J., Virmani, A., Wistuba, I., Sekido, Y., Bader, S. A., et al. (1997) *FHIT* and FRA3B allele loss are common in lung cancer and preneoplastic bronchial lesions and are associated with cancer-related *FHIT* cDNA splicing aberrations. *Cancer Res.* **57**, 2256–2267.

49. Sundaresan, V., Chung, G., Heppell-Parton, A., Xiong, J., Grundy, C., Roberts, I., et al. (1998) Homozygous deletions at 3p12 in breast and lung cancer. *Oncogene* **17**, 1723–1729.

50. Loeb, L. A. (1994) Microsatellite instability: marker of a mutator phenotype in cancer. *Cancer Res.* **54**, 5059–5063.

51. Baylin, S. B., Herman, J. G., Graff, J. R., Vertino, P. M., and Issa, J. P. (1998) Alterations in DNA methylation: a fundamental aspect of neoplasia. *Adv. Cancer Res.* **72**, 141–196.

52. Costello, J. F., Fruhwald, M. C., Smiraglia, D. J., Rush, L. J., Robertson, G. P., Gao, X., et al. (2000) Aberrant CpG-island methylation has non-random and tumour-type-specific patterns. *Nat. Genet.* **24**, 132–138.

53. Esteller, M., Sanchez-Cespedes, M., Rosell, R., Sidransky, D., Baylin, S. B., and Herman, J. G. (1999) Detection of aberrant promoter hypermethylation of tumor suppressor genes in serum DNA from non-small cell lung cancer patients. *Cancer Res.* **59**, 67–70.

54. Tang, X., Khuri, F. R., Lee, J. J., Kemp, B. L., Liu, D., Hong, W. K., and Mao, L. (2000) Hypermethylation of the death-associated protein (DAP) kinase promoter and aggressiveness in stage I non-small-cell lung cancer. *J. Natl. Cancer Inst.* **92**, 1511–1516.

55. Virmani, A. K., Rahti, A., Z^chbauer-M,ller, S., Sacchi, N., Fukuyama, Y., Bryant, D., et al. (2000) Promoter methylation and silencing of the retinoic acid receptor beta gene in lung carcinomas. *J. Natl. Cancer Inst.* **92**, 1303–1307.

56. Zochbauer-Muller, S., Fong, K. M., Virmani, A. K., Geradts, J., Gazdar, A. F., and Minna, J. D. (2001) Aberrant promoter methylation of multiple genes in non-small cell lung cancers. *Cancer Res.* **61**, 249–255.

57. Toyooka, K. O., Toyooka, S., Virmani, A. K., Sathyanatayan, U. G., Euhus, D. M., Gilcrease, M., et al. Loss of expression and aberrant methylation of the CDH13 (H-Cadherin) gene in breast and lung carcinomas. *Clin. Cancer Res.* In press.

58. Shivapurkar, N., Virmani, A. K., Wistuba, II, Milchgrub, S., Mackay, B., Minna, J. D., and Gazdar, A. F. (1999) Deletions of chromosome 4 at multiple sites are frequent in malignant mesothelioma and small cell lung carcinoma. *Clin. Cancer Res.* **5**, 17–23.

59. Betticher, D. C., Heighway, J., Thatcher, N., and Hasleton, P. S. (1997) Abnormal expression of CCND1 and RB1 in resection margin epithelia of lung cancer patients. *Br. J. Cancer* **75**, 1761–1768.

60. Nuorva, K., Soini, Y., Kamel, D., Autio-Harmainen, H., Risteli, L., Risteli, J., et al. (1993) Concurrent p53 expression in bronchial dysplasias and squamous cell lung carcinomas. *Am. J. Pathol.* **142**, 725–732.

61. Smith, A. L., Hung, J., Walker, L., Rogers, T. E., Vuitch, F., Lee, E., and Gazdar, A. F. (1996) Extensive areas of aneuploidy are present in the respiratory epithelium of lung cancer patients. *Br. J. Cancer* **73**, 203–209.
62. Westra, W. H., Baas, I. O., Hruban, R. H., Askin, F. B., Wilson, K., Offerhaus, G. J., and Slebos, R. J. (1996) K-ras oncogene activation in atypical alveolar hyperplasias of the human lung. *Cancer Res.* **56**, 2224–2228.
63. Sundaresan, V., Ganly, P., Hasleton, P., Rudd, R., Sinha, G., Bleehen, N. M., and Rabbitts, P. (1992) p53 and chromosome 3 abnormalities, characteristic of malignant lung tumours, are detectable in preinvasive lesions of the bronchus. *Oncogene* **7**, 1989–1997.
64. Mao, L., Lee, J. S., Kurie, J. M., Fan, Y. H., Lippman, S. M., Lee, J. J., et al. (1997) Clonal genetic alterations in the lungs of current and former smokers. *J. Natl. Cancer Inst.* **89**, 857–862.
65. Franklin, W. A., Gazdar, A. F., Haney, J., Wistuba, I. I., La Rosa, F. G., Kennedy, T., et al. (1997) Widely dispersed *p53* mutation in respiratory epithelium. *J. Clin. Invest.* **100**, 2133–2137.
66. Belinsky, S. A., Nikula, K. J., Palmisano, W. A., Michels, R., Saccomanno, G., Gabrielson, E., et al. (1998) Aberrant methylation of p16(INK4a) is an early event in lung cancer and a potential biomarker for early diagnosis. *Proc. Natl. Acad. Sci. USA* **95**, 11891–11896.
67. Palmisano, W. A., Divine, K. K., Saccomanno, G., Gilliland, F. D., Baylin, S. B., Herman, J. G., and Belinsky, S. A. (2000) Predicting lung cancer by detecting aberrant promoter methylation in sputum. *Cancer Res.* **60**, 5954–5958.
68. Mao, L., Hruban, R. H., Boyle, J. O., Tockman, M., and Sidransky, D. (1994) Detection of oncogene mutations in sputum precedes diagnosis of lung cancer. *Cancer Res.* **54**, 1634–1637.
69. Mills, N. E., Fishman, C. L., Scholes, J., Anderson, S. E., Rom, W. N., and Jacobson, D. R. (1995) Detection of K-ras oncogene mutations in bronchoalveolar lavage fluid for lung cancer diagnosis. *J. Natl. Cancer Inst.* **87**, 1056–1060.
70. Ahrendt, S. A., Chow, J. T., Xu, L. H., Yang, S. C., Eisenberger, C. F., Esteller, M., et al. (1999) Molecular detection of tumor cells in bronchoalveolar lavage fluid from patients with early stage lung cancer. *J. Natl. Cancer Inst.* **91**, 332–339.
71. Gazdar, A. F., Lam, S., and Wistuba, I. I. (2000) Molecular and cytologic techniques of early detection, in *Lung Cancer. Principles and Practice* (Pas, H. I., Mitchell, J. B., Johnson, D. H., Turrisi, A. T., and Minna, J. D., eds.), Lippincott Williams & Wilkins, Philadelphia, PA, pp. 407–424.

II

ETIOLOGY AND CLASSIFICATION OF LUNG TUMORS

2

Clinical and Biological Relevance of Recently Defined Categories of Pulmonary Neoplasia

Edward Gabrielson

1. Introduction

The clinical management of lung neoplasia now involves considerations of several diagnostic categories that were not in common use only a few years ago. In particular, there is now an increased recognition of neuroendocrine differentiation in lung cancer, including acknowledgment of large-cell neuroendocrine cancer as a distinct class of lung cancer. In addition, there is growing awareness of various form of early neoplasia in the lung, particularly *in situ* squamous cell proliferations and atypical adenomatous proliferations. With an emphasis on implications for clinical management, this review will discuss the biology of these important categories of lung neoplasia and compare them to other commonly recognized forms of lung tumors.

2. Neuroendocrine Differentiation and Classification of Lung Neoplasia

Other than the distinction between benign and malignant, the distinction between small cell cancer (SCLC) and non-small cell cancer (NSCLC) is perhaps considered to be the most important diagnostic decision made by the pathologist in the evaluation of lung neoplasms. SCLC is well-recognized to be highly aggressive and, because it is most often widely disseminated by the time a diagnosis is made, it is usually treated by chemotherapy rather than surgery.

SCLC is well-recognized as a highly malignant form of lung cancer, with neuroendocrine differentiation among its distinguishing characteristics. Carcinoid tumors, with an even greater degree of neuroendocrine differentia-

From: *Methods in Molecular Medicine, vol. 74: Lung Cancer, Vol. 1: Molecular Pathology Methods and Reviews*
Edited by: B. Driscoll © Humana Press Inc., Totowa, NJ

tion, typically have a low malignant potential and thus represent the other end of the clinical spectrum of lung tumors. These two types of neoplasia, which are clinically diverse, are frequently thought to represent different ends of a single biological class of tumors, based on the neuroendocrine differentiation common to these types of neoplasms. However, as discussed below, there is significant evidence to suggest that SCLC and carcinoid tumors are fundamentally different disease processes. In addition to these common forms of pulmonary neoplasia, a class of tumors known as large cell neuroendocrine carcinoma has been recently recognized. The accurate classification of lung tumors with neuroendocrine differentiation is thus more complex than previously recognized.

2.1. Small Cell Lung Cancer

Small cell lung cancers are distinctive tumors, with a characteristic cellular morphology that includes scant cytoplasm (thus resulting in an overall relatively small size of the cells), finely granular chromatin, absent or conspicuous nucleoli, and frequent mitoses (*see* **Fig. 1**). In actuality, the nuclear morphology, chromatin distribution, and high mitotic rate are more important than cell size in establishing the diagnosis, and variants of SCLC, all with similarly poor prognosis, are recognized (*1*). Although small cell lung cancers usually have only vague semblance to the usual neuroendocrine architecture in terms of nesting of cells and vacularity, electron microscopy has demonstrated that many SCLCs have dense-core granules typical of neuroendocrine cells. Dense-core granules in SCLC are occasionally situated in cell processes that resemble dendrites (*2*) but are generally few and small (100 to 13 nm). Moreover, approximately one-third of SCLCs do not have dense core granules, and cytoplasmic structures of other differentiation pathways, such as glandular structures or cytokeratin bundles, are also occasionally seen (*3*). Immunohistochemical studies of small cell lung cancer have confirmed the expression of markers of neuroendocrine differentiation but, again, these markers are not expressed in about 20% of small cell lung cancers (*4*). Furthermore, epithelial (cytokeratin) markers are expressed at variable levels (*5*), suggesting that many small cell cancers share differentiation phenotypes with non-small cell cancers. Thus, when classifying SCLC on the basis of neuroendocrine differentiation, it must be remembered that the association between small cell lung cancer and neuroendocrine differentiation is not absolute. Importantly, the diagnosis of SCLC is established by the characteristic microscopic morphology, and not by immunohistochemical or ultrastructural demonstration of neuroendocrine differentiation.

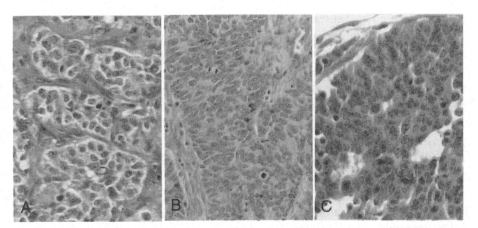

Fig. 1. Representative histology of pulmonary carcinoid (**A**), small cell lung cancer (**B**), and large cell neuroendocrine cancer (**C**). Note the "organoid architecture," lack of nuclear atypia, and low mitotic rate that distinguish carcinoid from the highly malignant forms of lung cancer. Small cell lung cancer has fewer and smaller nucleoli, as well as generally smaller cells, than the large cell neuroendocrine cancer. Other distinguishing characteristics are discussed in the text and references.

2.2. Pulmonary Carcinoid Tumors

Another common class of lung neoplasms with neuroendocrine differentiation is that of pulmonary carcinoid tumors, which are relatively uncommon (about 8% of all lung tumors) but distinctive neoplasms (*6*). Although these tumors have been previously classified as bronchial adenomas, they are now considered to be neoplasms of variable malignant potential. Most carcinoid tumors (typical carcinoids) are relatively well-circumscribed and have an "organoid" microscopic appearance similar to carcinoid tumors of other organs (*see* **Fig. 1**). Consistent with their nonaggressive nature, mitoses are infrequent and lymphatic or vascular invasion are rare in tumors classified as "typical carcinoid" (*6*).

A subset of pulmonary carcinoid tumors does have morphological and clinical features consistent with a relatively aggressive clinical biology (*7*). These tumors, termed atypical carcinoids, have increased numbers of mitoses compared to typical carcinoids and frequently manifest other morphological characteristics of malignancy, such as necrosis, lymphatic invasion, and vascular invasion. The prognosis of atypical carcinoid is intermediate between that of typical carcinoid and small cell lung cancer, and is related to the morphological characteristics of malignancy (*8,9*). These neoplasms are generally treated by aggressive surgery, including lymph-node dissection (10), and benefits of chemotherapy for treatment are still uncertain.

For many years, typical carcinoids and atypical carcinoids have been considered to represent the benign and intermediate levels of the spectrum of neuroendocrine lung tumors (respectively), with SCLC representing the malignant end of the spectrum of this group of tumors. A common progenitor cell, the Kulchitsky cell (11), has been proposed for all of these forms of neoplasia although, as discussed below, there is substantial evidence to suggest that SCLC and pulmonary carcinoid are fundamentally different classes of neoplasia.

Interestingly, carcinoid tumors typically show a much higher degree of neuroendocrine differentiation than small cell cancers. Electron microscopy almost invariably demonstrates numerous dense-core granules and immuno-histochemical markers of neuroendocrine differentiation typically stain these neoplasms with high intensity. These findings argue against a direct link between the extent of neuroendocrine differentiation and aggressive clinical biology.

2.3. Large Cell Neuroendocrine Cancer and Neuroendocrine Features in NSCLC

Neuroendocrine differentiation in pulmonary neoplasms extends beyond SCLC and carcinoid tumors. Recognizing that all non-small cell lung cancers with neuroendocrine differentiation cannot be neatly classified as atypical carcinoids or as SCLC, Travis and colleagues proposed large-cell neuroendo-crine cancer (LCNEC) as a new category of lung cancer (12). This category of lung cancer is defined by light microscopic evidence of neuroendocrine differentiation (e.g., organoid, palisading, trabecular or rosette-like growth patterns), large cell size, prominent nucleoli, high mitotic rate, coagulative necrosis, and neuroendocrine differentiation by electron microscopy or immu-nohistochemistry (see Fig. 1).

LCNEC occurs most frequently in the seventh decade of life and, similar to SCLC, occurs almost exclusively in smokers (13). More than half of LCNEC patient present with at least stage II disease and 5- and 10-yr survival rates for this cancer are only 27% and 9%, respectively (8). Thus, survival for this cancer is significantly worse that for atypical carcinoid and is not significantly different than that of SCLC of comparable stage. Because this category of lung cancer is relatively rare and only recently recognized, there is insufficient data to determine whether LCNEC has a response to chemotherapy comparable to SCLC.

Distinguishing LCNEC from atypical carcinoid is important from the standpoint of prognosis and, as discussed below, from the standpoint of studying the biology of these different forms of neoplasia. Yet, the diagnosis of these tumors can be difficult, even in the hands of pathologists with expertise in pulmonary neoplasia *(14)*.

Finally, a discussion of neuroendocrine differentiation in lung tumors should acknowledge that a significant percentage of non-small cell lung cancers have subtle characteristics of neuroendocrine differentiation, but not of a sufficient extent to warrant a diagnosis of SCLC or NLNEC. For example, one study reported that 12 % of non-small cell lung cancers stained immunohistochemically for two or more markers of a neuroendocrine panel (neuron-specific enolase (NSE), chromogranin A, Leu-7, gastrin-releasing peptide) *(15)*. These tumors were not found to have any difference in clinical outcome, however, suggesting that neuroendocrine features in NSCLC may not be clinically significant.

2.4. Neuroendocrine Differentiation in Classification of Pulmonary Neoplasia

Although pulmonary carcinoid tumors are often considered to be a part of the same spectrum of lung neoplasms as SCLC and LCNEC by virtue of neuroendocrine differentiation, there is significant molecular evidence that pulmonary carcinoid tumors are distantly related to these more aggressive forms of lung cancer. For example, while carcinoid tumors, SCLC, and LCNEC share a number of loci where loss of heterozygosity (LOH) is common, the patterns of p53 mutations are different between atypical carcinoids and SCLC or LCNEC *(16)*. Additional molecular evidence to separate carcinoid tumors from high-grade neuroendocrine cancers comes from analysis of the *MEN1* (multiple endocrine neoplasia type 1) gene, which is frequently mutated in typical and atypical carcinoid tumors *(17)*. In a study of small cell cancer, no mutations of this gene were found in any of the 45 SCLC samples (primary tumors and cell lines) analyzed and mutation of the gene was found in only 1 of 13 LCNEC samples studied *(18)*. Although it is possible that mutation of this gene represents a link between LCNEC and carcinoid, the possible misclassification of this single sample also remains a possibility. Finally, cDNA array studies have found little similarity in overall gene-expression patterns between carcinoid tumors and SCLC *(19)*.

More compelling evidence to classify carcinoids as distinct from SCLC or NCNEC, as opposed to a part of a continuous spectrum of neuroendocrine tumors, comes from clinical data. Notably, there is no evidence that tobacco smoking is a significant cause of pulmonary carcinoid *(13)*, although tobacco is clearly implicated as a cause of most cases of SCLC and NCNEC. Furthermore, clinical progression from typical carcinoid to high-grade neuorendocrine cancer (SCLC or LCNEC) has not been documented. Thus, while typical carcinoid, atypical carcinoid, LCNEC, and SCLC all share properties of neuroendocrine differentiation, there are substantial biological differences that separate the carcinoid tumors from high-grade neuroendocrine cancers.

Thus, many aspects of possible developmental relationships among SCLC, LCNEC, and carcinoid tumors are still unknown. It appears that there are fundamental and important differences between SCLC and carcinoid tumors on biological and molecular levels, yet these tumors still share the distinctive neuorendocrine properties. A common molecular link on this level may be expression at high levels of the human achaete-scute homolog-1 (HASH) gene, a basic helix-loop-helix transcription factor, in both SCLC and carcinoid tumors *(20)*. While expression of this transcription factor may be a common link between various forms of lung neoplasms with neuroendocrine differentiation, there is also clearly differential regulation of other molecular pathways in these various forms of lung tumors, which define the extent to which different tumors are malignant.

3. Early Neoplasia in the Lung

Another important area of pulmonary neoplasia that will be discussed in this chapter is that of early neoplasia in the lung. Currently, there is a great deal of interest in understanding the development of cancer and developing therapeutic interventions to halt or reverse the progression of lung cancer. As early forms of neoplasia are being recognized more frequently in patients, there is a need to have a sufficient understanding of the biology of these lesions to make reasonable treatment decisions.

It is probably appropriate to first note that in light of the evidence discussed above, there is no rationale for considering pulmonary carcinoid tumors, or the related "carcinoid tumorlets" to be precursors to SCLC or LCNEC. The precursor lesion for these tumors remains elusive and, because of the rapid growth rate usually seen in these highly malignant forms of cancer, may be difficult to find in analysis of lung cancer tissue.

3.1. Squamous Cell In Situ Proliferations

Squamous carcinoma *in situ* of the bronchial tree, the first form of early neoplasia to be described in the lung, was recognized by Oscar Auerbach and colleagues in an autopsy study of lungs from individuals who had smoked cigarettes *(21)*. Historically, this study was an important link in establishing cigarettes as a cause of lung cancer and it still has relevance today because molecular studies support the role of these *in situ* lesions in the multistage development of invasive lung cancer *(22)*.

In situ squamous cell cancers (and *in situ* dysplastic lesions) do not present with radiographically detectable lesions, but squamous dysplasia or carcinoma *in situ* can often be detected during endoscopic examination of bronchi, particularly when fluorescent lighting is used *(23)*. The recognition of *in situ* squamous cell cancers poses some complex patient management dilemmas. Although it is clear that many, and probably most, *in situ* squamous cell cancers will never progress to invasive cancer, it is not possible to predict in which lesions, or even in which individuals, will invasive cancer develop.

Logically, treatment of *in situ* squamous cell lesions should result in a decreased frequency of invasive squamous cell cancer in treated individuals. However, because individuals who have these lesions usually have multiple lesions, it is not feasible to treat *in situ* squamous cell carcinoma of the lung by surgical resection. Moreover, initial chemoprevention attempts for lung cancer have also been unsuccessful in decreasing lung cancer incidence (and possibly even increased lung cancer incidence) *(24,25)* and thus it is not clear that the chemopreventative agents with favorable activity in the squamous mucosa of the upper aerodigestive tract will help prevent the progression of squamous cell cancer in the lung. However, there remains hope that more specific interventions of lung cancer development will be found, and monitoring these *in situ* squamous lesions is likely to become important in the clinical management of pulmonary neoplasia.

3.2. Early Neoplasia in the Lung: Atypical Adenomatous Lesions

Only relatively recently has a lesion thought to be an early precursor for adenocarcinoma been recognized. In 1988, Miller and colleagues described a finding of discrete foci of atypical bronchioalveolar cells in lungs resected for adenocarcinoma *(26)*. These lesions, known as atypical adenomatous hyperplasia (AAH), can be recognized by routine microscopy as well as molecular studies to have similarities to adenocarcinoma and are thus thought to represent glandular carcinoma *in situ*.

AAH lesions present as 1- to 7-mm nodules with thickened alveolar septae lined by epithelial cells with varying degrees of atypia (*see* **Fig. 2**). Unlike most lung adenocarcinomas, there is no disruption of normal lung architecture and no stromal reaction typical of a host response to an invasive cancer. There are commonly (25%) multiple AAH lesions in lungs resected for pulmonary adenocarcinoma, particularly in those lungs of patients who smoke tobacco *(26,27)*. In contrast, AAH has been observed in only 2% of postmortem lungs from patients without lung neoplasms *(28)*.

The link between AAH and adenocarcinoma has been strengthened by molecular studies. In particular, *K-ras* mutations are found at approximately the same frequency in AAH and adenocarcinoma and the predominant type of mutation in both lesions is a G→T transversion at position 1 or 2 of codon 12 *(29)*. Interestingly, however, synchronous AAH and lung adenocarcinoma

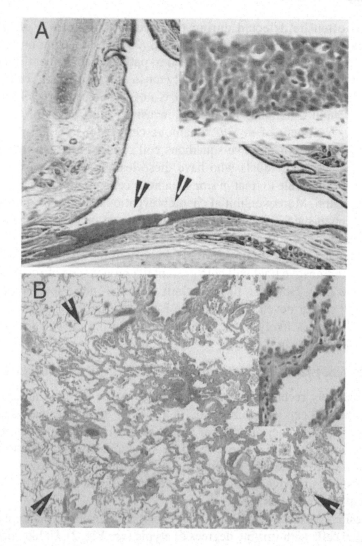

Fig. 2. Early, pre-invasive neoplasia in the lung. Squamous cell carcinoma *in situ* (**A**, arrows and inset) has lack of cellular maturation, and atypical cells with frequent mitoses, confined to the normal confines of the metaplastic stratified squamous epithelium. Atypical adenomatous hyperplasia (**B**, arrows and inset) has thickened alveolar septae lined by atypical epithelial cells. The lesion shown has a diameter of 7 mm, considered to be near the upper limits for classifying a lesion as atypical adenomatous hyperplasia as opposed to adenocarcinoma.

lesions often do not share the same *K-ras* base changes, suggesting that independent lesions can be arising simultaneously in subsets of high-risk patients *(29)*. Molecular characteristics that distinguish AAH from adenocarcinoma include lower allelic loss frequencies for chromosomal arms (3p, 9p, and 17p) that are commonly affected in adenocarcinoma *(30)*. In addition, no activation of telomerase activity has been observed in AAH, whereas activation of telomerase in nearly universal in adenocarcinoma *(31)*.

The clinical significance of AAH is still unknown. Because AAH is a multifocal process, it is reasonable to assume that patients with AAH found in a surgical resection specimen have many additional unresected lesions in others portions of their lungs. Yet, the presence of AAH does not appear to unfavorably affect prognosis and may, in fact, be associated with a somewhat better prognosis *(32,33)*. Thus, as for bronchial squamous cell carcinoma *in situ*, AAH does not inexorably progress to invasive cancer.

Because AAH is not as accessible by bronchoscopy as are squamous *in situ* lesions, it is not likely that AAH will be monitored as an intermediate endpoint in lung cancer chemoprevention trials. However, understanding the natural history of these lesions will become increasingly important as small pulmonary lesions are recognized more frequently by high-resolution imaging techniques, such as spiral computerized tomography (CT).

4. Concluding Remarks

The recognition of new classes of pulmonary neoplasia has contributed to our understanding of lung cancer biology, and will hopefully lead to improved clinical management of pulmonary neoplasia. One important area of progress is that of an increased understanding of neuroendocrine differentiation in lung tumors. While it appears that neuroendocrine differentiation itself does not confer an aggressive clinical behavior on a tumor, the NCNEC class of lung cancer does have a distinctively poor prognosis. Recognition of this class of cancers is an important first step in developing effective treatment for patients with this disease.

Additional progress has been made in the recognition of early, pre-invasive neoplasia with squamous or glandular differentiation. Again, our understanding of the biology of *in situ* squamous lesions and AAH is incomplete, compromising our ability to manage patients with these lesions. However, recognizing and monitoring these lesions during chemoprevention trials may help to gauge the effectiveness of various protocols in preventing lung cancer.

References

1. Colby, T. V., and Travis, W. D. (1995) Small cell carcinoma and large cell neuroendocrine carcinoma, in *Atlas of Tumor Pathology, Third Series: Tumors of*

the Lower Respiratory Tract (Colby, T. V., K., M. N., and Travis, W. D., eds.), Armed Forces Institute of Pathology, Washington, DC, pp. 235–257.

2. Mackay, B., Ordonez, N. G., Bennington, J. L., and Dugan, C. C. (1989) Ultrastructural and morphometric features of poorly differentiated and undifferentiated lung tumors. *Ultrastruct. Pathol.* **13**, 561–571.

3. Nomori, H., Shimosato, Y., Kodama, T., Morinaga, S., Nakajima, T., and Watanabe, S. (1986) Subtypes of small cell carcinoma of the lung: morphometric, ultrastructural, and immunohistochemical analyses. *Hum. Pathol.* **17**, 604–613.

4. Guinee, D. G., Jr., Fishback, N. F., Koss, M. N., Abbondanzo, S. L., and Travis, W. D. (1994) The spectrum of immunohistochemical staining of small-cell lung carcinoma in specimens from transbronchial and open-lung biopsies. *Am. J. Clin. Pathol.* **102**, 406–414.

5. Tabatowski, K., Vollmer, R. T., Tello, J. W., Iglehart, J. D., Shelburne, J. D., Schlom, J., and Johnston, W. W. (1988) The use of a panel of monoclonal antibodies in ultrastructurally characterized small cell carcinomas of the lung. *Acta Cytol.* **32**, 667–674.

6. Colby, T. V. and Travis, W. D. (1995) Carcinoid and other neuroendocrine tumors, In *Atlas of Tumor Pathology, Third Series: Tumors of the Lower Respiratory Tract* (Colby, T. V. and Travis, W. D., eds.), Armed Forces Institute of Pathology, Washington, DC, pp. 287–318

7. Arrigoni, M. G., Woolner, L. B., and Bernatz, P. E. (1972) Atypical carcinoid tumors of the lung. *J. Thorac. Cardiovasc. Surg.* **64**, 413–421.

8. Travis, W. D., Rush, W., Flieder, D. B., Falk, R., Fleming, M. V., Gal, A. A., and Koss, M. N. (1998) Survival analysis of 200 pulmonary neuroendocrine tumors with clarification of criteria for atypical carcinoid and its separation from typical carcinoid. *Am. J. Surg. Pathol.* **22**, 934–944.

9. Beasley, M. B., Thunnissen, F. B., Brambilla, E., Hasleton, P., Steele, R., Hammar, S. P., et al. (2000) Pulmonary atypical carcinoid: predictors of survival in 106 cases. *Hum. Pathol.* **31**, 1255–1265.

10. Wilkins, E. W., Jr., Grillo, H. C., Moncure, A. C., and Scannell, J. G. (1984) Changing times in surgical management of bronchopulmonary carcinoid tumor. *Ann. Thorac. Surg.* **38**, 339–344.

11. Cutz, E. (1982) Neuroendocrine cells of the lung. An overview of morphologic characteristics and development. *Exp. Lung Res.* **3**, 185–208.

12. Travis, W. D., Linnoila, R. I., Tsokos, M. G., Hitchcock, C. L., Cutler, G. B., Jr., Nieman, L., et al. (1991) Neuroendocrine tumors of the lung with proposed criteria for large-cell neuroendocrine carcinoma. An ultrastructural, immunohistochemical, and flow cytometric study of 35 cases. *Am. J. Surg. Pathol.* **15**, 529–553.

13. Flieder, D. B. and Vazquez, M. F. (2000) Lung tumors with neuroendocrine morphology. A perspective for the new millennium. *Radiol. Clin. North Am.* **38**, 563–577, ix.

14. Travis, W. D., Gal, A. A., Colby, T. V., Klimstra, D. S., Falk, R., and Koss, M. N. (1998) Reproducibility of neuroendocrine lung tumor classification. *Hum. Pathol.* **29**, 272–279.

15. Linnoila, R. I., Piantadosi, S., and Ruckdeschel, J. C. (1994) Impact of neuroendocrine differentiation in non-small cell lung cancer. The LCSG experience. *Chest* **106,** 367S–371S.
16. Onuki, N., Wistuba, I. I., Travis, W. D., Virmani, A. K., Yashima, K., Brambilla, E., et al. (1999) Genetic changes in the spectrum of neuroendocrine lung tumors. *Cancer* **85,** 600–607.
17. Debelenko, L. V., Brambilla, E., Agarwal, S. K., Swalwell, J. I., Kester, M. B., Lubensky, I. A., et al. (1997) Identification of MEN1 gene mutations in sporadic carcinoid tumors of the lung. *Hum. Mol. Genet.* **6,** 2285–2290.
18. Debelenko, L. V., Swalwell, J. I., Kelley, M. J., Brambilla, E., Manickam, P., Baibakov, G., et al. (2000) MEN1 gene mutation analysis of high-grade neuroendocrine lung carcinoma. *Genes Chromosomes Cancer* **28,** 58–65.
19. Anbazhagan, R., Tihan, T., Bornman, D. M., Johnston, J. C., Saltz, J. H., Weigering, A., et al. (1999) Classification of small cell lung cancer and pulmonary carcinoid by gene expression profiles. *Cancer Res.* **59,** 5119–5122.
20. Ball, D. W., Azzoli, C. G., Baylin, S. B., Chi, D., Dou, S., Donis-Keller, H., et al. (1993) Identification of a human achaete-scute homolog highly expressed in neuroendocrine tumors. *Proc. Natl. Acad. Sci. USA* **90,** 5648–5652.
21. Auerbach, O., Hammond, E. C., and Garfinkel, L. (1979) Changes in bronchial epithelium in relation to cigarette smoking, 1955–1960 vs. 1970–1977. *N. Engl. J. Med.* **300,** 381–385.
22. Wistuba, I. I., Behrens, C., Milchgrub, S., Bryant, D., Hung, J., Minna, J. D., and Gazdar, A. F. (1999) Sequential molecular abnormalities are involved in the multistage development of squamous cell lung carcinoma. *Oncogene* **18,** 643–650.
23. Lam, S., Kennedy, T., Unger, M., Miller, Y. E., Gelmont, D., Rusch, V., et al. (1998) Localization of bronchial intraepithelial neoplastic lesions by fluorescence bronchoscopy. *Chest* **113,** 696–702.
24. The Alpha-Tocopheral, B.-C.C.P.S.G. (1994) The effect of vitamin E and beta carotene on the incidence of lung cancer and other cancers in male smokers. The Alpha-Tocopherol, Beta Carotene Cancer Prevention Study Group. *N. Engl. J. Med.* **330,** 1029–1035.
25. Omenn, G. S., Goodman, G. E., Thornquist, M. D., Balmes, J., Cullen, M. R., Glass, A., et al. (1996) Risk factors for lung cancer and for intervention effects in CARET, the Beta-Carotene and Retinol Efficacy Trial. *J. Natl. Cancer Inst.* **88,** 1550–1559.
26. Miller, R. R., Nelems, B., Evans, K. G., Muller, N. L., and Ostrow, D. N. (1988) Glandular neoplasia of the lung. A proposed analogy to colonic tumors. *Cancer* **61,** 1009–1014.
27. Rao, S. K. and Fraire, A. E. (1995) Alveolar cell hyperplasia in association with adenocarcinoma of lung. *Mod. Pathol.* **8,** 165–169.
28. Sterner, D. J., Mori, M., Roggli, V. L., and Fraire, A. E. (1997) Prevalence of pulmonary atypical alveolar cell hyperplasia in an autopsy population: a study of 100 cases. *Mod. Pathol.* **10,** 469–473.

29. Westra, W. H., Baas, I. O., Hruban, R. H., Askin, F. B., Wilson, K., Offerhaus, G. J., and Slebos, R. J. (1996) K-ras oncogene activation in atypical alveolar hyperplasias of the human lung. *Cancer Res.* **56,** 2224–2228.
30. Kitaguchi, S., Takeshima, Y., Nishisaka, T., and Inai, K. (1998) Proliferative activity, p53 expression and loss of heterozygosity on 3p, 9p and 17p in atypical adenomatous hyperplasia of the lung. *Hiroshima J. Med. Sci.* **47,** 17–25.
31. Yashima, K., Litzky, L. A., Kaiser, L., Rogers, T., Lam, S., Wistuba, I. I., et al. (1997) Telomerase expression in respiratory epithelium during the multistage pathogenesis of lung carcinomas. *Cancer Res.* **57,** 2373–2377.
32. Suzuki, K., Nagai, K., Yoshida, J., Yokose, T., Kodama, T., Takahashi, K., et al. (1997) The prognosis of resected lung carcinoma associated with atypical adenomatous hyperplasia: a comparison of the prognosis of well-differentiated adenocarcinoma associated with atypical adenomatous hyperplasia and intrapulmonary metastasis. *Cancer* **79,** 1521–1526.
33. Takigawa, N., Segawa, Y., Nakata, M., Saeki, H., Mandai, K., Kishino, D., et al. (1999) Clinical investigation of atypical adenomatous hyperplasia of the lung. *Lung Cancer* **25,** 115–121.

3

Molecular Epidemiology of Human Cancer Risk

Gene–Environment Interactions and p53 Mutation Spectrum in Human Lung Cancer

Kirsi Vähäkangas

1. Introduction

Epidemiology has identified several etiological factors in lung cancer, of which the most important are exposure to cigarette smoke and other uses of tobacco products *(1,2)*. Epidemiological studies also have proved the synergistic effects between many of these factors, for example smoking and radon, and smoking and asbestos *(3)*. Owing to the long latency of the carcinogenic effect, the multietiology of cancer, and the interindividual differences in cancer risk, molecular studies are now being used in conjunction with epidemiological methods in order to gain a deeper understanding of cancer causation at an individual level *(4)*. In molecular epidemiology, the mechanistic hypotheses are tested in studies with epidemiological design. Family cancer syndromes, chromosomal instability syndromes, and the genes identified as causes for them *(5,6)*, as well as a better understanding of the mechanism of chemical carcinogenesis with the key role of xenobiotic metabolism *(7)*, have opened new avenues for hypothesis development in individual susceptibility *(8)*. Current challenges in molecular epidemiology include the establishment of good epidemiological designs and the development and validation of laboratory methods for such studies.

Understanding the role of genetic damage and its repair in the mechanism of lung cancer are providing ideas for new treatment options and better diagnostics as well as clues of etiology *(9–13)*. Recent studies have established

From: *Methods in Molecular Medicine, vol. 74: Lung Cancer, Vol. 1: Molecular Pathology Methods and Reviews*
Edited by: B. Driscoll © Humana Press Inc., Totowa, NJ

the molecular heterogeneity of tumors and tumor cells *(14–16)*. Of the many known genes mutated in lung cancer, mutations in the p53 tumor-suppressor gene are the most frequent and differ from mutations in other tumor-suppressor genes by being mostly missense mutations *(9,17)*. p53 protein and the whole p53 network *(18)* seem to be central players in lung carcinogenesis induced by environmental factors, especially smoking *(19)*.

Finally, most molecular epidemiology studies include genetic research among healthy people. Therefore, discussion of the ethical implications of such studies is necessary not only to protect those involved, but also to increase understanding of the positive implications of such studies *(20–22)*.

2. Genetic and Epigenetic Changes in Lung Cancer

2.1. Multiplicity of Genetic Defects in Lung Tumors

Multiple genetic changes are typical in cancer cells and are commonly found in oncogenes and tumor suppressor genes. In lung cancer, frequent gene defects and mutations have been shown to occur in chromosomes 3p (FHIT), 5q, 8p, 9p (p16/CDKN2), 9q, 11p, 11q, 13q (Rb), 17p (p53), and 17q, at sites of known or putative tumor-suppressor genes *(23–26)*. One tumor always contains a multitude of genetic defects, which has lead to a hypothesis of a mutator phenotype, which allows mutations to accumulate *(27)*. Of the known (over 100) oncogenes, those with most frequent aberrations in lung cancer are K-ras (up to 20% of lung cancers mutated) and C-myc (up to 30% incidence of overexpression or amplification) *(25)*. Of the tumor-suppressor genes, by far the most frequently mutated is p53 *(9,28)*. Other major genetic alterations in lung cancer detected so far are the inactivation of the Rb pathway (Rb and p16^{INK4} mutations) and the disruption of *fragile histidine triad* (FHIT) sequences *(25)*. According to recent studies, P14^{ARF}, an alternatively spliced product of the same gene that codes for p16^{INK4}, is also frequently altered in lung cancer (*29* and references therein).

2.2. The Role of Promoter Methylation

Lately, promoter hypermethylation of genes as a possible epigenetic mechanism for blocking the function of tumor suppressor genes in lung cancer has attracted interest *(30)*. Aberrant promoter methylation of several genes, including p16^{INK4}, has been found in NSCLC, both in malignant and nonmalignant tissue *(31)* with association to smoking (*32* and references therein). Hypermethylation of the p16^{INK4} promoter found in nonmalignant tissue and frequently in premalignant bronchial lesions *(33)* and also supported by other data (*see* **ref.** *30*) implicates methylation as an early marker for lung cancer.

This is further supported by the findings of Palmisano et al. *(34)* who describe methylation of p16^{INK4} in all 11 studied sputum samples taken up to 35 mo before the diagnosis of lung cancer, while among 123 noncancer patients less than 20% of sputum samples were positive for the methylation. On the other hand, the study of Seike and coworkers *(35)* suggests that it may also be a late change and an alternative carcinogenic mechanism in tumors with wild-type p53.

2.3. Differences Between SCLC and NSCLC

Molecular comparison of small cell lung cancer (SCLC) and non-small cell lung cancer (NSCLC) has revealed a different frequency of events at the genetic and protein levels *(25)*. High rates of C-myc amplification (up to 30%) and bcl-2 expression (up to 95%) are typical of SCLC, while the incidence of these events is much lower in NSCLC (5–10% and 10–35%, respectively). Also, SCLC frequently harbors p53 mutations and RB is almost always absent, while in NSCLC, p53 mutations are not as frequent and RB is absent in less than 30% of the tumors. Apoptotic capacity of the cells representing these two types of lung tumors also differ. SCLC cells are more prone to undergo apoptosis *(36)*. Unexpectedly, using SCLC and NSCLC cell lines, Joseph and coworkers *(37)* showed that regardless of the propensity to undergo spontaneous apoptosis, SCLC are deficient in several caspases and have a higher ratio of the anti-apoptotic bcl-2 to the pro-apoptotic Bax than NSCLC cells.

2.4. Molecular Heterogeneity Within Tumor Subtypes

The complexity does not end at the level of SCLC vs NSCLC. Within each of the histological subtypes, there exists molecular heterogeneity. In a recent paper, Sanchez-Cespedes and coworkers *(38)* also showed that adenocarcinoma of lung is molecularly a heterogenous group of tumors that develop probably through at least two distinct pathways. Allelic losses or gains were more frequent in several chromosomal arms (3p, 6q, 9p, 16p, 17p, 19p) in smokers than in nonsmokers. Tobacco-related adenocarcinoma could be further divided into two groups with high or low levels of chromosomal abnormalities. In keeping with the role of p53 as the guardian of the genome *(39)*, p53 mutations were more frequent among the tumors with a high level of abnormalities. Similar findings were reported by Ahrendt and coworkers *(40)*. Heterogeneity within lung cancer histological subtypes with a higher frequency of p53 mutations was found in lung cancers with a high level of microsatellite instability at tetranucleotide repeats. For p53-related markers (*see* **Table 1**) and FHIT *(50)* evidence already exists that a better molecular categorization of lung tumors would be of clinical significance.

Table 1
Possible p53-Associated Molecular Markers in Lung Cancer

P53 event	Marker for	Reference
P53 mutation spectrum	Exposure at population level	Greenblatt et al., 1994 *(9)*
		Hainaut and Pfeifer, 2001 *(19)*
Hypermethylation of p53 exons 5–8 in PBL of male smokers	Increased risk	Woodson et al., 2001 *(41)*
MspI polymorphism in intron 6	Increased risk	Biros et al., 2001 *(42)*
P53 mutation in bronchial lavage cells	Early detection	Ahrendt et al., 1999 *(43)*
P53 mutation in sputum smears	Early detection	Mao et al., 1994 *(44)*
		Chen et al., 2000 *(45)*
P53 mutation in bronchial biopsy	Early detection	Lang et al., 2000 *(46)*
Negative p53 IHC	Response to chemotherapy	Tanaka et al., 2001 *(47)*
P53 overexpression (in NSCLC)	Survival	Hanaoka et al., 2001 *(48)*
p53 antibodies in serum	Early detection	Soussi, 2000 *(49)*
	Poor prognosis	
	Better survival after radiotherapy	

3. Gene–Environment Interactions in Lung Cancer Risk

Lung cancer is a typical example of a cancer with known links to environmental factors. Gene-environment interactions can be recognized at several levels.

3.1. The Role of Cytochrome P450 (CYP) Catalyzed Reactions

The first gene-environment interaction that may occur in the development of lung cancer is carcinogen activation through cytochrome P450 (CYP) catalyzed reactions.

Genetic differences in these enzymes determine partly the extent of the activation and, consequently, the following amount of DNA-binding and the probability of mutagenic events *(51)*. The genes associated with lung cancer risk (*see* **Table 2**) include CYP1A1, microsomal epoxide hydrolase, and GSTM1, which all take part in the metabolism of benzo(a)pyrene (BP), the most studied tobacco carcinogen *(57)*. CYP1A1 and mEH (microsomal epoxide hydrolase) catalyze the activation of BP to BP-diolepoxide (BPDE) and GSTM1 deactivates epoxides created through the activation pathways. Support for the in vivo significance of the metabolism polymorphisms comes

Table 2
Susceptibility Factors for Lung Cancer Among Polymorphic
Xenobiotic Metabolizing Enzymes

Enzyme	Substrates	Change in activity	Risk	Reference
CYP1A1	PAH, AFB1	Increased	Increased in Japanese	Bartsch et al., 2000 *(52)*
CYP2A6	Nitrosamines, Heterocyclic Amines, AFB1	Decreased	Decreased in Japanese	Miyamoto et al., 1999 *(53)*
MEH	PAH, Aromatic amines, Styrene oxide, Benzene	Increased	Increased	Benhamou et al., 1998 *(54)*, Persson et al., 1999 *(55)*
GSTM1	Epoxides (PAH, AFB1)	Absent	Increased	Houlston, 1999 *(56)*

from studies showing that a genetically high CYP1A1 activity, combined with a genetically absent GSTM1, leads to higher BPDE adduct levels in blood *(58,59)*. As suggested by these findings, a lower level of BPDE-adducts were found in patients with two polymorphic slow alleles of mEH compared with those harboring wild-type alleles by Pastorelli and co-workers *(58)*. In our recent study we found that nonsmokers homozygous for GSTM1 null genotype have a greater risk from environmental tobacco smoke than people with other genotypes *(60)*.

3.2. Induction of Xenobiotic Metabolizing Enzymes

Another level of gene-environment interactions is the induction of the expression of xenobiotic metabolizing genes by environmental chemicals affecting carcinogen activation. CYP genes are regulated by ligand-activated nuclear receptors, e.g., induction of CYP1A1 gene expression through the binding of polycyclic aromatic hydrocarbons (PAH) to the Ah receptor *(61)*. The Ah-receptor-PAH complex, in association with the AhR nuclear translocator (Arnt), is translocated into the nucleus and binds to xenobiotic response elements, which turn on CYP gene transcription. So far, however, no polymorphisms in Ah receptor or the Arnt protein have been found that would explain the variation in inducibility of CYP1A1 *(62)*.

3.3. The Role of DNA Damage Repair Enzymes

Repair of carcinogen-DNA-adducts induced by carcinogen activation can be regarded as the third level of interaction. DNA-repair enzymes display a large interindividual variation, which makes the induction of smoking on these activities difficult to study *(63)*. Lung cancer risk is increased by lower activity of the repair functions, especially in females and in those with a family history of lung cancer *(64)*. Sequence variations occur in DNA-repair genes and recent data on XPD and XRCC1 genes support their clinical significance in lung cancer risk. Studies on lung cancer cases and controls suggest that XPD polymorphisms have a modulating effect on DNA repair capacity *(65)* and increase the risk of lung cancer *(66)*. XRCC1 polymorphisms seem to similarly influence lung cancer risk *(67)*, especially the risk for adenocarcinoma *(68)*.

3.4. Direct Action of Activated Carcinogens on Genes

The fourth level of gene-environment interactions in lung cancer involves the direct action of the activated carcinogens on targeted genes. Carcinogen-DNA adducts, if not corrected, may lead to mutations. The most serious of these occur in certain tumor-suppressor genes. The p53 tumor-suppressor gene, which is mutated the most in human lung cancer, is more prone to missense mutations when compared with other tumor-suppressor genes *(5)*.

4. P53 Mutations

4.1. p53 as a Molecular Marker

The p53 gene is located in chromosome 17p13.1 and encodes a multifunctional nuclear phosphoprotein. This protein has attracted interest in connection with chemical carcinogenesis for two reasons *(69)*: 1) in some cases the p53 gene shows a peculiar, carcinogen-specific mutation spectrum *(9,28)*; and 2) p53 protein expression is induced in cells in response to DNA damage and is involved in DNA repair and apoptosis *(70–72)*. The p53 protein plays an interesting role at the crossroads of the cellular pathways leading to cell-cycle arrest or apoptosis (*see* **Fig. 1**) *(11,18)*. This has lead to an explosion of p53 studies. Although the major result up to this point has been much confusion as to the usefulness of p53 as a molecular marker, this uncertainty should be resolved with better and more specific methodologies and bigger studies to validate the markers. In lung cancer, p53-related markers have been studied for various clinical purposes (*see* **Table 1**) and these preliminary studies implicate the usefulness of p53 for early diagnosis, therapeutic strategies, and prognosis *(11,13,73)*. Existing controversies are well-illustrated by the results of p53 serum antibodies as a marker for survival. Three papers report poor survival of NSCLC patients with p53 antibodies, especially patients with SCC, and one paper reports such an association in SCLC *(49)*. On the other hand, contradictory results have been reported both in SCLC *(74)* and in NSCLC *(75)*.

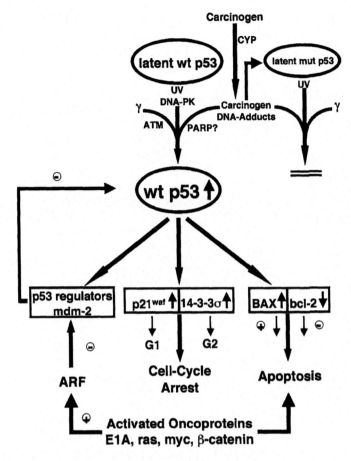

Fig. 1. Cellular pathways for p53.

4.2. Significance of p53 Mutations in Lung Cancer

p53 mutations reduce the rates of DNA repair and make cells more susceptible to further DNA-damage. For example, removal of BPDE-DNA-adducts is
slower from a human fibroblast cell line with defective p53 when compared with
the cell line with wild-type p53 *(76)*. Also, other genetic damage, like allelic
imbalance within the FHIT locus *(77)* and high levels of other chromosomal
abnormalities *(7,78)* often coexist with a p53 mutation. Alteration of TP53 gene,
as with any cancer-related mutation, represents a combination of the interaction
of carcinogens with DNA, failure of DNA-repair, and the selection of mutations
that provide premalignant cells with a growth advantage *(11,18,21)*. The
frequency, timing, and mutational spectrum of TP53 mutations provide insight
into the etiology and molecular pathogenesis of lung cancer *(9,11,17)*. Because

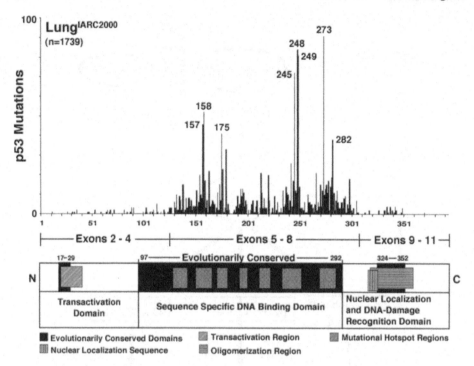

Fig. 2. p53 gene and protein with the mutation spectrum in lung cancer.

TP53 mutations are more common in cancers than any other mutations in cancer-related genes, more than 10,000 different mutations in human cancers have been reported and listed in the IARC-based database (http://www.iarc.fr/p53/homepage.html). For lung cancer, close to 2,000 mutations are listed (*see* **Fig. 2**) *(19)*.

4.3. The Relationship Between p53 Mutations and Smoking

Smoking is a well-known risk factor for lung cancer, and the incidence of all different histological types of lung cancers is increased because of it. Experimental studies have implied that carcinogens in cigarette smoke may be related to specific mutations in the mutation spectrum. Benzo(a)pyrene (BP), a polycyclic aromatic hydrocarbon (PAH), that is the most well-known of cigarette smoke-related carcinogens, typically induces $G:C-T:A$ transversions in genes *(69)*. These transversions are also quite common in smoking-related lung cancer, with a dose-response relationship *(5)*. Pfeifer and coworkers *(79–81)* have shown that the codons 157, 248, and 273 in the p53 gene, most often mutated in lung cancer (*see* **Fig. 2**), are also targets for DNA-adduct formation by BP and more prone to mutations by it. Slow repair of these adducts *(82)*, and the preferential BPDE adduct formation at methylated CpG sites *(83,84)*, probably contribute to the mutation spectrum in smoking-related lung cancer, where G to T mutations at CpG sites are the most common single-mutation type *(19)*. The same group *(81)* also studied other PAH-compounds and found a similar preference for adduct formation in codons 157, 158, 245, 248, and 273. These studies strongly support PAHs, especially BP, in cigarette smoke as contributing to the known cigarette-smoke-associated p53 mutation spectrum in lung cancer.

4.3.1. Comparison of p53 Mutations in Smokers vs Nonsmokers

However, the proof for a specific p53 mutation spectrum related to smoking requires the comparison of the mutation spectrum in lung cancers from smokers to that in nonsmokers. Such studies are difficult to carry out because of the rarity of lung cancer in nonsmokers. A further difficulty is that most smokers and smoking-related lung cancers are found in men and most nonsmokers are women. Consequently, the possible gender-difference, as well as a possible geographical difference *(5)* have to be taken into account in such studies. The few existing studies on nonsmokers can be interpreted as supporting the hypothesis of smoking-related TP53 mutations with an incidence of 10–26% in nonsmokers when compared with the incidence of about 60% in smokers *(85* and references therein). In recalculations based on the most recent edition of the IARC-based p53 mutation database, Hainaut and Pfeifer *(19)* confirmed the suggested statistically significant difference in G to T transversions between smokers and nonsmokers *(5,86)*.

4.3.2. The Effect of Former or Passive Smoking on p53 Mutations

Even fewer papers exist on the effect of former or passive smoking on p53 mutations. Husgafvel-Pursiainen and co-workers *(87)* showed that lung cancers from passive smokers have an increased risk for p53 mutations. In our own recent study *(85)*, the few cases of former smokers had a significantly higher frequency of p53 mutations than the ones with no smoking history. Also, sites of mutations seemed to differ from the typical smoking-related cases. Thus, the existing molecular epidemiology studies on different aspects of smoking-related lung cancer support the current mechanistic hypotheses, including carcinogen activation leading to mutations through DNA-adducts at specific inactivating sites of p53 tumor-suppressor gene, and this sequence of events opening the gates to accumulation of mutations *(5,8,19,39)*.

5. Ethical Aspects of Molecular Epidemiology

Molecular epidemiology deals with both healthy people and individual risk and is largely genetic by nature. Consequently, there are important ethical aspects to consider before the execution of studies *(21,22)*. At best, the analysis for individual susceptibility, e.g., analysis of drug-metabolism polymorphisms, protects individuals by warning of potential risks. Past discrimination has been known to occur based on the mere fact that a genetic test was performed, even without knowledge of the gene studied or the result of the test. The principle of informed consent is central in the Declaration of Helsinki *(88,89)* and is meant to ensure that no individual is misused in scientific research. Consideration of research subjects more as collaborators than mere "subjects" and education of the public to understand scientific principles aid in creating a good working relationship between scientists and the research subjects.

Health issues are regarded as sensitive and entitled to privacy *(21)*. In molecular epidemiology, both computerized databases and the storage of samples may endanger privacy. Samples with identifiers from older studies exist throughout research institutions and present a challenge for the guardians of these archives. Whether and how these sample collections can be used for purposes other than originally planned is only one of the unresolved questions for molecular epidemiologists. On one hand, there is a general feeling that coded samples without possibilities for identification could be used for validation of molecular epidemiology markers. On the other, in genetic studies, the possibility of a link to disease revealed by future studies has been presented as an argument for retaining personal information.

Ethics involves principles of conduct governing an individual or a group, conforming to accepted professional standards of conduct, and usually regarded as morally sufficient. However, ethics can also be understood as reconsideration of existing moral principles. If this is accepted, laws and moral principles are necessary but not sufficient for good ethics. Since personal thinking grows from personal values, ethics cannot be value-free. This applies also to research ethics. Molecular epidemiology, especially, is a field where risk of false conclusion about the hypothesis may have social consequences, and thus nonepistemic values should be taken into consideration *(90)*. For instance, molecular epidemiology of smoking and lung cancer *(19)* has direct social consequences depending on whether authorities in different countries regard the evidence convincing enough to ban smoking.

6. Summary

Molecular epidemiology of cancer risk utilizes knowledge of both the genetic changes in cancer and the current hypothesis of chemical carcinogenesis when selecting possible markers for individual susceptibility, early disease, and biologically significant exposure. Polymorphisms of drug-metabolizing enzymes, especially CYP enzymes, and mutations in the p53 tumor-suppressor gene have been in the center of interest for the past decade. Both have shown promise, CYP polymorphisms as markers for individual susceptibility and p53 mutation spectrum at population level for specific exposure. However, it is probable that very few markers, if any, are sufficient alone. Future challenges for molecular epidemiology in the lung cancer field include pursuing ethically the best performance in applying that knowledge, in addition to the development of reliable and well-validated markers.

Acknowledgments

Dr. Curtis C. Harris has given valuable comments to the manuscript. I also greatly appreciate the help of Ms. Judith A. Welsh in the search for references and in drawing the figures.

References

1. IARC (1986) IARC monographs on the evaluation of the carcinogenic risk of chemicals to man: tobacco smoking. *IARC Sci. Publ.* **38**, 1–397.
2. Hackshaw, A. K., Law, M. R., and Wald, N. J. (1997) The accumulated evidence on lung cancer and environmental tobacco smoke. *BMJ* **315**, 980–988.
3. Burkart, W. (2001) Combined effect of radiation and other agents: is there a synergism trap? *J. Environ. Pathol. Toxicol. Oncol.* **20**, 53–58.
4. Perera, F. P. (1996) Molecular epidemiology: Insights into cancer susceptibility, risk assessment, and prevention. *J. Natl. Cancer Inst.* **88**, 496–509.
5. Bennett, W. P., Hussain, S. P., Vahakangas, K. H., Khan, M. A., Shields, P. G., and Harris, C. C. (1999) Molecular epidemiology of human cancer risk: gene-environment interactions and p53 mutation spectrum in human lung cancer. *J. Pathol.* **187**, 8–18.
6. Wright, E. G. (1999) Inherited and inducible chromosomal instability: a fragile bridge between genome integrity mechanisms and tumourigenesis. *J. Pathol.* **187**, 19–27.
7. Pelkonen, O., Raunio, H., Rautio, A., and Lang, M. (1999) Chapter 8. Xenobiotic-metabolizing enzymes and cancer risk: correspondence between genotype and phenotype. *IARC Sci. Publ.* **148**, 77–88.
8. Shields, P. G. and Harris, C. C. (2000) Cancer risk and low-penetrance susceptibility genes in gene-environment interactions. *J. Clin. Oncol.* **18**, 2309–2315.
9. Greenblatt, M. S., Bennett, W. P., Hollstein, M., and Harris, C. C. (1994) Mutations in the p53 tumor suppressor gene: clues to cancer etiology and molecular pathogenesis. *Cancer Res.* **54**, 4855–4878.
10. Sidransky, D. and Hollstein, M. (1996) Clinical implications of the p53 gene. *Annu. Rev. Med.* **47**, 285–301.
11. Harris, C. C. (1996) Structure and function of the p53 tumor suppressor gene: clues for rational cancer therapeutic strategies. *J. Natl. Cancer Inst.* **88**, 1442–1455.
12. Fahraeus, R., Fischer, P., Krausz, E., and Lane, D. P. (1999) New approaches to cancer therapies. *J. Pathol.* **187**, 138–146.

13. Hupp, T. R., Lane, D. P., and Ball, K. L. (2000) Strategies for manipulating the p53 pathway in the treatment of human cancer. *Biochem. J.* **352 (Pt 1)**, 1–17.
14. Soues, S., Wiltshire, M., and Smith, P. J. (2001) Differential sensitivity to etoposide (VP-16)-induced S phase delay in a panel of small-cell lung carcinoma cell lines with G1/S phase checkpoint dysfunction. *Cancer Chemother. Pharmacol.* **47**, 133–140.
15. Shin, S. W., Breathnach, O. S., Linnoila, R. I., Williams, J., Gillespie, J. W., Kelley, M. J., and Johnson, B. E. (2001) Genetic changes in contralateral bronchioloalveolar carcinomas of the lung. *Oncology* **60**, 81–87.
16. Tanaka, F., Otake, Y., Yanagihara, K., Yamada, T., Miyahara, R., Kawano, Y., et al. (2001) Apoptosis and p53 status predict the efficacy of postoperative administration of UFT in non-small cell lung cancer. *Br. J. Cancer* **84**, 263–269.
17. Hainaut, P. and Hollstein, (2000) M. p53 and human cancer: the first ten thousand mutations. *Adv. Cancer Res.* **77**, 81–137.
18. Vogelstein, B., Lane, D., and Levine, A. J. (2000) Surfing the p53 network. *Nature* **408**, 307–310.
19. Hainaut, P. and Pfeifer, G. P. (2001) Patterns of p53 G→T transversions in lung cancers reflect the primary mutagenic signature of DNA-damage by tobacco smoke. *Carcinogenesis* **22**, 367–374.
20. Schulte, P. A., Hunter, D., and Rothman, N. (1997) Ethical and social issues in the use of biomarkers in epidemiological research. *IARC Sci. Publ.* **142**, 313–318.
21. Hainaut, P. and Vahakangas, K. (1999) Chapter 24. Genetic analysis of metabolic polymorphisms in molecular epidemiological studies: social and ethical implications. *IARC Sci. Publ.* **148**, 395–402.
22. Vahakangas, K. (2001) Ethical implications of genetic analysis of individual susceptibility to diseases. *Mutat. Res.* **482**, 105–110.
23. Viallet, J. and Minna, J. D. (1990) Dominant oncogenes and tumor suppressor genes in the pathogenesis of lung cancer. *Am. J. Respir. Cell Mol. Biol.* **2**, 225–232.
24. Gazdar, A. F. (1994) The molecular and cellular basis of human lung cancer. *Anticancer Res.* **14**, 261–267.
25. Sekido, Y., Fong, K. M., and Minna, J. D. (1998) Progress in understanding the molecular pathogenesis of human lung cancer. *Biochim. Biophys. Acta* **1378**, F21–F59.
26. Kohno, T. and Yokota, J. (1999) How many tumor suppressor genes are involved in human lung carcinogenesis? *Carcinogenesis* **20**, 1403–1410.
27. Loeb, L. A. (2001) A mutator phenotype in cancer. *Cancer Res.* **61**, 3230–3239.
28. Hollstein, M., Sidransky, D., Vogelstein, B., and Harris, C. C. (1991) p53 mutations in human cancers. *Science* **253**, 49–53.
29. Gao, N., Hu, Y. D., Cao, X. Y., Zhou, J., and Cao, S. L. (2001) The exogenous wild-type p14ARF gene induces growth arrest and promotes radiosensitivity in human lung cancer cell lines. *J. Cancer Res. Clin. Oncol.* **127**, 359–367.
30. Baylin, S. B. and Herman, J. G. (2001) Promoter hypermethylation: can this change alone ever designate true tumor suppressor gene function? *J. Natl. Cancer Inst.* **93**, 664–665.

31. Zöchbauer-Muller, S., Fong, K. M., Virmani, A. K., Geradts, J., Gazdar, A., F., and Minna, J. D. (2001) Aberrant promoter methylation of multiple genes in non-small cell lung cancers. *Cancer Res.* **61,** 249–255.

32. Kim, D.-H., Nelson, H. H., Wiencke, J. K., Zheng, S., Christiani, D., C., Wain, J. C., et al. (2001) p16^{INK4a} and histology-specific methylation of CpG islands by exposure to tobacco smoke in non-small cell lung cancer. *Cancer Res.* **61,** 3419–3424.

33. Belinsky, S. A., Nikula, K. J., Palmisano, W. A., Micheles, R., Saaccomanno, G., Gabrielsson, E., et al. (1998) Aberrant methylation of p16INK4a is an early event in lung cancer and a potential marker for early diagnosis. *Proc. Natl. Acad. Sci. USA* **95,** 11891–11896.

34. Palmisano, W. A., Divine K. K., Saccomanno, G., Gilliland, F. D., Baylin, S. B., Herman, J. G., and Belinsky, S. A. (2000) Predicting lung cancer by detecting aberrant promoter methylation in sputum. *Cancer Res.* **60,** 5954–5958.

35. Seike, M., Gemma, A., Hosoya, Y., Hemmi, S., Taniguchi, Y., Fukuda, Y., et al. (2000) Increase in the frequency of p16^{INK4} gene inactivation by hypermethylation in lung cancer during the process of metastasis and its relation to the status of p53. *Clin. Cancer Res.* **6,** 4307–4313.

36. Sirzen, F., Zhivotovsky, B., Nilsson, A., Bergh, J., and Lewensohn, R. (1998) Higher spontaneous apoptotic index in small cell compared with non-small cell lung carcinoma cell lines; lack of correlation with Bcl-2/Bax. *Lung Cancer* **22(1),** 1–13.

37. Joseph, B., Ekedahl, J., Sirzen, F., Lewensohn, R., and Zhivotovsky, B. (1999) Differences in expression of pro-caspases in small cell and non-small cell lung carcinoma. *Biochem. Biophys. Res. Commun.* **262(2),** 381–387.

38. Sanchez-Cespedes, M., Ahrendt, S. A., Piantadosi, S., Rosell, R., Monzo, M., Wu, L., et al. (2001) Chromosomal alterations in lung adenocarcinoma from smokers and nonsmokers. *Cancer Res.* **61,** 1309–1313.

39. Lane, D. P. (1992) Cancer. p53, guardian of the genome. *Nature* **358,** 15–16.

40. Ahrendt, S. A., Decker, P. A., Doffek, K., Wang, B., Xu, L., Demeure, M. J., et al. (2000) Microsatellite instability at selected tetranucleotide repeats is associated with p53 mutations in non-small cell lung cancer. *Cancer Res.* **60,** 2488–2491.

41. Woodson, K., Mason, J., Choi, S. W., Hartman, T., Tangrea, J., Virtamo, J., et al. (2001) Hypomethylation of p53 in peripheral blood DNA is associated with the development of lung cancer. *Cancer Epidemiol. Biomarkers Prev.* **10,** 69–74.

42. Biros, E., Kalina, I., Kohut, A., Stubna, J., and Salagovic, J. (2001) Germ line polymorphisms of the tumor suppressor gene p53 and lung cancer. *Lung Cancer* **31,** 157–162.

43. Ahrendt, S. A., Chow, J. T., Xu, L. H., Yang, S. C., Eisenberger, C. F., Esteller, M., et al. (1999) Molecular detection of tumor cells in bronchoalveolar lavage fluid from patients with early stage lung cancer. *J. Natl. Cancer Inst.* **91,** 332–339.

44. Mao, L., Hruban, R. H., Boyle, J. O., Tockman, M., and Sidransky, D. (1994) Detection of oncogene mutations in sputum precedes diagnosis of lung cancer. *Cancer Res.* **54,** 1634–1637.

45. Chen, J. T., Ho, W. L., Cheng, Y. W., and Lee, H. (2000) Detection of p53 mutations in sputum smears precedes diagnosis of non-small cell lung carcinoma. *Anticancer Res.* **20,** 2687–2690.
46. Lang, S. M., Stratakis, D. F., Freudling, A., Ebelt, K., Oduncu, F., Hautmann, H., and Huber, R. M. (2000) Detection of K-ras and p53 mutations in bronchoscopically obtained malignant and non-malignant tissue from patients with non-small cell lung cancer. *Eur. J. Med. Res.* **5,** 341–346.
47. Tanaka, F., Otake, Y., Yanagihara, K., Yamada, T., Miyahara, R., Kawano, Y., et al. (2001) Apoptosis and p53 status predict the efficacy of postoperative administration of UFT in non-small cell lung cancer. *Br. J. Cancer* **84,** 263–269.
48. Hanaoka, T., Nakayama, J., Mukai, J., Irie, S., Yamanda, T., and Sato, T. A. (2001) Association of smoking with apoptosis-regulated proteins (Bcl-2, bax and p53) in resected non-small-cell lung cancers. *Int. J. Cancer* **91,** 267–269.
49. Soussi, T. (2000) p53 Antibodies in the sera of patients with various types of cancer: a review. *Cancer Res.* **60(7),** 1777–1788.
50. Burke, L., Khan, M. A., Freedman, A. N., Gemma, A., Rusin, M., Guinee, D. G., et al. (1998) Allelic deletion analysis of the FHIT gene predicts poor survival in non-small cell lung cancer. *Cancer Res.* **58,** 2533–2536.
51. Pelkonen, O. and Raunio, H. (1997) Metabolic activation of toxins: tissue-specific expression and metabolism in target organs. *Environ. Health Perspect.* **105 (Suppl. 4),** 767–774.
52. Bartsch, H., Nair, U., Risch, A., Rojas, M., Wikman, H., and Alexandrov, K. (2000) Genetic polymorphism of CYP genes, alone or in combination, as a risk modifier of tobacco-related cancers. *Cancer Epidemiol. Biomarkers Prev.* **9,** 3–28.
53. Miyamoto, M., Umetsu, Y., Dosaka Akita, H., Sawamura, Y., Yokota, J., et al. (1999) CYP2A6 gene deletion reduces susceptibility to lung cancer. *Biochem. Biophys. Res. Commun.* **261,** 658–660.
54. Benhamou, S., Reinikainen, M., Bouchardy, C., Dayer, P., and Hirvonen, A. (1998) Association between lung cancer and microsomal epoxide hydrolase genotypes. *Cancer Res.* **58,** 5291–5293.
55. Persson, I., Johansson, I., Lou, Y. C., Yeu, Q. Y., Duan, L. S., Bertilsson, L., and Ingelman Sundberg, M. (1999) Genetic polymorphism of xenobiotic metabolizing enzymes among Chinese lung cancer patients. *Int. J. Cancer* **81,** 325–329.
56. Houlston, R. S. (1999) Glutathione S-transferase M1 status and lung cancer risk: a meta-analysis. *Cancer Epidemiol. Biomarkers Prev.* **8,** 675–682.
57. Vahakangas, K. and Pelkonen, O. (1989) Host variations in carcinogen metabolism and DNA repair, in *Genetic Epidemiology of Cancer* (Lynch, H. T. and Hirayama, T., eds.), CRC Press, Boca Raton, FL, pp. 35–54.
58. Pastorelli, R., Guanci, M., Cerri, A., Negri, E., La Vecchia, C., Fumagalli, F., et al. (1998) Impact of inherited polymorphisms in glutathione S-transferase M1, microsomal epoxide hydrolase, cytochrome P450 enzymes on DNA, and blood protein adducts of benzo(a)pyrene-diolepoxide. *Cancer Epidemiol Biomarkers Prev.* **7(8),** 703–709.

59. Rojas, M., Cascorbi, I., Alexandrov, K., Kriek, E., Auburtin, G., Mayer, L., et al. (2000) Modulation of benzo[a]pyrene diolepoxide-DNA adduct levels in human white blood cells by CYP1A1, GSTM1 and GSTT1 polymorphism. *Carcinogenesis* **21**, 35–41.

60. Bennett, W. P., Alavanja, M. C. R., Blomeke, B., Vahakangas K. H., Castren, K., Welsh, J. A., et al. (1999) Environmental tobacco smoke, genetic susceptibility, and risk of lung cancer in never-smoking women. *J. Natl. Cancer Inst.* **91**, 2009–2014.

61. Honkakoski, P. and Negishi, M. (2000) Regulation of cytochrome P450 (CYP) genes by nuclear receptors. *Biochem. J.* **347**, 321–337.

62. Anttila, S., Lei, X. D., Elovaara, E., Karjalainen, A., Sun, W., Vainio, H., and Hankinson, O. (2000) An uncommon phenotype of poor inducibility of CYP1A1 in human lung is not ascribable to polymorphisms in the AHR, ARNT, or CYP1A1 genes. *Pharmacogenetics* **10**, 741–751.

63. Vahakangas, K., Trivers, G. E., Plummer, S., Hayes, R. B., Krokan, H., Rowe, M., et al. (1991) O(6)-methylguanine-DNA methyltransferase and uracil DNA glycosylase in human broncho-alveolar lavage cells and peripheral blood mononuclear cells from tobacco smokers and non-smokers. *Carcinogenesis* **12**, 1389–1394.

64. Wei, Q., Cheng, L., Amos, C. I., Wang, L. E., Guo, Z., Hong, W. K., and Spitz, M. R. (2000) Repair of tobacco carcinogen-induced DNA adducts and lung cancer risk: a molecular epidemiologic study. *J. Natl. Cancer Inst.* **92**, 1764–1772.

65. Spitz, M. R., Wu, X., Wang, Y., Wang, L. E., Shete S., Amos, C. I., et al. (2001) Modulation of nucleotide excision repair capacity by XPD polymorphisms in lung cancer patients. *Cancer Res.* **61**, 1354–1357.

66. Butkiewicz, D., Rusin, M., Enewold, L., Shields, P., Chorazy, M., and Harris, C. C. (2001) Genetic polymorphisms in DNA repair genes and risk of lung cancer. *Carcinogenesis* **22**, 593–597.

67. Ratnasinghe, D., Yao, S. X., Tangrea J. A., Qiao, Y. L., Andersen, M. R., Barrett, M. J., et al. (2001) Polymorphisms of the DNA repair gene XRCC1 and lung cancer risk. *Cancer Epidemiol. Biomarkers Prev.* **10**, 119–123.

68. Divine, K. K., Gilliland, F. D., Crowell, R. E., Stidley, C. A., Bocklage, T. J., Cook, D. L., and Belinsky, S. A. (2001) The XRCC1 399 glutamine allele is a risk factor for adenocarcinoma of the lung. *Mutat. Res.* **461**, 273–278.

69. Hainaut, P. and Vahakangas, K. (1997) p53 as a sensor of carcinogenic exposures: mechanisms of p53 protein induction and lessons from p53 gene mutations. *Pathol. Biol. (Paris)* **45**, 833–844.

70. Ko, L. J. and Prives, C. (1996) p53: puzzle and paradigm. *Genes Dev.* **10**, 1054–1072.

71. Levine, A. J. (1997) p53, the cellular gatekeeper for growth and division. *Cell* **88**, 323–331.

72. Colman, M. S., Afshari, C. A., and Barrett, J. C. (2000) Regulation of p53 stability and activity in response to genotoxic stress. *Mutat. Res.* **462(2–3)**, 179–188.

73. Wright, G. S. and Gruidl, M. E. (2000) Early detection and prevention of lung cancer. *Curr. Opin. Oncol.* **12,** 143–148.
74. Jassem, E., Bigda, J., Dziadziuszko, R., Schlichtholz, B., Le Roux, D., Grodzki, T., et al. (2001) Serum p53 antibodies in small cell lung cancer: the lack of prognostic relevance. *Lung Cancer* **31,** 17–23.
75. Mitsudomi, T., Suzuki, S., Yatabe, Y., Nishio, M., Kuwabara, M., Gotoh, K., et al. (1998) Clinical implications of p53 autoantibodies in the sera of patients with non-small-cell lung cancer. *J. Natl. Cancer Inst.* **90,** 1563–1568.
76. Wani, M. A., Zhu, Q., El Mahdy, M., Venkatachalam, S., and Wani, A. A. (2000) Enhanced sensitivity to anti-benzo(a)pyrene-diol-epoxide DNA damage correlates with decreased global genomic repair attributable to abrogated p53 function in human cells. *Cancer Res.* **60,** 2273–2280.
77. Garinis, G. A., Gorgoulis, V. G., Mariatos, G., Zacharatos, P., Kotsinas, A., Liloglou, T., et al. (2001) Association of allelic loss at the FHIT locus and p53 alterations with tumour kinetics and chromosomal instability in non-small cell lung carcinomas (NSCLCs). *J. Pathol.* **193,** 55–65.
78. Zienolddiny, S., Ryberg, D., Arab, M. O., Skaug, V., and Haugen, A. (2001) Loss of heterozygosity is related to p53 mutations and smoking in lung cancer. *Br. J. Cancer* **84,** 226–231.
79. Denissenko, M. F., Pao, A., Tang, M., and Pfeifer, G. P. (1996) Preferential formation of benzo[a]pyrene adducts at lung cancer mutational hotspots in P53. *Science* **274,** 430–432.
80. Pfeifer, G. P. and Denissenko, M. F. (1998) Formation and repair of DNA lesions in the p53 gene: relation to cancer mutations? *Environ. Mol. Mutagen.* **31,** 197–205.
81. Smith, L. E., Denissenko, M. F., Bennett, W. P., Li, H., Amin, S., Tang, M., and Pfeifer, G. P. (2000) Targeting of lung cancer mutational hotspots by polycyclic aromatic hydrocarbons. *J. Natl. Cancer Inst.* **92,** 803–811.
82. Denissenko, M. F., Pao, A., Pfeifer, G. P., and Tang, M. (2000) Slow repair of bulky DNA adducts along the nontranscribed strand of the human p53 gene may explain the strand bias of transversion mutations in cancers. *Oncogene* **16,** 1241–1247.
83. Denissenko, M. F., Chen, J. X., Tang, M. S., and Pfeifer, G. P. (1997) Cytosine methylation determines hot spots of DNA damage in the human P53 gene. *Proc. Natl. Acad. Sci. USA* **94,** 3893–3898.
84. Tang, M. S., Zheng, J. B., Denissenko, M. F., Pfeifer, G. P., and Zheng, Y. (1999) Use of UvrABC nuclease to quantify benzo[a]pyrene diol epoxide-DNA adduct formation at methylated versus unmethylated CpG sites in the p53 gene. *Carcinogenesis* **20,** 1085–1089.
85. Vahakangas, K., Bennett, W. P., Castren, K., Welsh, J. A., Khan, M. A., Blomeke, B., et al. (2001) p53 gene and K-ras mutations in lung cancers from ex-, passive or never smoking females in a population-based case-controlled study. *Cancer Res.* **61,** 4350–4356.
86. Hernandez-Boussard, T. M. and Hainaut, P. (1998) A specific spectrum of p53 mutations in lung cancer from smokers: review of mutations compiled in the IARC p53 database. *Environ. Health Perspect.* **106,** 385–391.

87. Husgafvel-Pursiainen, K., Boffetta, P., Kannio, A., Nyberg, F., Pershagen, G., Mukeria, A., et al. (2000) p53 mutations and exposure to environmental tobacco smoke in a multicenter study on lung cancer. *Cancer Res.* **60,** 2906–2911.
88. Christie, B. A. (2000) Doctors revise Declaration of Helsinki. *BMJ* **321,** 913.
89. Reynolds, T. (2000) Declaration of Helsinki revised. *J. Natl. Cancer Inst.* **92,** 1801–1803.
90. Douglas, H. (2000) Inductive risk and values in science. *Philosophy Sci.* **67,** 559–579.

4

Neuroendocrine Phenotype of Small Cell Lung Cancer

Judy M. Coulson, Marta Ocejo-Garcia, and Penella J. Woll

1. Lung Cancer

Human lung cancers are divided into small cell lung cancer (SCLC) and non-small cell lung cancer (NSCLC), the two types having distinct clinical, histological, and biological features. Clinically, SCLC tends to present as a disseminated cancer that is not amenable to surgical resection and is treated with systemic chemotherapy and/or radiotherapy. SCLC cells typically contain dense neurosecretory granules measuring 80–90 nm in diameter. The granules contain hormones and neuropeptides that biologically characterize the neuroendocrine phenotype of SCLC. Specific neuropeptides and other neuroendocrine markers are discussed here, both in the context of their biological implications in SCLC, and for their potential as specific markers of disease and neuroendocrine progression.

All classes of lung cancer, along with most other tumors, share common molecular changes that contribute to their oncogenicity and may distinguish them from "normal" cells. Such traits include: 1) overexpression of oncogenes; 2) genetic changes, such as loss of heterozygosity at tumor-suppressor loci; and 3) epigenetic changes, such as methylation of genomic DNA that can modulate gene expression. Certain changes at specific loci are now being described that are more closely associated with specific lung tumor types; for example, RASSF1 promoter methylation is particularly high in SCLC *(1)*. In addition, as data emerge from more global approaches, such as genome-wide *(2)* or transcriptome-wide *(3)* analyses, profiles that typify distinct tumor subtypes are being characterized (e.g., within the classification of NSCLC) and may allow treatments to be more individually tailored to patients. Despite these recent

From: *Methods in Molecular Medicine, vol. 74: Lung Cancer, Vol. 1: Molecular Pathology Methods and Reviews*
Edited by: B. Driscoll © Humana Press Inc., Totowa, NJ

advances, the long-established co-expression of both common neuroendocrine and epithelial markers remains the defining biological feature of SCLC, allowing distinction of these tumor cells from the majority of other normal and neoplastic lung cell types.

2. Neuropeptides

Small cell lung cancers produce a variety of mitogenic neuropeptides and growth factors. They can also express receptors for these signaling peptides, leading to the hypothesis that multiple autocrine and paracrine loops promote tumor proliferation and progression. These neuropeptides include gastrin releasing peptide (GRP) *(4)*, gastrin *(5)*, cholecystokinin (CCK) *(6)*, neurotensin *(7)*, and arginine vasopressin (AVP) *(8)*. The receptors for these neuropeptides are members of the large family of G-protein-coupled seven-transmembrane-spanning receptors. In contrast to SCLC, the major growth factors for NSCLC are polypeptides that act through tyrosine kinase receptors. These lung tumors are not characteristically neuroendocrine *(9)* although some NSCLC may display neuroendocrine features *(10,11)*. Other growth factors may play a common role across the spectrum of lung cancer types. For example, we have recently shown that endothelin-1, which can promote tumorigenesis through paracrine effects on other cell types including endothelial cells, can be produced and processed by both SCLC and NSCLC *(12)*.

The expression of neuropeptides and their receptors in SCLC is of interest for several reasons. Firstly, many neuropeptides can bind to lung cancer cells via their cognate receptors, stimulating specific signal-transduction pathways, and are postulated to act as autocrine growth factors. As different SCLC cell lines express a variety of peptides and receptors, it has been suggested that multiple autocrine and paracrine growth loops operate, constituting one mechanism by which these cells escape normal growth control *(9,13–16)*.

Secondly, neuropeptides and their receptors may represent therapeutic targets. A GRP antibody has been shown to cause SCLC regression in vitro *(4)* and is being evaluated in vivo *(17)*. Other specific antagonists have been unsuccessful, although one targeted against neurotensin has recently been described to inhibit SCLC growth *(18)*. Broad-spectrum neuropeptide receptor antagonists were shown to have anti-proliferative effects several years ago *(19)* and one of these substance P analogs is now in clinical trial. Interestingly, in addition to acting as a broad-spectrum antagonist, this analog can act as a biased agonist, stimulating alternative G-protein coupling and signal transduction-promoting apoptosis *(20,21)*. Another way in which the neuroendocrine phenotype may be exploited is the use of neuropeptide promoters to direct specific gene therapy in SCLC *(22–24)*.

Thirdly, the expression of neuropeptides and their receptors may be of diagnostic or prognostic importance. The expression of neuron specific enolase (NSE) and neural cell adhesion molecule (NCAM) are already used to distinguish SCLC from NSCLC *(25)*. In future, the neuroendocrine phenotype may be used to distinguish different prognostic groups and select patients for the most appropriate treatment. These same gene products are of interest as potential markers for the early detection of lung cancer *(26–29)* and examples of candidates are discussed below.

2.1. Vasopressin

AVP is a nonapeptide physiologically produced by the hypothalamus and secreted from the posterior pituitary *(30)*, but is one of the neuropeptides most commonly expressed ectopically in SCLC. It has a number of physiological functions mediated through different subtypes of receptor, including vasoconstriction, neuromodulation and an antidiuretic role. The overexpression of AVP in SCLC is clinically important, as it can result in the syndrome of inappropriate secretion of anti-diuretic hormone (SIADH) leading to hyponatremia *(31)*. AVP is detectable in 65–100% of SCLC *(16,32)* but in contrast is rarely present in NSCLC *(33)*. However, it is now becoming apparent that AVP is also expressed in some breast cancers *(34,35)*.

AVP stimulates mobilization of intracellular calcium stores via the V1a receptor *(16)* and has been shown to be mitogenic for SCLC *(13)*. All the known subtypes of vasopressin receptor are expressed by SCLC, implying that there is a multifaceted role for this peptide *(36,37)*. Our studies on the transcriptional regulation of AVP in SCLC *(23,38,39)* are beginning to elucidate how ectopic AVP expression is achieved by specific promoter activation *(40,41)* and may be exploited to target gene therapy to SCLC *(23,42)*. However, as vasopressin is synthesized as a precursor peptide, it is key to an autocrine growth model that the relevant processing enzymes are also produced to generate biologically active peptides. It has been shown that both correctly and novel processed forms of AVP are seen in SCLC *(32,43,44)*. More recently, it was shown that even in variant forms of SCLC (with reduced neuroendocrine capacity) there is the potential to process neuropeptides as the key classes of enzymes are all produced (prohormone convertases, carboxypeptidases, and peptidylglycine ac-amidating monooxygenases) *(45)*.

2.2. Gastrin-Releasing Peptide

Gastrin-releasing peptide (GRP; a larger peptide of 27 amino acids) and neuromedin B are human homologs of bombesin. GRP is normally expressed in the gastrointestinal tract and was one of the first neuropeptides proposed to have a role as an autocrine growth factor in SCLC *(4)*. It is now becoming clear that GRP also plays a similar role in other cancers with some neuroendocrine potential, such as prostate, colorectal, and primitive neuroectodermal tumors *(46)*. Recent studies have shown that the GRP receptor (GRPR) is more highly expressed in women and can be induced by tobacco exposure *(47)*. GRP exerts its effects through G-protein-coupled receptors such as the GRPR, the neuromedin B receptor, and the bombesin receptor subtype 3 (BRS-3), which can all be detected in SCLC *(48)*. The peptide has been demonstrated to function as a mitogen in vitro in some human bronchial epithelial cells, SCLC cell lines and in vivo nude mouse models *(49,50)*. Recently, the GRP promoter has been utilized to target gene therapy to SCLC *(24)*.

2.3. Gastrin and Cholecystokinin

The structurally related peptides cholecystokinin (CCK) and gastrin are less classically associated with SCLC than GRP, but have been implicated in the growth of gastrointestinal tumors *(51)*. There are two main subtypes of receptor: the cholecystokinin A receptor (CCK-AR), which shows selectivity for processed CCK and is quite widely distributed, and the CCK-BR, which binds both peptides with similar affinity, but shows a more highly restricted distribution. Other receptor isoforms also exist and could be particularly associated with tumors *(52)*. CCK is expressed and correctly processed in SCLC *(6)*, the receptors have been reported and the peptides shown to be mitogenic in SCLC cell lines *(15,53,54)*. The CCK-BR has previously been suggested as a marker for the diagnosis of SCLC in biopsy material *(27)* and is being investigated as a target for radiolabeled ligands in medullary thyroid cancer and SCLC *(55)*.

2.4. Neurotensin

Neurotensin is most widely known as a tumor-associated neuropeptide in prostate cancer *(56)*. However, it has also been shown to be expressed by SCLC and a Ca^{2+} mobilizing receptor for neurotensin has been demonstrated on SCLC cell lines *(53,54)*. A recent study shows co-expression of neurotensin mRNA with prohormone convertases implying that biologically active processed peptide is generated in SCLC *(57)*. A third subtype of neurotensin receptor (NTR) has been identified as being of importance in human tumors *(58)* and neurotensin receptors have generated recent interest as drug targets for specific antagonists *(18)*.

3. Neuroendocrine Markers

We recently conducted a systematic study into the neuroendocrine pheno-type, examining the expression of neuropeptides in a panel of lung cancer cell lines. Previous authors have used radioimmunoassays to study individual

Table 1
Summary of Results for Expression of Neuropeptides and Receptors in a Panel of Lung Cancer Cell Lines[a]

Neuropeptides and Receptors	SCLC							NSCLC				Blood	Bronchial Epithelium		% Positivity	
	H-345	Lu165	H-69	GLC19	H-711	COR-L88	COR-L24	COR-L23	H-460	A549	MOR/P	HL-60	NHBE	SV40-HBE	SCLC	NSCLC
GRP	+	+	+	+	+	+	+	−	−	−	−	−	−	+	100	0
GRPR	+	+	+	−	+	+	−	+	+	−	−	−	−	−	71	50
CCK	−	+	−	−	−	+	+	+	−	+	+	−	+	+	43	75
GASTRIN	−	−	−	−	−	−	−	+	−	−	+	−	+	−	0	50
CCK-AR	+	+	+	+	−	−	−	−	−	−	+	−	+	−	57	25
CCK-BR	+	+	+	−	+	+	+	−	−	−	−	−	−	−	86	0
NT	+	−	+	−	+	+	+	+	+	+	−	−	−	−	71	75
NTR	+	+	−	+	+	−	+	+	+	−	+	+	−	−	71	75
AVP	+	+	+	+	+	nd	nd	−	−	−	−	−	−	−	100	0
V1a	+	+	+	+	+	nd	nd	−	−	−	−	−	−	−	100	0
ET-1	+	+	−	+	+	+	+	+	+	+	+	+	+	+	86	100
ETAR	−	+	−	+	+	−	−	−	−	+	−	−	+	+	43	25
ETBR	+	+	+	+	+	+	+	+	+	+	+	+	+	+	100	100

[a](+), positive expression; (−), no expression; (nd), not done; and the percentage of cell lines positive in SCLC or NSCLC is also shown. Reprinted with permission from **ref. 59**.

neuropeptide expression; instead, we applied reverse transcriptase polymerase chain reaction (RT-PCR) to allow evaluation of both peptides and receptors with increased sensitivity *(59)*. We studied the expression of a range of neuropeptides, including GRP, gastrin, CCK, neurotensin, and some of the corresponding receptors (GRPR, CCK-AR, CCK-BR, NTR). These findings are shown in **Table 1**, including comparison with our previous data for AVP *(23)*, V1a receptor *(16)*, endothelin-1 (ET-1), and the endothelin A and B type receptors (ETAR and ETBR) *(12)* expression in the same panel of cells.

Although no SCLC line expressed all markers, it was clear that co-expression of neuropeptides and their receptors is common in SCLC, but uncommon in NSCLC. From this study, we identified several neuroendocrine markers that are selectively and frequently expressed in SCLC, but not in NSCLC, or in cell line models of bronchial epithelium or white blood cells *(59)*. These are currently being investigated as potential SCLC markers in studies of dysplasia in bronchial epithelium *(60)* and detection of micrometastases in blood samples *(61–63)*. In particular, we observed that AVP and the CCK-BR were exclusively expressed in SCLC, being detected in 100% and 86% of SCLC lines, respectively *(59)*. These are potential markers for both studies. We also found two other markers, GRP and V1a, to be highly selective for SCLC over NSCLC and expressed in 100% of the SCLC lines investigated. However, GRP may be expressed in normal bronchial epithelium *(59,64)* and may therefore not be a useful marker for detection of dysplastic areas within bronchial epithelium. Similarly, the V1a receptor has been described in normal rat bronchial epithelium *(65)*, and we also demonstrated V1a expression in 3 out of 4 blood samples taken from normal volunteers *(66)*, limiting its use as a marker.

Interestingly, GRP precursors were recently identified as the most successful of a panel of potential SCLC markers in both an enzyme-linked immunosorbent assay (ELISA)-based serum screen *(67)* and a RT-PCR based screen of peripheral blood and sputum *(68)*. Another recent study of neuropeptide receptor expression across a panel of tumor types found CCK-BR to be expressed in SCLC and a pancreatic cancer line, with CCK-AR more common in pancreatic cancer *(69)*.

4. The Neuroendocrine Phenotype

Because SCLC cells express both neuroendocrine and epithelial antigens, the cell type of origin has long been debated. This question is of relevance in the context of using neuroendocrine markers for early detection. It has been suggested that these tumors arise from pockets of cells of the dispersed neuroendocrine system within the lung, known as amine precursor uptake and decarboxylase (APUD) cells. However, opinion is now swinging in favor of an endodermal origin *(10)*. It was recently proposed that neuropeptide production by certain tumors was an important part of a special process of oncogenic transformation rather than a pre-existing condition of progenitor cells, in a concept named Selective Tumor gene Expression of Peptides essential for Survival (STEPS) *(37)*. Interestingly, this is supported by data from a high-density cDNA array analysis comparing gene expression in SCLC against that for neuroendocrine carcinoids and normal lung epithelium. From statistical analyses of the data, the authors conclude that SCLC is much more closely related to epithelial cells than carcinoids, which themselves are closely related to neural crest-derived brain tumors *(70)*.

If the STEPS hypothesis is correct, then neuroendocrine differentiation would be an early event in the establishment of SCLC, where acquired neuropeptide growth factors and other neuroendocrine characteristics promote tumor growth. Results from our recent work indirectly support such a mechanism. For example, the use of RT-PCR for AVP and GRP as markers of SCLC micrometastases in the peripheral blood of lung cancer patients revealed a trend towards increased survival for those patients positive for both neuroendocrine markers *(62,63)*. Although this was not statistically significant, it could be interpreted as consistent with the hypothesis that neuroendocrine features are early markers of SCLC, which may be followed later in disease by the de-differentiation more generally characteristic of tumors.

Studies on the transcriptional regulation of AVP, which identified the minimal promoter and transcription factor binding sites that are required for expression in SCLC *(23,38,39)*, also provide support for this theory. We recently described two transcription factors, which contribute to the ectopic expression of AVP in these tumors. These are upstream stimulatory factor (USF) *(38,41)* and an isoform of the neuron-restrictive silencer factor (sNRSF) *(40)*. USF is simplistically regarded as a ubiquitous factor, but is being described as playing a role in an increasing number of tissue-specific gene expression patterns, including that of surfactant A in the lung *(71)*. As USF appears to be important in regulating the AVP promoter, we performed immunohistochemistry on lung sections. Preliminary data suggest USF to be specifically associated with differentiated epithelium but not other normal cell types. However, it was retained in preneoplastic lesions, upregulated in SCLC and lost in NSCLC *(72)*.

In contrast, NRSF is expressed in all non-neuronal cells *(73,74)*, while the isoform we described in SCLC (sNRSF) *(40)* may be a marker of neuronal cells *(75,76)* and hence a potential marker of neuroendocrine differentiation in SCLC. In a pair of cell lines we found sNRSF to be most highly expressed in cells established early in disease, but less highly expressed in the post-treatment cell line *(40)*. Interestingly, expression of other epithelial and neuronal-associated transcription factors is also characteristic of SCLC, including TTF-1 *(77,78)* and hASH-1 *(79,80)*. Thus SCLC express transcription factors characteristic of both lung epithelial cells (USF) and neuronal cells (sNRSF) that are involved in regulation of at least one neuropeptide gene promoter. The former appears to be retained, and if the latter is acquired then this may be an early event in the pathogenesis of SCLC.

5. Summary

In conclusion, we have identified several neuroendocrine markers of SCLC and it is likely that for a successful screening program a small panel would need to be employed. From our studies AVP, CCK-BR, and GRP would be the most appropriate of the classical markers, while certain transcription factors such as sNRSF will also prove useful. Although SCLC may not originate from neuro-endocrine cells, these genes appear to be expressed early in disease. The application of neuroendocrine markers for screening clinical samples is discussed in detail in Chapter 20 of the companion to this volume: Detection of small cell lung cancer by RT-PCR for neuropeptides, neuropeptide receptors, or a splice variant of the neuron restrictive silencer factor, Coulson, J. M., et al.

References

1. Dammann, R., Takahashi, T., and Pfeifer, G. P. (2001) The CpG island of the novel tumor suppressor gene RASSF1A is intensely methylated in primary small cell lung carcinomas. *Oncogene* **20(27)**, 3563–3567.
2. Girard, L., Zochbauer-Muller, S., Virmani, A. K., Gazdar, A. F., and Minna, J. D. (2000) Genome-wide allelotyping of lung cancer identifies new regions of allelic loss, differences between small cell lung cancer and non-small cell lung cancer, and loci clustering. *Cancer Res.* **60(17)**, 4894–4906.
3. Hellmann, G. M., Fields, W. R., and Doolittle, D. J. (2001) Gene expression profiling of cultured human bronchial epithelial and lung carcinoma cells. *Toxicol Sci.* **61(1)**, 154–163.
4. Cuttitta, F., Carney, D. N., Mulshine, J., Moody, T. W., Fedorko, J., Fischler, A., and Minna, J. D. (1985) Bombesin-like peptides can function as autocrine growth factors in human small-cell lung cancer. *Nature* **316(6031)**, 823–826.
5. Reubi, J. C., Schaer, J. C., and Waser, B. (1997) Cholecystokinin(CCK)-A and CCK-B/gastrin receptors in human tumors. *Cancer Res.* **57(7)**, 1377–1386.
6. Geijer, T., Folkesson, R., Rehfeld, J. F., and Monstein, H. J. (1990) Expression of the cholecystokinin gene in a human (small-cell) lung carcinoma cell-line. *FEBS Lett.* **270(1–2)**, 30–32.
7. Moody, T. W., Carney, D. N., Korman, L. Y., Gazdar, A. F., and Minna, J. D. (1985) Neurotensin is produced by and secreted from classic small cell lung cancer cells. *Life Sci.* **36(18)**, 1727–1732.
8. Sausville, E., Carney, D., and Battey, J. (1985) The human vasopressin gene is linked to the oxytocin gene and is selectively expressed in a cultured lung cancer cell line. *J. Biol. Chem.* **260(18)**, 10236–10241.
9. Woll, P. J. (1996) Growth factors and lung cancer, in *Lung Cancer: Principles and Practice.* (Pass H. I., Mitchell, J. B., Johnson, D. M., and Turrisi, A. T., eds.), Lippincott-Raven, Philadelphia, PA, pp. 123–131.
10. Brambilla, E., Lantuejoul, S., and Sturm, N. (2000) Divergent differentiation in neuroendocrine lung tumors. *Semin. Diagn. Pathol.* **17(2)**, 138–148.
11. Graziano, S. L., Tatum, A., Herndon, J. E., Box, J., Memoli, V., Green, M. R., and Kern, J. A. (2001) Use of neuroendocrine markers, p53, and HER2 to predict response to chemotherapy in patients with stage III non-small cell lung cancer: a cancer and leukemia group B study. *Lung Cancer* **33(2–3)**, 115–123.
12. Ahmed, S. I., Thompson, J., Coulson, J. M., and Woll, P. J. (2000) Studies on the expression of endothelin, its receptor subtypes, and converting enzymes in lung cancer and in human bronchial epithelium. *Am. J. Resp. Cell Mol. Biol.* **22**, 422–431.
13. Sethi, T. and Rozengurt, E. (1991) Multiple neuropeptides stimulate clonal growth of small-cell lung-cancer—effects of bradykinin, vasopressin, cholecystokinin, galanin, and neurotensin. *Cancer Res.* **51(13)**, 3621–3623.

14. Tallett, A., Chilvers, E. R., Hannah, S., Dransfield, I., Lawson, M. F., Haslett, C., and Sethi, T. (1996) Inhibition of neuropeptide-stimulated tyrosine phosphorylation and tyrosine kinase activity stimulates apoptosis in small cell lung cancer cells. *Cancer Res.* **56(18)**, 4255–4263.

15. Sethi, T., Herget, T., Wu, S. V., Walsh, J. H., and Rozengurt, E. (1993) CCK(A) and CCK(B) receptors are expressed in small-cell lung-cancer lines and mediate Ca²⁺ mobilization and clonal growth. *Cancer Res.* **53(21)**, 5208–5213.

16. Coulson, J. M., Stanley, J., Staff, D., and Woll, J. P. (1997) Evaluation of vasopressin (AVP) and V1a receptor expression in SCLC cell lines: potential for an autocrine growth loop? *Lung Cancer* **18**, A599.

17. Chaudhry, A., Carrasquillo, J. A., Avis, I. L., Shuke, N., Reynolds, J. C., Bartholomew, R., et al. (1999) Phase I and imaging trial of a monoclonal antibody directed against gastrin-releasing peptide in patients with lung cancer. *Clin. Cancer Res.* **5(11)**, 3385–3393.

18. Moody, T. W., Chiles, J., Casibang, M., Moody, E., Chan, D., and Davis, T. P. (2001) SR48692 is a neurotensin receptor antagonist which inhibits the growth of small cell lung cancer cells. *Peptides* **22(1)**, 109–115.

19. Woll, P. J. and Rozengurt, E. (1990) A neuropeptide antagonist that inhibits the growth of small-cell lung-cancer in vitro. *Cancer Res.* **50(13)**, 3968–3973.

20. MacKinnon, A. C., Waters, C., Rahman, I., Harani, N., Rintoul, R., Haslett, C., and Sethi, T. (2000) [Arg(6), D-Trp(7,9), N(me)Phe(8)]-substance P (6-11) (antagonist G) induces AP-1 transcription and sensitizes cells to chemotherapy. *Br. J. Cancer* **83(7)**, 941–948.

21. MacKinnon, A. C., Waters, C., Jodrell, D., Haslett, C., and Sethi, T. (2001) Bombesin and substance P analogues differentially regulate G-protein coupling to the bombesin receptor—direct evidence for biased agonism. *J. Biol. Chem.* **276(30)**, 28083–28091.

22. Woll, P. J., and Hart, I. R. (1995) Gene-therapy for lung-cancer. *Ann. Oncology* **6(S1)**, 73–77.

23. Coulson, J. M., Stanley, J., and Woll, P. J. (1999) Tumour-specific arginine vasopressin promoter activation in small- cell lung cancer. *Br. J. Cancer* **80(12)**, 1935–1944.

24. Inase, N., Horita, K., Tanaka, M., Miyake, S., Ichioka, M., and Yoshizawa, Y. (2000) Use of gastrin-releasing peptide promoter for specific expression of thymidine kinase gene in small-cell lung carcinoma cells. *Int. J. Cancer* **85(5)**, 716–719.

25. Niklinski, J. and Furman, M. (1995) Clinical tumour markers in lung cancer. *Eur. J. Cancer Prev.* **4(2)**, 129–138.

26. Bork, E., Hansen, M., Urdal, P., Paus, E., Holst, J. J., Schifter, S., et al. (1988) Early detection of response in small cell bronchogenic-carcinoma by changes in serum concentrations of creatine-kinase, neuron specific enolase, calcitonin, ACTH, serotonin and gastrin releasing peptide. *Euro. J. Cancer Clin. Oncol.* **24(6)**, 1033–1038.

27. Matsumori, Y. e. a. (1995) Cholecystokinin-B/gastrin receptor: a novel molecular probe for human small cell lung cancer. *Cancer Res.* **55**, 276–279.

28. North, W., Maurer, H., Valtin, H., and O'Donnell, J. (1980) Human neurophysins as potential tumour markers for small cell carcinoma of the lung: application of specific radioimmunoassays. *J. Clin. Endocrinol. Metab.* **51,** 892–896.

29. Wallach, S., Royston, I., Taetle, R., Wohl, H., and Deftos, L. (1981) Plasma calcitonin as a marker of disease activity in patients with small cell carcinoma of the lung. *J. Clin. Endocrinol. Metab.* **53,** 602–606.

30. Burbach, J. P., Luckman, S. M., Murphy, D., and Gainer, H. (2001) Gene regulation in the magnocellular hypothalamo-neurohypophysial system. *Physiol. Rev.* **81(3),** 1197–1267.

31. Johnson, B. E., Chute, J. P., Rushin, J., Williams, J., Le, P. T., Venzon, D., and Richardson, G. E. (1997) A prospective study of patients with lung cancer and hyponatremia of malignancy. *Am. J. Respir. Crit. Care Med.* **156(5),** 1669–1678.

32. Fay, M. J., Friedmann, A. S., Yu, X. M., and North, W. G. (1994) Vasopressin and Vasopressin-receptor immunoreactivity in small-cell lung-carcinoma (SCCL) cell-lines: disruption in the activation cascade of V-1a-receptors in variant SCCL. *Cancer Lett.* **82(2),** 167–174.

33. Friedmann, A. S., Memoli, V. A., and North, W. G. (1993) Vasopressin and oxytocin production by non-neuroendocrine lung carcinomas—an apparent low incidence of gene-expression. *Cancer Lett.* **75(2),** 79–85.

34. North, W. G., Pai, S., Friedmann, A., Yu, X. M., Fay, M., and Memoli, V. (1995) Vasopressin gene-related products are markers of human breast-cancer. *Breast Cancer Res. Treatment* **34(3),** 229–235.

35. North, W. G., Fay, M. J., and Du, J. L. (1999) MCF-7 breast cancer cells express normal forms of all vasopressin receptors plus an abnormal V2R. *Peptides* **20(7),** 837–842.

36. North, W. G., Fay, M. J., Longo, K. A., and Du, J. L. (1998) Expression of all known vasopressin receptor subtypes by small cell tumors implies a multifaceted role for this neuropeptide. *Cancer Res.* **58(9),** 1866–1871.

37. North, W. G. (2000) Gene regulation of vasopressin and vasopressin receptors in cancer. *Exp. Physiol.* **85,** 27S–40S.

38. Coulson, J. M., Fiskerstrand, C. E., Woll, P. J., and Quinn, J. P. (1999) E-box motifs within the human vasopressin gene promoter contribute to a major enhancer in small-cell lung cancer. *Biochem. J.* **344,** 961–970.

39. Coulson, J. M., Fiskerstrand, C. E., Woll, P. J., and Quinn, J. P. (1999) Arginine vasopressin promoter regulation is mediated by a neuron- restrictive silencer element in small cell lung cancer. *Cancer Res.* **59(20),** 5123–5127.

40. Coulson, J. M., Edgson, J. L., Woll, P. J., and Quinn, J. P. (2000) A splice variant of the neuron-restrictive silencer factor repressor is expressed in small cell lung cancer: a potential role in derepression of neuroendocrine genes and a useful clinical marker. *Cancer Res.* **60(7),** 1840–1844.

41. Coulson, J. M., Quinn, J. P., Edgson, J. L., Mulgrew, R. J., and Woll, P. J. Upstream stimulatory factor is an initiator of the vasopressin promoter in lung cancer cells. *In press.*

42. Coulson, J. M., Edgson, J., Stanley, J., and Woll, P. J. (1998) Tumor-specific gene therapy for small cell lung cancer (SCLC). *Proc. Amer. Assoc. Cancer Res.* **39,** 397.

43. North, W. G., and Yu, X. M. (1993) Forms of neurohypophyseal peptides generated by tumors, and factors regulating their expression. *Regul. Peptides* **45(1–2),** 209–216.

44. Friedmann, A. S., Malott, K. A., Memoli, V. A., Pai, S. I., Yu, X. M., and North, W. G. (1994) Products of vasopressin gene-expression in small-cell carcinoma of the lung. *Br. J. Cancer* **69(2),** 260–263.

45. North, W. G., and Du, J. L. (1998) Key peptide processing enzymes are expressed by a variant form of small-cell carcinoma of the lung. *Peptides.* **19(10),** 1743–1747.

46. Heasley, L. E. (2001) Autocrine and paracrine signaling through neuropeptide receptors in human cancer. *Oncogene* **20(13),** 1563–1569.

47. Shriver, S. P., Bourdeau, H. A., Gubish, C. T., Tirpak, D. L., Davis, A. L., Luketich, J. D., and Siegfried, J. M. (2000) Sex-specific expression of gastrin-releasing peptide receptor: relationship to smoking history and risk of lung cancer. *J. Natl. Cancer Inst.* **92(1),** 24–33.

48. Toi-Scott, M., Jones, C. L., and Kane, M. A. (1996) Clinical correlates of bombesin-like peptide receptor subtype expression in human lung cancer cells. *Lung Cancer* **15(3),** 341–354.

49. Carney, D. N., Cuttita, F., Moody, T. W., and Minna, J. D. (1987) Selective stimulation of small-cell lung-cancer clonal growth by bombesin and gastrin-releasing peptide. *Regul. Peptides* **19(1–2),** 103.

50. Siegfried, J. M., Guentert, P. J., and Gaither, A. L. (1993) Effects of bombesin and gastrin-releasing peptide on human bronchial epithelial-cells from a series of donors—individual variation and modulation by bombesin analogs. *Anat. Record* **236(1),** 241–247.

51. Dockray, G. J. (1999) Topical review. Gastrin and gastric epithelial physiology. *J. Physiol.* **518(Pt 2),** 315–324.

52. McWilliams, D. F., Watson, S. A., Crosbee, D. M., Michaeli, D., and Seth, R. (1998) Coexpression of gastrin and gastrin receptors (CCK-B and delta CCK-B) in gastrointestinal tumour cell lines. *Gut* **42(6),** 795–798.

53. Woll, P. J. and Rozengurt, E. (1989) Multiple neuropeptides mobilise calcium in small cell lung cancer: effects of vasopressin, bradykinin, cholecystokinin, galanin and neurotensin. *Biochem. Biophys. Res. Commun.* **164(1),** 66–73.

54. Bunn, P. A., Dienhart, D. G., Chan, D., Puck, T. T., Tagawa, M., Jewett, P. B., and Braunschweiger, E. (1990) Neuropeptide stimulation of calcium flux in human lung-cancer cells: delineation of alternative pathways. *Proc. Natl. Acad. Sci. USA* **87(6),** 2162–2166.

55. Behr, T. M., Behe, M., Angerstein, C., Gratz, S., Mach, R., Hagemann, L., et al. (1999) Cholecystokinin-B/gastrin receptor binding peptides: preclinical development and evaluation of their diagnostic and therapeutic potential. *Clin. Cancer Res.* **5(10 Suppl.),** 3124s–3138s.

56. Seethalakshmi, L., Mitra, S. P., Dobner, P. R., Menon, M., and Carraway, R. E. (1997) Neurotensin receptor expression in prostate cancer cell line and growth effect of NT at physiological concentrations. *Prostate* **31(3)**, 183–192.

57. Rounseville, M. P., and Davis, T. P. (2000) Prohormone convertase and autocrine growth factor mRNAs are coexpressed in small cell lung carcinoma. *J. Mol. Endocrinol.* **25(1)**, 121–128.

58. Dal Farra, C., Sarret, P., Navarro, V., Botto, J. M., Mazella, J., and Vincent, J. P. (2001) Involvement of the neurotensin receptor subtype NTR3 in the growth effect of neurotensin on cancer cell lines. *Int. J. Cancer* **92(4)**, 503–509.

59. Ocejo-Garcia, M., Ahmed, S. I., Coulson, J. M., and Woll, P. J. (2001) Use of RT-PCR to detect co-expression of neuropeptides and their receptors in lung cancer. *Lung Cancer* **33(1)**, 1–9.

60. Ocejo-Garcia, M., Coulson, J. M., and Woll, P. J. (2000) Mapping study of a post-mortem lung shows genetic changes of cancer in adjacent bronchial epithelium. *Br. J. Cancer* **83**, 53.

61. Ahmed, S. I., Coulson, J. M., and Woll, P. J. (1999) Optimisation of an RNA extraction method from blood for use in detection of micrometastases by RT-PCR in solid tumours. *Br. J. Cancer* **80(S2)**, 16.

62. Ahmed, S. I., Coulson, J. M., and Woll, P. J. (2000) Detection of small cell lung cancer cells in the peripheral blood by RT-PCR for expressed neuropeptides. *Proc. Am. Soc. Clin. Oncol.* **19**, 1901.

63. Ahmed, S. I., Coulson, J. M., and Woll, P. J. Detection of small cell lung cancer cells in the peripheral blood by RT-PCR for expressed neuropeptides. Manuscript in preparation.

64. Yamaguchi, K., Abe, K., Kameya, T., Adachi, I., Taguchi, S., Otsubo, K., and Yanaihara, N. (1983) Production and molecular size heterogeneity of immunoreactive gastrin-releasing peptide in fetal and adult lungs and primary lung tumors. *Cancer Res.* **43(8)**, 3932–3939.

65. Tahara, A., Tomura, Y., Wada, K., Kusayama, T., Tsukada, J., Ishii, N., et al. (1998) Characterization of vasopressin receptor in rat lung. *Neuropeptides* **32(3)**, 281–286.

66. Ahmed, S. I. (2000) The clinical significance of neuroendocrine differentiation in lung cancer. MD Thesis, University of Nottingham, UK.

67. Lamy, P., Grenier, J., Kramar, A., and Pujol, J. L. (2000) Pro-gastrin-releasing peptide, neuron specific enolase and chromogranin A as serum markers of small cell lung cancer. *Lung Cancer* **29(3)**, 197–203.

68. Lacroix, J., Becker, H. D., Woerner, S. M., Rittgen, W., Drings, P., and von Knebel Doeberitz, M. (2001) Sensitive detection of rare cancer cells in sputum and peripheral blood samples of patients with lung cancer by preproGRP-specific RT-PCR. *Int. J. Cancer* **92(1)**, 1–8.

69. Petit, T., Davidson, K. K., Lawrence, R. A., von Hoff, D. D., and Izbicka, E. (2001) Neuropeptide receptor status in human tumor cell lines. *Anticancer Drugs* **12(2)**, 133–136.

70. Anbazhagan, R., Tihan, T., Bornman, D. M., Johnston, J. C., Saltz, J. H., Weigering, A., et al. (1999) Classification of small cell lung cancer and pulmonary carcinoid by gene expression profiles. *Cancer Res.* **59(20)**, 5119–5122.

71. Gao, E. W., Wang, Y., Alcorn, J. L., and Mendelson, C. R. (1997) The basic helix-loop-helix-zipper transcription factor USF1 regulates expression of the surfactant protein-A gene. *J. Biol. Chem.* **272(37)**, 23398–23406.

72. Ocejo-Garcia, M., Coulson, J. M., Soomro, I. and Woll, P. J. USF-2 expression during bronchial carcinogenesis: upregulation in bronchial dysplasia, small cell and squamous cell lung cancers. Manuscript submitted.

73. Chong, J. H. A., Tapiaramirez, J., Kim, S., Toledoaral, J. J., Zheng, Y. C., Boutros, M. C., et al. (1995) REST: a mammalian silencer protein that restricts sodium-channel gene-expression to neurons. *Cell* **80(6)**, 949–957.

74. Schoenherr, C. J. and Anderson, D. J. (1995) The neuron-restrictive silencer factor (NRSF): a coordinate repressor of multiple neuron-specific genes. *Science* **267(5202)**, 1360–1363.

75. Palm, K., Belluardo, N., Metsis, M., and Timmusk, T. (1998) Neuronal expression of zinc finger transcription factor REST/NRSF/XRB gene. *J. Neurosci.* **18(4)**, 1280–1296.

76. Palm, K., Metsis, M., and Timmusk, T. (1999) Neuron-specific splicing of zinc finger transcription factor REST/NRSF/XBR is frequent in neuroblastomas and conserved in human, mouse and rat. *Mol. Brain Res.* **72(1)**, 30–39.

77. Agoff, S. N., Lamps, L. W., Philip, A. T., Amin, M. B., Schmidt, R. A., True, L. D., and Folpe, A. L. (2000) Thyroid transcription factor-1 is expressed in extra-pulmonary small cell carcinomas but not in other extrapulmonary neuroendocrine tumors. *Mod. Pathol.* **13(3)**, 238–242.

78. Ordonez, N. G. (2000) Value of thyroid transcription factor-1 immunostaining in distinguishing small cell lung carcinomas from other small cell carcinomas. *Am. J. Surg. Pathol.* **24(9)**, 1217–1223.

79. Linnoila, R. I., Zhao, B., DeMayo, J. L., Nelkin, B. D., Baylin, S. B., DeMayo, F. J., and Ball, D. W. (2000) Constitutive achaete-scute homologue-1 promotes airway dysplasia and lung neuroendocrine tumors in transgenic mice. *Cancer Res.* **60(15)**, 4005–4009.

80. Ito, T., Udaka, N., Ikeda, M., Yazawa, T., Kageyama, R., and Kitamura, H. (2001) Significance of proneural basic helix-loop-helix transcription factors in neuroendocrine differentiation of fetal lung epithelial cells and lung carcinoma cells. *Histol. Histopathol.* **16(1)**, 335–343.

5

AIDS-Associated Pulmonary Cancers

Kushagra Katariya and Richard J. Thurer

1. Introduction

Neoplastic disease occurs more frequently in immunocompromised patients than in the general population. It may be the presenting condition in patients with acquired immune deficiency syndrome (AIDS). The appearance of Kaposi's sarcoma (KS) in young men in the United States in the early 1980s and the increasing incidence of KS in Africa were among the first observations to suggest the emergence of a new disease (1). Individuals with human immunodeficiency virus (HIV) infection and those with AIDS represent a large segment of the group of patients with compromised immune status. These patients, on the whole, are more susceptible to the development of malignant neoplasms. KS and malignant lymphoma are the two most widely recognized neoplasms in patients with AIDS (2–5). The relationship between bronchogenic carcinoma and HIV infection is somewhat less clear and subject to ongoing study. Several other malignant neoplasms may also occur more frequently in this population.

2. Mechanisms of Development of Neoplasms in Immunocompromised Hosts

Certain tumors are more common in the immunocompromised state in both humans and animals. The development of malignant neoplasms in immunodeficient states has been well-documented in various primary immunodeficiency diseases (Wiskott-Aldrich syndrome, ataxia telangiectasia, X-linked lymphoproliferative syndrome), and secondary immunodeficiency states induced by immunosuppressive drugs (organ transplantation, cytotoxic cancer chemotherapy) (6–9).

From: *Methods in Molecular Medicine, vol. 74: Lung Cancer, Vol. 1: Molecular Pathology Methods and Reviews*
Edited by: B. Driscoll © Humana Press Inc., Totowa, NJ

Kaposi's sarcoma, B-cell high-grade non-Hodgkin's lymphoma, primary central nervous system lymphoma, and invasive cervical carcinoma are the four types of malignant neoplasms considered as AIDS-defining conditions *(1,6,10)*. The increased frequency of malignancies in this population appears to be related to immunosuppression secondary to HIV infection, which may allow tumor cells to escape T-cell immuno-surveillance. This hypothesis may parallel the finding that Epstein-Barr virus (EBV) infection is associated with a variety of malignancies, including Burkitt's lymphoma and post-transplant lymphoproliferative disorders *(11)*. The immune deficiency seen in EBV infection, which is associated with an increase in T helper 2 (Th2)-type cytokine profile that plays a central role in EBV-associated lymphoproliferative disorders, has recently been described in HIV-infected patients with lymphoma *(11–13)*. There are other viruses that are found coincidentally with HIV and their role in oncogenesis is currently being investigated. The role of HIV infection in the development of central nervous system lymphoma, when found coincidentally with EBV, in cervical carcinoma when found with human papilloma virus (HPV), in KS when found with the newly described KS-associated herpes virus-like virus is controversial *(1,11)*. Despite this direct and indirect evidence, the development of a particular malignant neoplasm in a patient with AIDS does not necessarily suggest a viral cause. Other factors that contribute to the development of malignancies in the general population, such as genetic and environmental, may be operative as well. The immunocompromised status of these patients may, however, make them more susceptible to these influences.

3. Incidence of Malignant Neoplasms in AIDS Patients

As many as 36% of patients with HIV-AIDS will develop a malignant neoplasm during the course of their illness *(6,13)*. Until recently, 95% of these malignancies have consisted of KS or B-cell lymphoma *(6)*. It is expected that the development of malignant disease will become even more prominent as these infected individuals live longer. There are recent reports in the literature documenting increasing numbers of patients with squamous cell carcinoma of the oral cavity, cloacogenic carcinoma of the anal canal, and basal cell carcinoma of the skin in the AIDS population. Apart from the four malignancies in the AIDS-defining group mentioned earlier, there are other non-AIDS-defining malignancies associated with AIDS. These are listed in **Table 1**.

Albu et al. from the Bronx Lebanon Hospital Center reviewed the incidence of malignancy in 3,578 patients with HIV-AIDS treated between 1993–1998 *(14)*. Of these 3,578 patients, 245 had one or more malignancies. Thirty-nine patients had malignancies located in the lung and 5 more in the pleura.

Table 1
Malignancies in the AIDS Population

AIDS-defining
  Kaposi's Sarcoma
  B-cell high-grade non-Hodgkin's lymphoma
  Primary central nervous system lymphoma
  Invasive cervical carcinoma
Non-AIDS-defining
  Hodgkin's lymphoma
  Squamous cell carcinoma
    Anal canal squamous cell carcinoma
    Squamous cell carcinoma of the skin
  Lung cancer
  Gastric carcinoma
  Testicular cancer
    Teratocarcinoma
    Seminoma
  Malignant melanoma
  Leiomyosarcoma

Nineteen of these patients with pulmonary malignancies had non-AIDS-defining neoplasms.

4. Kaposi's Sarcoma

KS is the most common tumor associated with HIV infection and AIDS *(1,6,15)*. Cutaneous lesions are the most common presentation of KS. Cutaneous KS is characterized by flat, plaque-like, or nodular lesions that vary in size from a few millimeters to several centimeters. Patients may present with lesions in the lymph nodes or visceral KS only.

The cell of origin of KS is uncertain. KS spindle cells display features of mesenchymal cells, particularly endothelial cells, and KS is almost always associated with evidence of infection with human herpes virus-8 (HHV-8), or KS herpes-like virus (KSHV) *(16–18)*. Kaposi's sarcomas produce a variety of autocrine and paracrine growth factors. These include oncostatin M, interleukin-6 (IL-6), tumor necrosis factor-α (TNF-α) and IL-1β *(1)*. They enhance tumor, but not normal, endothelial cell proliferation and may serve as targets for therapy *(17)*.

The clinical course varies from indolent to rapidly progressive, with eventual progression in nearly all cases. Visceral involvement occurs in 50% of cases, with involvement of the lung in 20% *(1)*. The pulmonary form of the disease is perhaps the most life-threatening, with a median survival generally less than 6 mo *(1)*. The hallmark of KS is an aberrant, diffuse proliferation of vascular structures. The various growth factors may play a role in the increased angiogenesis. The preponderance of KS in men suggests a role for sex steroid hormones in KS associated with HIV-AIDS; however, no data has been reported to support this view. The role of glucocorticoids in furthering the progression of existing KS or promoting its development is well-documented, and it is thus important to limit the use of glucocorticoids in its management *(1,16)*.

The actual frequency of pulmonary KS in patients with known mucocutaneous and respiratory symptoms probably is higher than the reported 21–49% *(19–21)*, since lung involvement may be silent. Autopsy reports have found evidence of pulmonary KS in 47–75% in patients with AIDS who had KS documented antemortem *(20,22)*. Pulmonary involvement in the absence of mucocutaneous involvement is infrequent, with the incidence of isolated pulmonary KS ranging from 0–11% *(19–21)*. In a report by Huang et al. 15.5% of their 136 patients had isolated pulmonary KS diagnosed at bronchoscopy *(20)*. One half of these patients developed other lesions of KS within a median period of 3 mo, whereas the other half died without ever developing disseminated KS. Pulmonary KS can involve the tracheobronchial tree, parenchyma, or pleura. Pleural involvement does not occur without parenchymal involvement *(20)*, but is common in those with parenchymal involvement Approximately 50% of patients with pulmonary KS have pleural effusions *(23)*. Many believe that the appearance of characteristic tracheobronchial KS lesions is sufficient to make a presumptive diagnosis of pulmonary KS *(20)*. KS is the most common endobronchial lesion associated with HIV-AIDS and has a characteristic appearance, with erythematous or violaceous macules or papules typically located at bifurcations of the airway. Bronchoscopically assisted biopsies of these lesions are helpful but not 100% sensitive. Huang's study also suggests that pulmonary KS occurs at levels of profound immunosuppression *(20)*. The median CD-4 cell count was 19 cells/microliter in patients affected by pulmonary KS, a finding noted in other reports as well. No specific symptoms or signs were noted in these patients that would differentiate them from others with non-KS pulmonary complications. Serum LDH levels seemed to be higher in patients with pulmonary KS associated with opportunistic infections as compared to those with pulmonary KS alone.

Treatment for AIDS-related KS is, for the most part, palliative. However, since the introduction of protease inhibitors in combination with anti-retroviral agents, the possibility of long-term survival in a subset of patients exists. Decisions regarding treatment should be based on parameters predictive of survival, including tumor burden, immunologic status, especially the CD4 count, the viral load history of opportunistic infections, and performance status. Treatment can be divided into local and systemic therapy. Local therapy is well-suited for those individuals with few lesions or those with a slowly progressive form of the disease. Surgery, radiation therapy, cryotherapy, photodynamic therapy, intralesional vinblastine, intralesional sclerosing agents, and human chorionic gonadotropin are among the choices of local therapy *(16)*. Surgery has a role most commonly in patients with pleural involvement who have large pleural effusions *(23)*. These patients may need a lung biopsy to establish the diagnosis, since the parietal and visceral pleura may be free of the characteristic lesions *(23)*. Treatment of the pleural effusion may require tube thoracostomy and talc pleurodesis *(23)*. Radiation therapy has a high response rate with reduction in tumor size and resolution of pain. Mucosal tissues in patients with AIDS are at a higher risk of local toxicity such as mucositis, and thus a low daily dose of radiation may be appropriate. For advanced mucocutaneous disease and visceral involvement, a variety of more aggressive forms of therapy including some investigational protocols are available. Interferon-α (IFN-α) is approved for use in AIDS-associated KS. Response rates of 30–50% have been reported with lasting response in a minority of patients. The best predictor of a good response is a high (>400 cells/microliter) CD4 count. Patients with constitutional symptoms, prior or concurrent opportunistic infections and elevated β-2 microglobulin levels do not respond well to IFN therapy *(1)*. Synergism is seen with anti-retroviral agents and protease inhibitors. Systemic cytotoxic chemotherapy produces a rapid response in some patients and is useful in patients with progressive visceral involvement. Vinblastine, doxorubicin, and bleomycin are some of the agents that have showed response rates from 25–70%. More recently, liposomal encapsulation of doxorubicin has been used in an effort to reduce toxicity and achieve higher doses with better tolerance. Liposomal agents enhance the delivery of the drug in KS tissue by as much as 5–50 times compared with surrounding normal tissue *(16)*. Paclitaxel has also been studied, both as a single agent and as part of combination chemotherapy.

To combat the effect of factors being produced by KS cells, including angiogenic factors and cytokines, pathogenesis-based therapies are also being studied. Anti-angiogenic compounds such as tecogalan are being evaluated for treatment of progressive visceral and pulmonary KS *(1)*. Thalidomide, which inhibits angiogenesis and blocks TNF-α, is also undergoing clinical trials in treatment of KS. Because of the isolation and association of HHV-8 with KS, there has been a great deal of interest in using agents active against HHV-8.

Other areas of current interest include evaluation of the immune response to the viral infection and augmentation of specific immune response.

5. Lung Cancer

Recently, lung cancer has been reported with increasing frequency in the AIDS population *(1,10,13,14,22)*. Lung cancer is the most frequent cause of cancer deaths in men and women in the United States and tobacco smoking is accepted as the major cause.

Although the association of HIV-AIDS and lung cancer is rare, multiple reports have documented their coexistence *(1,10,15)*. In their epidemiologic study, Parker et al. *(15)* identified primary lung cancer in 36 patients with HIV-AIDS. Without adjusting for age at onset or smoking history, the observed to expected ratio for primary lung cancer in this population as compared with that of the US population was 6.5. As with AIDS-defining malignancies, lung cancer in these patients appears to be more aggressive and associated with a shortened survival compared to HIV-indeterminate patients.

In a study by Flores et al. *(25)*, 19 patients, all male, with HIV infection and primary lung cancer were studied and compared to historic controls. Of these, 17 patients were found to have lung cancer after having been diagnosed with HIV infection, the median interval being less than 1 mo. Two patients were diagnosed with HIV infection after being diagnosed with lung cancer, within an average of 1 mo. Fifteen of the nineteen (79%) were smokers. Three patients had stage I disease, one had stage II, five had stage III, and ten patients had stage IV disease. Adenocarcinoma was the most common cell type. Four patients were deemed to have operable disease and underwent standard surgical therapy. All others underwent chemotherapy and radiation therapy only. The median survival for all 19 patients was 3 mo, with a range of 1–10 mo. The longest survivor had the highest pre-operative CD4 cell count. The mean CD4 cell count for all patients was 217 and the median 121. The mean CD4 count for those with stage IV disease was 216, no different than the others.

Thurer et al. *(26)* reported on 20 patients with HIV infection and bronchogenic carcinoma. Four of these patients underwent surgical resection with curative intent. All 4 had stage Ia disease. The three patients with CD4 counts less than 200/microliter had survivals of 5, 3, and 5 mo, respectively and died of complications of AIDS without clinical evidence of recurrent carcinoma. The fourth patient had a CD4 count of 963/microliter and was alive 12 mo after surgery.

Alshafie et al. compared 11 patients with HIV infection and lung cancer with 116 patients with lung cancer and indeterminate HIV status *(11)*. The mean age in the HIV-infected group was 49.7 yr compared to 62.7 yr for the HIV-indeterminate group. Almost 90% of patients in both groups were cigarette smokers. Most patients in both groups had stage III or IV disease. No correlation was seen between the CD4 count and the stage of the disease at presentation in the HIV infected group. The median survival in the HIV group was 3 mo, the longest survival being 10 mo.

Parker et al. *(15)* identified 36 patients with primary lung cancers among 26,181 patients with HIV-AIDS followed by the Texas Department of Health between 1990 and 1995. Forty other patients had malignant tumors in the lung other than primary lung cancer. Twenty-two of these 40 were KS, 12 were lymphomas, and 6 were reticulosarcomas. Of the 36 primary lung cancers, various histologies were represented with equal numbers of adenocarcinomas and squamous cell carcinomas. There were 3 patients with small cell lung cancer and 1 with a mesothelioma. Thirty-five of these patients (97.2%) were male, 24 (66.7%) were white, and 10 (27.8%) were African-Americans. The median age at the time of HIV-AIDS diagnosis was 48 yr and the median age at the time of diagnosis of the lung cancer was 49 yr. The observed to expected ratio for all malignant lung neoplasms compared to the US population was 13.6 and that for primary lung cancer was 6.5. This is one of the few reports that provides strong epidemiologic data to link HIV-AIDS and primary lung cancer.

Tirelli et al. from Italy *(22)* reviewed the data from 1986–1998 collected by the Italian Cooperative Group on AIDS and Tumors (GICAT). Thirty-six patients presented with lung carcinoma and HIV-AIDS. These were compared to a control group of 102 patients younger than 60 yr of age of HIV-indeterminate status. Patients with HIV-AIDS and lung carcinoma were younger (38 yr vs 53 yr) and smoked more than the control group. TNM stage III/IV was observed in 53% patients from this group and their median CD4 cell count was 150/mm^3. The median overall survival was significantly shorter in the HIV-AIDS patients compared with the control group (5 mo vs 10 mo, $p = 0.0001$).

Lung cancer pathogenesis is characterized by multiple molecular changes, including the activation of oncogenes and loss of known and putative tumor-suppressive genes (TSGs). Microsatellites are highly polymorphic short tandem repeat DNA sequences *(27)*. Because they are abundantly and evenly distributed throughout the genome and are easily analyzed by polymerase chain reaction (PCR)-based methods, they are frequently used for studies of allelic loss in tumors. Change in microsatellite size is another genetic alteration seen in many cancers. Wistuba et al. *(27)* investigated the molecular changes in HIV-associated lung cancers and compared them to lung cancers in HIV-indeterminate subjects. Analysis of the frequency of loss of heterozygosity

(LOH) and microsatellite alterations (MA) using PCR and 16 microsatellite markers at eight chromosomal regions frequently deleted in lung cancer was performed. The overall frequency of LOH in all chromosomal regions was similar in both groups. Frequency of the MA present in HIV-associated tumors (O.18) was sixfold higher than in sporadic tumors. At least 1 MA was present in 10 of 11 (91%) HIV-associated tumors as compared to 17 of 35 (48%) sporadic tumors ($p = 0.02$). An increased rate of MAs was described in 7 of 13 other HIV-associated malignancies including KS and non-Hodgkins lymphoma.

The prevalence of lung cancer in this population may be underestimated, as shown by reports documenting that 22% of HIV-positive patients with focal lung disease undergoing transthoracic needle biopsies were found to have lung cancer *(2,25)*. Survival of HIV-AIDS patients who develop lung cancer is poor despite appropriate therapy. The shorter survival in these patients raises the question of whether progression of the underlying disease process of HIV-AIDS plays a role in the early death of these patients. Multiple reports *(11,28)* have suggested that progression of the viral infection has a synergistic or additive effect in producing an increased mortality rate. In addition, the shorter survival may also be influenced by the poor condition of these patients, which may preclude conventional surgical and/or chemoradiation therapy.

6. Non-Hodgkin's Lymphoma

Intermediate and high-grade non-Hodgkin's lymphoma (NHL) are AIDS-defining illnesses. The incidence of systemic NHL and primary central nervous system NHL is increased 104 times in the HIV-AIDS population when compared to the HIV-indeterminate population. More than two-thirds of AIDS-associated NHL have extranodal presentation *(1,6,29)*. Bone marrow involvement is seen in approx 30% of patients and meningeal involvement is seen in 10–40% of patients at presentation. Autopsy studies show a much higher incidence and prevalence of the disease in this population *(29)*. Rarely, primary extranodal NHL may present as pleural or pericardial effusions. Cesarman et al. reported eight such patients, all of whom had clonal rearrangement of the immune globulin heavy-chain gene, indicating a B-cell type lymphoma *(30)*. All cases showed presence of clonal EBV genome by PCR, indicating EBV infection and genomic integration prior to clonal expansion. All cases also had evidence of DNA sequences from the recently described HHV-8 by PCR, Southern blot or both. Whereas post-transplant large cell lymphomas are nearly always associated with EBV and probably represent the end result of an EBV-driven lymphoproliferation in the absence of effective antiviral T-cell immunity, only about 50% of AIDS associated large cell lymphomas are positive for EBV *(31)*. AIDS-associated large cell lymphomas occur late in the disease when CD4 cell counts are low. Their frequency increases with age *(32)*.

Several cases of the newly described large cell lymphoma were seen in HIV-AIDS patients *(33)*. These lymphomas are characterized by bizarre, pleomorphic malignant cells that resemble the Reed-Sternberg cells seen in Hodgkin's disease. Most of those seen in this population are of the B-cell type, although occasionally the T-cell type may also be seen. With increased survival becoming more frequent in the AIDS population due to the recent improvements in therapy, NHL are becoming more common. Patients usually present with disseminated disease, with pulmonary involvement seen in 20–30% of these patients. The clinical picture is one of a pneumonia often with hemoptysis. Patients are initially treated for opportunistic infections before a diagnosis can be made. Usually the diagnosis is made by bronchoscopy and biopsy *(1)*.

Chow et al. first reported a case of primary esophageal lymphoma in a patient with AIDS in 1995 *(34)*. Multiple endoscopic biopsies of a large, flat, nonhealing ulcer in the esophagus were performed on a patient presenting with dysphagia unresponsive to antifungal and antiviral therapy. Secondary superinfection with opportunistic infectious agents makes diagnosis difficult and causes significant delays in initiating appropriate therapy. Atypical locations of lymphomas, such as in the orophaynx and esophagus, are common in patients with AIDS and must be considered *(35)*. Despite a 50% remission rate with standard chemotherapy regimens, most patients relapse within a short period of time. The median survival is 5–8 mo with visceral involvement *(32)*. In a select group of patients with CD4 cell counts greater than 200/microliter and no constitutional symptoms and good performance status, lasting remission may be possible, thus making aggressive therapy a valid choice. New treatments using IL-6 antibody and IL-2 with zidovudine have shown promising early results *(29)*.

7. Other Thoracic Malignancies

Moysset et al. *(36)* recently reported the occurrence of a thymoma associated with KS and cytomegalovirus infection in a patient with HIV infection and low CD4 counts. The patient was a 76-yr-old female who presented with disseminated KS and a large anterior mediastinal mass. She died 9 mo after initial presentation. Autopsy revealed a large medullary thymoma. Thymomas can occur with a variety of immune disorders and it was suggested that the complex interaction of an immunocompromised state along with the presence of disseminated KS may have led to its development in this patient.

Schreiner et al. reported a case of pseudomesotheliomatous adenocarcinoma of the lung in a patient with HIV infection *(37)*. This tumor is a relatively rare form of lung cancer with a poor prognosis and an overall survival of 6 mo when found in the general population. This patient was a 33-year-old male and survived 32 mo after initial diagnosis.

Multiple other malignant tumors have been reported with increasing frequency in the HIV-AIDS population. All these may involve the intrathoracic organs. The immunocompromised state is thus a major risk factor for the development of malignant tumors. Whether the tumor cells escape normal tumor-surveillance detection or destruction mechanisms due to the underlying immunosuppression or whether the viral particle itself influences the development of a malignant neoplasm has not yet been clearly defined. Both scenarios, along with the immunomodulating therapies used, may play a role. Malignant tumors in these patients are more aggressive than in the general population. Opportunistic infections may be blamed for the clinical picture due to the tumors and may lead to delay in appropriate therapy. Prognosis is generally poor after diagnosis of such tumors in this population, although aggressive therapy is still warranted in view of the improved survival seen with new treatment programs.

References

1. Katariya, K. and Thurer, R. J. (1999) Malignancies associated with the immunocompromised state. *Chest Surg. Clin. North Am.* **9**, 63–77.
2. Haverkos, H. W. and Drotman, D. P. (1985) Prevalence of Kaposi's sarcoma among patients with AIDS. *N. Engl. J. Med.* **213**, 1518–1522.
3. Heitzman, E. R. (1990) Pulmonary neoplastic and lymphoproliferative disease in AIDS: a review. *Radiology* **17**, 347–351.
4. CDC. (1982) Diffuse undifferentiated non-Hodgkin's lymphoma among homosexual males—United States. *MMWR* **31**, 277–279.
5. Moore, R. D., Kessler, H., Richmann, D. D., et al. (1991) Non-Hodgkin's lymphoma in patients with advanced HIV infection treated with Zidovudine. *JAMA* **65**, 2208–2211.
6. Katariya, K. and Thurer, R. J. (2000) Thoracic malignancies associated with AIDS. *Semin. Thorac. Cardiovasc. Surg.* **12**, 148–153.
7. Levine, A. M. Non-Hodgkin's lymphoma and other malignancies in the acquired immune deficiency syndrome. *Semin. Oncol.* **14**, 34–39.
8. Nguyen, V. Q., Osorio, M. A., and Roy, T. M. (1991) Bronchogenic carcinoma and the acquired immune deficiency syndrome. *J. Ky. Med. Assoc.* **89**, 322–324.
9. Penn, I. (1988) Tumors in the immunocompromised patient. *Annu. Rev. Med.* **39**, 63–73.
10. Serraino, D., Pezzotti, P., Dorrucci, M., et al. (1997) Cancer incidence in a cohort of human immunodeficiency virus seroconverters. *Cancer* **79**, 1004–1007.
11. Alshafie, M. T., Donaldson, B., and Oluwole, S. F. (1997) Human immunodeficiency virus and lung cancer. *Br. J. Surg.* **84**, 1068–1071.

12. Emilie, D., Touitou, R., Raphael, M., et al. (1992) In vivo production of interleu-kin-10 by malignant cells in AIDS lymphomas. *Eur. J. Immunol.* **22,** 2937–2942.
13. Pallesen, G., Hamilton-Dutiot, S. J., Rowe, M., et al. (1991) Expression of Epstein-Barr replicative proteins in AIDS-related non-Hodgkin's lymphoma cells. *J. Pathol.* **165,** 289–299.
14. Albu, E., Reed, M., Pathak, R., et al. (2000) Malignancy in HIV/AIDS: a single hospital experience. *J. Surg. Oncol.* **75,** 11–18.
15. Parker, M. S., Leveno, D. M., Campbell, T. J., et al. (1998) AIDS-related broncho-genic carcinoma, fact or fiction. *Chest* **113,** 154–161.
16. Jie, C., Tulpule, A., Zheng, T., et al. (1997) Treatment of epidemic (AIDS-related) Kaposi's sarcoma. *Curr. Opin. Oncol.* **9,** 433–439.
17. Curiel, T. J., Piche, A., Kasono, K., et al. (1997) Gene therapy strategies for AIDS-related malignancies. *Gene Ther.* **4,** 1284–1288.
18. Karp, J. E., Pluda, J. M., and Yarchoan, R. (1996) AIDS-related Kaposi's sarcoma. A template for the translation of molecular pathogenesis into targeted therapeutic approaches. *Hematol. Oncol. Clin. North Am.* **10,** 1031–1049.
19. Fouret, P. J., Touboul, J. L., Mayaud, C. M., et al. (1987) Pulmonary Kaposi's sarcoma in patients with acquired immune deficiency syndrome. A clinicopatho-logical study. *Thorax* **42,** 262–268.
20. Huang, A., Schnapp, L. M., Gruden, J. F., et al. (1996) Presentation of AIDS-related pulmonary Kaposi's sarcoma diagnosed by bronchoscopy. *Am. J. Resp. Crit. Care Med.* **153,** 1385–1390.
21. Stover, D. E., White, D. A., Romano, P. A., et al. (1985) Spectrum of pulmonary diseases associated with acquired immune deficiency syndrome. *Am. J. Med.* **78,** 429–437.
22. Tirelli, U., Spina, M., Sandri, S., et al. (2000) Lung carcinoma in 36 patients with human immunodeficiency virus infection. *Cancer* **88,** 563–569.
23. Welch, K., Finkbeiner, W., Alpers, C. E., et al. (1984) Autopsy findings in the acquired immune deficiency syndrome. *JAMA* **252,** 1152–1159.
24. DiMaio, J. M. and Wait, M. A. (1999) The thoracic surgeon's role in the manage-ment of patients with HIV infection and AIDS. *Chest Surg. Clin. North Am.* **9,** 97–111.
25. Flores, M. R., Sridhar, K. S., Thurer, R. J., et al. (1995) Lung cancer in patients with human immunodeficiency virus infection. *Am. J. Clin. Oncol.* **18,** 59–66.
26. Thurer, R. J., Jacobs, J. P., Holland, F. W., et al. (1995) Surgical treatment of lung cancer in patients with human immunodeficiency virus. *Ann. Thorac. Surg.* **60,** 599–602.
27. Wistuba, I. I., Behrens, C., Milchgrub, S., et al. (1998) Comparison of molecular changes in lung cancer in HIV-positive and HIV-indeterminate subjects. *JAMA* **279,** 1554–1559.
28. Chan, T. K., Aranda, C. P., and Rom, W. N. (1993) Bronchogenic carcinoma in young patients at risk of acquired immune deficiency syndrome. *Chest* **103,** 862–864.
29. Straus, D. J. (1997) HIV-associated lymphomas. *Curr. Opin. Oncol.* **9,** 450–454.

30. Miles, S. A. (1996) Pathogenesis of AIDS-related Kaposi's sarcoma. *Hematol. Oncol. Clin. North Am.* **10**, 1011–1021.
31. Herndier, B. G., Kaplan, L. D., and McGrath, M. S. (1992) Pathogenesis of AIDS lymphomas. *AIDS* **8**, 1025–1049.
32. Schulz, T. F. and Boshoff, C. H. (1996) HIV infection and neoplasia. *Lancet* **348**, 587–591.
33. Moore, P. S., Boshoff, C. H., Weiss, R. A., et al. (1996) Molecular mimicry of human cytokine and cytokine response pathway genes by KSHV. *Science* **274**, 1739–1744.
34. Chow, D. C., Sheikh, S. H., Eickhoff, L., et al. (1996) Primary esophageal lymphoma in AIDS presenting as a nonhealing esophageal ulcer. *Am. J. Gastroenterol.* **91**, 602–603.
35. Heise, W., Arasteh, K., Mostertz, P., et al. (1997) Malignant gastrointestinal lymphomas in patients with AIDS. *Digestion* **58**, 218–224.
36. Moysset, I., Lloreta, J., Miguel, A., et al. (1997) Thymoma associated with CD4+ lymphopenia, cytomegalovirus infection and Kaposi's sarcoma. *Hum. Pathol.* **28**, 1211–1213.
37. Schreiner, S. R., Kirkpatrick, B. D., and Askin, T. B. (1998) Pseudoepitheliomatous adenocarcinoma of the lung in a patient with HIV infection. *Chest* **113**, 839–841.

III

MOLECULAR ABNORMALITIES IN LUNG CANCER

A. DETECTION OF ALTERATIONS IN THE CELL CYCLE

6

Abrogation of the RB-p16 Tumor Suppressor Pathway in Human Lung Cancer

Joseph Geradts

1. Introduction

There is compelling evidence that human lung cancers are characterized by disruption of several important physiological pathways that govern proliferation, apoptosis, intracellular signaling, and cell-cell interactions. Uncontrolled cellular proliferation is one of the hallmarks of malignant tumors, and it is usually owing to abrogation of one or more checkpoints that regulate the cell cycle. The best-characterized checkpoint controls progression from G1 to S phase. The most important component of this late G1 restriction point is the protein product of the retinoblastoma gene, pRB *(1)*. In its hypophosphorylated form, pRB binds E2F-family transcription factors. Functional inactivation of pRB leads to release of these transcription factors which then activate a program that moves the cell into S phase *(1)*. The most effective way to abrogate the late G1 checkpoint is a hemizygous mutation in the *RB* gene, with concomitant loss of the second allele—the prototypic mechanism of tumor suppressor gene inactivation. This occurs in almost all small cell lung cancers (SCLC), as well as in 15–25% of non-small cell lung cancers (NSCLC) *(2–5)*.

Alternatively, pRB function can be abrogated by increased phosphorylation of the protein. pRB phosphorylation is catalyzed by cyclin-dependent kinases (CDK) activated by their respective cyclins *(1)*. CDK amplification occurs at significant rates in some human tumors such as sarcomas, but is uncommon in lung cancer. However, overexpression of D-type cyclins, which activate CDK4 and CDK6, has been reported in 10–45% of NSCLC *(6,7)*. The kinases are inactivated by cyclin-dependent kinase inhibitors (CDKN) including $p15^{INK4b}$, $p16^{INK4a}$, $p21^{WAF1}$, and $p27^{KIP1}$ *(1)*, which therefore are functional

From: *Methods in Molecular Medicine, vol. 74: Lung Cancer, Vol. 1: Molecular Pathology Methods and Reviews*
Edited by: B. Driscoll © Humana Press Inc., Totowa, NJ

pRB agonists. Downregulation of these CDKN occurs in many malignancies including lung cancer and is significantly more common than mutations in the *RB* gene. It is associated with continuous phosphorylation of pRB and loss of cell-cycle control. Inactivation of p16^{INK4a} is one of the most prevalent molecular abnormalities in human neoplasia, rivalling *p53* mutations in importance *(8)*. In NSCLC, loss of p16^{INK4a} appears to occur in 40–50% of cases *(2,4,7)*.

We have developed immunohistochemical assays to detect inactivation of pRB or p16^{INK4a} in archival tissues as an alternative to conventional molecular genetic analyses. *RB* is a large gene spanning 200kb and comprising 27 exons, and mutations in the gene are not clustered *(9)*. Molecular analysis of *CDKN2/INK4a*, the gene encoding p16^{INK4a}, is complicated by the fact that this gene can be abrogated by one of three mechanisms. Homozygous deletion of the gene and transcriptional silencing by promoter methylation are the predominant mechanisms of inactivation, while hemizygous mutations with loss of the second allele occur at significant rates in certain types of tumors, such as esophageal and pancreatic adenocarcinomas but less commonly in lung cancer *(10,11)*. Furthermore, an important problem associated with molecular genetic methods using tissue homogenates is the invariable contamination of the tumor cells by non-neoplastic cells containing four normal alleles of the gene. We reasoned that these problems could be circumvented by studying the expression of pRB and p16^{INK4a} at the protein level *in situ*, i.e., by immunohistochemistry (IHC). This technique can detect the absence of immunoreactive protein specifically in the cells of interest, whatever the underlying mechanism of inactivation. As pRB and p16^{INK4a} are expressed in at least some non-neoplastic cells, IHC stains of tumor sections benefit from the presence of admixed positive internal controls. This technique has additional advantages. It can highlight intratumoral heterogeneity and allows the examination of marker expression in small precursor lesions. Importantly, it can be performed comparatively easily and inexpensively in most pathology laboratories. We originally described our IHC staining protocols for the detection of pRB and p16^{INK4a} in 1994 and 1995, respectively, using commercially available reagents in formalin-fixed paraffin-embedded (FFPE) tissue sections *(12,13)*.

We reported on the loss of pRB and p16^{INK4a} expression in two different series of resected NSCLC. The first group of patients (n = 100) was from The VA Medical Center in Minneapolis, MN *(2)*, and the second group (n = 103) was from The Prince Charles Hospital in Brisbane, Australia *(4)*. Interestingly, the immunohistochemical staining results were very similar (*see* **Table 1**). Only 35–40% of tumors expressed both pRB and p16^{INK4a}. Thirteen to fourteen percent were negative for pRB, and 45–50% were negative for p16^{INK4a}. Only

Table 1
pRB and p16^{INK4a} IHC Staining Patterns in Two Reported Series of NSCLC

Origin of NSCLC	Number	pRB+/p16+	pRB−/p16+	pRB+/p16−	pRB−/p16−	p
Minnesota (Kratzke) (2)	100	35	14	50	1	0.0002
Australia (Fong) (4)	103	43	13	46	1	0.0019
Total	203 (100%)	78 (38.4%)	27 (13.3%)	96 (47.3%)	2 (1.0%)	<0.0001

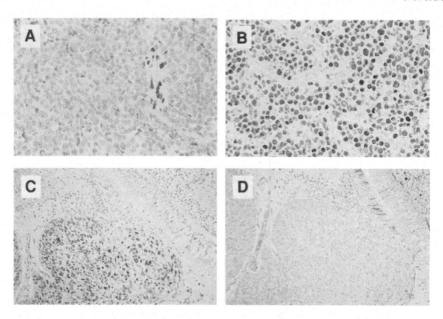

Fig. 1. Abnormal pRB and p16^INK4a staining patterns in human lung cancer. Left panels, RB stains; right panels, p16 stains. **A, B:** RB−/p16+ SCLC. Note admixed pRB positive endothelial and inflammatory cells in **A. C, D:** RB+/p16− NSCLC. Note the p16 positive bronchial epithelium and stroma in D. Original magnifications 400× **(A,B)**, 200× **(C,D)**.

1% of NSCLC showed loss of both tumor suppressor proteins. As in almost all other reported studies on pRB and p16^INK4a expression in human tumors, the inverse relationship between the two proteins was statistically highly significant ($p < 0.0001$). This association is expected because pRB and p16^INK4a are components of the same regulatory pathway, and their inactivation is functionally redundant. **Figure 1** illustrates aberrant pRB/p16^INK4a staining patterns in human lung cancer. Although there are exceptions, we generally observed that pRB and p16^INK4a immunoreactivity was strongest in tumors that demonstrated downregulation of the other tumor suppressor protein. Other studies showed that this probably is due to loss of reciprocal negative feedback mechanisms *(14,15)*. The earlier study confirmed previous reports that the rate of p16 inactivation in NSCLC increases with stage of disease *(16)*, but no such correlation was found in the Australian cohort. The Minnesota study also was the first to show that loss of p16^INK4a is an adverse prognostic factor in NSCLC *(2)*, and this was subsequently confirmed by other groups *(17,18)*. In our second study, p16^INK4a negative tumors also were associated with shortened survival, but the difference did not reach statistical significance ($p = 0.13$) *(4)*. Combining the data from both studies, it is evident that bronchogenic

Table 2
Loss of p16^{INK4a} Expression in Pulmonary Adenocarcinoma vs Squamous Cell Carcinoma (SqCCa)[a]

Histologic type	p16^{INK4a} IHC	
	+	−
Adenoca	55	36
SqCCa	35	47

[a]NB: The numbers in this table are aggregates of two published studies *(2,4)*. The higher rate of p16^{INK4a} loss in SqCCa is statistically significant ($p = 0.023$).

squamous cell carcinomas have a higher rate of p16^{INK4a} downregulation than pulmonary adenocarcinomas (57.3 vs 39.6%; *see* **Table 2**). This difference is statistically significant ($p = 0.023$).

2. Materials

2.1. Immunohistochemical Staining Protocol for pRB

1. One strongly and one weakly positive external control, plus an external negative control. Either FFPE tissues or paraffin-embedded cell buttons may be used (*see* **Note 1**).
2. Endogenous peroxidase block: methanol containing 0.3% H_2O_2.
3. Antigen retrieval buffer: 0.01 *M* citrate buffer, pH 6.0.
4. Protein block: 1% horse serum in PBS.
5. Anti-RB monoclonal antibody 3C8 (QED, San Diego, CA) *(19)* (*see* **Note 2**). Follow manufacturers' antibody storage recommendations.
6. Nonspecific mouse IgG used for negative antibody control.
7. Phosphate-buffered saline (PBS).
8. Vectastain Elite ABC Kit (Vector Laboratories, Burlingame, CA).
9. Diaminobenzidine (DAB) Kit from Vector (other sources of DAB are equally acceptable).
10. Hematoxylin (any vendor).
11. Snowcoat X-tra slides from Surgipath (Richmond, IL), Superfrost Plus slides from BDH (Northampton, UK), or normal glass slides coated with Vectabond (from Vector Laboratories). (Any type of coated microscope slides are suitable for IHC analysis.)

2.2. Immunohistochemical Staining Protocol for p16^{INK4a}

1. One strongly and one weakly positive external control, plus an external negative control. Either FFPE tissues or paraffin-embedded cell buttons may be used (*see* **Note 1**).

2. Anti-p16 monoclonal 16P07 (NeoMarkers, Fremont, CA) *(20)*. Follow manufacturers' antibody storage recommendations (*see* **Note 2**).
3. 0.1 *M* EDTA buffer, pH 8.0.

4–11. As above (**Subheading 2.1., steps 4–11**).

3. Methods

3.1. Immunohistochemical Staining Protocol for pRB

1. Cut 5-μm sections from the paraffin blocks of interest and place them onto coated glass slides. Dry the slides in a 60°C oven for 20 min (*see* **Notes 3–5**).
2. De-wax and rehydrate the paraffin sections (*see* **Note 6**).
3. Quench endogenous peroxidase activity in methanol containing 0.3% H_2O_2 for 20 min at room temperature (RT). Wash in running water, transfer to distilled water (*see* **Note 7**).
4. Antigen retrieval step: place slides in preheated 0.01 *M* citrate buffer, pH 6.0, keep at 95–100°C for 20 min. Wash in running water, transfer to distilled water (*see* **Note 8**).
5. Protein block: cover sections with 1% horse serum in PBS for 20 min at room temperature. Drain slides.
6. Primary antibody incubation: cover sections with monoclonal antibody (MAb) 3C8 (2 μg/mL in PBS) for 2 h at RT. Wash in PBS for 5 min × 3 (*see* **Notes 1 and 9**).
7. Add secondary antibody as per Vectastain Kit for 30 min at RT. Wash in PBS for 5 min × 3 (*see* **Note 10**).
8. Add ABC conjugate as per Vectastain Kit for 30 min at RT. Wash in PBS for 5 min × 3 (*see* **Note 10**).
9. Cover slides in DAB chromogen as per Vector Kit. Rinse in distilled and then in running water (*see* **Note 10**).
10. Counterstain with hematoxylin. Dehydrate, mount, and coverslip slides.
11. Interpretation of stains: look for nuclear staining in the neoplastic cells of interest. Cytoplasmic staining, if any, should be disregarded. If there is nuclear reactivity in a mosaic or diffuse pattern throughout the lesion, it is considered "positive." If there is no nuclear staining in the tumor cells, but preserved reactivity in admixed non-neoplastic cells, the lesion is considered "negative." If there is complete absence of nuclear staining only in certain areas of the tumor, whereas the normal cells in these areas react positively, the neoplasm should be scored as heterogeneous (*see* **Notes 11, 12**).

3.2. Immunohistochemical Staining Protocol for p16INK4a

1–3. As above (**Subheading 3.1., steps 1–3**).
4. Antigen retrieval step: place slides in preheated 0.1 *M* EDTA buffer, pH 8.0, keep at 95–100°C for 20 min. Wash in running water, transfer to distilled water (*see* **Note 8**).
5. As above (**Subheading 3.1., step 5**).

6. Primary antibody incubation: cover sections with monoclonal antibody 16P07 (1 μg/mL in PBS) overnight at 4°C. Wash in PBS for 5 min × 3 (*see* **Notes 1** and **13**).

7–10. As above (**Subheading 3.1., steps 7–10**).

11. As above (**Subheading 3.1., step 6**). The significance of cytoplasmic reactivity on p16 immunostains is uncertain (*see* **Notes 11, 12, 14**).

4. Notes

1. For both RB and p16^{INK4a} IHC runs, it is recommended to include one strongly and one weakly positive external control. To ensure specificity of the assay, an external negative control may be added. Either FFPE tissues or paraffin-embedded cell buttons may be used. Specimens that have high levels of pRB and which typically are negative for p16^{INK4a} include pancreatic adenocarcinomas, mesotheliomas, and cell lines derived from these tumors. Conversely, SCLC and derivative cell lines are pRB-negative but have high levels of p16^{INK4a}. Non-neoplastic tissues show intermediate immunoreactivity for pRB and low reactivity for p16^{INK4a}, although the expression levels of these two proteins appear to be cell-type dependent. In addition, non-neoplastic elements in tumor sections serve as positive internal controls. pRB is expressed in a mosaic pattern in almost all cell types. p16^{INK4a} staining usually is observed in a small subset of fibroblasts, endothelial cells, lymphocytes, and many epithelia.

2. Alternative antibodies that give satisfactory staining results include anti-RB monoclonal PMG3-245 and the anti-p16 polyclonal and monoclonal (clone G175-405) antibodies from PharMingen (San Diego, CA) *(21)*.

3. For IHC, it is important to place the tissue sections on slides that have been coated with an adhesive material, otherwise they will detach. Old slides may lose some of their adhesive properties.

4. The protocols described here were designed for tissues that have been fixed in 10% buffered formalin for 24–48 h. Longer fixation times reduce the antigenicity, and overfixed tissues may give completely negative staining results. Other types of fixatives may enhance or diminish the immunoreactivity.

5. The paraffin sections should be used shortly after they are cut. If this is not possible, they should be stored at 4°C. We have noted extensive nonspecific loss of p16 reactivity in sections that had been stored at RT for several weeks or months. Sections stored at 4°C appear to preserve their p16 immunoreactivity for at least 1 yr. pRB seems to be more stable in paraffin sections. Interestingly, both proteins are stable in paraffin blocks. We have been able to obtain good RB and p16 staining results in freshly cut paraffin sections from blocks that were 10–20 yr old.

6. In addition to paraffin sections, these protocols can also be adapted to frozen section analysis. Frozen sections may not require an antigen retrieval step (**step 4**), and it may be possible to use lower antibody concentrations and/or shorter primary incubation times.

7. The protocols described here may be performed by hand or with a (semi-) automated immunostainer. The RB stains can be performed on any type of machine. The p16 stains require equipment that permits overnight incubation of the slides at 4°C. We routinely use the Shandon Sequenza system and the fully automated immunostainer from Tecan (Crailsheim, Germany) which uses the same coverplate technology.

8. Several different antigen retrieval protocols may work equally well. We use citrate buffer for pRB and EDTA for p16, but either buffer can be used for either protocol with relatively small differences in staining quality. In addition, there are a number of commercial reagents (typically rather more expensive) that may be equally or more effective. It is important to keep the solution at 95–100°C for at least 20 min. If the buffer boils, there is an increased risk that the tissue sections detach from the slide. This is a problem particularly with fatty tissues such as breast. If the temperature falls below 95°C, the epitopes are not optimally restored. It does not seem to matter how the sub-boiling temperature is achieved. We have used microwave ovens, pressure cookers, and waterbaths with similar success. Autoclaves have been used by other groups. In our experience, a cool-down period after the antigen-retrieval step is not necessary.

9. Different anti-RB antibodies have different performance characteristics. We found MAb 3C8 to be very sensitive, but it also reacts with mutant RB proteins, which are very rare *(19,22)*. Monoclonal PMG3-245 is slightly less sensitive but more specific for wild-type pRB *(22)*. It is highly recommended to establish sensitivity and specificity for anti-RB antibodies whose immunohistochemical performance characteristics have not been described in detail.

10. The protocols described here are indirect immunohistochemical assays that are based on avidin-biotin conjugation and that utilize horseradish peroxidase to convert diaminobenzidine into a brown precipitate, which indicates the presence of pRB or p16. Other detection systems may work equally well, and other chromogens may be used. Similarly, we routinely use hematoxylin counterstaining, but other counterstains such as methyl green are equally acceptable.

11. Beware of certain staining artifacts. The "edge artifact" is common to many IHC assays. It refers to the nonspecific staining that can be seen at the edge of a tissue section. Thus, it is prudent to evaluate the whole section and to ignore the staining pattern at the extreme periphery of the tissue if it differs from that of the remainder of the section. If pRB or p16 is present in the cells of interest, the staining in a positive nucleus will be diffuse and uniform. Partial or irregular nuclear staining is artifactual. Cytoplasmic cross-reactivity usually is not a problem in RB assays, but is an issue for p16 analysis (*see* **Note 14**).

12. There is no universally agreed upon scoring system for pRB IHC. We have used a simple dichotomous system based on the premise that most neoplasms are monoclonal and have either two normal *RB* alleles or a mutation in one with loss of the other. Tumors with a normal *RB* gene will display nuclear immunoreactivity. Because the intranuclear level of pRB is variable and partly cell-cycle phase-dependent, often only a subset of nuclei will stain, yielding a

mosaic pattern of reactivity. In tumors with inactivated p16, pRB staining tends to be stronger and more uniform due to loss of negative feedback *(15)*. This is the basis for some authors to diagnose "RB overexpression," which often is a reflection of p16 loss. "Overexpression" of a tumor suppressor protein is far more difficult to define, and it implies a cut off that distinguishes two biologically different groups of immunoreactive tumors. However, the percentage of positive cells and the staining intensity depend on a large number of variables including tissue fixation, antibody use, detection reaction, and so on, casting doubt on any arbitrary cut-off. I do not suggest that any positive staining pattern is indicative of normal functional pRB. As outlined earlier (*see* **Note 7**), rare mutant proteins may create false-positive staining. Moreover, the current anti-RB antibodies do not distinguish active pRB from hyperphosphorylated and inactive pRB in IHC assays. Lastly, immunoreactivity may be preserved in cells in which pRB is inactivated by binding to viral oncoproteins. On the other hand, complete absence of nuclear reactivity is a definite indication of an abnormal *RB* gene. Of course, external and internal positive controls should react appropriately to demonstrate the presence of an *RB* abnormality specifically in the neoplastic cells.

13. Different anti-p16 antibodies have different immunohistochemical performances characteristics. For example, the PharMingen polyclonal antibody (PAb) has good sensitivity but reacts with p16 mutant proteins, while MAb G175-405 is rather specific for wild-type p16 but is less sensitive and yields substantial cytoplasmic staining. These two antibodies require a modified detection reaction *(21)*. At present, we routinely use MAb 16P07, which is very sensitive, and p16 stains obtained with this antibody have a markedly improved signal-to-noise ratio. Although the specificity of this antibody remains to be formally demonstrated, thus far we have not seen nuclear staining in cells known to be p16-negative. Like for RB, investigators should establish the immunohistochemical performance characteristics of any anti-p16 antibody that has not been adequately described.

14. With all anti-p16 antibodies, cytoplasmic staining is a problem. It is observed even in cells that are known to have a *CDKN2/INK4a* deletion and thus may be nonspecific *(21)*. However, the possibility cannot be ruled out that in certain instances, cytoplasmic reactivity reflects aberrant subcellular localization of p16. To resolve this issue, IHC stains of frozen tissues or immunofluorescent studies on cytologic preparations may be considered. In general, p16 stains of normal and neoplastic tissues are weaker than pRB stains. Usually, a smaller percentage of cells stain, and the average staining intensity is weaker. Tumors with inactivation of the *RB* gene tend to have a higher level of p16 reactivity, probably due to loss of negative feedback *(14)*. Again, some authors attempt to subclassify p16 positive tumors into low and high expressors, but this distinction is very problematic for reasons mentioned earlier (*see* **Note 10**). Absence of nuclear p16 immunoreactivity, in the presence of appropriate external and especially internal positive controls, on the other hand, practically is diagnostic of functional inactivation of the gene.

References

1. Sherr, C. J. (1996) Cancer cell cycles. *Science* **6**, 1672–1677.
2. Kratzke, R. A., Greatens, T. M., Rubins, J. B., Maddaus, M. A., Niewohner, D. E., Niehans, G. A. and Geradts, J. (1996) Rb and p16^{INK4A} expression in resected non-small cell lung tumors. *Cancer Res.* **56**, 3415–3420.
3. Cagle, P. T., El-Naggar, A. K., Xu, H.-J., Hu, S.-X., and Benedict, W. F. (1997) Differential retinoblastoma protein expression in neuroendocrine tumors of the lung. *Am. J. Pathol.* **150**, 393–400.
4. Geradts, J., Fong, K. M., Zimmerman, P. V., Maynard, R. and Minna, J. D. (1999) Correlation of abnormalities of RB, p16^{ink4a}, and p53 expression with 3p loss of heterozygosity, other genetic abnormalities and clinical features in 103 primary non-small cell lung cancers. *Clin. Cancer Res.* **5**, 791–800.
5. Yuan, J., Knorr, J., Altmannsberger, M., Goeckenjan, G., Ahr, A., Scharl, A., and Strebhardt, K. (1999) Expression of p16 and lack of pRB in primary small cell lung cancer. *J. Pathol.* **189**, 358–362.
6. Mishina, T., Dosaka-Akita, H., Konoshita, I., Hommura, F., Morikawa, T., Katoh, H., and Kawakami, Y. (1999) Cyclin D1 expression in non-small-cell lung cancers: its association with altered p53 expression, cell proliferation and clinical outcome. *Br. J. Cancer* **80**, 1289–1295.
7. Brambilla, E., Moro, D., Gazzeri, S. and Brambilla, C. (1999) Alterations of expression of Rb, p16^{INK4a} and cyclin D1 in non-small cell lung carcinoma and their clinical significance. *J. Pathol.* **188**, 351–360.
8. Kamb, A., Gruis, N. A., Weaver-Feldhaus, J., Liu, Q., Harshman, K., Tavtigian, S. V., et al. (1994) A cell cycle regulator potentially involved in genesis of many tumor types. *Science* **264**, 436–440.
9. Weinberg, R. A. (1992) The retinoblastoma gene and gene product. *Cancer Surv.* **12**, 43–57.
10. Zhou, X., Tarmin, L., Yin, J., Jiang, H.-Y., Suzuki, H., Rhyu, M.-G., et al. (1994) The MTS1 gene is frequently mutated in primary human esophageal tumors. *Oncogene* **9**, 3737–3741.
11. Schutte, M., Hruban, R. H., Geradts, J., Maynard, R., Hilgers, W., Rabindran, S. K., et al. (1997) Abrogation of the RB/p16 tumor-suppressive pathway in virtually all pancreatic carcinomas. *Cancer Res.* **57**, 3126–3130.
12. Geradts, J., Hu, S.-X., Lincoln, C. E., Benedict, W. F., and Xu, H.-J. (1994) Aberrant RB gene expression in routinely processed, archival tumor tissues determined by three different anti-RB antibodies. *Int. J. Cancer* **58**, 161–167.
13. Geradts, J., Kratzke, R. A., Niehans, G. A., and Lincoln, C. E. (1995) Immunohistochemical detection of the cyclin-dependent kinase inhibitor 2/multiple tumor suppressor gene 1 (CDKN2/MTS1) product p16^{INK4A} in archival human solid tumors: correlation with retinoblastoma protein expression. *Cancer Res.* **55**, 6006–6011.
14. Li, Y., Nichols, M. A., Shay, J. W., and Xiong, Y. (1994) Transcriptional repression of the D-Type cyclin-dependent kinase inhibitor p16 by the retinoblastoma susceptibility gene product pRb. *Cancer Res.* **54**, 6078–6082.

15. Fang, X., Jin, X., Xu, H.-J., Lui, L., Peng, H.-Q., Hogg, D., et al. (1998) Expression of p16 induces transcriptional downregulation of the *RB* gene. *Oncogene* **16,** 1–8.

16. Nakagawa, K., Conrad, N. K., Williams, J. P., Johnson, B. E., and Kelley, M. J. (1995) Mechanism of inactivation of *CDKN2* and *MTS2* in non-small cell lung cancer and association with advanced stage. *Oncogene* **11,** 1843–1851.

17. Volm, M., Koomägi, R., and Mattern, J. (1998) Prognostic value of p16[INK4A] expression in lung adenocarcinoma. *Anticancer Res.* **18,** 2309–2312.

18. Kawabuchi, B., Moriyama, S., Hironaka, M., Fujii, T., Koike, M., Moriyama, H., Nishimura, Y., et al. (1999) p16 inactivation in small-sized lung adenocarcinoma: its association with poor prognosis. *Int. J. Cancer (Pred. Oncol).* **84,** 49–53.

19. Wen, S.-F., Nodelman, M., Nareed-Hood, K., Duncan, J., Geradts, J., and Shepard, H. M. (1994) Retinoblastoma protein monoclonal antibodies with novel characteristics. *J. Immunol. Methods* **169,** 231–240.

20. Maitra, A., Roberts, H., Weinberg, A. G., and Geradts, J. (2001) Loss of p16(INK4a) expression correlates with decreased survival in pediatric osteosarcomas. *Int. J. Cancer* **95,** 34–38.

21. Geradts, J., Hruban, R., Schutte, M., Kern, S., and Maynard, R. (2000) Immunohistochemical p16[INK4a] analysis of archival tumors with deletion, hypermethylation, or mutation of the CDKN2/MTS1 gene: a comparison of four commercial antibodies. *Appl. Immunohistochem. Mol. Morphol.* **81,** 71–79.

22. Geradts, J., Kratzke, R. A., Crush-Stanton, S., Wen, S.-F., and Lincoln, C. E. (1996) Wild-type and mutant retinoblastoma protein in paraffin sections. *Mod Pathol.* **9,** 339–347.

7

Sensitive Detection of Hypermethylated p16^{INK4a} Alleles in Exfoliative Tissue Material

Marcus Schuermann and Michael Kersting

1. Introduction

Epigenetic DNA modification by aberrant methylation of cytosine residues is thought to be an important mechanism contributing to tumorigenesis. Methylation of cytosines normally occurs at distinct sites of the genome containing stretches of repeated CpG (CpG islands) often found within promoter areas of transcribed genes. The cytosine methylation pattern is established very early in development by a continuous process of demethylation and *de novo* methylation (for review *see* **refs.** *1,2*). Normally, methylation patterns are faithfully maintained through all subsequent cell divisions and are dependent on DNA methyltransferase activity *(3)*. It has been observed, however, that tumour cells often show extensive upregulation of DNA methyltransferase and at the same time hypomethylation of CpG sites *(4)*. The mechanism of this apparent deregulation in cancer cells is not clear but is generally thought that *de novo* methylation of otherwise nonmethylated genes is the active component of functional disturbance in cancer *(4–6)*. Methylated islands will recruit special methyl-binding proteins and in conjunction with histone deacetylases are then thought to form repressive chromatin states around the promoter regions, leading to transcriptional loss of genes residing downstream *(7)*. If important genes reside within this region loss of functional control in cell proliferation will ensue. It is therefore not surprising that *de novo* methylation found in cancer includes many tumor-suppressor genes known to date, thus forming an alternative to gene silencing by inactivating deletions *(8)*.

Gene silencing by promoter methylation is now a generally accepted mechanism involved in the pathogenesis of solid tumors and leukemias *(6)*.

From: *Methods in Molecular Medicine, vol. 74: Lung Cancer, Vol. 1: Molecular Pathology Methods and Reviews*
Edited by: B. Driscoll © Humana Press Inc., Totowa, NJ

This accounts also for lung cancer, a tumor with growing incidence and the leading cause of cancer-related deaths in industrial nations. The majority of lung cancer cases are smoking-related, and commonly preceded by multifocal preneoplastic changes in the entire tracheobronchial tract, caused by cumulative genetic damage *(9)*. While it has been clearly shown that chronic smoking leads to oncogene mutations, e.g., *p53*-mutations in non-neoplastic tissue *(10–13)*. It might be now equally important to look for early changes in the methylation pattern of distinct genes and correlate these with gradual neoplastic transformation of respiratory epithelium.

One of the first genes shown to be systematically methylated in lung cancer was the *p16^{INK4a}* tumor-suppressor gene *(14)*. This gene resides on a critical region of the short arm of chromosome 9, which is commonly deleted in lung cancer in up to 25% of all tumors examined. It was found that epigenetic modification of CpG-islands in the *p16^{INK4a}* promoter region could be detected likewise in approximately as many cases *(14,15)* and at early stages of tumor development *(16,17)*. Other candidate genes frequently inactivated by methylation were subsequently discovered, and comprise the genes coding for estrogen receptor *(18)*, HIC (hypermethylated in cancer) *(19)*, H-cadherin *(20)*, O^6-methylguanine-DNA-methyltransferase *(21)*, death-associated protein (DAP) kinase *(22)*, and retinoic acid receptor-β (RAR-β) *(23)*. The increasing number of emerging methylation markers *(24)* has now broadened the view that many more genes may be alternatively involved in lung cancer pathogenesis. It is hoped that the increasing number of promoter areas subject to cancer-specific methylation could serve as biomarkers useful for the early detection of cancer *(25)*.

Methylation-specific polymerase chain reaction (MSP), developed by Herman et al. *(26)*, has provided the means of determining the methylation status of individual genes in a rapid and sensitive fashion. The method is based on the principle that methylated cytosines in CpG islands of promoters are resistant to bisulfite treatment, which chemically converts cytosines to uracil. The modified DNA is then analyzed in two parallel PCR reactions, one containing a 5′-primer designed to amplify only nonconverted cytosines in CpG positions (methylation-sensitive primer, M-primer) and a second with primers specifically designed to detect unmethylated alleles (U-primer). The resulting fragments are then separated on nondenaturing polyacrylamide gels and DNA bands visualized by ethidium bromide staining are checked for size and taken as indicators for either methylated or unmethylated allele-status.

MSP as described earlier is rapid and sufficiently sensitive for screening purposes. The method is "mutation selective," in that the choice of primers differentiates between bisulfite-converted nonmethylated and methylated alleles. This method is limited, however, when the number of methylated alleles is critically small. We therefore performed a modification of this protocol, enabling detection of individual, hypermethylated *p16^{INK4a}* alleles, present in only nanogram quantities within nonclonal DNA material, while retaining the sensitivity achieved by MSP *(27)*. This is mainly achieved by introducing a nonspecific amplification step for total genomic DNA, which amplifies bisulfite-converted DNA (a step that often leaves tiny amounts of amplifiable DNA available). As in conventional MSP, the specific detection of methylated alleles is then achieved by analogous methylation-sensitive primers.

Using this protocol we were able to identify hypermethylated *p16^{INK4a}*-alleles in sputum and bronchial lavage samples with as little as 10–200 ng of total DNA input. Thus, this protocol can be used to detect methylated alleles from sources containing very small quantities of DNA, even if the majority of alleles are nonmethylated.

2. Materials

2.1. DNA-Preparation

1. Qiagen Tissue Kit.
2. Scalpels.
3. Brush cytology material lysis buffer: 10 mM Tris-HCl, pH 8.3, 50 mM KCl, 2.5 mM MgCl$_2$, 0.5% Tween-20, containing proteinase K at 0.5 mg/mL.
4. 10 mM Tris-HCl, pH 8.3.

2.2. Bisulfite Conversion

1. Poly(dA-dT)•Poly(dA-dT) copolymers (Pharmacia-Biotech).
2. 1 N NaOH.
3. 10 mM hydroquinone (Sigma).
4. 3 M sodium bisulfite, pH 5.0 (Sigma).
5. Mineral oil.
6. Wizard DNA Clean-up System (Promega).
7. 10 mM Tris-HCl, 1 mM EDTA (TE), pH 7.6.
8. 3 M Sodium acetate.
9. 70% ethanol.

2.3. Primer Extension Preamplification (PEP)

1. N15 primers, 400 µM, gel-filtrated (TIB, Berlin) (*see* **Note 1**).
2. dNTPs (each at 20 mM).
3. 10X PCR-Buffer (Qiagen).
4. *Taq* polymerase (Qiagen).
5. PCR-quality H$_2$O (Merck).
6. Perkin-Elmer 9600 or 9700 thermocycler allowing linear ramping.

2.4. Semi-Nested Methylspecific PCR (snMSP)

2.4.1. M-Sensitive PCR

1. MSP primers for methylated *p16^INK4a*-alleles (M-primers):
   First PCR: p16Mf   5′-TTA TTA GAG GGT GGG GCG GAT CG
                    p16M2r   5′-CCA CCT AAA TCG ACC TCC GAC CG
   Second PCR: p16Mf   5′-TTA TTA GAG GGT GGG GCG GAT CG
                    p16Mr   5′-GAC CCC GAA CCG CGA CCG TAA
2. 1X PCR buffer (Qiagen).

2.4.2. U-Sensitive PCR

1. MSP primers for nonmethylated *p16^INK4a*-alleles (U-primers):
   First PCR: p16Uf   5′-TTA TTA GAG GGT GGG GTG GAT TG
                    p16U2r   5′-CCA CCT AAA TCA ACC TCC AAC
   Second PCR: p16Uf   5′-TTA TTA GAG GGT GGG GTG GAT TG
                    p16Ur   5′-CAA CCC CAA ACC ACA ACC ATAA)
2. 1X solution Q (Qiagen).

2.5. Gel Analysis

1. 2% agarose gels.
2. TAE electrophoresis buffer working solution: 40 m*M* Tris acetate, 2 m*M* EDTA, pH 8.5, diluted from 50X stock.

3. Method

3.1. DNA-Preparation: see Enriched PCR-RFLP Protocol

1. For DNA analysis of sputum or bronchial lavage fluid, extract DNA from 50 µL homogenized material following the Qiagen Tissue Kit-DNA preparation protocol according to the manufactors' specifications.
2. The method was tested for brush cytology samples in a few cases with results being comparable preparations from sputum and bronchial lavage fluid (BALF). To prepare DNA from brush cytology samples, remove cell debris from the glass by scratching with a scalpel, transfer to Eppendorf tubes and incubate in 500 µL lysis buffer containing proteinase K overnight at 56°C with regular shaking. Then extract DNA using the Qiagen Tissue Kit-DNA preparation protocol.
3. DNA can be stored frozen for up to 1 yr or as a solution in 50 µL 10 m*M* Tris-HCl, pH 8.3, for 4–6 wk at 4°C.

3.2. Bisulfite Conversion

Existing bisulfite conversion protocols *(26,28,29)* were modified to allow for small DNA quantities. Protocols are adapted from a protocol by James Herman *(26)* (*see* **Note 2**).

1. Denature 1/10 of prepared DNA (10–200 ng) and 2 µg Poly(dA-dT)•Poly(dA-dT) copolymers for 20 min at 42°C by adding 1 N NaOH in a volume of 50 µL (to a final concentration of 0.3 M).
2. Add fresh solutions of 10 mM hydroquinone (30 µL) and 3 M sodium bisulfite, pH 5.0 (520 µl), gently mix the solution, overlayed with mineral oil, and incubated in the dark for 12–13 h at 50°C.
3. Recover the aqueous phase using the Wizard DNA Clean-up System according to manufacturer's instructions.
4. The elution efficiency of small DNA quantities is significantly improved by successive elution of bound DNA using prewarmed (80°C) TE, pH 7.6.
   a. Add 50 µL TE and incubate 15 min.
   b. Add another 30 µL aliquot of pre-warmed TE and incubate 1 min.
   c. Centrifuge at 9000g for 20 s (13,000 rpm desk top centrifuge).
5. The purified DNA is subsequently mixed with 1 N NaOH to a final concentration of 0.3 M and incubated for 20 min at 37°C to ensure complete desulfonisation.
6. Ethanol precipitate DNA in the presence of 1/10 vol 3 M sodium acetate at –20°C overnight, spin down at 9000g for 20 min (13,000 rpm desk-top centrifuge).
7. Wash the resulting pellet with 70% ethanol and resuspended in 50 µL H$_2$O. Store at –20°C.

3.3. Primer Extension Preamplification (PEP) (see Note 3)

The genomic amplification is performed following a protocol by Zhang et al. *(30)*.

1. Add 20 µL bisulfite-treated DNA to 5 µL N15 primers, 0.6 µL of each dNTP, 6 µL of 10X PCR-Buffer, 5 U *Taq* polymerase, and H$_2$O (Merck) to yield a total volume of 60 µL (whereby the quality of random primer synthesis proved to be of special importance).
2. After initial denaturation at 94°C for 3 min, 50 primer extension cyles are performed using the following parameters: 1 min denaturation at 92°C, 2 min annealing at 37°C, followed by a 3 min linear ramping to 55°C, and 4 min elongation at 55°C. Protocols with a faster ramping rate or stepwise temperature progression result in inefficient PEP-amplification.
3. Store product DNAs at –20°C.

3.4. Semi-Nested Methylspecific PCR (snMSP) (see Note 4)

This step is done in parallel using either M-primers and U-primers to detect both methylated and unmethylated p16 alleles. Each step of the semi-nested PCR protocol is performed in a 25 µL reaction volume.

3.4.1. M-Sensitive PCR

1. In the first PCR, a 5-µL aliquot of the PEP-product is added to 200 µM dNTPs, 0.4 µM of primers p16Mf and p16M2r, 1X PCR buffer, and 0.65 U *Taq* Polymerase.

2. The second PCR contains 5 μL of the product of the first PCR, diluted 1:10, 200 μ*M* dNTPs, 0.4 μ*M* of primers p16Mf and p16Mr, 1X PCR buffer, and 0.65 U *Taq* Polymerase.
3. Both reactions run for 25 cycles at 95°C 30 s, 65°C 30 s, 72°C 40 s, with initial denaturation at 95°C for 3 min and a final elongation at 72°C for 10 min.

3.4.2. U-Sensitive PCR

To control for complete bisulfite conversion and subsequent PEP amplification, the semi-nested PCR is also performed for the nonmethylated alleles.

1. Use the same protocol as in **Subheading 3.4.1.**, but include 1X solution Q to optimize buffer conditions.
2. Use primers p16Uf and p16U2r in the first reaction and primers p16Uf and in the second.
3. Lower the annealing temperature to 58°C.

3.5. Gel Analysis

1. Resolve products from the second PCR step by gel electrophoresis on 2% agarose gels. Fragments of the U- and M-PCR migrate at around 150 bp.

4. Notes

1. Genomic amplification by random primers is a way to preserve enough DNA for multiplex or repeated analysis. A critical parameter is the quality of random primers as automated oligonucleotide synthesis may not provide equal representation of all degenerate sequences. We found products synthesized by TIB MolBiol to give best DNA yields. 50 linear primer extension cycles resulted in an approx 100-fold amplification of the genomic material.
2. All steps involving bisulfite treatment, primers and PCR conditions for MSP are essentially adopted from the original publication by Herman et al. *(26)*. A detailed description is also available at the following web site: *http://www3.mdanderson .org/leukemia/methylation/*. This web site gives very detailed technical information on bisulfite treatment and conventional MSP so that the reader can easily follow this protocol step by step.
3. A unique advantage feature of this protocol is the generation of sufficient DNA by primer extension pre-amplification. This step is added directly following bisulfite modification and provides a basis for simultaneous or repetitive determination of methylation patterns at multiple sites working with one source of DNA-material. As it becomes evident that aberrant methylation affects many genes, it will be more and more important to determine a specific perhaps individual methylation pattern. Amplification by PEP will therefore allow for the simultaneous analysis of multiple hypermethylated sites and could provide a starting platform for future array technology.
4. A two-stage nested MSP approach has recently published by Palmisano et al. *(31)* for the analysis of *p16* and *MGMT* methylation. As noted by the authors,

this allowed a roughly 50-fold increase in sensitivity over conventional MSP (up to one methylated allele in >50,000 unmethylated alleles). We tested the SN-MSP for optimal sensitivity by serial dilution of DNA isolated from a cell line positive for *p16* methylation into normal genomic DNA and could detect up to a 1 methylated allele detected in 5,000 normal alleles. Compared to the approach by Palmisano et al. we noted only a moderate increase in sensitivity, with respect to conventional MSP by a factor of about 5. However, it should be noted that any increase in sensitivity will have to be evaluated for its diagnostic impact. As with many "mutant-enriched" PCR protocols, drastically increased sensitivity will either yield false-positive results or variant alleles will be detected in a normal "unsuspicious" background. The empirical determination of cut-off values will therefore be equally important to critically evaluate any improvement in technology.

References

1. Bird, A. P. (1986) CpG-rich islands and the function of DNA methylation. *Nature* **321,** 209–213.
2. Turker, M. S. and Bestor, T. H. (1997) Formation of methylation patterns in the mammalian genome. *Mutat. Res.* **386,** 119–130.
3. Holliday, R. (1990) DNA methylation and epigenetic inheritance. *Philos. Trans. R. Soc. Lond. B. Biol. Sci.* **326,** 329–338.
4. Schmutte, C. and Fishel, R. (1999) Genomic instability: first step to carcinogenesis. *Anticancer Res.* **19,** 4665–4696.
5. Baylin, S. B., Esteller, M., Rountree, M. R., Bachman, K. E., Schuebel, K., and Herman, J. G. (2001) Aberrant patterns of DNA methylation, chromatin formation and gene expression in cancer. *Hum. Mol. Genet.* **10,** 687–692.
6. Issa, J. P. (2000) CpG-island methylation in aging and cancer. *Curr. Top. Microbiol. Immunol.* **249,** 101–118.
7. Rountree, M. R., Bachman, K. E., Herman, J. G., and Baylin, S. B. (2001) DNA methylation, chromatin inheritance, and cancer. *Oncogene* **20,** 3156–3165.
8. Baylin, S. B., Herman, J. G., Graff, J. R., Vertino, P. M., and Issa, J. P. (1998) Alterations in DNA methylation: a fundamental aspect of neoplasia. *Adv. Cancer Res.* **72,** 141–196.
9. Gazdar, A. F. (1994) The molecular and cellular basis of human lung cancer. *Anticancer. Res.* **14,** 261–267.
10. Fontanini, G., Vignati, S., Bigini, D., Merlo, G. R., Ribecchini, A., Angeletti, C. A., et al. (1994) Human non-small cell lung cancer: p53 protein accumulation is an early event and persists during metastatic progression. *J. Pathol.* **174,** 23–31.
11. Sozzi, G., Miozzo, M., Donghi, R., Pilotti, S., Cariani, C. T., Pastorino, U., et al. (1992) Deletions of 17p and p53 mutations in preneoplastic lesions of the lung. *Cancer Res.* **52,** 6079–6082.
12. Walker, C., Robertson, L. J., Myskow, M. W., Pendleton, N., and Dixon, G. R. (1994) p53 expression in normal and dysplastic bronchial epithelium and in lung carcinomas. *Br. J. Cancer* **70,** 297–303.

13. Tockman, M. S. (2000) Advances in sputum analysis for screening and early detection of lung cancer. *Cancer Control* **7**, 19–24.

14. Merlo, A., Herman, J. G., Mao, L., Lee, D. J., Gabrielson, E., Burger, P. C., et al. (1995) 5′ CpG island methylation is associated with transcriptional silencing of the tumour suppressor p16/CDKN2/MTS1 in human cancers. *Nat. Med.* **1**, 686–692.

15. Shapiro, G. I., Park, J. E., Edwards, C. D., Mao, L., Merlo, A., Sidransky, D., et al. (1995) Multiple mechanisms of p16INK4A inactivation in non-small cell lung cancer cell lines. *Cancer Res.* **55**, 6200–6209.

16. Ahrendt, S. A., Chow, J. T., Xu, L. H., Yang, S. C., Eisenberger, C. F., Esteller, M., et al. (1999) Molecular detection of tumor cells in bronchoalveolar lavage fluid from patients with early stage lung cancer. *J. Natl. Cancer Inst.* **91**, 332–339.

17. Belinsky, S. A., Nikula, K. J., Palmisano, W. A., Michels, R., Saccomanno, G., Gabrielson, E., et al. (1998) Aberrant methylation of p16(INK4a) is an early event in lung cancer and a potential biomarker for early diagnosis. *Proc. Natl. Acad. Sci. USA* **95**, 11891–11896.

18. Issa, J. P., Baylin, S. B., and Belinsky, S. A. (1996) Methylation of the estrogen receptor CpG island in lung tumors is related to the specific type of carcinogen exposure. *Cancer Res.* **56**, 3655–3658.

19. Eguchi, K., Kanai, Y., Kobayashi, K., and Hirohashi, S. (1997) DNA hypermethylation at the D17S5 locus in non-small cell lung cancers: its association with smoking history. *Cancer Res.* **57**, 4913–4915.

20. Sato, M., Mori, Y., Sakurada, A., Fujimura, S., and Horii, A. (1998) The H-cadherin (CDH13) gene is inactivated in human lung cancer. *Hum. Genet.* **103**, 96–101.

21. Esteller, M., Sanchez-Cespedes, M., Rosell, R., Sidransky, D., Baylin, S. B., and Herman, J. G. (1999) Detection of aberrant promoter hypermethylation of tumor suppressor genes in serum DNA from non-small cell lung cancer patients. *Cancer Res.* **59**, 67–70.

22. Tang ,X., Khuri, F.R., Lee, J.J., Kemp, B.L., Liu, D., Hong, W.K., and Mao, L. (2000) Hypermethylation of the death-associated protein (DAP) kinase promoter and aggressiveness in stage I non-small-cell lung cancer. *J. Natl. Cancer Inst.* **92**, 1511–1566.

23. Virmani, A. K., Rathi, A., Zochbauer-Muller, S., Sacchi, N., Fukuyama, Y., Bryant, D., et al. (2000) Promoter methylation and silencing of the retinoic acid receptor-beta gene in lung carcinomas. *J. Natl. Cancer Inst.* **92**, 1303–1307.

24. Zochbauer-Muller, S., Fong, K. M., Virmani, A. K., Geradts, J., Gazdar, A. F., and Minna, J. D. (2001) Aberrant promoter methylation of multiple genes in non-small cell lung cancers. *Cancer Res.* **61**, 249–255.

25. Tockman, M. S. and Mulshine, J. L. (2000) The early detection of occult lung cancer. *Chest Surg. Clin. North Am.* **10**, 737–749.

26. Herman, J. G., Graff, J. R., Myohanen, S., Nelkin, B. D., and Baylin, S. B. (1996) Methylation-specific PCR: a novel PCR assay for methylation status of CpG islands. *Proc. Natl. Acad. Sci. USA* **93**, 9821–9826.

27. Kersting, M., Friedl, C., Kraus, A., Behn, M., Pankow, W., and Schuermann, M. (2000) Differential frequencies of p16(INK4a) promoter hypermethylation, p53 mutation, and K-ras mutation in exfoliative material mark the development of lung cancer in symptomatic chronic smokers. *J. Clin. Oncol.* **18,** 3221–3229.

28. Frommer, M., McDonald, L. E., Millar, D. S., Collis, C. M., Watt, F., Grigg, G. W., et al. (1992) A genomic sequencing protocol that yields a positive display of 5- methylcytosine residues in individual DNA strands. *Proc. Natl. Acad. Sci. USA* **89,** 1827–1831.

29. Stöger, R., Kajimura, T. M., Brown, W. T., and Laird, C. D. (1997) Epigenetic variation illustrated by DNA methylation patterns of the fragile-X gene FMR1. *Hum. Mol. Genet.* **6,** 1791–1801.

30. Zhang, L., Cui, X., Schmitt, K., Navidi, W., and Arnheim, N. (1992) Whole genome amplification from a single cell: implications for genetic analysis. *Proc. Natl. Acad. Sci. USA* **89,** 5847–5851.

31. Palmisano, W. A., Divine, K. K., Saccomanno, G., Gilliland, F. D., Baylin, S. B., Herman, J. G., and Belinsky, S. A. (2000) Predicting lung cancer by detecting aberrant promoter methylation in sputum. *Cancer Res.* **60,** 5954–5958.

III

MOLECULAR ABNORMALITIES IN LUNG CANCER

B. DETECTION OF ALTERATIONS IN SIGNAL TRANSDUCTION PATHWAYS

8

Role of Receptor Tyrosine Kinases in Lung Cancer

Gautam Maulik, Takashi Kijima, and Ravi Salgia

1. Introduction

Lung cancer cells express receptor tyrosine kinases (RTKs) that may be important targets for therapies. RTKs are proto-oncogenes, which are key regulators for cell growth, differentiation, survival, or motility. More than 50 RTKs, in both lung and other tissues, have been identified *(1)*. The receptors contain an N-terminal extracellular ligand-binding domain, a single transmembrane α helix, and a cytosolic C-terminal domain with tyrosine kinase activity. The binding of growth factors to the RTKs extracellular domain activates the cytosolic kinase domain. Growth factor activation of the RTK results in dimerization of the receptor, with phosphorylation of the receptor and downstream targets. Upon activation of RTKs, various biological functions are altered in lung cancer cells, including cell growth, migration/motility, alterations of reactive oxygen species (ROS), and activation of downstream signal-transduction events.

Lung cancer is mainly subdivided into non-small cell lung cancer (NSCLC, approx 75% of all lung cancers) and small cell lung cancer (SCLC, approx 20% of all lung cancers). It has been shown that lung cancer cells overexpress various RTKs *(2)*. With the novel therapeutics available against these RTKs, excitement has been generated for testing these compounds against lung cancer. Based on these new findings, we will describe three such RTKs in lung cancer: epidermal growth factor receptor (EGFR), c-Kit, and c-Met. These receptors play an important role in lung cancer (EGFR and c-Met for NSCLC; c-Kit and c-Met for SCLC) and will be detailed in terms of their structure, role in transformation, expression, role in biological and biochemical functions, and finally, their use as potential therapeutic targets.

From: *Methods in Molecular Medicine, vol. 74: Lung Cancer, Vol. 1: Molecular Pathology Methods and Reviews*
Edited by: B. Driscoll © Humana Press Inc., Totowa, NJ

2. EGFR

2.1. Structure, Role in Transformation, Expression

EGFR (also known as HER1 or c-erbB-1) belongs to a family that includes HER2/neu, HER3, and HER4. EGFR is a 170 kDa glycoprotein with an extracellular domain containing two cysteine-rich repeats, a catalytic domain, and a C-terminus with multiple tyrosines that can bind the SH2 domains of adapter molecules. EGFR ligands include EGF, transforming growth factor-α (TGF-α), betacellulin, and epiregulin. Initially, the role of EGFR in oncogenesis was tested in NIH3T3 cells by overexpression of the receptor itself, stimulation by manipulation of expression of the ligand, EGF, and examination of its role in tumor formation in nude mice *(3)*.

EGFR has been shown to be overexpressed in a variety of solid tumors, including glioblastomas, breast, prostate, ovary, stomach, colon, larynx, and lung. In NSCLC, expression of EGFR has been correlated with a poor prognosis and also correlated with stage of disease. As an example, Volm et al. *(4)* have determined the median survival for 121 patients with squamous cell lung cancer and determined that those whose tumors express EGFR have a shorter survival time. The mean EGFR concentration in tumors has also been shown to be lower in pathological stage I–II disease as compared to stage IV disease.

2.2. EGFR Role in Motility, Migration, Metastasis

There are intrinsic abnormalities of cell motility, migration, and the ability to metastasize in lung cancer cells. Most cell motility processes are tightly regulated by tyrosine kinases and protein tyrosine phosphatases. In malignant lung cancer cells, activation of receptor tyrosine kinases is an important pathway towards alteration of a cell's motility and its ability to migrate, invade, and metastasize. Cell motility is dependent on the actin structure in the cell, involves various cytoskeletal proteins (especially, in the focal adhesion, such as tensin, talin, p125FAK, and paxillin), and is dependent on PI3-K and Rho family members (Rho, Rac, Cdc42). EGF stimulation of human breast cancer cells overexpressing EGFR has been shown to induce cell migration *(5)*. In SKBR3 breast cancer cells overexpressing EGFR, EGF causes increased motility and invasion, and also induces the expression of extracellular matrix (ECM)-targeting proteases, including type I and type IV collagenases, uPA, and its receptor *(6)*.

2.3. EGFR Role in Regulation of Reactive Oxygen Species

Reactive oxygen species (ROS), such as $O_2^{\cdot-}$, $OH^{\cdot-}$, $NO^{\cdot}$, and H_2O_2, have recently begun to be appreciated for their role in regulation of signal transduction, gene expression, proliferation, and motility *(7,8)*. Cigarette smoke, an important pathogen in terms of lung cancer, contains more than 10^{14} free radicals per puff *(9)*. Generation of ROS in lung cancer cells can lead to alteration of multiple downstream signal-transduction pathways. Activation of EGFR can lead to generation of ROS, and the modulation of ROS can lead to phosphorylation of EGFR. The EGFR signaling mechanism involves the generation of H_2O_2 *(10)*, and modification of a reduced cysteine residue in EGFR may reversibly affect its activation *(11)*. Goldkorn et al. *(12)* have shown that H_2O_2 increases tyrosine phosphorylation of EGFR, and the receptor has a slower rate of turnover and altered downstream phosphorylation in its presence.

2.4. EGFR Role in Signal Transduction

EGFR signal transduction is a classic pathway through which many novel signal-transduction cascades have been identified. We obviously cannot report all the pathways, such as PI3K, Stats, MAPK, SHC, and ras, which are affected by this pathway, but will refer to general references. In the context of the aforementioned effects on cell motility, we will restrict ourselves to how EGFR activation can affect cytoskeletal proteins. EGF ligation of EGFR can lead to F-actin rearrangement, with phosphorylation of focal adhesion proteins, such as p125FAK and paxillin *(13)*.

2.5. EGFR Tyrosine Kinase Inhibition

Several strategies have been utilized to inhibit EGFR in lung cancer, including neutralizing antibodies, tyrosine kinase inhibitors, ligand conjugates, immunoconjugates, and antisense oligonucleotides. Currently, there are several oral tyrosine kinase inhibitors against EGFR being utilized, as well as specific antibody therapy, in clinical trials. Of the oral inhibitors, ZD1839 (a quinazoline targeting the EGFR ATP tyrosine kinase domain) has shown activity against NSCLC, and various Phase II and Phase III trials are being conducted *(14,15)*. Interestingly, ZD1839 is already being used in clinical trials in combination with standard therapy for NSCLC, carboplatin, and paclitaxel. There are also monoclonal antibodies (MAbs) against the extracellular domain of EGFR being utilized in clinical trials. MAb-C225, a human/murine chimeric antibody, binds to EGFR in a similar fashion as the EGF ligand, and is currently being utilized in NSCLC, and head and neck cancer. MAb-C225 is also being combined with radiation therapy in most recent trials *(16)*.

3. c-Kit

3.1. Structure, Role in Transformation, Expression

c-Kit, a proto-oncogene with a molecular weight of 145kDa, is a type III receptor tyrosine kinase (similar to c-Fms and PDGF-R), containing

5 immunoglobulin-like domains, a single transmembrane domain, and a cytoplasmic domain with a split kinase domain and a hydrophilic kinase insert sequence *(17,18)*. c-Kit ligand is stem cell factor (SCF, also known as steel factor).

In normal tissues, c-Kit is expressed in mast cells, melanocytes, testis, and in bone marrow *(18)*. c-Kit, along with SCF, is aberrantly expressed in approximately 70% of SCLC tumors (primary tissues and cell lines) *(19)*, and 40% of NSCLC. There is also overexpression of c-Kit in breast, cervical, ovarian, melanoma, and GI stromal tumors (GIST) *(20,21)*. Activating mutations in the catalytic domain have been described in GIST *(21)*. A constitutively active form of c-Kit (D816V) has been found in mastocytosis *(20)*.

In SCLC, the SCF/c-Kit autocrine loop is functional and causes cell growth. As shown by Krystal et al. *(22)*, when a dominant negative kinase defective c-Kit (a frame-shift mutation in the extracellular domain of c-Kit) was introduced into c-Kit/SCF expressing cell line, there was growth suppression. Most recently, we *(23)* and Krystal's group *(24)* have shown that inhibiting c-Kit by the novel TK inhibitor, STI571, leads to growth suppression of SCLC cell lines.

3.2. c-Kit Role in Motility, Migration, and Metastases

In hematopoietic cells, SCF is a chemotactic agent and promotes cell adhesion. SCF upregulates hematopoietic stem cell avidity of β_1 integrins, VLA-4 ($\alpha_4\beta_1$), and VLA-5 ($\alpha_5\beta_1$), for fibronectin *(25)*. SCF, in synergy with the chemokine SDF-1α (ligand for G-protein coupled chemokine receptor CXCR4), can mobilize hematopoietic CD34+ stem cells from the bone marrow to other organs such as the spleen *(26,27)*. In SCLC, utilizing transwell assays, SCF has been shown to act as a chemotactic signal *(28)*. The role of SCF/c-Kit in normal and tumor cells with respect to cell motility and metastasis has not been elucidated.

3.3. c-Kit Role in Regulation of Reactive Oxygen Species

Recently, we have shown that ROS can be generated by growth factor stimulation *(29)*. We initially utilized the hematopoietic cell model, since c-Kit/SCF pathways have been well characterized in Mo7e, a megakaryocytic cell line. We have shown, in Mo7e cells, that stimulation with SCF leads to a rapid increase in ROS. Using exposure to H_2O_2 as a model to increase ROS, we found increased tyrosine phosphorylation of multiple proteins, including STAT5 (a viability signaling molecule). H_2O_2 also induced expression of early response gene c-Fos and a G1-to-S-phase transition. And, by using the antioxidants pyrrolidine dithiocarbonate (PDTC), N-acetyl cysteine, and 2-mercaptoethanol, we observed decreased viability of M07e cells.

3.4. c-Kit Role in Signal Transduction

A plethora of downstream signal-transduction intermediates, including those of the cytoskeleton, have been identified in response to SCF stimulation *(25)*. In hematopoietic cells, focal adhesion proteins such as paxillin, p125FAK, and PYK2 (also known as RAFTK) are phosphorylated in response to c-Kit stimulation *(30)*. The role of c-Kit/SCF stimulation of the cytoskeletal protein in SCLC has thus far not been elucidated.

3.5. c-Kit Tyrosine Kinase Inhibition

The development of small molecules that inhibit the tyrosine kinase receptor c-Kit offers a way of potentially inhibiting autocrine growth loops in SCLC. This is a novel approach towards therapeutic agents in SCLC.

A tyrosine kinase inhibitor, STI 571, was developed as an ATP competitive inhibitor of the Abl protein kinase *(31)*. This inhibitor (formerly known as CGP57148B and currently as Gleevec, Novartis Pharmaceuticals) was initially shown to inhibit BCR/ABL kinase activity, and therefore, chronic myelogenous leukemia cell growth and the viability of cells transformed by Abl oncogenes *(32–34)*. This drug has most recently been shown to be effective in a phase I trial for patients with chronic-phase chronic myclogenous leukemia (CML) for whom treatment with interferon-α (IFN-α) failed. With administration of STI 571, 53 of 54 patients attained complete hematologic responses for at least 4 wk at doses of 300 mg or greater *(35)*. STI 571 inhibits not only the kinase activity of Abl, but also the kinase activity of PDGF-receptor (PDGFR) and c-Kit as well *(36)*. Interestingly, though STI 571 can inhibit the kinase activity of c-Kit, it has no effect on the related receptor tyrosine kinases c-Fms and Flk2/Flt3 *(37)*. We have determined the effect of STI 571 on SCLC cell line growth and viability *(23)*, and have shown dramatic inhibition of SCLC by STI 571. Based on this, clinical trials are underway for the role of STI571 in SCLC.

4. c-Met
4.1. Structure, Role in Transformation, Expression

c-Met is a proto-oncogene belonging to the family of heterodimeric tyrosine kinases that includes Ron, Ryk, Sea, and Sex *(1,38,39)*. The p190c-Met protein consists of an extracellular α-chain plus a β-subunit composed of a ligand-binding extracellular domain, a membrane-spanning region, and an intracellular tyrosine kinase catalytic domain *(40,41)*. Both subunits are derived by glycosylation and proteolytic cleavage of a common precursor of 170 kDa. The major autophosphorylation site for c-Met is Y1235, located in the catalytic domain *(42–44)*. This tyrosine residue is part of a three-tyrosine motif containing Y1230, Y1234 and Y1235. Two more tyrosines, Y1349 and Y1356, are located within multidocking sites and are phosphorylated upon ligand binding. Mutations of these residues abrogate all receptor activity. The *met* proto-oncogene efficiently transforms NIH/3T3 cells *(45)* and co-expression of c-Met and HGF was shown to have oncogenic potential *(38)*.

c-Met itself has been shown to be expressed in epithelial cells and in a variety of tumor tissues. The oncogene is overexpressed in tumors, including thyroid, pancreatic carcinoma, and lung cancer *(46)*. Germ-line missense mutations in the tyrosine kinase domain are detected in the majority of hereditary papillary renal cell carcinomas (HPRCC) *(47)*, whereas somatic mutations have been found in some sporadic papillary renal carcinomas *(48)*.

Overexpression of c-Met has been detected in SCLC and NSCLC cells. In a study by Olivero et al. *(49)*, c-Met was found to be increased 2–10-fold in 25% of NSCLC tumor tissue as compared to adjacent normal tissue. In a further study by Ichimura et al. *(50)*, the expression of c-Met was determined by immunoblotting and shown to be positive in 11/11 NSCLC cell lines studied, demonstrated in 34/47 (72%) adenocarcinoma, and 20/52 (38.5%) squamous cell carcinoma tumor tissues. c-Met protein expression tended to correlate with higher pathological tumor stage and a worse clinical outcome. c-Met expression, at both mRNA and protein levels, have been described in 22/25 SCLC cell lines and nude mouse xenografts *(51)*.

The ligand for c-Met is hepatocyte growth factor (HGF), also known as scatter factor, since it stimulates cellular motility and functions as a morphoregulatory molecule *(52)*. HGF is a heterodimer composed of a 69 kDa and a 34 kDa subunit *(53)*. HGF is believed to be expressed by stromal cells, and HGF stimulation of the c-Met receptor in a paracrine fashion leads to activation of cellular motility, migration, and signal-transduction pathways in target cells. Elevated levels of HGF have also been implicated in the more aggressive biology of NSCLC *(54,55)*.

4.2. c-Met Role in Motility, Migration, and Metastases

The mechanism whereby HGF stimulation of c-Met leads to increased motility, migration, and invasion is not well-understood. c-Met stimulation promotes cell movement, causes epithelial cells to disperse ("scatter") and endothelial cells to migrate, and promotes chemotaxis. Evidence exists that enhanced cell motility and invasion may be an important consequence of c-Met signaling. For example, examination of mutant mice nullizygous for Met shows that muscles in the limb, diaphragm, and tip of the tongue, which normally originate from migrating dermomyotome cells, fail to develop *(56)*.

Cell motility has been shown to be tightly controlled by the lipid kinase PI3-K and the p21GTPases, including Ras, Rac, and Rho *(57,58)*. PI3-K appears to be an important molecule in HGF-induced mito-, moto-, and morpho-genesis, since inhibition of PI3-K by wortmannin leads to decreased branching formation on collagen matrix and chemotaxis of renal cells *(59,60)*. Microinjection of activated H-Ras stimulates cell spreading and actin reorganization, whereas inhibition of endogenous Ras abolishes spreading, actin reorganization, and scattering *(61–63)*. In A549 NSCLC cells, HGF stimulation increases the level of Ras-GTP by 50% *(64)*. Dominant-negative Rac microinjection abolishes HGF-induced spreading and actin reorganization. Finally, microinjection of Rho inhibits HGF-induced spreading and scattering, though not motility *(65)*.

4.3. c-Met Role in Regulation of Reactive Oxygen Species

In a recent study from Arakaki et al. *(66)*, it was shown that N-acetylcysteine (NAC) prevented HGF-suppressed growth of Sarcoma 180 and Meth A cells, and HGF-induced apoptosis. ROS was measured by the peroxide sensitive fluorescent probe DCF-DA (2′,7′-dichlorofluoroscein-diacetate). As mentioned in the previous section, there is a fine balance between ROS and anti-oxidants. Anti-oxidants include the scavengers NAC, vitamin E, and the free-radical spin traps N-t-butyl-a-phenylnitrone and 3,3,5,5-tetramethyl-1-pyrroline-1-oxide. Enzymatic anti-oxidants include superoxide dismutase (SOD) and catalase. What is interesting about this study is that HGF stimulation inhibited cellular growth, whereas, in lung cancer cells, HGF induces proliferation. However, the study does point out that HGF/c-Met is important in ROS regulation.

4.4. c-Met Role in Signal Transduction

Stimulation of c-Met leads to its association with multiple proteins, as well as activation of several pathways *(67)*. An innumerable number of signal-transduction pathways have been identified in HGF signaling, and reviewed exhaustively by Furge et al. *(68)*. There have also been reports of phosphorylation of cytoskeletal proteins paxillin and p125FAK in response to HGF stimulation *(69)*.

4.5. Inhibitors of c-Met

c-Met is an attractive target for inhibition in SCLC, however no small molecules such as STI 571 have been identified that can act against the c-Met tyrosine kinase. Recently, Bardelli et al. *(70)* have reported using neutralizing peptides against the tyrosines located in the c-Met kinase activation loop. Sequences were obtained from the Antennapedia protein for internalization: Ant-Y1234-1235-*RQIKIWFQNRRHKWKK*GLARDMYDKEYYSVHNKTG) as well as from the carboxy-tail of c-Met Ant-Y1349-1356 *RQIKIWFQNRRH KWKK*-IGEHYVHVNATYVNVKCVA). Peptides derived from the c-Met receptor tail, and not from the kinase domain, bind the receptor, inhibit kinase activity and HGF-mediated invasive growth of A549 cells by approx 50% (as assayed by examining invasion, cell migration, and branched morphogenesis).

HGF also leads to plasmin activation, and Webb et al. *(71)* have reported that administration of geldanamycins, belonging to the ansamycin family of antibiotics, leads to decreased plasmin activation at femtomolar concentrations. Using the geldanamycins at nanomolar concentrations led to downregulation of c-Met, inhibition of HGF-mediated cell motility and invasion in MDCK-2 cells, and reversion of Met-transformed NIH3T3 cells.

5. Summary

Receptor tyrosine kinases are important in normal cellular physiology as well in the pathogenesis of a variety of tumors, including lung cancer. RTKs are a target for novel therapies currently being investigated. In the clinics, EGFR inhibitors and c-Kit inhibitors are already being utilized, and c-Met inhibitors are in development. Even though the RTK inhibitors provide a novel mechanism, it is important to realize that lung cancer etiology is a complex process, and eventually standard chemotherapy may need to be used in conjunction with these novel therapies to make an important difference in response rates.

References

1. Porter, A. C. and Vaillancourt, R. R. (1998) Tyrosine kinase receptor-activated signal transduction pathways which lead to oncogenesis. *Oncogene* **17,** 1343–1352.
2. Salgia, R. and Skarin, A. T. (1998) Molecular abnormalities in lung cancer. *J. Clin. Oncol.* **16,** 1207–1217.
3. Velu, T. J., Beguinot, L., Vass, W. C., Willingham, M. C., Merlino, G. T., Pastan, I., and Lowy, D. R. (1987) Epidermal-growth-factor-dependent transformation by a human EGF receptor proto-oncogene. *Science* **238,** 1408–1410.
4. Volm, M., Rittgen, W., and Drings, P. (1998) Prognostic value of ERBB-1, VEGF, cyclin A, FOS, JUN and MYC in patients with squamous cell lung carcinomas. *Br. J. Cancer* **77,** 663–669.
5. Verbeek, B. S., Adriaansen-Slot, S. S., Vroom, T. M., Beckers, T., and Rijksen, G. (1998) Overexpression of EGFR and c-erbB2 causes enhanced cell migration in human breast cancer cells and NIH3T3 fibroblasts. *FEBS Lett.* **425,** 145–150.
6. Watabe, T., Yoshida, K., Shindoh, M., Kaya, M., Fujikawa, K., Sato, H., et al. (1998) The Ets-1 and Ets-2 transcription factors activate the promoters for invasion-associated urokinase and collagenase genes in response to epidermal growth factor. *Int. J. Cancer* **77,** 128–137.
7. Adler, V., Yin, Z., Tew, K. D., and Ronai, Z. (1999) Role of redox potential and reactive oxygen species in stress signaling. *Oncogene* **18,** 6104–6111.
8. Kamata, H. and Hirata, H. (1999) Redox regulation of cellular signalling. *Cell Signal.* **11,** 1–14.

9. Rahman, I. and MacNee, W. (1996) Role of oxidants/antioxidants in smoking-induced lung diseases. *Free Radic. Biol. Med.* **21**, 669–681.

10. Bae, Y. S., Kang, S. W., Seo, M. S., Baines, I. C., Tekle, E., Chock, P. B., and Rhee, S. G. (1997) Epidermal growth factor (EGF)-induced generation of hydrogen peroxide. Role in EGF receptor-mediated tyrosine phosphorylation. *J. Biol. Chem.* **272**, 217–221.

11. Woltjer, R. L. and Staros, J. V. (1997) Effects of sulfhydryl modification reagents on the kinase activity of the epidermal growth factor receptor. *Biochemistry* **36**, 9911–9916.

12. Goldkorn, T., Balaban, N., Matsukuma, K., Chea, V., Gould, R., Last, J., et al. (1998) EGF-Receptor phosphorylation and signaling are targeted by H_2O_2 redox stress. *Am. J. Respir. Cell Mol. Biol.* **19**, 786–798.

13. Sattler, M., Pisick, E., Morrison, P. T., and Salgia, R. (2000) Role of the cytoskeletal protein paxillin in oncogenesis. *Crit. Rev. Oncol.* **11**, 63–76.

14. Baselga, J. and Averbuch, S. D. (2000) ZD1839 ('Iressa') as an anticancer agent. *Drugs* **60**, 33–40; discussion 41–42.

15. Ciardiello, F. (2000) Epidermal growth factor receptor tyrosine kinase inhibitors as anticancer agents. *Drugs* **60**, 25–32; discussion 41–42.

16. Harari, P. M. and Huang, S. M. (2001) Head and neck cancer as a clinical model for molecular targeting of therapy: combining EGFR blockade with radiation. *Int. J. Radiat. Oncol. Biol. Phys.* **49**, 427–433.

17. Galli, S. J., Tsai, M., and Wershil, B. K. (1993) The c-kit receptor, stem cell factor, and mast cells. What each is teaching us about the others. *Am. J. Pathol.* **142**, 965–974.

18. Ashman, L. K. (1999) The biology of stem cell factor and its receptor C-kit. *Int. J. Biochem. Cell. Biol.* **31**, 1037–1051.

19. Hibi, K., Takahashi, T., Sekido, Y., Ueda, R., Hida, T., Ariyoshi, Y., and Takagi, H. (1991) Coexpression of the stem cell factor and the c-kit genes in small-cell lung cancer. *Oncogene* **6**, 2291–2296.

20. Boissan, M., Feger, F., Guillosson, J. J., and Arock, M. (2000) c-Kit and c-kit mutations in mastocytosis and other hematological diseases. *J. Leukoc. Biol.* **67**, 135–148.

21. Hirota, S., Isozaki, K., Nishida, T., and Kitamura, Y. (2000) Effects of loss-of-function and gain-of-function mutations of c-kit on the gastrointestinal tract. *J. Gastroenterol.* **35**, 75–79.

22. Krystal, G. W., Hines, S. J., and Organ, C. P. (1996) Autocrine growth of small cell lung cancer mediated by coexpression of c-kit and stem cell factor. *Cancer Res.* **56**, 370–376.

23. Wang, W. L., Healy, M. E., Sattler, M., Verma, S., Lin, J., Maulik, G., et al. (2000) Growth inhibition and modulation of kinase pathways of small cell lung cancer cell lines by the novel tyrosine kinase inhibitor STI 571. *Oncogene* **19**, 3521–3528.

24. Krystal, G. W., Honsawek, S., Litz, J., and Buchdunger, E. (2000) The selective tyrosine kinase inhibitor STI571 inhibits small cell lung cancer growth. *Clin. Cancer Res.* **6**, 3319–3326.

25. Linnekin, D. (1999) Early signaling pathways activated by c-Kit in hematopoietic cells. *Int. J. Biochem. Cell Biol.* **31**, 1053–1074.
26. Aiuti, A., Webb, I. J., Bleul, C., Springer, T., and Gutierrez-Ramos, J. C. (1997) The chemokine SDF-1 is a chemoattractant for human CD34+ hematopoietic progenitor cells and provides a new mechanism to explain the mobilization of CD34+ progenitors to peripheral blood. *J. Exp. Med.* **185**, 111–120.
27. Peled, A., Grabovsky, V., Habler, L., Sandbank, J., Arenzana-Seisdedos, F., Petit, I., et al. (1999) The chemokine SDF-1 stimulates integrin-mediated arrest of CD34(+) cells on vascular endothelium under shear flow. *J. Clin. Invest.* **104**, 1199–1211.
28. Sekido, Y., Takahashi, T., Ueda, R., Takahashi, M., Suzuki, H., Nishida, K., et al. (1993) Recombinant human stem cell factor mediates chemotaxis of small-cell lung cancer cell lines aberrantly expressing the c-kit protooncogene. *Cancer Res.* **53**, 1709–1714.
29. Sattler, M., Winkler, T., Verma, S., Byrne, C. H., Shrikhande, G., Salgia, R., and Griffin, J. D. (1999) Hematopoietic growth factors signal through the formation of reactive oxygen species. *Blood* **93**, 2928–2935.
30. Takahira, H., Gotoh, A., Ritchie, A., and Broxmeyer, H. E. (1997) Steel factor enhances integrin-mediated tyrosine phosphorylation of focal adhesion kinase (pp125FAK) and paxillin. *Blood* **89**, 1574–1584.
31. Buchdunger, E., Zimmermann, J., Mett, H., Meyer, T., Muller, M., Druker, B. J., and Lydon, N. B. (1996) Inhibition of the Abl protein-tyrosine kinase in vitro and in vivo by a 2-phenylaminopyrimidine derivative. *Cancer Res.* **56**, 100–104.
32. Druker, B. J., Tamura, S., Buchdunger, E., Ohno, S., Segal, G. M., Fanning, S., et al. (1996) Effects of a selective inhibitor of the Abl tyrosine kinase on the growth of Bcr-Abl positive cells. *Nat. Med.* **2**, 561–566.
33. Druker, B. J. and Lydon, N. B. (2000) Lessons learned from the development of an abl tyrosine kinase inhibitor for chronic myelogenous leukemia. *J. Clin. Invest.* **105**, 3–7.
34. Sawyers, C. L. and Druker, B. (1999) Tyrosine kinase inhibitors in chronic myeloid leukemia. *Cancer J. Sci. Am.* **5**, 63–69.
35. Druker, B. J., Talpaz, M., Resta, D. J., Peng, B., Buchdunger, E., Ford, J. M., et al. (2001) Efficacy and safety of a specific inhibitor of the BCR-ABL tyrosine kinase in chronic myeloid leukemia. *N. Engl. J. Med.* **344**, 1031–1037.
36. Carroll, M., Ohno-Jones, S., Tamura, S., Buchdunger, E., Zimmermann, J., Lydon, N. B., et al. (1997) CGP 57148, a tyrosine kinase inhibitor, inhibits the growth of cells expressing BCR-ABL, TEL-ABL, and TEL-PDGFR fusion proteins. *Blood* **90**, 4947–4952.
37. Heinrich, M. C., Griffith, D. J., Druker, B. J., Wait, C. L., Ott, K. A., and Zigler, A. J. (2000) Inhibition of c-kit receptor tyrosine kinase activity by STI 571, a selective tyrosine kinase inhibitor. *Blood* **96**, 925–932.
38. Rong, S., Bodescot, M., Blair, D., Dunn, J., Nakamura, T., Mizuno, K., et al. (1992) Tumorigenicity of the met proto-oncogene and the gene for hepatocyte growth factor. *Mol. Cell Biol.* **12**, 5152–5158.

39. Muraoka, R. S., Sun, W. Y., Colbert, M. C., Waltz, S. E., Witte, D. P., Degen, J. L., and Friezner Degen, S. J. (1999) The Ron/STK receptor tyrosine kinase is essential for peri-implantation development in the mouse. *J. Clin. Invest.* **103**, 1277–1285.

40. Weidner, K. M., Sachs, M., and Birchmeier, W. (1993) The Met receptor tyrosine kinase transduces motility, proliferation, and morphogenic signals of scatter factor/hepatocyte growth factor in epithelial cells. *J. Cell Biol.* **121**, 145–154.

41. Weidner, K. M., Hartmann, G., Sachs, M., and Birchmeier, W. (1993) Properties and functions of scatter factor/hepatocyte growth factor and its receptor c-Met. *Am. J. Respir. Cell Mol. Biol.* **8**, 229–237.

42. Jeffers, M., Schmidt, L., Nakaigawa, N., Webb, C. P., Weirich, G., Kishida, T., et al. (1997) Activating mutations for the met tyrosine kinase receptor in human cancer. *Proc. Natl. Acad. Sci. USA* **94**, 11445–11450.

43. Jeffers, M., Fiscella, M., Webb, C. P., Anver, M., Koochekpour, S., and Vande Woude, G. F. (1998) The mutationally activated Met receptor mediates motility and metastasis. *Proc. Natl. Acad. Sci. USA* **95**, 14417–14422.

44. Jeffers, M. F. (1999) Activating mutations in the Met receptor overcome the requirement for autophosphorylation of tyrosines crucial for wild type signaling. *Oncogene* **18**, 5120–5125.

45. Iyer, A., Kmiecik, T. E., Park, M., Daar, I., Blair, D., Dunn, K. J., et al. (1990) Structure, tissue-specific expression, and transforming activity of the mouse met protooncogene. *Cell Growth Differ.* **1**, 87–95.

46. To, C. T. and Tsao, M. S. (1998) The roles of hepatocyte growth factor/scatter factor and met receptor in human cancers (Review). *Oncol. Rep.* **5**, 1013–1024.

47. Olivero, M., Valente, G., Bardelli, A., Longati, P., Ferrero, N., Cracco, C., et al. (1999) Novel mutation in the ATP-binding site of the MET oncogene tyrosine kinase in a HPRCC family. *Int. J. Cancer* **82**, 640–643.

48. Di Renzo, M. F., Olivero, M., Martone, T., Maffe, A., Maggiora, P., Stefani, A. D., et al. (2000) Somatic mutations of the MET oncogene are selected during metastatic spread of human HNSC carcinomas. *Oncogene* **19**, 1547–1555.

49. Olivero, M., Rizzo, M., Madeddu, R., Casadio, C., Pennacchietti, S., Nicotra, M. R., et al. (1996) Overexpression and activation of hepatocyte growth factor/scatter factor in human non-small-cell lung carcinomas. *Br. J. Cancer* **74**, 1862–1868.

50. Ichimura, E., Maeshima, A., Nakajima, T., and Nakamura, T. (1996) Expression of c-met/HGF receptor in human non-small cell lung carcinomas in vitro and in vivo and its prognostic significance. *Jpn. J. Cancer Res.* **87**, 1063–1069.

51. Rygaard, K., Nakamura, T., and Spang-Thomsen, M. (1993) Expression of the proto-oncogenes c-met and c-kit and their ligands, hepatocyte growth factor/scatter factor and stem cell factor, in SCLC cell lines and xenografts. *Br. J. Cancer* **67**, 37–46.

52. Bottaro, D. P., Rubin, J. S., Faletto, D. L., Chan, A. M., Kmiecik, T. E., Vande Woude, G. F., and Aaronson, S. A. (1991) Identification of the hepatocyte growth factor receptor as the c-met proto-oncogene product. *Science* **251**, 802–804.

53. Stella, M. C. and Comoglio, P. M. (1999) HGF: a multifunctional growth factor controlling cell scattering. *Int. J. Biochem. Cell Biol.* **31**, 1357–1362.

54. Siegfried, J. M., Weissfeld, L. A., Singh-Kaw, P., Weyant, R. J., Testa, J. R., and Landreneau, R. J. (1997) Association of immunoreactive hepatocyte growth factor with poor survival in resectable non-small cell lung cancer. *Cancer Res.* **57,** 433–439.

55. Siegfried, J. M., Weissfeld, L. A., Luketich, J. D., Weyant, R. J., Gubish, C. T., and Landreneau, R. J. (1998) The clinical significance of hepatocyte growth factor for non-small cell lung cancer. *Ann. Thorac. Surg.* **66,** 1915–1918.

56. Bladt, F., Riethmacher, D., Isenmann, S., Aguzzi, A., and Birchmeier, C. (1995) Essential role for the c-met receptor in the migration of myogenic precursor cells into the limb bud. *Nature* **376,** 768–771.

57. Nobes, C. D., Hawkins, P., Stephens, L., and Hall, A. (1995) Activation of the small GTP-binding proteins rho and rac by growth factor receptors. *J. Cell Sci.* **108,** 225–233.

58. Nobes, C. D. and Hall, A. (1995) Rho, rac, and cdc42 GTPases regulate the assembly of multimolecular focal complexes associated with actin stress fibers, lamellipodia, and filopodia. *Cell* **81,** 53–62.

59. Derman, M. P., Cunha, M. J., Barros, E. J., Nigam, S. K., and Cantley, L. G. (1995) HGF-mediated chemotaxis and tubulogenesis require activation of the phosphatidylinositol 3-kinase. *Am. J. Physiol.* **268,** F1211–F1217.

60. Derman, M. P., Chen, J. Y., Spokes, K. C., Songyang, Z., and Cantley, L. G. (1996) An 11-amino acid sequence from c-met initiates epithelial chemotaxis via phosphatidylinositol 3-kinase and phospholipase C. *J. Biol. Chem.* **271,** 4251–4255.

61. Ridley, A. J., Paterson, H. F., Johnston, C. L., Diekmann, D., and Hall, A. (1992) The small GTP-binding protein rac regulates growth factor-induced membrane ruffling. *Cell* **70,** 401–410.

62. Ridley, A. J. and Hall, A. (1992) Eye development. Function for Ras in sight. *Nature* **355,** 497–498.

63. Ridley, A. J., Comoglio, P. M., and Hall, A. (1995) Regulation of scatter factor/hepatocyte growth factor responses by Ras, Rac, and Rho in MDCK cells. *Mol. Cell Biol.* **15,** 1110–1122.

64. Graziani, A., Gramaglia, D., dalla Zonca, P., and Comoglio, P. M. (1993) Hepatocyte growth factor/scatter factor stimulates the Ras-guanine nucleotide exchanger. *J. Biol. Chem.* **268,** 9165–9168.

65. Takaishi, K., Sasaki, T., Kato, M., Yamochi, W., Kuroda, S., Nakamura, T., et al. (1994) Involvement of Rho p21 small GTP-binding protein and its regulator in the HGF-induced cell motility. *Oncogene* **9,** 273–279.

66. Arakaki, N., Kajihara, T., Arakaki, R., Ohnishi, T., Kazi, J. A., Nakashima, H., and Daikuhara, Y. (1999) Involvement of oxidative stress in tumor cytotoxic activity of hepatocyte growth factor/scatter factor. *J. Biol. Chem.* **274,** 13541–13546.

67. Stuart, K. A., Riordan, S. M., Lidder, S., Crostella, L., Williams, R., and Skouteris, G. G. (2000) Hepatocyte growth factor/scatter factor-induced intracellular signalling. *Int. J. Exp. Pathol.* **81,** 17–30.

68. Furge, K. A., Zhang, Y. W., and Vande Woude, G. F. (2000) Met receptor tyrosine kinase: enhanced signaling through adapter proteins. *Oncogene* **19,** 5582–5589.

69. Nakaigawa, N., Weirich, G., Schmidt, L., and Zbar, B. (2000) Tumorigenesis mediated by MET mutant M1268T is inhibited by dominant-negative Src. *Oncogene* **19,** 2996–3002.

70. Bardelli, A., Longati, P., Williams, T. A., Benvenuti, S., and Comoglio, P. M. (1999) A peptide representing the carboxyl-terminal tail of the met receptor inhibits kinase activity and invasive growth. *J. Biol. Chem.* **274,** 29274–29281.

71. Webb, C. P., Hose, C. D., Koochekpour, S., Jeffers, M., Oskarsson, M., Sausville, E., et al. (2000) The geldanamycins are potent inhibitors of the hepatocyte growth factor/scatter factor-met-urokinase plasminogen activator-plasmin proteolytic network. *Cancer Res.* **60,** 342–349.

9

Relationship of EGFR Signal-Transduction Modulation by Tyrosine Kinase Inhibitors to Chemosensitivity and Programmed Cell Death in Lung Cancer Cell Lines

Wendong Lei, Patrick P. Koty, and Mark L. Levitt

1. Introduction

Epidermal growth factor receptor (EGFR) is a transmembrane glycoprotein of 170 kDa with an extracellular EGF-binding domain and intracellular domain possessing intrinsic tyrosine kinase activity *(1–3)*. Overexpression of the EGFR has been reported in a wide range of human malignancies, including non-small cell lung cancer (NSCLC) *(4–6)*. One early consequence of the binding of EGFR ligands (EGF or transforming growth factor-α [TGF-α]) to EGFR is the induction of receptor dimerization with the subsequent activation of tyrosine kinase activity and trans-phosphorylation at several tyrosine residues in the intracellular domain of the receptor *(2,7)*. The activated receptor transduces signals through tyrosine phosphorylation of itself and other adaptor proteins that mediate the activation of its downstream signal molecules such as mitogen-activated protein (MAP) kinase and phosphatidylinositol 3-kinase (PI3K) *(8,9)*. These cascades can then regulate nuclear and cytoplasmic events controlling transformation, mitogenesis, and cell survival *(10)*. Because overexpression of EGFR is a common occurrence in many human cancers, including lung, and increased receptor levels are associated with metastasis and poor clinical prognosis, EGFR represents an attractive therapeutic target.

A number of approaches to inhibiting either EGFR activity or its ligands themselves have been investigated *(11,12)*, and inhibition of EGFR tyrosine kinase activity by tyrosine kinase inhibitors is currently in preclinical and clinical development *(13)*. We have used a selective EGFR tyrosine kinase

From: *Methods in Molecular Medicine, vol. 74: Lung Cancer, Vol. 1: Molecular Pathology Methods and Reviews*
Edited by: B. Driscoll © Humana Press Inc., Totowa, NJ

inhibitor, tyrphostin AG 1478, and performed a series of studies to elucidate whether EGFR is correlated with chemoresistance and to determine the role of EGFR in the regulation of programmed cell death in lung cancer cells *(14)*. NCI-H596 is a NSCLC cell line that expresses high levels of EGFR. When cells were treated with EGF, the EGFR was tyrosine phosphorylated as determined by immunoprecipitation in combination with Western blotting. The phosphorylation of EGFR was rapid and peaked at 20 min *(see* **Fig. 1A**). The addition of tyrphostin AG 1478 completely abrogated the effect of EGF-stimulated EGFR tyrosine phosphorylation *(see* **Fig. 1B**). NCI-H358, another NSCLC cell line, expresses very low levels of EGFR, and was more sensitive to the chemotherapeutic drugs cisplatin, doxorubicin, and etoposide than NCI-H596 *(14)*. When cells were treated with any of the three chemotherapeutic reagents in combination with tyrphostin AG 1478, the antiproliferative effect was significantly increased in NCI-H596 cells, whereas no such increase was observed in NCI-H358 cells. These results indicate that high levels of EGFR may confer chemoresistance in lung cancer cells and that the EGFR-specific tyrosine kinase inhibitor tyrphostin AG 1478 can sensitize cells that express high levels of EGFR to the chemotherapeutic drugs cisplatin, doxorubicin, and etoposide.

To determine whether programmed cell death (apoptosis) was part of the mechanism by which enhancement of chemosensitivity by tyrphostin AG 1478 occurred, DNA fragmentation was analyzed by agarose gel electrophoresis. Tyrphostin AG 1478 in combination with any of the three chemotherapeutic reagents resulted in the appearance of DNA fragmentation—considered a hallmark for programmed cell death *(15,16)*—in NCI-H596 cells. No such effect was observed in NCI-H358 cells *(14)*, indicating that the enhancement of chemosensitivity by tyrphostin AG 1478 in NCI-H596 cells may be due to the induction of programmed cell death when chemotherapeutic drugs combined with tyrphostin AG 1478.

Tyrphostin AG 1478 can not only sensitize chemotherapeutic drugs to induce programmed cell death in NCI-H596 cells, but also induces DNA fragmentation itself. As shown in **Fig. 2**, tyrphostin AG 1478 induces DNA fragmentation as detected by agarose gel electrophoresis in a time-dependent manner.

In this chapter, we will describe in detail the protocols for immunoprecipitation, Western blotting, DNA fragmentation by gel electrophoresis, and a ^{3}H-thymidine incorporation assay that we have been using in the investigation of the role of tyrphostin AG 1478 in chemosensitivity and programmed cell death in lung cancer cell lines.

1.1. Immunoprecipitation

Immunoprecipitation is one of the most useful immunochemical techniques to detect and quantitate target antigens in mixtures of proteins *(17)*. When

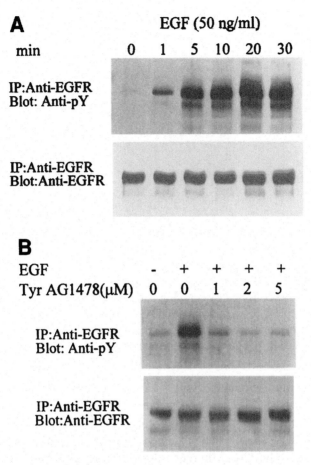

Fig. 1. Tyrosine phosphorylation of EGFR induced by EGF and abrogated by tyrphostin AG 1478 in NCI-H596 NSCLC cells as determined by immunoprecipitation in combination with Western blotting. Cells were stimulated with 50 ng/mL EGF (Collaborative Biomedical Products, Bedford, MA) alone for the indicated time periods (**A**), or treated with 50 ng/mL EGF alone or 50 ng/mL EGF plus increasing concentrations of tyrphostin AG 1478 (Calbiochem, La Jolla, CA) for 10 min (**B**). Cells were then collected, lysed in NP-40 cell lysis buffer, and immunoprecipitated with 1 µg MAb against EGFR (AB-5, Oncogene Research Products, Cambridge, MA). Immunoprecipitates of EGFR from whole-cell lysates were resolved by 6% SDS-PAGE, transferred to nitrocellulose membranes, blocked with 2% horse serum, immunoblotted with an anti-phosphotyrosine (PY99) (Santa Cruz), and detected with chemiluminescence reagents (Amersham Pharmacia Biotech) (upper panel). The blots were then stripped in 62.5 mM Tris-HCl, pH 6.7, 2% SDS, and 100 mM β-mercaptoethanol at 50°C with agitation for 30 min and reblotted with a MAb against EGFR (Sigma, Cat. no. 3138) (lower panel).

Tyrphostin AG1478 (10μM)

0   24 48 72 96   (hour)

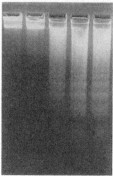

Fig. 2. DNA fragmentation by agarose gel electrophoresis. NCI-H596 NSCLC cells were treated with the EGFR tyrosine kinase inhibitor Tyrphostin AG 1478 for the time indicated. Cells were collected by scraping and lysed in a buffer containing 1% SDS, 50 m*M* Tris-HCl, pH 8.0, and 50 m*M* EDTA. DNA was purified by extracting once with phenol:chloroform:isoamyl alcohol (25:24:1) and separated on a 1.5% agarose gel electrophoresis with 1 μg/mL ethidium bromide.

immunoprecipitation is coupled with sodium dodecyl sulfate-polyacrylamide gel electrophoresis (SDS-PAGE), it is a very sensitive method for the analysis of protein synthesis and processing of foreign antigens expressed in prokaryotic and eukaryotic cells *(18)*. It can determine a number of important characteristics of a target antigen that are difficult to determine using other techniques. The advantages of this technique when compared to Western blotting followed by SDS-PAGE include: 1) high specificity and efficiency; 2) the potential use of radiolabeled material for detection; 3) relatively mild denaturing conditions; and 4) further biochemical analysis of isolated proteins is feasible. The immunoprecipitation procedure involves the following basic steps: lysis of the cells to release the antigen, binding of the antigen to the antibody, and purification of the antigen-antibody complex. The antigen is usually extracted from the cells by adding an appropriate cell lysis buffer that will disrupt cells and lead to the release of proteins to the solution. This is perhaps the most important step in immunoprecipitation. The purpose of this step is to solubilize the target antigen in an immunoreactive and undegraded state in order to subsequently form an immune complex with a specific antibody (or antibodies). The addition of a specific antibody directed against the target protein (antigen) in the cell lysate results in the formation of an antigen-antibody complex. Then, a solid-phase matrix containing protein A (or protein G) is added, and the immune complex is allowed to bind by adsorption of the antibody to proteins A or G. Protein A is a bacterial protein that binds the F_c domain of many immunoglobulins. It has high affinity to most IgG isotypes from human, pig, mouse, rabbit, goat, and sheep. Protein G has a broader species specificity and binds certain rat IgGs better than protein A. After protein A-antibody complex formation occurs, the unbound proteins are removed by washing the solid phase and the protein of interest is subsequently isolated by centrifugation. The purified antigen-antibody complex is often analyzed by gel electrophoresis, or used in combination with a number of other techniques such as immunoblotting, ligand binding, and measurement of enzymatic activities. The combination of immunoprecipitation together with these additional techniques can greatly enhance the amount of information gathered regarding the target antigen.

1.2. Western Blotting

A specific technique and the term "blotting" were first used in 1975 when Southern described the transfer of electrophoretically separated single-strand DNA from agarose gels to an immobilized state on a nitrocellulose membrane *(19)*. "Blotting" refers to the transfer procedure because the appearance of bands on the membrane is an exact replica of the pattern in the original gel and therefore the technique for analysis of DNA became known as the "Southern blotting." The approach was soon applied to analysis of RNA *(20)* and protein *(21,22)* that were termed as "Northern blotting" and "Western blotting," respectively, by a somewhat dubious geographical analogy. Western blotting has become a very powerful method for the identification and quantification of specific antigens in complex mixtures of proteins. The proteins are usually prepared by lysing cells in a cell lysis buffer, separated by electrophoresis through SDS-polyacrylamide gels, and then transferred electrophoretically from the gel to a membrane that binds the protein nonspecifically. After blocking of nonspecific binding sites on the membrane, the immobilized proteins are reacted with a specific monoclonal or polyclonal antibody (MAb/PAb) to allow the formation of antigen-antibody complex. The antigen-antibody complex is finally detected by radiographic, chromogenic, or chemiluminescent reactions.

1.3. DNA Fragmentation by Gel Electrophoresis

Intranucleosomal fragmentation of nuclear DNA that occurs during the process of programmed cell death is now considered a specific hallmark of apoptosis *(15,16)*. Cells undergoing programmed cell death are typified by the appearance of a 180–200 bp ladder, which reflects the organized degradation of chromatin during the apoptotic process *(15,16,23)* as determined by agarose gel electrophoresis. DNA fragmentation into oligonucleosomal length fragments was first identified in glucocorticoid-induced death of thymocytes *(15)* and has been extensively used as the most reliable biochemical marker for programmed cell death. Although the molecular mechanisms by which the DNA is fragmented during programmed cell death are not well-elucidated, the involvement of a Ca^{2+}- and Mg^{2+}-dependent endonuclease activity has been speculated *(24)*. Recent studies revealed that a heterodimeric protein termed DNA fragmentation factor, or DFF, was capable of causing chromosomal DNA fragmentation in the presence of an activated caspase 3 *(25)*. It has been reported that the appearance of apoptotic intranucleosomal DNA fragmentation is not due to double-strand cleavage, but is the consequence of frequent single-strand breaks *(26,27)*. The individual bands of the ladder as detected by agarose gel electrophoresis represent oligonucleosomes of different length produced by the intranucleosomal cleavage of nuclear DNA. This laddering is usually not found when looking at DNA from intact cells that contain only high molecular-weight DNA or a smear of randomly degraded DNA. Because of its technical simplicity, the detection of DNA fragmentation by agarose gel electrophoresis has become one of the most important techniques in determining programmed cell death. This technique is basically composed of the following steps: 1) homogenization of the cells in detergent; 2) extraction and purification of DNA; 3) DNA concentration by precipitation in ethanol; 4) size fractionation by agarose gel electrophoresis; and 5) visualization of the DNA in the presence of ethidium bromide.

1.4. ³H-thymidine Incorporation Assay

Quantitative assessment of tritiated (^3H)-thymidine incorporation is by far the most widely used technique for the determination of DNA synthesis that reflects cell proliferation. The spread of this technique has benefited from the development of labeled precursors of macromolecules and detection techniques for radiolabeled materials. This technique involves incorporation of ^3H-thymidine into proliferating cultured cells, precipitation and solubilization of the DNA, and detection of the radioactivity. In the first step, ^3H-thymidine is added to the media of cell cultures for a variable time period. Thymidine can enter the cells readily and incorporate into replicating DNA. Total DNA is then precipitated, solubilized, and the radioactivity from ^3H is measured by liquid-scintillation counting. The principle of liquid scintillation counting is to convert the radioactivity emitted from a sample to photons of visible light that can be detected by a photomultiplier tube. To begin this process, solubilized DNA is transferred to a vial containing scintillation fluid. The liquid contains an organic solvent and a fluor. The energy of the beta particles emitted from tritium is transferred to the solvent, causing ionization or excitation of solvent molecules. Then the energy is further transferred to the fluor resulting in the excitation of the fluor. A fluor is a compound that fluoresces proportional to the amount of radioactivity that is being emitted. Thus, the invisible radioactivity is converted into visible light. A liquid scintillation counter can count the bursts of light resulting from the radioactive emissions exciting the fluor, and records them as counts per minute (cpm).

2. Materials

2.1. Immunoprecipitation

1. Phosphate-buffered saline (PBS), pH 7.4: 0.8% NaCl, 0.02% KCl, 0.144% Na_2HPO_4 and 0.024% KH_2PO_4. PBS can be stored at 4°C.
2. Cell lysis buffer: 1% NP-40, 20 mM Tris-HCl, pH 7.4, 150 mM NaCl, 2 mM EDTA, 1 mM sodium orthovanadate, 1 mM phenylmethylsulfonyl fluoride (PMSF), 1 μg/mL aprotinin, 1 μg/mL pepstatin A, and 1μg/ml leupeptin. The cell lysis buffer is diluted from stock solutions of 100% NP-40, 1 M Tris-HCl, 5 M NaCl, 0.5 M EDTA, pH 8.0, 100 mM sodium orthovanadate, 100 mM PMSF in isopropanol, 10 mg/mL aprotinin in 0.01 M HEPES, pH 8.0, 1 mg/mL pepstatin A in ethanol, and 10 mg/mL leupeptin in water. Stock solutions of NP-40, Tris-HCl, NaCl, and EDTA are stored at room temperature; sodium orthovanadate stored at 4°C; aprotinin, PMSF, pepstatin A and leupeptin are stored at –20°C. Cell lysis buffer without PMSF, sodium orthovanadate, aprotinin, pepstatin A, and leupeptin can be stored at room temperature. **Caution:** PMSF is extremely destructive to the mucous membranes of the respiratory tract, eyes, and skin. PMSF may be fatal if inhaled, swallowed, or absorbed through the skin. Wear gloves when manipulating PMSF and flush eyes or skin with copious amounts of water in case of contact.
3. Washing buffer: 0.1% Triton X-100, 20 mM Tris-HCl, pH 7.4, 150 mM NaCl, 2 mM EDTA, 1 mM sodium orthovanadate, 1 mM PMSF, and 1 μg/mL aprotinin. The washing buffer without sodium orthovanadate, PMSF, and aprotinin can be stored at room temperature.
4. Protein A-Sepharose CL-4B (Pharmacia Biotech, Piscataway, NJ, or Sigma, St. Louis, MO), store at 4°C.
5. Protein concentration determination reagents (Bio-Rad, Hercules, CA), store at 4°C.
6. Primary antibody: Antibody may be degraded when stored inappropriately. Most antibodies should be stored at either 4°C or –20°C. Refer to the manufacturer's recommendations for storage and stability of a specific antibody.

2.2. Western Blotting

1. 1X SDS gel-loading buffer: 50 mM Tris-HCl, pH 6.8, 2% SDS (electrophoresis-grade), 0.1% bromophenol blue, 10% glycerol, and 100 mM dithiothreitol (DTT). 1X SDS gel-loading buffer lacking DTT can be stored at room temperature. DTT is stored at –20°C at 1 M concentration and should be added to the buffer just before use.

2. Acrylamide and bis-acrylamide. **Caution:** Acrylamide is a potent cumulative neurotoxin that is absorbed through the skin. Wear gloves and a mask when weighting acrylamide and bis-acrylamide. Powdered acrylamide and bis-acrylamide can be stored at room temperature. Solutions should be stored at 4°C.

3. Tris-glycine electrophoresis buffer: 25 mM Tris-HCl, 250 mM glycine, pH 8.3, and 0.1% SDS. One liter of 5X stock electrophoresis buffer can be made by dissolving 15.1 g of Tris base, 94 g of glycine, and 50 mL of 10% SDS, and the volume is adjusted with ddH2O. The buffer can be stored at room temperature.

4. Transfer buffer: 39 mM glycine, 48 mM Tris-HCl, 0.037% SDS, and 20% methanol. One liter of transfer buffer can be made by mixing 2.9 g of glycine, 5.8 g of Tris base, 0.37 g of SDS, and 200 mL of methanol. Use ddH$_2$O to adjust the volume. The buffer can be stored at room temperature.

5. TBS buffer: 10 mM Tris-HCl, pH 7.4, 150 mM NaCl. The buffer can be stored at room temperature.

6. TBS-Tween buffer: 10 mM Tris-HCl, pH 7.4, 150 mM NaCl, and 0.05% Tween-20. The buffer can be stored at room temperature.

7. Blocking reagents: Horse or goat serum. Serum should be stored at –20°C. Diluted serum can be stored at 4°C.

8. Primary antibody: Antibody may be degraded when stored inappropriately. Most antibodies should be stored at either 4°C or –20°C. Refer to the manufacturer's recommendations for storage and stability of a specific antibody.

9. Horseradish peroxidase (HRP)-conjugated secondary antibody (New England BioLabs, Beverly, MA): The antibody should be stored at –20°C and is stable for up to 1 yr.

10. Enhanced chemiluminescence (ECL) Western blotting detection reagents (Amersham Pharmacia Biotech, Piscataway, NJ, Cat no. RPN2106): The reagents are stable for at least 6 mo when stored at 4°C. **Caution:** Certain components in the reagents may cause bleaching on contact with skin. Wash immediately with water in case of contact with skin or eyes.

2.3. DNA Fragmentation by Gel Electrophoresis

1. Cell lysis buffer: 50 mM Tris-HCl, pH 8.0, 50 mM EDTA, pH 8.0, 1% SDS. The buffer is prepared from stock solutions of 1 M Tris-HCl, pH 8.0, 0.5 M EDTA, and 20% SDS and can be stored at room temperature.

2. Proteinase K: Store at –20°C at 20 mg/mL in sterile distilled water.

3. 1X PBS, pH 7.4: 0.8% NaCl. 0.02% KCl, 0.144% Na$_2$HPO$_4$, and 0.024% KH$_2$PO$_4$. PBS can be stored at room temperature.

4. Phenol:chloroform:isoamyl alcohol (25:24:1) (Gibco BRL): store at 4°C in a brown bottle. **Caution:** Phenol is highly corrosive and can cause severe burns. Wear gloves, goggles, and protective clothing. All manipulations should be carried out in a chemical hood. Dispose of used phenol in a glass receptacle. Do not pour down drain.

5. 5 M NaCl: Store at room temperature.

6. Isopropanol: Store at room temperature.

7. DNase-free RNase A: Store at –20°C at 10 mg/mL in 10 mM Tris-HCl, pH 7.5 and 15 mM NaCl. RNase A solutions should be boiled for 15 min prior to use.

8. TE buffer: 10 mM Tris-HCl, pH 8.0, 1 mM EDTA. Store at room temperature.

9. 70% ethanol: Store at room temperature.

10. Agarose (molecular biology-grade): Store at room temperature.

11. TAE buffer: 40 mM Tris-acetate and 1 mM EDTA. TAE is usually stored as 50X solution at room temperature. 50X TAE buffer: 242 g of Tris base, 57.1 mL of glacial acetic acid, and 100 mL 0.5 M EDTA, pH 8.0 in 1 L of sterile distilled water.

12. Loading buffer: 40% sucrose, 0.25% bromophenol blue, and 0.25% xylene cyanol FF. The buffer is at 6X concentration.

13. Ethidium bromide (EB): Store at 10 mg/mL in distilled water at room temperature in light-tight container completely wrapped in aluminum foil. **Caution:** EB is a powerful mutagen and is moderately toxic. Gloves should be worn when working with solutions containing it.

2.4. ³H-thymidine Incorporation

1. RPMI-1640 culture medium (Gibco BRL, Grand Island, NY): Store at 4°C.

2. Fetal bovine serum (FBS) (Gibco BRL): Store at –20°C.

3. Penicillin (Gibco BRL): Store at 4°C.

4. Streptomycin (Gibco BRL): Store at 4°C.

5. Amphotericin B (Gibco BRL): Store at 4°C.

6. ³H-thymidine (NEN-Dupont, Boston, MA). **Caution:** ³H-thymidine is a radioactive material and should be stored and handled as specified by the institutional Radiation Safety committee.

7. PBS, pH 7.4: 0.8% NaCl, 0.02% KCl, 0.144% Na_2HPO_4, and 0.024% KH_2PO_4. PBS can be stored at room temperature.

8. 10% trichloroacetic acid (TCA): Store at room temperature.

9. 0.25 N NaOH: Store at room temperature.

10. Scintillation fluid: Store at room temperature. The scintillation fluid contains three major components: an organic solvent constituting the bulk of the mass, a primary solute (fluor), and a secondary solute (fluor). The scintillation fluid can be stored at room temperature.

3. Methods

3.1. Immunoprecipitation

1. Culture cells as monolayers, in 6-well culture plates or 35-mm culture dishes, and start by rinsing twice with PBS (*see* **Notes 1** and **2**).

2. Aspirate PBS and add 1 mL of fresh ice-cold PBS. Collect cells by scraping with a rubber policeman and transfer the cell suspension to a 1.5-ml microcentrifuge tube (*see* **Note 3**).

3. Centrifuge at 1000g for 2 min at 4°C to pellet cells.

4. Pour off the supernatant, add 120 µL cell lysis buffer, and triturate until the cells are homogenized (*see* **Note 4**).
5. Leave on ice for 20 min.
6. Centrifuge at 12,000*g* for 15 min at 4°C.
7. Transfer the supernatant to a clean 1.5-mL microcentrifuge tube and discard tube pellet.
8. Determine the protein concentration by the Bradford assay *(28)* using reagents from Bio-Rad (*see* **Note 5**).
9. Incubate 200 µg of protein with 1 µg of primary antibody in 0.5 mL of cell lysis buffer with constant agitation at 4°C for 1 h (*see* **Note 6**).
10. Add 2 mg of protein A-Sepharose CL-4B and continue to incubate with agitation at 4°C overnight (*see* **Note 7**).
11. Spin at 12,000*g* for 2 min at 4°C to pellet sepharose beads.
12. Aspirate supernatant and rinse three times with washing buffer, 1 mL/well with constant agitation at 4°C for 10 min.
13. Aspirate the washing buffer. The immunoprecipitate can be stored at –20°C, or used immediately, for Western blotting.

3.2. Western Blotting

1. To the above immunoprecipitate add 25 µL of 1X SDS gel-loading buffer and boil for 3 min. This step is to separate the target protein from sepharose beads and also denature the protein.
2. Cool down the denatured protein to room temperature. Centrifuge at 12,000*g* for 2 min. Electrophorese the denatured protein on a SDS-PAGE gel with subsequent transfer onto a nitrocellulose membrane.
3. Rinse the nitrocellulose membrane once with TBS buffer and block in either 2% horse serum (for MAbs) or 2% goat serum (for PAbs), which is diluted with TBS-Tween buffer at room temperature with agitation for 1 h (*see* **Note 8**).
4. Save the blocking solution. Briefly rinse the membrane using two changes of TBS-Tween buffer for 5 min each.
5. Incubate the membrane with appropriate concentration of the primary antibody diluted in TBS buffer at 4°C overnight. This will allow the formation of the antigen-antibody complex (*see* **Note 9**).
6. Save the diluted primary antibody. Wash the membrane with three changes of TBS-Tween buffer for 20 min each at room temperature (*see* **Note 10**).
7. Add a 1:2000 dilution of HRP-conjugated secondary antibody in TBS buffer and incubate with constant agitation at room temperature for 1 h (*see* **Note 11**).
8. Save the diluted secondary antibody. Wash the membrane four times with TBS-Tween buffer at 15-min intervals (*see* **Note 12**).
9. Mix an equal volume of ECL detection solution 1 and solution 2 to provide a sufficient amount to cover the membrane. The final volume required is 0.125 mL/cm^2 membrane.
10. Drain the excess buffer from the washed membrane and put the membrane on a piece of Saran Wrap, leaving protein side up. Add the detection solution mixture

to the surface of the membrane, so that the mixed solution is held by surface tension on the membrane surface (*see* **Note 13**).

11. Incubate for 1 min at room temperature (*see* **Note 14**).
12. Drain the detection solution off the surface of the membrane by holding the membrane vertically and leaving the lower edge of the membrane against a piece of tissue paper until there is no free detection solution on the membrane (*see* **Note 15**).
13. Wrap the membrane with Saran Wrap and expose to a Hyperfilm ECL (Amersham Pharmacia Biotech) in a darkroom (*see* **Note 16**).

3.3. Intranucleosomal DNA Fragmentation by Gel Electrophoresis

1. Culture cells in 6-well culture plates or 35 mm culture dishes. After treatment with experimental agents, harvest the cells by scraping with a rubber policeman. Transfer the cell suspension to a 15-mL plastic disposable centrifuge tube. Rinse the dish once with 2 mL of PBS and pool with the cell suspension (*see* **Note 17**).
2. Centrifuge at 250g for 5 min at room temperature.
3. Pour off supernatant. Add 3 mL of PBS to rinse cell pellet by gently pipetting up and down five times, and recover by centrifugation as in **step 2**.
4. Pour off supernatant. Resuspend the cell pellet in 1 mL of PBS, pipet up and down five times, and transfer the cell suspension to a 1.5-mL microcentrifuge tube.
5. Centrifuge at 1,000g for 2 min.
6. Pour off the supernatant and resuspend the cell pellet in 0.6 mL of cell lysis buffer. Pipet up and down with a wide-bore pipet until the cells are homogenously dispersed (*see* **Note 18**).
7. Add 3 μL of 20 mg/mL Proteinase K, pipet up and down with a wide-bore pipet for 5 times, and incubate at 37°C overnight in a water bath (*see* **Note 19**).
8. Cool the solution to room temperature. Add an equal volume (0.6 mL) of phenol:chloroform:isoamyl alcohol (25:24:1) and seal the tube with parafilm. Mix by repeatedly inverting the tube for 5 min (*see* **Note 20**).
9. Centrifuge at 6,000g for 10 min.
10. Transfer the aqueous phase with a wide-bore pipet to a new 1.5-mL microcentrifuge tube (*see* **Note 21**).
11. Precipitate the DNA by adding 0.05 volume (30 μL) of 5 M NaCl, and 0.7 volume (420 μL) of isopropanol at –20°C overnight (*see* **Note 22**).
12. Centrifuge at 13,000g for 30 min at 4°C.
13. Pour off the supernatant and add 1 mL of 70% ethanol to remove precipitated salt. Mix by pipetting up and down five times.
14. Centrifuge at 13,000g for 15 min at 4°C (*see* **Note 23**).
15. Repeat **steps 14** and **15**.
16. Pour off supernatant. Dry the pellet in the open tube at room temperature until the last visible traces of ethanol have evaporated (*see* **Note 24**).
17. Dissolve pellet DNA in 150 μL TE buffer and add 2 μL of 20 mg/mL RNase A to digest RNA at 37°C overnight in a water bath.

18. Take 30 μL of dissolved DNA and mix with 3 μL of gel loading buffer.
19. Electrophorese the sample in a 1.5% agarose gel with 1 μg/mL EB in 1X TAE buffer for 3 h at 40V.
20. Photograph the gel.

3.4. ^{3}H-thymidine Incorporation

1. Cell-culture conditions: 24-well plates are used as the culture vessels and all subsequent operations are carried out in the wells. Cells are maintained in RPMI-1640 medium supplemented with 10% fetal bovine serum (FBS), 50 U/mL penicillin, 50 μg/mL streptomycin, and 2.5 μg/mL Amphotericin B at 37°C in a humidified atmosphere containing 5% CO_2 (*see* **Notes 25** and **26**).
2. Labeling conditions: cells are seeded at a density of 5×10^5 per well in 1 mL of culture medium and are allowed to grow for at least 16 h before treatment with any agent and labeling. After treatment, the culture medium and agents are removed by aspiration and cells are washed twice with fresh serum-free medium. Then ^{3}H-thymidine is added to the serum-free medium at a final concentration of 0.4 μCi/mL and incubated at 37°C for 90 min (*see* **Note 27**).
3. Pour off the radioactive medium and wash twice with PBS to remove residual radioactive material.
4. Pour off the PBS and add 0.5 mL of cold 10% TCA for 10 s.
5. Pour off the TCA and add 0.8 mL of 0.25 *N* NaOH to solubilize the ^{3}H-thymidine-containing DNA. Pipet up and down five times (*see* **Notes 28** and **29**).
6. Take 0.6 mL of each sample to a 4 mL scintillation vial with 3 mL scintillation fluid. Vortex vigorously for 10 s (*see* **Note 30**).
7. Radioactivity is quantified by a liquid-scintillation counter.

4. Notes

1. Many protocols suggest the preparation of relatively large quantities of cultured cells for immunoprecipitation. Thus, 100-mm plates are the most commonly used culture vessels for this purpose. This will ensure that there are enough proteins to immunoprecipitate, but, in our experience, is a waste of supplies, culture medium, and reagents. Sufficient protein for a single immunoprecipitation can be generated when monolayer cultures on 6-well plates or 35-mm culture dishes reach 70% or more of confluence, if extracted properly. The expression level of the target protein in the experimental cells is often a big factor that should be considered when determining the quantity of cells required.
2. From the point of view of manipulation, a 35-mm culture dish is easier for individual handling than a 6-well plate.
3. Always collect cells by scraping for immunoprecipitation purposes. Do not try to collect them by trypsinization due to the fact that trypsin may disrupt cells and result in the release of cytoplasmic proteins. Trypsin digestion may also damage cell membrane proteins like EGFR.
4. Protease inhibitors are commonly included in cell lysis buffer and should be prepared fresh. The detergent NP-40 can be replaced by Triton X-100.

5. The Bradford method is a colorimetric assay based upon color change caused by the binding of Coomassie Brilliant Blue to protein. The protein concentration is measured by monitoring absorption at 595 nm using a plate reader. For cultures on a 35-mm culture dish, the amount of lysis buffer should not exceed 150 µL since over-diluted protein may result in inaccuracy by a plate reader.

6. One µg antibody is sufficient to immunoprecipitate target antigen in most cases. However, this quantity should be optimized for each antibody used.

7. Protein A-Sepharose should be hydrated in lysis buffer before use and withdrawn using a wide-bore pipet.

8. The blocking of nonspecific binding sites on the blot is essential for increasing the sensitivity of Western blotting. Along with serum, nonfat dry milk (22) and bovine serum albumin (BSA) (29) are another two commonly used blocking reagents and suitable for both MAbs and PAbs. The diluted serum is reusable for up to 1 wk when stored at 4°C.

9. Alternatively, the incubation of the membrane with primary antibody can be performed at room temperature with agitation for 1 h. Longer incubation times may increase the sensitivity to detect the target antigen, but the background of nonspecific binding also increases as a function of the time and temperature. The optimal concentration of the primary antibody varies depending on the source and the quality of the antibody and dilution should be as per the manufacturer's recommendations. For most antibodies from Santa Cruz, a dilution of 0.1–1 µg/mL is recommended by the manufacturer. We used a working dilution of 0.5 µg/mL of anti-phosphotyrosine (PY99) from Santa Cruz to detect the tyrosine phosphorylation of EGFR stimulated by EGF (*see* **Fig. 1**). Diluted primary antibody is reusable for up to 5 d in most cases when stored at 4°C in TBS buffer.

10. This step should last for at least 30 min or more (e.g., for 2 h), in order to reduce the background.

11. The incubation period of the membrane with the secondary antibody should be as per the manufacturer's recommendations with individual optimization since a longer time of incubation may result in a high background and insufficient incubation in a weak signal. The diluted secondary antibody can be used for up to 5 d when stored at 4°C in TBS buffer.

12. Thorough washing of the membrane before incubating with ECL detection solutions is a very important step to minimize background. The washing period can be longer if desired.

13. Make sure that the surface of the membrane is well covered. It is not necessary to immerse the membrane in the detection solutions.

14. A 1-min incubation is enough to produce a strong signal. Longer incubation times may result in high background.

15. Free detection solution will definitely result in very high background; therefore, there must be no visible residual on the membrane before exposure to film. In another words, the membrane can be moist, but not wet.

16. This is the last step for a Western blotting. A film with sharp bands and little background should be obtained if the procedure has been performed correctly.

The exposure time varies from blot to blot. A strong signal can usually be imaged within several seconds. Practically, the membrane may be exposed to film at four time intervals of 2, 5, 10, and 15 s. For a mini-blot, these four exposures can be accomplished on a single film by exposing different areas of the film to the blot sequentially. The optimal exposure should be chosen for photographing. A good blot rarely needs more than a minute of exposure since prolonged exposure also increases the background proportionally. When the background is high, continued washing of the membrane usually does not work. Remember, the best way to solve this problem is to redo the procedure from the beginning.

17. Fragmented DNA may be released into the culture medium from apoptotic cells. Therefore, it is important to combine the harvested cells together with their medium for centrifugation to reduce the chance of loss of low molecular-weight DNA. It is also necessary in this method to collect cells by scraping. Do not recover monolayer cultures by trypsinization when isolating low molecular weight DNA since cells may be disrupted by trypsin digestion.

18. SDS is a detergent that can solubilize nuclear membranes and result in release of nuclear DNA that will make the solution very viscous. Practically, we usually add premixed Tris-HCl and EDTA first to disaggregate the cell pellet by pipetting up and down five times and only then add the SDS. This allows the cells to disintegrate more easily and minimize the formation of intractable clumps of DNA.

19. Optionally, digestion with Proteinase K can be employed at 50°C for 3 h. The mixture should be reasonably clear and viscous at the end of the incubation. More Proteinase K may be added as required.

20. Phenol extraction is an essential step to purify DNA. However, sequential extraction with phenol will result in loss of low molecular-weight DNA with each purification, especially when it is processed in a relatively small volume (e.g., in a 1.5-mL microcentrifuge tube). Unlike most protocols in which DNA is purified with phenol at least three times, the DNA is extracted only once with phenol in this protocol and it is of adequate quality for agarose gel electrophoresis (*see* **Fig. 2**).

21. At this stage, the aqueous phase can be very viscous because of the high viscosity of high molecular-weight DNA. Care must be taken when transferring the aqueous phase so not to disturb the interface. In most cases, the aqueous phase can be transferred safely. However, it is sometimes hard to remove the aqueous phase even with a wide-bore pipet due to the viscosity of the DNA that sticks to the orifice of the pipet and cannot be withdrawn. In this case, the DNA that is adherent to the orifice of the pipet should simply be carefully transferred to a new microcentrifuge tube by holding the pipet up. If failed to transfer safely, take both of the organic and aqueous phases to a larger tube, add more lysis buffer to dilute it, and re-extract with equal volume of phenol:chloroform:isoamyl alcohol (25:24:1).

22. High molecular-weight DNA will form a precipitate immediately. However, low molecular-weight DNA may not form a visible precipitate after the addition of isopropanol.

23. The sample can be centrifuged at room temperature if desired to remove precipitated salt more thoroughly.
24. Care must be taken not to overdry the DNA pellet since desiccated DNA is very difficult to dissolve.
25. The cell lines used in this protocol are human NSCLC cell lines NCI-H596 and NCI-H358 that are known to grow well in RPMI-1640 medium. The culture medium should be selected depending on individual cell type.
26. Each treatment should be performed in duplicate or triplicate to minimize experimental bias.
27. Pre-mix ^{3}H-thymidine with fresh culture medium at concentration of 0.4 µCi/mL and pre-warm the mixture to 37°C before labeling the cultured cells because cold medium influences DNA synthesis and reduces the incorporation of ^{3}H-thymidine into replicating DNA. Also, make sure to add equal volumes of ^{3}H-thymidine-containing medium to each well because we have noticed the cpm was higher when adding 1 mL of 0.4 µCi/mL ^{3}H-thymidine than adding 0.5 mL of the same mixture. This may be due to the concentration of ^{3}H-thymidine not being saturating. Thus, equal volumes of ^{3}H-thymidine containing media should be added to each well.
28. Cells may detach from the bottom of the wells when precipitated with TCA. Therefore, attention should be paid to avoid cell loss when discarding TCA.
29. The addition of 0.25 N NaOH to each well must be precisely the same volume.
30. The volume of each sample taken for scintillation counting must be exactly the same. Since investigators often do not wish to contaminate their newest pipettor with radioactive materials and usually use old ones for this purpose, make sure the pipettor is in good condition. The accuracy of the pipettor may be a problem, especially when pipetting up and down again and again in order to solubilize 3H-thymidine incorporated DNA before removing a sample to add to the scintillation vial. This issue is frequently neglected.

References

1. Carpenter, G. (1987) Receptors for epidermal growth factor and other polypeptide mitogens. *Annu. Biochem.* **56**, 881–914.
2. Fantl, W. J., Johnson, D. E., and Williams, L. T. (1993) Signalling by receptor tyrosine kinases. *Annu. Rev. Biochem.* **62**, 453–481.
3. Carpenter, G. and Cohen, S. (1990) Epidermal growth factor. *J. Biol. Chem.* **265**, 7709–7712.
4. Salmon, D. S., Brandt, R., Ciardiello, F., and Normanno, N. (1995) Epidermal growth factor-related peptides and their receptors in human malignancies. *Crit. Rev. Oncol. Haematol.* **19**, 183–232.
5. Tateishi, M., Ishida, T., Mitsudomi, T., Kaneko, S., and Sugimachi, K. (1990) Immunohistochemical evidence of autocrine growth factors in adenocarcinoma of the human lung. *Cancer Res.* **50**, 7077–7080.
6. Gorgoulis, V., Aninos, D., Mikou, P., Kanavarous, P., Karameris, A., Joardanoglu, J., et al. (1992) Expression of EGF, TGF-alpha, and EGFR in squamous cell lung carcinomas. *Anticancer Res.* **12**, 1183–1187.

7. Kazlauskas, A. and Cooper, J. A. (1989) Autophosphorylation of the PDGF receptor in the kinase insert region regulates interactions with cell proteins. *Cell* **58,** 1121–1133.

8. Takishima, K., Griswold-Prenner, I., Ingebritsen, T., and Rosner, M. R. (1991) Epidermal growth factor (EGF) receptor T669 peptide kinase from 3T3-L1 cells is an EGF-stimulated "MAP" kinase. *Proc. Natl. Acad. Sci. USA* **88,** 2520–2524.

9. Soltoff, S. P., Carraway, K. L., Prigent, S. A., Gullick, W. G., and Cantley, L. C. (1994) ErbB3 is involved in activation of phosphatidylinositol 3-kinase by epidermal growth factor. *Mol. Cell. Biol.* **14,** 3550–3558.

10. Pawson, T. and Schlessinger, J. (1993) Signal transduction by receptor tyrosine kinases. *Curr. Biol.* **3,** 434–442.

11. Ennis, B. W., Lippman, M. E., and Dickson, R. B. (1991) The EGF receptor system as a target for antitumor therapy. *Cancer Invest.* **9,** 553–562.

12. Davies, D. E. and Chamberlin, S. G. (1996) Targeting the epidermal growth factor receptor for therapy of carcinomas. *Biochem. Pharmacol.* **51,** 1101–1110.

13. Levitt, M. L. and Koty, P. P. (1999) Tyrosine kinase inhibitors in preclinical development. *Invest. New Drugs* **17,** 213–226.

14. Lei, W., Mayotte, J. E., and Levitt, M. L. (1999) Enhancement of chemosensitivity and programmed cell death by tyrosine kinase inhibitors correlates with EGFR expression in non-small-cell lung cancer cells. *Anticancer Res.* **19,** 221–228.

15. Wyllie, A. H. (1980) Glucocorticoid-induced thymocyte apoptosis is associated with endogenous endonuclease activation. *Nature* **248,** 555–556.

16. Wyllie, A. H., Morris, R. G., Smith, A. L., and Dunlop, D. (1984) Chromatin cleavage in apoptosis: association with condensed chromatin morphology and dependence on macromolecular synthesis. *J. Pathol.* **142,** 67–77.

17. Harlow, E. and Lane, D. (1988) *Antibodies: A Laboratory Manual.* Cold Spring Harbor Laboratory Press, Cold Spring Harbor, NY, pp. 421–470.

18. Sambrook, J., and Russell, D. W. (2001) *Molecular Cloning: A Laboratory Manual,* 3rd ed. Cold Spring Harbor Laboratory Press, Cold Spring Harbor, NY, pp. A9–A29.

19. Southern, E. M. (1975) Detection of specific sequences among DNA fragments separated by gel electrophoresis. *J. Mol. Biol.* **98,** 503–517.

20. Alwine, J. C., Kemp, D. J., Parker, B. A., Reiser, J., Renard, J., Stark, G. R., and Wahl, G. M. (1979) Detection of specific RNAs for specific fragments of DNA by fractionation in gels and transfer to diazobenzyloxymethyl paper. *Methods Enzymol.* **68,** 220–242.

21. Renart, J., Reiser, J., and Stark, G.R. (1979) Transfer of proteins from gels to diazobenzyloxymethyl-paper and detection with antisera: a method for studying antibody specificity and antigen structure. *Proc. Natl. Acad. Sci. USA* **76,** 3116–3120.

22. Towbin, H., Staehelin, T., and Gordon, J. (1979) Electrophoretic transfer of proteins from polyacrylamide gels to nitrocellulose sheets: procedure and some applications. *Proc. Natl. Acad. Sci. USA* **76,** 4350–4354.

23. Arends, M. J. and Wyllie, A. H. (1991) Apoptosis: mechanisms and roles in pathology. *Int. Rev. Exp. Pathol.* **32,** 223–254.

24. Peitsch, M.C., Polzar, B., Stephan, H., Compton, T., Robson McDonald, H., Mannherz, H. G., and Tschopp, J. (1993) Characterization of the endogenous deoxyribonuclease involved in nuclear DNA fragmentation during apoptosis (programmed cell death). *EMBO J.* **12,** 371–377.

25. Liu, X., Zou, H., Slaughter, C., and Wang, X. (1997) DFF, a heterodimeric protein that functions downstream of caspase-3 to trigger DNA fragmentation during apoptosis. *Cell* **89,** 175–184.

26. Peitsch, M. C., Muller, C., and Tschopp, J. (1993) DNA fragmentation during apoptosis is caused by frequent single-strand cuts. *Nucleic Acids Res.* **21,** 4206–4209.

27. Tomei, L. D., Shapiro, J. P., and Cope, F. O. (1993) Apoptosis in C3H/10T1/2 mouse embryonic cells: evidence for internucleosomal DNA modification in the absence of double-strand cleavage. *Proc. Natl. Acad. Sci. USA* **90,** 853–857.

28. Bradford, M. M. (1976) A rapid and sensitive method for the quantitative of microgram quantities of protein utilizing the principle of protein-dye binding. *Anal. Biochem.* **72,** 248–254.

29. Johnson, D. A., Gautsch, J. W., Sportsman, J. R., and Elder, J. H. (1984) Improved technique utilizing nonfat dry milk for analysis of proteins and nucleic acids transferred to nitrocellulose. *Gene Anal. Tech.* **1,** 3–8.

10

Detection of the Transcripts and Proteins for the Transforming Growth Factor-β Isoforms and Receptors in Mouse Lung Tumorigenesis Using *In Situ* Hybridization and Immunohistochemistry in Paraffin-Embedded Tissue Sections

Sonia B. Jakowlew and Jennifer Mariano

1. Introduction

Several critical polypeptide growth factors have been identified for the lung, including transforming growth factor-beta (TGF-β). The three mammalian TGF-β isoforms, TGF-β1, TGF-β2, and TGF-β3, are homologous growth mediators that have been shown to participate in multiple biological processes, including cellular proliferation, tissue repair, embryogenesis, hematopoiesis and immune response, and extracellular matrix (ECM) production (reviewed in **refs. *1*** and *2*). TGF-β1 is the most prevalent among the three TGF-β isoforms in mammals. The TGF-βs are potent growth inhibitors of most normal epithelial cell types, although many cancer cells are resistant to their growth-inhibitory effects *(3–5)*. The biological activities of TGF-β are mediated by binding to a heteromeric receptor complex consisting of two subunits, designated type I (TGF-β RI) and type II (TGF-β RII) (reviewed in **ref. *6***). Molecular cloning and functional analyses have demonstrated that TGF-β RI and TGF-β RII are serine/threonine kinases that are essential elements for TGF-β-mediated signal transduction *(7,8)*. The cooperativity of TGF-β RI and TGF-β RII in signal transduction suggests that loss of functional TGF-β RI and/or TGF-β RII expression could have an impact on the ability of TGF-β to inhibit proliferation. It has been demonstrated that there is an association between inactivation of TGF-β RII and a decrease in TGF-β-mediated growth inhibition in several

From: *Methods in Molecular Medicine, vol. 74: Lung Cancer, Vol. 1: Molecular Pathology Methods and Reviews*
Edited by: B. Driscoll © Humana Press Inc., Totowa, NJ

human tumor cell lines *(9–11)*. In addition, a dysfunctional TGF-β-mediated signal-transduction pathway, resulting from loss of TGF-β RII function, has been linked to the development of several human malignancies, including breast, prostate, colorectal, colon, and hepatocellular cancer *(12–16)*.

Multiple molecular biological techniques have been developed to examine expression of various growth factors, including TGF-β, in normal and malignant tissues. These include Southern blot and polymerase chain reaction (PCR) amplification analyses to investigate sequence variation in the different genes, Northern blot and reverse transcription-polymerase chain reaction (RT-PCR) amplification analyses to investigate changes in mRNA transcripts of these genes, and Western blot and immunoprecipitation analyses to investigate alterations in expression of the protein products translated from these mRNA transcripts. At the single cell level, the need to identify the cell type in tissue samples that contains a particular RNA transcript has resulted in the development of *in situ* hybridization techniques, which represent the histochemical counterparts to Northern-blot analysis in molecular biology. Because it is the protein products of these genes that ultimately represent the functionality of these genes, immunohistochemical methods employing monoclonal and polyclonal antibodies (MAbs/PAbs) generated against these protein products have also been developed to identify the cell type in tissue samples that express the protein products that correspond to the different mRNA transcripts. Using these techniques, we have the ability to delineate which cells in a mixed population express the mRNA and protein of interest. Although not rigorously quantitative, with appropriate controls and simultaneous analysis of normal and diseased tissues, in situ hybridization and immunohistochemical staining analyses can provide semiquantitative information about the relative amounts of specific mRNAs and proteins in tissues. Utilizing *in situ* hybridization and immunohistochemical staining analyses, it is possible to examine the localization and pattern of expression of TGF-β and its receptors in normal tissues, and to determine its possible alteration during tumorigenesis and malignancy.

In order to define the mechanism by which the TGF-β signaling system participates in tumorigenesis in a tissue such as the lung, it is necessary to employ a model system in which the appearance and localization of TGF-β shows similarities to the human system, and in which alterations in the appearance and localization of TGF-β can be easily examined. In contrast to human lung cancer, where the majority of patients present in advanced stages of the disease, mouse model systems of lung cancer offer a means of understanding the molecular pathways involved in the development of human lung cancer. Histologically early lesions such as hyperplasias and adenomas can be observed in many mouse models of lung cancer *(17)*. In addition, the more advanced mouse tumors resemble human papillary and bronchioalveolar adenocarcinomas *(18–20)*. Although mouse models are not exact representations of human lung cancer in that they metastasize only infrequently, these model systems are similar enough to provide information to be able to deduce pivotal changes that are shared by mouse and human lung cancer. Several molecular alterations have been identified in mouse lung tumors that are shared with human lung cancer specimens, including K-ras activating mutations in 80–90% of tumors; $p16^{INK4a}$ deletion or reduced expression through promoter methylation in 50% of adenocarcinomas; p53 mutations in advanced adenocarcinomas; as well as loss of heterozygosity (LOH) at chomosomes 4, 11, and 14, known to involve $p16^{INK4a}$, p53, and Rb *(21–23)*. Current mouse models for lung cancer include strains that are susceptible to spontaneous and chemically induced lung tumor development, and several transgenic mouse strains that express viral and cellular oncogenes. Chemical agents, such as 4-(methylnitrosoamino)-1-(3-pyridyl)-1-butanone, ethylnitrosourea, and ethyl carbamate enhance lung tumor development by inducing more tumors than those that would have spontaneously occurred, and by reducing the latency period before tumor appearance. Mouse strains that are resistant to carcinogens, such as the C57BL6 mouse, develop few lung tumors. However, some mouse strains are sensitive to these carcinogens, including the strain A mouse, and develop increased lung tumors in response to administered carcinogens. The immunocompetent A/J mouse, a substrain of strain A, has been used extensively to determine the carcinogenic potency of synthetic and natural compounds (reviewed in **ref. 24**). In addition, chemically induced lung tumors in A/J mice have been reported to be histologically similar to human lung adenocarcinomas and develop in a time-dependent manner, progressing from hyperplasia to benign adenoma, and ultimately to malignancy *(20,25,26)*. These sequential morphological changes correlate with multistep genetic aberrations, involving activation of protooncogenes and inactivation of tumor-suppressor genes, induced by environmental carcinogens superimposed on genetic factors, which confer susceptibility to malignant transformation in this inbred mouse strain *(21,27–29)*. By utilizing these mice and *in situ* hybridization and immunohistochemical staining analyses to detect the mRNAs and proteins for TGF-β and its receptors, it may be possible to determine the pattern of expression of TGF-β and its receptors during the progression that occurs between the various stages that lead to malignancy in lung cancer.

2. Materials

2.1. Preparation of Tissues for In Situ Hybridization

1. A/J mouse lungs from animals treated with ethyl carbamate and from control mice.

2. Phosphate-buffered saline (PBS), pH 7.4: 4.3 mM Na$_2$HPO$_4$, 1.4 mM KH$_2$PO$_4$, 137 mM NaCl, and 2.7 mM KCl.
3. 10% phosphate-buffered formalin (Sigma Chemical Co., St. Louis, MO; Cat. no. HT50-1-12B).

2.2. Total RNA Purification from Mouse Lung Tissues

1. 100–500 mg of adult mouse lung tissue from animals treated with ethyl carbamate and from control mice.
2. Guanidine isothiocyanate (GIT) (Fluka, Ronkonkoma, NY; Cat. no. 50990).
3. 3 M Sodium acetate, pH 5.2.
4. β-mercaptoethanol (Sigma).
5. Guanidine isothiocyanate buffer: 472.6 g GIT, 0.83 mL β-mercaptoethanol, and 0.83 mL 3 M sodium acetate, pH 5.2, to 100 mL with H$_2$O.
6. Cesium chloride (Invitrogen, Carlsbad, CA; Cat. no. 15507-023).
7. Cesium chloride buffer: 95.97 g CsCl and 0.83 mL 3 M sodium acetate, pH 5.2, to 100 mL with H$_2$O.
8. Sterile H$_2$O (diethylpyrocarbonate (DEPC)-treated).
9. 100% (200-proof) ethyl alcohol (Warner-Graham Co., Cockeysville, MD).

2.3. Preparation of TGF-β Hybridization Probes

2.3.1. cDNA Synthesis

1. SuperScript Preamplification System (Invitrogen; Cat. no. 18089-011): Oligo dT$_{12-18}$ (0.5 µg/L), 10X PCR buffer: 200 mM Tris-HCl, pH 8.4, 500 mM KCl, 25 mM MgCl$_2$, 0.1 M dithiothreitol (DTT) and Superscript II reverse transcriptase (200 U/µL).
2. Random hexamers (10 mg/mL) (Invitrogen).
3. RNA template: 10 µg/µL.
4. d(CGAT)TP mix: 20 mM each of dCTP, dGTP, dATP, and dTTP (Invitrogen).
5. RNase H (Promega, Madison, WI; Cat. no. M4281).
6. Sterile H$_2$O (DEPC-treated).
7. G-50 sephadex columns (Three Prime-Five Prime, Boulder, CO; 5302-224424).

2.3.2. PCR Amplification of TGF-β

1. Sense and antisense specific primers (25 mM) (Bioserve, Laurel, MD).
   TGF-β1 (mature coding region): 620-bp product (nucleotides 782-1401).
     Sense: 5′-GTGCCCGAACCCCCATTGCTGTCC-3′.
     Antisense: 5′-GCGCCCGGGTTGTGTTGGTTGTAG-3′.
   TGF-β1 (5′ untranslated region): 469-bp product (nucleotides 935-467).
     Sense: 5′-CTAGCAGCCCAGGCACTCATCAGC-3′.
     Antisense: 5′-AGTGCCCCCGACAGTCCAAACAGT-3′.
   TGF-β2 (mature coding region):443-bp product (nucleotides 2121-2563).
     Sense: 5′-CGCGCTTTGGATGCTGCCTACT-3′.
     Antisense: 5′-ATCAAAACTCCCTCCCTCCTGTCA-3′.

TGF-β2 (3′ untranslated region): 407-bp product (nucleotides 2472-2878).
Sense: 5′-CTTTCGGTCCTGTGCTTTTAGTGC-3′
Antisense: 5′-GAAATGCGGGCTGGAAACAATACG-3′.

TGF-β3 (mature coding region): 446-bp product (nucleotides 616-1061).
Sense: 5′-GTGCGCGAGTGGCTGTTGAGGAGA-3′.
Antisense: 5′-GTGTCTGCGCTGCGGAGGTATGG-3′.

TGF-β RI (extracellular coding region): 488-bp product (nucleotides 34-521).
Sense: 5′-GTCCGCAGCTCCTCATCGTGTTG-3′.
Antisense: 5′-GGTGGTGCCCTCTGAAATGAAAG-3′.

TGF-β RI (intracellular coding region): 551-bp product (nucleotides 436-986).
Sense: 5′-GCCATAACCGCACTGTCA-3′.
Antisense: 5′-ATGGGCAATAGCTGGTTTTC-3′.

TGF βRII (intracellular coding region): 437-bp (nucleotides 1101-1537).
Sense: 5′-CCCGGGGGCATCGCTCATCTC-3′.
Antisense: 5′-AATTTCTGGGCGCCCTCGGTCTCT-3′.

2. 10X PCR buffer: 100 mM Tris-HCl, pH 8.3, 500 mM KCl, and 15 mM MgCl$_2$ (Roche, Indianapolis, IN).
3. 20 µM dNTP mix: 20 µM each of dATP, dGTP, dCTP, and dTTP (Roche).
4. Sterile H$_2$O (DEPC-treated).
5. Ampli Taq 5 U/mL (Roche; Cat. no. 1146165).
6. GeneAmp PCR system 9600 machine from Perkin Elmer/Cetus (Norwalk, CT).
7. 100-bp DNA ladder (New England Biolabs, Cambridge, MA).

2.3.3. Ligation into Vector and Transformation

1. TA cloning kit (Invitrogen; cat. no. K2000-01): 10X ligation buffer: 60 mM Tris-HCl, pH 7.5, 60 mM MgCl$_2$, 50 mM NaCl, 1 mg/mL bovine serum albumin (BSA), 70 mM β-mercaptoethanol, 1 mM ATP, 20 mM DTT, and 10 mM spermidine.
2. PCRII vector (25 ng/µL) (Invitrogen; Cat. no. 2050-01).
3. Sterile H$_2$O (DEPC-treated).
4. T4 DNA ligase (5 U/µL) (Invitrogen; Cat. no. 15224-017).
5. SOC medium: 2% tryptone, 0.5% yeast extract, 10 mM NaCl, 2.5 mM KCl, 10 mM MgCl$_2$, 10 mM MgSO$_4$, and 20 mM glucose (Invitrogen; Cat. no. 5544SA).
6. INVαF′ competent *Escherichia coli* cells (Invitrogen; Cat. no. C658-03).
7. Large-scale plasmid prep kit (Qiagen, Chatsworth, CA).

2.3.4. Linearization

1. Restriction enzyme *Bam*HI (Invitrogen).
2. Restriction enzyme *Eco*RV (Invitrogen).

2.3.5. Labeling with Digoxigenin-UTP by In Vitro Transcription

1. DIG RNA labeling kit (SP6/7) (Roche; Cat. no. 1-175-025): pSPT18 DNA (0.25 mg/mL), pSPT19 DNA (0.25 mg/mL), 10X NTP containing 10 mM ATP,

10 mM CTP, 6.5 mM UTP, and 3.5 mM DIG-UTP, pH 7.5, 10X transcription buffer, RNase-free DNase (10 U/μL), RNase inhibitor (20 U/μL), SP6 RNA polymerase (20 U/μL), and T7 RNA polymerase (20 U/μL).
2. Elutip columns (Schleicher & Schuell; Keene, NH; Cat. no. 020/2).
3. 100% ethyl alcohol.
4. 4 M LiCl (Sigma).
5. 0.2 M EDTA, pH 8.0.
6. Sterile H$_2$O (DEPC-treated).

2.4. Detection of TGF-β Transcripts by In Situ Hybridization

2.4.1. Preparation of Glass Slides for In Situ Hybridization

1. Superfrost Plus glass microscope slides (Fisher Scientific, Pittsburgh, PA).
2. 10% HCl.
3. 70% and 95% ethyl alcohol.
4. 3-aminopropyltriethoxysilane (Sigma).
5. Acetone (Malinckrodt Baker, Paris, KY).
6. Sigmacote (Sigma).
7. Sterile H$_2$O (DEPC-treated).

2.4.2. Tissue Sectioning

1. Microtome.
2. RNase-free blades.
3. Xylene (Malinckrodt Baker).
4. 30, 50, 70, 95, and 100% ethyl alcohol.
5. Hematoxylin and eosin solution (Fisher).
6. Sterile H$_2$O (DEPC-treated).

2.4.3. Tissue Pretreatment

1. Xylene.
2. 100% and 70% ethyl alcohol.
3. Phosphate buffered saline.
4. Sterile H$_2$O (DEPC-treated).

2.4.4. Proteinase K Digestion

1. Proteinase K (Sigma; Cat. no. P-0390): 1 μg/μL in 0.1 M Tris-HCl, pH 8.0, and 50 mM EDTA.
2. 0.1 M glycine (Sigma).
3. Sterile H$_2$O (DEPC-treated).

2.4.5. Tissue Fixation

1. 4% paraformaldehyde (Fisher).
2. 0.25% acetic anhydride (Sigma).

3. 0.1 M triethanolamine (Sigma).
4. Sterile H_2O (DEPC-treated).

2.4.6. Hybridization of Riboprobe to Tissue

1. Hybridization Buffer: 0.5 M phosphate buffer, pH 7.4, 7% sodium dodecyl sulfate (SDS), and 1 mM EDTA, pH 7.0, 1% BSA (Pentex, Kankakee, IL; Cat. no. 81-003-4).
2. Sterile H_2O (DEPC-treated).
3. Humid chamber.
4. Rubber cement.

2.4.7. Stringency Washing

1. Wash Buffer A: 0.04 M phosphate buffer, pH 7.4, 5% SDS, 1 mM EDTA, and 0.5% BSA.
2. Wash Buffer B: 0.04 M phosphate, pH 7.4, 1% SDS, and 1 mM EDTA.
3. RNase A solution (Ambion, Austin, TX; Cat. no. 2270): 10 µg/µL in 1 M NaH_2PO_4, pH 7.4.
4. Sterile H_2O (DEPC-treated).

2.4.8. Visualization of In Situ Hybridization

1. Digoxigenin (DIG) Detection kit (Roche; Cat. no. 1210-220). Anti-digoxigenin-alkaline phosphatase (750 U/mL), nitroblue tetrazolium chloride (NBT), 5-bromo-4-chloro-3-indolyl-phosphate (50 mg/mL), and blocking solution in Tris-buffered saline, pH 7.5.
2. Anti-digoxigenin-alkaline phosphatase substrate: Tris buffer, pH 9.5 (0.1 M Tris-HCl, pH 9.5, 0.1 M NaCl, 0.05 M $MgCl_2$), NBT (750 U/mL), nitroblue tetrazolium chloride (NBT), and 5-bromo-4-chloro-3-indolyl-phosphate (50 mg/mL).
3. Tris-buffered saline (ISH Buffer 1): 0.1 M Tris-HCl, pH 7.5, 0.1 M NaCl, 2 mM $MgCl_2$, and 3% BSA (Invitrogen).
4. Tris-buffered saline (ISH Buffer 2): 0.1 M Tris-HCl, pH 9.5, 0.1 M NaCl, and 50 mM $MgCl_2$ (Invitrogen).
5. Tris-buffered saline (ISH Buffer 3): 20 mM Tris-HCl, pH 7.5, and 50 mM EDTA (Invitrogen).
6. Dimethylformamide (Sigma).
7. Sterile H_2O (DEPC-treated).
8. Crystal Mount mounting medium.

2.5. Detection of TGF-β Proteins by Immunohistochemistry

2.5.1. Preparation of Tissues for Immunohistochemistry

1. PBS, pH 7.4.
2. 10% phosphate-buffered formalin (Sigma).
3. 70% ethyl alcohol.

2.5.2. Antibodies

1. TGFβ1(V) (Santa Cruz Biotechnology, Santa Cruz, CA; Cat. no. SC-146).
2. TGF-β2(V) (Santa Cruz Biotechnology; Cat. no. SC-090).
3. TGF-β3(III) (Santa Cruz Biotechnology; Cat. no. SC-83).
4. TGF-βRI(V-22) (Santa Cruz Biotechnology; Cat. no. SC-398).
5. TGF-βRII(L-21) (Santa Cruz Biotechnology; Cat. no. SC-400).

2.5.3. Preparation of Tissues on Slides for Immunohistochemical Staining Analysis

1. Xylene.
2. 100, 90, 70, and 30% ethyl alcohol.
3. 3% H_2O_2 in methyl alcohol (Fisher).
4. Citrate buffer: 1.8 mM citric acid and 8.6 mM sodium citrate.
5. PBS.

2.5.4. Immunohistochemical Staining Analysis

1. Vectastain ABC Elite kit (Vector Laboratories, Burlingame, CA; Cat. no. PK-4001). Biotinylated goat anti-rabbit IgG, avidin enzyme, and normal goat serum.
2. 0.1 M Tris-HCl, pH 7.6.
3. 3,3'-diaminobenzidine hydrochloride (DAB) (Sigma): DAB stock solution 3 g DAB in 100 mL 0.1 M Tris-HCl. Working solution: Add 100 mL stock solution to 200 mL 0.1 M Tris-HCl, pH 7.6. Add 120 µL of H_2O_2 to 200 mL DAB solution just before use.
4. H_2O_2.
5. Acid alcohol: 70% ethyl alcohol and 0.37% HCl.
6. Ammonia H_2O (Sigma).
7. Hematoxylin solution-Gill's Formulation #2 (Fisher; Cat. no. CS401-1D)).
8. Permount resinous mounting medium.

3. Methods

3.1. Preparation of Tissues for In Situ Hybridization

In situ hybridization procedures to localize mRNAs for the TGF-βs and TGF-β receptors can be performed using freshly frozen tissues or phosphate-buffered formalin-fixed and paraffin-embedded tissue sections. Superior morphological preservation of cellular structure is obtained with paraffin-embedded tissue compared to frozen tissue. Rapid fixation in formalin also inactivates endogenous tissue ribonucleases that are detrimental to mRNA transcripts. Unlike frozen tissues, formalin-fixed and paraffin-embedded lung tissue can be stored at room temperature with successful detection of the mRNAs for the TGF-β isoforms and TGF-β receptors possible for several years. We routinely use formalin-fixation and paraffin-embedding to prepare normal and tumorigenic mouse lungs for *in situ* hybridization. Note that because of the numerous steps that are involved in *in situ* hybridization, the procedure requires a significant investment of time and reagents to optimize.

3.2. Purification of Total RNA from Tissues

Total lung RNA is extracted from normal mouse lung tissue and is used as a template for reverse transcription and synthesis of cDNA for TGF-β and its receptors. The following is a modification of procedures by Chirgwin et al. *(31)* and Glisin et al. *(32)*.

1. Excise lung tissue from the mouse and quickly wash 2 times in cold PBS. Freeze lung tissue immediately in liquid nitrogen or process immediately.
2. Homogenize 100–500 mg of lung tissue with a Power Gen 35 homogenizer or a baked siliconized glass tissue grinder in 7 mL GIT buffer. If homogenate is too viscous, additional GIT buffer may be added and the process of homogenization continued.
3. Centrifuge lung tissue homogenate at 13,000g for 10 min at 4°C and discard the pellet.
4. Transfer the supernatant to a 50-mL tube and pass through an 18-gauge needle 12 times to shear genomic DNA (*see* **Note 1**).
5. Transfer the supernatant to a polyallomer centrifuge tube containing 4 mL CsCl buffer.
6. Centrifuge in an ultracentrifuge SW-41 rotor at 35,000g for 20 h at 20°C.
7. Discard the supernatant and allow the tube to drain for 5 min.
8. Dissolve the white RNA pellet in 300 µL DEPC-treated H_2O. Add 30 µL 3 M sodium acetate, pH 5.2, and 1 mL 100% ethyl alcohol. Allow RNA to precipitate at –20°C overnight.
9. Centrifuge the RNA at 13,000g at 4°C for 30 min. Decant and discard the supernatant. Wash the RNA pellet 2 times in 70% ethyl alcohol. Dry the RNA pellet briefly under vacuum. Dissolve the RNA pellet in 100–500 µL DEPC-treated H_2O. Determine the concentration of the RNA by spectrophotometry. Store RNA at –80°C.

3.3. Preparation of TGF-β Hybridization Probes

The choice of probes for *in situ* hybridization to localize transcripts for the TGF-βs and receptors includes oligonucleotide probes, cDNA probes, and cRNA (riboprobes) reagents. We have used cRNA probes generated from specific regions of the mouse TGF-βs and receptors, the sequence and usefulness of which were determined using Lasergene software (DNASTAR, Madison, WI). The cRNA probes are designed to be 400–600 base pairs in length (*see* **Note 2**).

Probe detection can be performed using several methods, including autoradiography, biotin, or digoxigenin. The following method outlines a cRNA-based *in situ* hybridization procedure which has been successfully used to detect transcripts for TGF-β and its receptors in formalin-fixed and paraffin-embedded lung tissue sections. Because mRNA is subject to degradation by ribonucleases, extreme care must be taken to prevent contamination by exogenous ribonucleases (RNases). Gloves and oven-baked glassware must be used throughout the procedure.

3.3.1. cDNA Synthesis

1. Mix 1 μL of total RNA (10 μg/μL) with 1 μL of oligo dT_{12-18} and 10 μL H_2O in a 1.5-mL tube. Incubate at 70°C for 10 min and then chill on ice for 2 min.
2. Add 2 μL 10X PCR buffer, 2 μL $MgCl_2$, 1 μL dNTP mix, and 2 μL DTT and mix. Incubate at 42°C for 5 min to anneal. Add 1 μL SuperScript II reverse transcriptase and incubate at 42°C for 50 min for cDNA synthesis. Terminate the reaction at 70°C for 15 min and place on ice.
3. Add 1 μL RNase H and incubate at 37°C for 20 min.
4. Store the cDNA at –20°C until needed.

3.3.2. Polymerase Chain Reaction (PCR) Amplification, Ligation into Vector, and Transformation of Cells

The DNA to be transcribed is cloned into the polylinker site of appropriate transcription vectors, including pCRII which contains promoters for T7 and SP6 RNA polymerases adjacent to the polylinker.

1. Mix 1 μL cDNA template, 1 μL sense primer, 1 μL antisense primer, 2 μL 10X PCR buffer, 2 μL 10X PCR buffer, 2 μL 20 μ*M* dNTP mix, 0.5 μL AmpliTaq, and 10.5 μL H_2O in a 0.5 mL thin-walled PCR tube. Perform PCR using the following parameters: 94°C for 20 s, 42°C for 20 s, 72°C for 30 s for 40 cycles at 72°C for 10 min.
2. Confirm the size of the PCR product by examining 5 μL of the reaction on a 1.5% agarose gel (*see* **Note 3**).
3. Mix 2 μL PCR product with 1 μL 10X ligation buffer, 2 μL pCRII vector, 4 μL H_2O, and 1 μL T4 DNA ligase in a 1.5-mL tube, and incubate at 14°C overnight. The pCRII plasmid vector contains promoters for T7 and SP6 RNA polymerases adjacent to the polylinker.
4. Transform into INVβF' competent *E. coli* cells or similar competent cells following the Invitrogen protocol. Spread transformants onto Luria-Bertani (LB) plates, and incubate at 37°C overnight.
5. Pick 12 white colonies for each PCR product and perform mini-preparations on each. Digest 5–10 μL of each DNA with *Eco*RI (*see* **Note 4**).
6. Perform a large-scale plasmid preparation of the positive clones and purify the DNA following the Qiagen protocol.
7. Determine the concentration of plasmid DNA using spectrophotometry. Confirm the identity and orientation of the TGF-β PCR product insert by sequencing analysis (*see* **Note 5**).

3.3.3. Linearization and RNA Labeling by In Vitro Transcription

After linearization of TGF-β template DNA at a suitable site, T7 and SP6 RNA polymerases are used to produce "run-off" transcripts. Digoxigenin (DIG)-UTP is used as a substrate and incorporated into the transcript (*see* **Note 6**).

1. Linearize 10 μg pCRII plasmid DNA containing TGF-β PCR product by incubating with either *Bam*HI or *Eco*RV to obtain the T7 promoter with antisense TGF-β PCR product insert or the SP6 promoter with sense TGF-β PCR product insert, respectively. Confirm the size of the linearized pCRII plasmid with insert by agarose gel electrophoresis (*see* **Note 7**).
2. RNA labeling by in vitro transcription is performed using Roche's DIG RNA labeling kit (SP6/T7). In a RNase-free microcentrifuge tube, add the following reagents on ice: 1 μg purified TGF-β DNA template, 2 μL NTP labeling mix, 2 μL 10X transcription buffer, 1 μL RNase inhibitor, 13 μL H₂O (DEPC-treated), and 2 μL RNA polymerase (T7 or SP6). Mix and incubate at 37°C for 2 h. After 2 h, add 2 μL RNase-free DNase I and incubate at 37°C for 15 min to remove the TGF-β DNA template. Add 2 μL EDTA, pH 8.0 to terminate the DNase I reaction.
3. For prolonged storage of the transcribed cRNA riboprobe, add 2.5 μL 4 *M* LiCl and 75 μL pre-chilled 100% ethyl alcohol. Mix and allow to precipitate at –20°C for at least 2 h. Centrifuge and wash the pellet with 50 μL cold 70% ethyl alcohol. Dry briefly under vacuum and dissolve in DEPC-treated H₂O. Store at –20°C.

3.4. Detection of TGF-β Transcripts by In Situ Hybridization

3.4.1. Preparation of Glass Slides for In Situ Hybridization

Glass slides should be pretreated as described for optimal retention of the lung tissue sections. All aqueous solutions should be made using DEPC-treated water that has been autoclaved for at least 20 min to inactivate RNases (*see* **Note 8**).

1. Microscope glass slides are dipped successively in 10% HCl in 70% ethyl alcohol, water, and then 95% ethyl alcohol.
2. Dry the slides at 150°C for 5 min.
3. Dip the slides in 2% 3-aminopropyltriethoxysilane in acetone for 10 s. Wash 2 times in acetone and 3 times in water.
4. Dry the slides overnight at 42°C.
5. Siliconize the cover slips in Sigmacote for 10 s and wash 2 times in 95% ethanol. Allow to air dry. Autoclave for 20 min.

3.4.2. Tissue Sectioning

Formalin-fixed and paraffin-embedded normal and tumor containing lung tissues are studied simultaneously (*see* **Note 9**).

1. Cut 5-μm lung sections using a microtome and float sections in a RNase-free water bath at 42°C.
2. Lift tissue sections onto pretreated microscope slides and dry at 42°C for 2 h.
3. Heat the slides at 60°C for 2 h in glass Coplin jars. The slides may be stored at room temperature.

3.4.3. Tissue Pretreatment

1. Deparaffinize the slides by 2 changes of xylene at room temperature for 20 min each (*see* **Note 10**).
2. Rehydrate the slides through a series of graded ethyl alcohol solutions, each made with DEPC-treated water, including 100% (10 min), 95% (10 min), 70% (5 min), 50% (5 min), 30% (5 min), and finally, H_2O (2 min) (*see* **Note 11**).

3.4.4. Proteinase K Digestion

1. Place the slides in RNase-free PBS (2 min) twice.
2. The sections are digested with 100–200 μL RNase-free Proteinase K solution, pre-warmed to 37°C. The concentration of Proteinase K and the length of the digestion time should be titrated (*see* **Note 12**). We use a final Proteinase K concentration of 10 μg/mL for adult mouse lung sections and digest for 10 min.

3.4.5. Tissue Fixation

1. Immerse the slides in 0.1 *M* glycine in RNase-free PBS at room temperature for 5 min.
2. Post-fix the tissue sections with 4% paraformaldehyde in RNase-free PBS for 3 min.
3. Wash the slides 2 times with RNase-free PBS for 2 min each.
4. Immerse the slides in freshly prepared 0.25% acetic anhydride in 0.1 *M* triethanolamine buffer, pH 8.0 for 10 min with gentle agitation.
5. Wash the slides in DEPC-treated H_2O 2 times for 5 min.
6. The slides are then dried at 37°C for 2 h.

3.4.6. Hybridization of Riboprobe to Tissue (see **Note 13**)

1. Pre-warm Hybridization Buffer to 65°C.
2. Add 2–4 μL TGF-β cRNA probe using equal amounts of sense and antisense probes to 40 μL Hybridization Buffer, mix, and apply slowly to the tissue section, dissipating all bubbles. A siliconized glass cover slip (24 × 30 mm) is slowly applied and sealed in position using rubber cement to prevent drying.
3. Incubate the slides horizontally in humid glass dishes at 65°C for 16 h.

3.4.7. Stringency Washing

1. Pre-warm Wash Buffer A and Wash Buffer B to 65°C, and 1 *M* phosphate buffer, pH 7.4, and RNase A solution to 37°C.
2. After hybridization, remove the rubber cement from the slides, and incubate slides in Wash A at room temperature for 10 min to remove cover slips.

3. Wash the slides with Wash Buffer A that has been pre-warmed to 65°C for 4 times for 5 min each time at 65°C with gentle agitation.
4. Wash the slides with Wash Buffer B that has been pre-warmed to 65°C for 2 times for 10 min each time at 65°C with gentle agitation.
5. Wash the slides with 1 *M* phosphate buffer, pH 7.4, that has been pre-warmed to 37°C for 5 min.
6. Incubate the slides in RNase A solution that has been pre-warmed to 37°C for 15 min.
7. Wash the slides with 1 *M* phosphate buffer, pH 7.4, that has been pre-warmed to 37°C for 2 min.

3.4.8. Visualization of In Situ Hybridization

1. Wash the slides in ISH Buffer 1 at room temperature for 1 min 2 times.
2. Incubate the slides in ISH Buffer 1 at room temperature for 10 min.
3. Prepare anti-DIG antibody (1/500) using 1 µL antibody in 0.5 mL ISH Buffer 1. Add 100 µL anti-DIG antibody to each section and incubate the slides in a humidified chamber at room temperature for 2 h.
4. Wash the slides in ISH Buffer 1 at room temperature 3 times for 3 min each time.
5. Incubate the slides in ISH Buffer 2 at room temperature for 10 min.
6. Prepare the digoxigenin substrate in ISH Buffer 2 just before use and add 100 µL to each section. Incubate at room temperature for 1–16 h in a dark humidified chamber (*see* **Note 14**).
7. Terminate the reaction by placing the slides in ISH Buffer 3 at room temperature for 5 min.
8. Wipe the slides of excess buffer and apply Crystal Mount mounting medium. Bake at 80°C for 20 min. Positive hybridization will be visible as a purple precipitate.

3.5. Detection of TGF-β Proteins in Adult Mouse Lungs by Immunohistochemistry

3.5.1. Preparation of Tissues for Immunohistochemistry

Immunohistochemical staining procedures to localize the proteins for the TGF-βs and TGF-β receptors can be performed using paraffin-embedded tissue sections that have been fixed in phosphate-buffered formalin or 70% ethyl alcohol. Superior morphology is obtained using fixation in phosphate-buffered formalin. We routinely use phosphate-buffered formalin to fix mouse lung tissue for immunohistochemical staining.

3.5.2. Antibodies

Rabbit polyclonal antibodies for the TGF-β isoforms and receptors are tested for specificity using Western-blot analysis with their respective blocking peptides. The synthetic peptides are interchanged to further validate the specificity (*see* **Note 15**).

3.5.3. Preparation of Tissues on Slides for Immunohistochemical Staining Analysis

As for *in situ* hybridization, formalin-fixed and paraffin-embedded normal and tumor-containing lung tissues are studied simultaneously.

1. Cut 5-µm lung sections using a microtome and float sections in a water bath at 42°C.
2. Lift tissue sections onto poly-L-lysine coated microscope slides and dry at 42°C for 2 h. The slides may be stored at room temperature.

3.5.4. Immunohistochemical Staining Analysis

TGF-β protein can be localized in tissue sections using immunohistochemical staining. The method that is described localizes the expression of TGF-β by the avidin-biotin complex (ABC) method on paraffin-embedded mouse lung tissues (*33*). Many of the reagents are commercially available as a kit (Vectastain ABC Elite, Vector Labs). We have used the following method to localize the expression of TGF-β and TGF-β receptors in normal and tumor containing adult mouse lung tissue (*34,35*).

1. Warm the slides to 60°C to partially melt the paraffin and facilitate its removal.
2. Deparaffinize the slides with 2 changes of xylene for 10 min each time (*see* **Note 10**).
3. Rehydrate the sections through a series of graded ethyl alcohol solutions (100%, 100% for 10 min each, 95%, 70%, 50%, and 30% for 5 min each), and 2 times in H_2O for 1 min each time (*see* **Note 11**).
4. Perform antigen retrieval if necessary (*see* **Note 16**). Place the hydrated slides into 500 mL citrate buffer at room temperature for 12 h. Alternatively, the slides can be heated in a microwave oven in citrate buffer at full power 2 times for 5 min each time. Allow slides to cool to room temperature.
5. Place the slides in PBS for 5 min.
6. Drain the slides and apply 100 µL blocking solution of normal goat serum (1/30 dilution in PBS) to cover the tissue section (*see* **Note 17**). Incubate in a humid chamber at room temperature for 1 h.
7. Drain the slides and apply anti-TGF-β antiserum. It is necessary to perform several dilutions of antibody in PBS to determine the correct dilution for each different lot of antibody (*see* **Note 18**). Place the slides in a humid chamber, close tightly, and incubate at 4°C for 16 h (*see* **Note 19**).
8. Wash the slides individually with PBS, and then place in PBS for 3 min 2 times.
9. Prepare biotinylated anti-rabbit IgG secondary antibody (1/200 dilution in PBS). Apply 100–200 µL secondary antibody to the slides and incubate at room temperature for 1 h in a humid chamber.

10. Prepare ABC complex (Vectastain ABC Elite) 30 min in advance. Dilute A and B reagents (1/50 dilution in PBS).
11. Wash the slides individually with PBS, and then place in PBS for 5 min.
12. Apply 100–200 μL ABC complex to the slides and incubate at room temperature for 1 h in humid chamber.
13. While the slides are incubating with the ABC complex, prepare DAB working solution.
14. Wash the slides in PBS for 5 min, and then in 0.1 M Tris-HCl, pH 7.6 for 5 min.
15. Place the slides in 200 mL DAB/H_2O_2 and incubate at room temperature for 3–10 min. Monitor the color development in the tissue sections with the microscope. Wash the slides 2 times in H_2O. Add bleach to the used DAB/H_2O_2 solution for 30 min and discard in the aqueous chemical waste container.
16. To counterstain the slides, incubate in Gill's hematoxylin at room temperature for 5 min.
17. Wash the slides briefly in tap water.
18. Dip the slides in acid alcohol 3 times.
19. Dip the slides in H_2O 3 times.
20. Dip the slides in ammonia water 3 times.
21. Dip the slides in H_2O 3 times.
22. Dehydrate the slides through a series of graded ethyl alcohol solutions, including 70% (5 min for 2 times), 95% (5 min for 2 times), 100% (5 min for 2 times), and xylene (10 min for 2 times). Mount the slides with Permount resinous mounting medium. Apply cover slips to the slides and allow them to dry at room temperature overnight (*see* **Note 20**).

4. Notes

1. For the preparation of mRNA from lung tissue, it is important to thoroughly shear the genomic DNA by passing the DNA and RNA mixture through an 18-gauge needle. The A260 : A280 ratio should be 1.6 to 1.8.
2. The optimal size range for cRNA *in situ* hybridization probes is 400–600 bp to permit sufficient labeling with DIG-UTP and to allow uptake into the tissues.
3. To determine the size of the PCR product DNA, compare to a molecular size marker loaded in a separate lane. **Figure 1A** shows a representative agarose gel containing PCR products for mouse TGF-β1, TGF-β RI, and TGF-β RII.
4. Confirm the size of the PCR DNA product by agarose gel electrophoresis as described previously. **Figure 1B** shows a representative agarose gel containing PCR products for mouse TGF-β1, TGF-β RI, and TGF-β RII that have been cloned into the pCRII plasmid Vector (full plasmid).
5. The sense and antisense TGF-β PCR products are cloned into the polylinker sites of the pCRII plasmid vector that contains promoters for T7 and SP6 RNA polymerases adjacent to the polylinker. Because the PCR products can be incorporated into the plasmid vector in both directions, it is helpful to sequence the positive clones and select those that have incorporated the antisense primer near the T7 promoter sequence to be used for the antisense cRNA hybridization

A   PCR Products   **B**   Full Plasmid   **C**   Linearized Plasmid

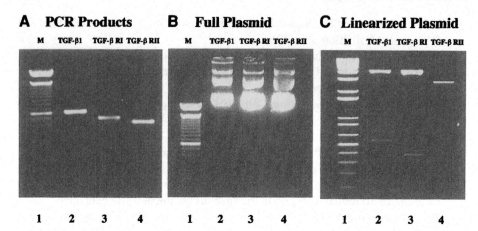

Fig. 1. Gel electrophoresis of reverse transcription polymerase chain reaction amplification of TGF-β1, TGF-β RI, and TGF-β RII mRNAs from normal mouse lung tissue. Total RNA was isolated from normal mouse lung tissue and cDNA was synthesized using reverse transcriptase. PCR amplification was performed on the cDNA using specific oligodeoxynucleotide primers for TGF-β1, TGF-β RI, and TGF-β RII. (**A**) PCR products for mouse TGF-β1 (620-bp), TGF-β RI (488-bp), and TGF-β RII (437-bp). (**B**) PCR products for mouse TGF-β1, TGF-β RI, and TGF-β RII cloned into the pCRII plasmid vector; full plasmid. (**C**) PCR products for mouse TGF-β1, TGF-β RI, and TGF-β RII cloned into the pCRII plasmid vector and linearized by digestion with *Bam*HI; linearized plasmid. M: DNA ladders.

probe, and those that have incorporated the sense primer near the SP6 promoter sequence to be used for the sense cRNA hybridization probe.

6. It is helpful to design and construct at least two cRNA hybridization probes, with one encompassing a section of the coding region of the transcript and the other encompassing a section of the 5'- or 3'-untranslated region of the transcript. Probes corresponding to the 5'- or 3'-untranslated region of the transcript are likely to be more specific than those corresponding to the coding region. However, because the 5'- or 3'-untranslated region of the transcripts are likely to be more GC-rich than the coding region, cRNA probes corresponding to the 5'- or 3'-untranslated region may not incorporate the digoxigenin-UTP label as efficiently as coding region cRNA probes. The two different cRNA probes should be used simultaneously and should validate one another.

7. **Figure 1C** shows a representative agarose gel containing PCR products for mouse TGF-β1, TGF-β RI, and TGF-β RII that have been cloned into the pCRII plasmid vector and linearized with *Bam*HI (linearized plasmid).

8. It is necessary to properly perform the silinization procedure on the microscope slides before the tissues are applied. Failure to do so will result in nonadherence of the tissues as they are used during the hybridization process.

9. cRNA probes are generated as pairs of antisense and sense constructs. *In situ* hybridization reactions should be routinely conducted using antisense and sense cRNA probes in parallel. This will help to determine the level of nonspecific background hybridization by these probes. In a similar fashion, *in situ* hybridization should be performed simultaneously on normal and tumorigenic tissues.

10. Paraffin must be completely and efficiently removed from the sections in order for the cRNA probes to hybridize with the fixed transcripts in the tissue sections. Warming the xylene to 60°C and allowing sufficient space between the slides improves the efficiency of removal of paraffin from the tissue sections. For optimal results, solutions should be changed and refreshed on a regular basis. Reagents, buffers, and solutions should be made with DEPC-treated RNase-free water and autoclaved for 20 min whenever possible.

11. The graded ethyl alcohol solutions should be always used in one direction only for optimal results.

12. The amount of Proteinase K that is used to digest the tissue sections should be titrated. Excessive amounts of Proteinase K are likely to result in degraded and suboptimal tissue morphology, while too little Proteinase K will result in the cRNA hybridization probe not being able to permeate the tissue well.

13. *In situ* hybridization of tissue sections should be performed on duplicate sections on the same slide whenever possible. Additionally, it is prudent to perform these reactions on at least three separate occasions in order to avoid any artifacts.

14. The time required for detection of the digoxigenin signal may vary with the cRNA hybridization probe and reflects the amount of transcript in the tissue. The time for the color to appear may range from 1 h to overnight. When the color appears, it is stable and maintains itself for at least 1 y. **Figure 2** shows representative *in situ* hybridization patterns of transcripts for TGF-β1, TGF-β RI, and TGF-β RII in normal and tumorigenic mouse lung tissue detected using TGF-β cRNA probes.

15. To establish the specificity of the antibody, serial tissue sections should be stained using a solution of the primary antibody that has been pre-incubated overnight with the antigenic peptide used to generate the antibody and with another "nonsense" nonhomologous peptide.

16. In situations where the amount of protein in the tissue is minimal or difficult to obtain, antigen retrieval methods can be used to increase protein staining. These methods include overnight incubation of the tissues in citrate buffer, and heating by microwave in citrate buffer. However, these methods for antigen retrieval are relatively harsh for the tissues and the tissues may not adhere well to the microscope slides. If antigen retrieval must be performed, overnight incubation of the tissues in citrate buffer is preferable to heating by microwave in citrate buffer.

17. Antibodies and reagents can be conserved with use of a hydrophobic marking pen (PAP pen, Research Products International, Mt. Prospect, IL) to draw a wax border around the tissue section. The antibody and other reagents are retained by surface tension close to the tissue section. This also permits the use of more than one antibody on a slide that contains multiple serial tissue sections.

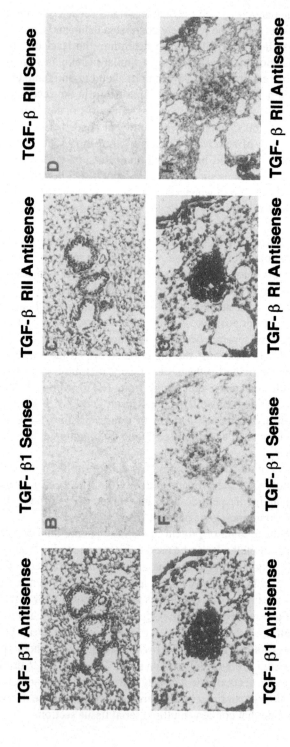

Fig. 2. In situ hybridization of TGF-β in mouse lung carcinogenesis. Lung sections isolated from (**A–D**) normal mouse lungs and (**E–H**) tumorigenic mouse lungs were hybridized with digoxigenin-labeled antisense (A, C, E, G, and H) and sense (B, D, and F) cRNA probes for TGF-β1 (A, B, E, and F), TGF-β RII (C, D, and H), TGF-β RI (G), and TGF-β RII (C, D, and H). Magnification, 40× in (A–D), 200× in panels (E–H).

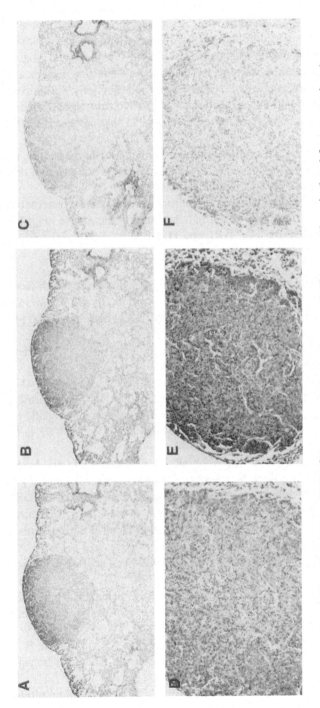

Fig. 3. Immunohistochemistry of TGF-β in mouse lung carcinogenesis. Lung sections isolated from tumorigenic mouse lungs were reacted with (**A** and **D**) anti-TGF-β1(V), (**B** and **E**) anti-TGF-βRI(V), and (**C** and **F**) anti-TGF-βRII(L-21) antibodies. Magnification, 40× in (A–C), 100× in (D–F).

18. In order to be able to semi-quantitatively compare the amounts of proteins in tissue sections, immunohistochemical staining should be performed on tissues at the same time in a coordinate fashion. Wherever possible, a positively stained tissue section should be established as a positive control, and used each time immunohistochemical staining is performed so that the relative amounts of staining in tissues can be assessed and compared. Similarly, a negatively stained tissue section should be established as a negative control, and used each time immunohistochemical staining is performed so that nonspecific staining can be determined.

19. In situations where the amount of protein in the tissue is substantial, incubation with the primary antibody may only require a few hours at room temperature than overnight at 4°C. This should be established.

20. **Figure 3** shows representative immunohistochemical staining patterns of TGF-β1, TGF-β RI, and TGF-β RII in normal and tumorigenic mouse lung tissue using antibodies for TGF-β1, TGF-β RI, and TGF-β RII.

References

1. Roberts, A. B. and Sporn, M. B. (1990) The transforming growth factor-β's, in *Handbook of Experimental Pharmacology. Peptide Growth Factors and Their Receptors* (Sporn, M. B. and Roberts, A. B., eds.), Springer-Verlag, Germany, pp. 419–772.

2. Massague', J., Cheifetz, S., Laiho, M., and Ralph, D. A. (1992) Transforming growth factor-beta. *Cancer Surv.* **12,** 81–103.

3. Manning, A., Williams, A., Game, S., and Paraskeva, C. (1991) Differential sensitivity of human colonic adenoma and carcinoma cells to transforming growth factor-β (TGF-β): Conversion of an adenoma cell line to a tumorigenic phenotype is accompanied by a reduced response to the inhibitory effects of TGF-β. *Oncogene* **6,** 1471–1476.

4. Geiser, A. G., Burmester, J. K., Webbink, R., Roberts, A. B., and Sporn, M. B. (1992) Inhibition of growth by transforming growth factor-β following fusion of two non-responsive human carcinoma cell lines. *J. Biol. Chem.* **267,** 2588–2593.

5. Filmus, J. and Kerbel, R. (1993) Development of resistance mechanisms to the growth-inhibitory effects of transforming growth factor-β during tumor progression. *Curr. Opin. Oncol.* **5,** 123–129.

6. Massague', J., Attisano, L., and Wrana, J. (1994) The TGF-β family and its composite receptors. *Trends Cell Biol.* **4,** 172–178.

7. Franzen, P., ten Dijke, P., Ichijo, H., Yamashita, H., Schulz, P., Heldin, C.-H., and Miyazono, K. (1993) Cloning of a receptor that forms a heteromeric complex with the TGF-β type II receptor. *Cell* **75,** 681–692.

8. Lin, H. Y., Wang, X.-F., Ng-Eaton, E., Weinberg, R. A., and Lodish, H. F. (1992) Expression cloning of the TGF-β type II receptor, a functional transmembrane serine/threonine kinase. *Cell* **68,** 775–785.

9. Laiho, M., Weiss, F. M. B., and Massague', J. (1990) Concomitant loss of transforming growth factor-β receptors type I and type II in TGF-β-resistant cell

mutants implicates both receptor types in signal transduction. *J. Biol. Chem.* **265,** 18518–18524.

10. Park, K., Kim, S.-J., Bang, Y.-J., Park, J.-G., Kim, N. K., Roberts, A. B., and Sporn, M. B. (1994) Genetic changes in the transforming β type II receptor gene in human gastric cells: correlation with sensitivity to TGF-β. *Proc. Natl. Acad. Sci. USA* **81,** 8772–8776.

11. Sun, L., Wu, G., Wilson, J. K., Zborowska, E., Yang, J., Raajka-Runanayeke, I., et al. (1994) Expression of transforming growth factor β type II receptor leads to reduced malignancy in human breast cancer MCF-7 cells. *J. Biol. Chem.* **269,** 26449–26455.

12. Chakravarthy, D., Green, A. R., Green, V. L., Kerin, M. J., and Speirs, V. (1999) Expression and secretion of TGF-β isoforms and expression of TGF-β-receptors I, II and III in normal and neoplastic human breast. *Int. J. Oncol.* **15,** 187–194.

13. Guo, Y., Jacobs, S. C., and Kyprianou, N. (1997) Down-regulation of protein and mRNA expression for transforming growth factor-β (TGF-β1) type I and type II receptors in human prostate cancer. *Int. J. Cancer* **71,** 573–579.

14. Matsushita, M., Matsuzaki, K., Date, M., Watanabe, T., Shibano, K., Nakagawa, T., et al. (1999) Down-regulation of TGF-β receptors in human colorectal cancer: implications for cancer development. *Br. J. Cancer* **80,** 194–205.

15. Grady, W. M, Rajput, A., Myerhof, L., Liu, D. F., Kwon, K., Willis J., and Markowitz, S. (1998) Mutation of the type II transforming growth factor-β receptor is coincident with the transformation of human colon adenomas to malignant carcinomas. *Cancer Res.* **58,** 3101–3104.

16. Furta, K., Misao, S., Takahashi K., Tagaya, T., Fukuzawa Y., Ishikawa, T., et al. (1999) Gene mutation of transforming growth factor β1 type II receptor in hepatocellular carcinoma. *Int. J. Cancer* **81,** 851–853.

17. Thaete, L. G. and Malkinson, A. M. (1991) Cells of origin of primary pulmonary neoplasms in mice: morphological and histochemical studies. *Exp. Lung Res.* **17,** 219–228.

18. Stewart, H. L., Dunn, T. B., Snell, K. C., and Deringer, M. K. (1979) Tumors of the respiratory tract, in *Pathology of Tumors in Laboratory Animals* (Turosov, V. S., ed.), IARC Press, Lyon, pp. 251–288.

19. Dixon, D., Horton, J., Haseman, J. K., Talley, F., Greenwall, A., Nettesheim, P., et al. (1991) Histomorphology and ultrastructure of spontaneous neoplasms in strain A mice. *Exp. Lung Res.* **17,** 131–155.

20. Foley, J. F., Anderson, M. W., Stoner, G. D., Gaul, B. W., Hardisty, J. F., and Maronpot, R. R. (1991) Proliferative lesions of the mouse lung: progression studies in strain A mice. *Exp. Lung Res.* **17,** 157–168.

21. You, M., Candrian, U., Moronpot, R., Stoner, G., and Anderson, M. (1989) Activation of the K-ras protooncogene in spontaneously occurring and chemically-induced lung tumors of the stain A mouse. *Proc. Natl. Acad. Sci. USA* **86,** 3070–3074.

22. Wiseman, R. W., Cochran, C., Dietrich, W., Lander, E. S., and Soderkvist, P. (1994) Allelotyping of butadiene-induced lung and mammary adenocarcinomas of

B6C3F1 mice: frequent losses of heterozygosity in regions homologous to human tumor-suppressor genes. *Proc. Natl. Acad. Sci. USA* **91**, 3759–3763.

23. Herzog, C. R., Wiseman, R. W., and You, M. (1994) Deletion mapping of a putative tumor suppressor gene on chromosome 4 in mouse lung tumors. *Cancer Res.* **54**, 4007–4010.

24. Stoner, G. (1991) Lung tumors in strain A mice as a bioassay for carcinogenicity of environmental chemicals. *Exp. Lung Res.* **17**, 157–168.

25. Malkinson, A.M. (1992) Primary lung tumors in mice: an experimentally manipulable model of human adenocarcinoma. *Cancer Res. (Suppl.)* **52**, 2670s–2767s.

26. Devesa, S. S., Shaw, G. L., and Blot, W. J. (1991) Changing patterns of lung cancer incidence by histological type. *Cancer Epidemiol. Biomarkers Prev.* **1**, 29–34.

27. Ohmori, H., Abe, T., Hirano, H., Murakami, T., Katoh, T., Gotoh, S., et al. (1992) Comparison of Ki-ras gene mutation among simultaneously occurring multiple urethan-induced lung tumors in individual mice. *Carcinogenesis* **13**, 851–855.

28. Festing, M. F. W., Yang, A., and Malkinson, A. M. (1994) At least four genes and sex are associated with susceptibility to urethane-induced pulmonary adenomas in mice. *Genet. Res.* **64**, 99–106.

29. Oreffo, V. I., Robinson, S., You, M., Wu, M.-C., and Malkinson, A. M. (1998) Decreased expression of the adenomatous polyposis coli (APC) and mutated in colorectal cancer (Mcc) genes in mouse lung neoplasia. *Mol. Carcinog.* **21**, 37–49.

30. Gibson, S. J. and Polak, J. M. (1990) Principles and applications of complementary RNA probes, in *In Situ Hybridization: Principles and Practice* (Polak, J. M. and McGee, J. O. D., eds.), Oxford University Press, New York, pp. 25–50.

31. Chirgwin, J. M., Przybyla, A. E., MacDonald, R. J., and Rutter, W. J. (1979) Isolation of biologically active ribonucleic acid from sources enriched in ribonuclease. *Biochemistry* **18**, 5294–5299.

32. Glisin, V., Crkvenjakov, R., and Byus, C. (1974) Ribonucleic acid isolated by cesium chloride centrifugation. *Biochemistry* **13**, 2633–2640.

33. Hsu, S.M., Raine, L., and Fanger, H. (1981) Use of avidin-biotin-peroxidase complex (ABC) in immunoperoxidase techniques: a comparison between ABC and unlabelled antibody (PAP) procedures. *J. Histochem. Cytochem.* **29**, 577–580.

34. Jakowlew, S. B., Moody, T. W., You, L., and Mariano, J. M. (1998) Transforming growth factor-beta expression in mouse lung carcinogenesis. *Exp. Lung Res.* **24**, 579–593.

35. Jakowlew, S. B., Moody, T. W., You, L., and Mariano, J. M. (1998) Reduction in transforming growth factor-β type II receptor in mouse lung carcinogenesis. *Mol. Carcinog.* **22**, 46–56.

11

Alterations in the Expression of Insulin-Like Growth Factors and Their Binding Proteins in Lung Cancer

Carrie M. Coleman and Adda Grimberg

1. Introduction

1.1. The Insulin-Like Growth Factor Axis

The insulin-like growth factors (IGF), named for their structural homology to proinsulin, are potent mitogens involved in the endocrine, paracrine, and autocrine regulation of growth. IGF bioactivity may be altered by changes to any level of the IGF axis. The IGF axis is comprised of IGF-I and IGF-II, two IGF receptors, six IGF binding proteins (IGFBPs), and at least nine IGFBP-related proteins (IGFBP-rPs).

1.2. IGFs

There are two IGFs: IGF-I and IGF-II. IGF-I is the main IGF in the circulation. IGF-I is made throughout the body, but the liver is the main source of circulating IGF-I *(1)*. Only one percent circulates in the free form, as the majority of circulating IGFs are found in a 150kDa complex composed of three subunits: IGF (1 or 2), IGFBP-3 and an acid labile subunit (ALS) *(2)*. This complex increases the serum half-life of IGF-I from 10 min to 15 h *(3)* and also helps to eliminate the hypoglycemic effects of free IGFs *(4)*. Binding of IGFs by IGFBPs limits the amount of bioavailable IGF, preventing IGF-receptor complexes. IGF-I expression is affected by hormones, cyclic adenosine monophosphate (cAMP), transforming growth factor-β (TGF-β) *(5)* and nutritional status *(6)*. The maximum concentration of IGF-II is found in fetal tissues *(7)* and remains at high levels post-natally in the central nervous system (CNS), skeletal muscle, and skin *(8)*.

From: *Methods in Molecular Medicine, vol. 74: Lung Cancer, Vol. 1: Molecular Pathology Methods and Reviews*
Edited by: B. Driscoll © Humana Press Inc., Totowa, NJ

1.3. IGF Receptors

The IGF receptors are known as types 1 and 2. IGF-IR is a tyrosine kinase receptor, similar to the insulin receptor, that mediates the growth-promoting effects of both IGF-I and IGF-II *(9)*. The roles of IGF-IR include cellular protection against apoptosis and stimulation of mitogenesis *(5)*. In addition to binding IGFs, IGF-IR can also bind insulin *(10)*. IGF-R type 2 is identical to the mannose-6-phosphate receptor *(11)*. Its main functions are to eliminate IGF-II from the circulation *(11)* and to limit the autocrine and paracrine actions of IGF-II *(12)*. In contrast to the type 1 receptor, type 2 binds IGF-II with a greater affinity than IGF-I and does not bind insulin *(10)*.

1.4. IGFBPs 1 Through 6

The six IGFBPs are defined by their high affinity binding to the IGFs and their cysteine-rich amino termini. Homology among the IGFBPs is limited to the N-terminus and C-terminus domains. The cysteine residues found in these two conserved regions form intradomain disulfide bonds and are an integral part of the IGF-binding capacity. A variable region, possibly accounting for the specificity amongst the IGFBPs, is found in the mid-region of all the IGFBPs *(13)*. **Table 1** provides a summary of the unique properties of these proteins.

IGFBPs play a general role as growth inhibitors, controlling IGF action as well as regulating cell growth and apoptosis in an IGF-independent fashion *(5)*. By binding IGF with greater affinity than does membrane-bound IGF-IR, IGFBPs competitively inhibit IGF activation of IGF-IR. The higher affinity of IGFBPs for IGF can be reversed by proteolysis of IGFBPs into fragments with reduced IGF-binding affinity. The IGF-I analog Des-(1-3)-IGF-I that binds the IGF-IR but cannot bind IGFBP-3, has been useful in determining the effects of IGFBP-3 on IGF actions *(14)*.

IGFBPs also have IGF-independent actions. IGFBP-3 inhibits growth in an IGF-independent fashion, as shown by experiments with IGF-IR knockout fibroblasts and with IGFBP-3 fragments that cannot bind IGF *(5)*. IGF-independent actions of IGFBP-3 are related to specific cell-surface IGFBP-3 association proteins and receptors *(15,16)*. IGFBP-3 interacts with regulatory molecules such as heparin, transferrin, type 1-alpha collagen, and latent TGF-β binding *(5)* and with the human papilloma virus (HPV) oncoprotein E7 *(17)*. IGF-independent actions of IGFBPs may also involve nuclear translocation, as both IGFBP-3 and IGFBP-5 contain nuclear localization sequences (NLS) *(18–20)*. IGFBP-3 binds to the retinoid X-receptor (RXR) and the complex relocates to the nucleus after treatment with retinoic acid *(21)*. Serum-free cultures of osteoblast clones from IGF-I knockout mice that were treated with

Table 1
IGFBPs and Their Characteristics[a]

Binding protein	Gene locus	Genebank accession number	Unmodified molecular weights (kDa)	Post-translational modifications and molecular weight (kDa)	Location in body	Significance
IGFBP-1	7p	S74080	25	Phosphorylated 29[b]	Main IGFBP in amniotic fluid	Serum levels regulated by insulin, glucose
IGFBP-2	2q	NM000597 (mRNA)	31	None	High levels found in cerebrospinal fluid (CSF) and seminal plasma	Concentration age-dependent; high levels during infancy and old age
IGFBP-3	7p	X64875	29	Glycosylated forms 40 and 44	Most abundant IGFBP in endocrine serum (mostly hepatic origin); made throughout the body (autocrine and paracrine)	IGF-dependent and IGF-independent effects on growth inhibition and apoptosis; regulated by growth hormone; peak serum levels at puberty
IGFBP-4	17q	Y12508	24	Glycosylated 28	High levels extracellularly and found in all biological fluids	Exists mostly as extracellular solute
IGFBP-5	2q	NM000599 (mRNA)	29	Several glycosylated forms ranging from 29 to 32	Binds to bone with high affinity; main IGFBP in kidney; high levels in CSF, connective tissues and fetal tissues	Only binding protein with nuclear localization other than IGFBP-3
IGFBP-6	12q	AJ006952	22	O-glycosylated 34	High levels in CSF and serum	Only IGFBP preferentially binding IGF-II

[a]For additional information, *see* **refs. 13** and **57.**
[b]For additional information, *see* **refs. 58** and **59.**

recombinant hIGFBP-5 showed IGFBP-5 can stimulate growth in an IGF-independent manner *(22)*. Nuclear transport of IGFBP-5, as well as IGFBP-3, requires the C-terminus region containing the NLS and is mediated by the importin-beta subunit *(23)*.

IGFBP-3 is not only an active member of the IGF axis, but also other cellular pathways including the tumor suppressor, p53 *(24)*. IGFBP-3 is induced by p53 *(25,26)*, WT-I *(27)*, retinoic acid *(28)*, and cytokines *(29)*. In addition, IGFBP-3 mediates p53-induced apoptosis during serum starvation *(30)*.

1.5. IGFBP-rPs

There are at least nine IGFBP-rPs. They are defined by the presence of a cysteine-rich N-terminal domain, homologous to that of the IGFBPs, yet low-affinity binding to IGFs, in contrast to the high-affinity binding of the IGFBPs *(13)*. Conservation of the N-terminal domain is seen among human, mammalian, and other vertebrate and Drosophila protein sequences and lends support for the proposed evolution of a common ancestoral gene among the IGFBP superfamily *(31)*. As the sequences near the C-terminus, a region thought to assist in high-affinity binding to IGFs, the similarity between IGFBPs and IGFBP-rPs decreases to 15% or less. It has been hypothesized that the lack of a C-terminus similar to IGFBPs may account for the low-affinity binding to IGFs exhibited by IGFBP-rPs. The IGFBP-rPs have been implicated in the regulation of cell growth and carcinogenesis in a variety of systems *(13)*.

1.6. Changes in the IGF Axis in Lung Cancer and Methods of Detection

1.6.1. Systemic Changes in Lung Cancer

Multiple large case-control studies have shown a correlation between serum concentrations of IGF-I positively and IGFBP-3 negatively to the risk of cancer. These relationships are associations and do not prove causation. In one hospital-based study, serum was collected from 204 consecutive patients whose primary lung cancer was histologically confirmed, and 218 control subjects matched to patients by age, sex, race, and smoking status. An enzyme-linked immunoabsorbent assay was used to measure plasma levels of IGF-I, IGF-II and IGFBP-3. Values were divided into quartiles, according to their distribution in the control subjects, and correlated to lung cancer risk by odds ratios (ORs). The highest quartile of IGF-I was associated with an increased risk of lung cancer (OR = 2.06; $p = 0.01$), but elevated plasma IGFBP-3 levels were linked to a lower risk of lung cancer (OR = 0.48; $p = 0.03$). Circulating levels of IGF-II did not correlate with the risk of lung cancer *(32)*.

A second study focused on the interactions of the IGF axis, intrinsic carcinogenic sensitivity, and lung cancer risk in 183 lung cancer patients and 227 matched control subjects. Carcinogen sensitivity was quantified using bleomycin- and benzo[a]pyrene diole poxide (BPDE)-induced chromatid breaks in peripheral blood lymphocyte cultures. Plasma IGF-I, IGF-II, and IGFBP-3 levels were measured by immunoassay. Increased IGF-I levels and carcinogen sensitivity were each linked to lung cancer (OR = 2.13 for IGF-I; OR = 2.50 for bleomycin sensitivity; OR = 2.95 for BPDE). Combining the IGF-I levels and the carcinogenic sensitivity further increased the risk of lung cancer (ORs up to 13.53) *(33)*.

Similar positive associations with IGF-I levels and negative associations with IGFBP-3 concentrations have also been found for prostate cancer *(34,35)* colorectal cancer *(36)*, leukemia *(37)*, and breast cancer *(38)*. These studies exemplify the importance of using correct techniques to quantify IGF-I levels. When IGF-I levels were measured by radioimmunoassay (RIA) following acid-ethanol extraction, a 28% increase was found among prostate cancer patients *(39)*. However, acid-ethanol extraction does not eliminate IGFBPs from the analysis. IGFBP-2, which is increased in prostate cancer *(40,41)*, can compete with the radiolabeled IGF-I trace and falsely raise the detected IGF-I level. This problem can be avoided by performing RIA after acid chromatography *(40)* or double antibody methods, like immuno-radiometric assay (IRMA) *(35)* and enzyme-linked immunosorbent assay (ELISA) *(34)*. Studies that employed these techniques concurred a 7–8% increase in IGF-I levels in patients with prostate cancer *(41)*.

1.6.2. Local Changes in Lung Cancer

Alterations of the IGF axis have been detected in in vitro studies of lung cancer biology. Conditioned medium of NSCLC and SCLC cell lines grown in serum- and hormone-free media, contained IGF-II and IGF-IR when isolated under acidic conditions and analyzed by Western ligand blot (WLB). NSCLC cell lines exhibited IGF-II expression in 8/10 cell lines and IGF-IR in 12/12. SCLC cell lines expressed IGF-II in 10/13 and IGF-IR in 14/14 *(42)*. The presence of both IGF-II and IGF-IR can facilitate autocrine and paracrine stimulation of cell growth.

Enhanced IGF mitogenic signaling can be achieved not only by increasing IGF production, but also by altering IGF-IR activity. NSCLC cell lines respond mitogenically to IGF-I and the enhanced growth can be blocked by an anti-IGF-IR antibody *(43)*. Stable transfection of a dominant negative IGF-IR into lung cancer cells resulted in suppressed tumorigenicity and increased sensitivity to apoptotic signals, such as UV radiation and proteasome inhibitors

(44). Antisense, shown to decrease the amount of IGF-IR by 50% in lung cancer cell lines, reduced soft agar clonogenicity by 84% *(45)*. In contrast, lung cancer cell lines transfected with a plasmid expressing a full-length human IGF-IR cDNA exhibited enhanced proliferation in response to IGF-I and acquired invasive potential *(46)*.

IGF action in lung cancer can be further modulated through changes in the IGFBPs. Lung cancer cell lines express all six IGFBPs *(47–50)*. IGFBP-1 has been detected in lung cancer cell lines using Northern-blot analysis and reverse transcriptase polymerase chain reaction (RT-PCR) *(51)*, however, some primary lung cancer tumors do not express IGFBP-1 *(48)*. In SCLC cell lines, both soluble and membrane-associated IGFBP-2 are the preferred binding sites for IGF-I and IGF-II *(52)*. Stable transfection of hIGFBP-3 cDNA into NSCLC cell lines was used to study the effects of IGFBP-3 on lung cancer cell growth. The transfected NSCLC cell lines, with a 20-fold increase in IGFBP-3 protein relative to control cell lines, grew more slowly in serum-containing medium and lost the growth response normally seen to IGF-I, IGF-II, Long R(3) IGF-I, or insulin. Furthermore, the transfected cell lines had absent or minimal tumor growth when xenotransplanted into nude mice *(53)*. Degradation of IGFBP-4 occurs in NSCLC cell lines with increased conditioned medium concentrations of IGFs, but not insulin or IGF-I analog *(50,54)*. IGFBP-5 transcripts of varied lengths, isolated from lambda gt10 libraries of SCLC cell lines, were found in both normal and cancerous lung cell lines *(49)*. Infection of a NSCLC cell line with an adenovirus expressing hIGFBP-6 activated programmed cell death. Intratumoral injection of the same hIGFBP-6 viral construct decreased the NSCLC xenograft size in nude mice by 45% *(55)*.

Alterations in IGFBP production in lung cancer or any other cellular system can be detected by western ligand blot (WLB) or Western immunoblot (IMB), two variations of the Western-blot technique *(56)*. WLBs utilize ^{125}I-labeled IGF-I and ^{125}I-labeled IGF-II to detect any and all proteins in the experimental system with high-affinity binding to IGFs. Using this method, multiple IGFBPs are detected and their identities can be inferred from the molecular weights of the respective bands visualized on the WLB film. Specific IMBs, utilizing primary antibodies unique to a particular IGFBP, confirm the identity of the IGFBPs. WLB and IMB can be equally effective for conditioned medium, to detect secreted IGFBPs, and cell pellets, for intracellular IGFBPs. **Figure 1** depicts a flow chart for WLB and IMB.

2. Materials

2.1. Lyophilization of Conditioned Medium (CM)

1. Commercial Integrated SpeedVac.
2. 1X Phosphate-buffered saline (PBS; Boehringer Mannheim, Indianapolis, IN).

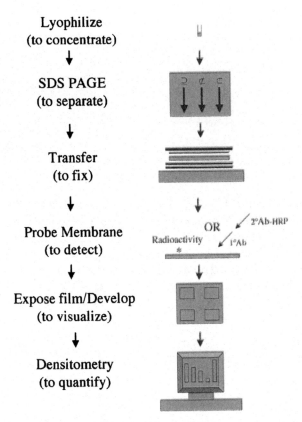

Fig. 1. Flow chart of Western-blot techniques. There are two probe variations of a Western-blot technique: radioactively labeled ligand probes (WLB) and antibody probes (IMB). Each variation can be carried out separately or in series. The initial steps of the techniques are identical. First, the CM samples are lyophilized to concentrate the proteins. Then, the resuspended samples are separated by electrophoresis. Thirdly, the proteins are permanently transferred from the SDS gel to a membrane, in this case nitrocellulose. Use of ligand or antibody probes detects the transferred proteins. The probed membranes expose X-ray film, which is developed, and the signal intensity quantified by densitometry.

2.2. 12.5% Sodium Dodecyl Sulfate Polyacrylamide Gel Electrophoresis (SDS-PAGE)

1. SDS-PAGE apparatus (methods described here for 16-cm apparatus) and power source.
2. 100% Ethanol.
3. 30% Acrylamide/Bis solution, 37:5:1 (2.6% C).
4. Distilled water.

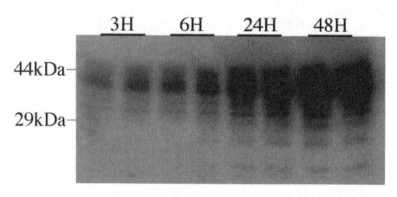

Fig. 2. WLB of CM of H460 cells in serum starvation. H460 cells were plated in 6-well culture plates. Complete medium was changed to serum-free medium. After periods of serum starvation, CM was collected up to 48 h and separated by 12.5% SDS-PAGE. The membranes were incubated overnight with ^{125}I-labeled IGF-I and ^{125}I-labeled IGF-2. Film was exposed for 5 d at –80°C. Bands are seen at 44, 40, 34, 31, 29, and 24 kDa. From our experience with other IMB (data not shown), these correspond to IGFBP-3 (doublet), 6, 2, 1, and 4, respectively. The position of the molecular-weight marker is shown at the left.

5. 10% Ammonium persulfate (APS).
6. 69% Glycerol.
7. N-Butanol.
8. TEMED.
9. Control specimen(s) are optional, but recommended.
10. Experimental samples.
    a. Conditioned medium.
    b. Cell pellets (collected in 1X sample buffer).
11. Rubber stopper.
12. Prestained molecular-weight marker.
13. Prewritten, asymmetrical gel plan.
14. 4X Lower gel buffer, pH 8.8: Tris-HCl 36.9 g, Tris Base 153.9 g, SDS 4.0 g, and 750 mL distilled water (store at 4°C).
15. 4X Upper gel buffer, pH 6.8: (pH 6.8) Tris Base 30.3g, SDS 2.0 g, and 500 mL distilled water (store at 4°C).
16. 4X SDS sample buffer: for 100 mL, 9.2 g SDS, 50 mL glycerol, 50 mL 4X upper gel buffer and 10 mg Bromophenol Blue (store at 4°C).
17. SDS running buffer: for 1 L of 10X buffer, 30.3 g Tris base, 144.0 g glycine, and 10.0 g SDS (store at 4°C).

2.3. Gel Transfer

1. Shallow, stackable plastic trays large enough to hold the SDS gels/membranes and the solutions for washing/antibody incubations.

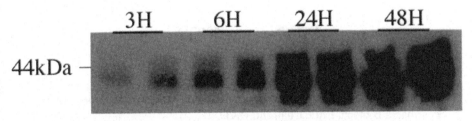

Fig. 3. IGFBP-3 IMB of CM of H460 cells in serum starvation. The NC membrane from **Fig. 2** was probed with a primary antibody (high-affinity purified polyclonal goat anti-hIGFBP-3 antibody from Diagnostic Systems Laboratories, Webster, TX) for 2 h, followed by a secondary antibody (HRP-linked rabbit anti-goat IgG from Chemicon International, Inc, Temecula, CA) incubation overnight. IGFBP-3 doublet results from gel separation of the two glycosylated forms of IGFBP-3. The position of the molecular-weight marker is shown at the left.

2. Nitrocellulose (NC) membranes ($5.5'' \times 6.5''$).
3. Blotting paper ($6'' \times 6.5''$).
4. Porous cellophane ($6.5'' \times 7''$).
5. Commercial semi-dry transfer cell and power source.
6. Transfer Buffer: 25 mM Tris base, 192 mM glycine, and 20% (v/v) methanol (store at 4°C).

2.4. Probing Blots

2.4.1. Western Ligand Blotting (WLB)

1. Radioisotopes are specific to the target of the experiment. Here, ^{125}I-IGF-I and ^{125}I-IGF-II were used.
2. Tris-buffered saline (TBS). For 1 L: 8.766 g NaCl, 1.322 g Tris-HCl, and 0.194 g Tris (store at 4°C).
3. TBS/0.1% Tween-II0 (TBS-T): add 1 mL of Tween-II0 per 1 L (store at 4°C).
4. TBS/3% IGEPAL CA-630: add 30.0 mL IGEPAL CA-630 to 1 L of TBS (store at 4°C).
5. TBS-T/1% bovine serum albumin (BSA): add 10.0 g BSA to 1 L TBS-T (store at 4°C).

2.4.2. Western Immunoblotting (IMB)

2.4.2.1. Antibody Labeling

1. Shallow, stackable plastic trays with lid.
2. Primary antibody.
3. HRP-linked secondary antibody for ECL reaction.
4. Blotting-grade blocker non-fat dry milk.
5. Rotary shaker.

6. TBS (store at 4°C).
7. TBS-T (store at 4°C).

2.4.2.2. CHEMILUMINESCENT (ECL) REACTION

1. Shallow, stackable plastic trays.
2. Western blotting detection reagents for ECL reaction (available from Amersham Pharmacia Biotech, Little Chalfont, UK).

2.5. Visualization

1. Scientific imaging film.
2. Autoradiography cassette.
3. Cellophane wrap.
4. Adhesive laboratory tape.
5. Dark room and commercial developing machine.

3. Methods
3.1. Lyophilization of Conditioned Medium (CM)

1. Lyophilize CM samples overnight to concentrate the proteins.
2. Resuspend the pellet in 150 µL of 1X PBS (one-tenth the original volume of CM collected) (*see* **Note 1**).

3.2. 12.5% SDS Polyacrylamide Gel Electrophoresis (PAGE)

1. Assemble the gel apparatus (*see* **Note 2**).
2. Refer to **Table 2** for SDS-PAGE reagent calculations.

3.2.1. Preparation of Lower Gel

1. According to the number of gels desired, mix the appropriate volumes of the following ingredients in a 250-mL beaker with a vacuum attachment: 30% Acrylamide/Bis solution, Distilled water, 4X lower gel buffer and 10% APS.
2. Stopper the flask, connect the vacuum hose to the vacuum extension of the flask, and de-gas the flask for at least 1 min.
3. Add 20 µL of TEMED per gel and gently swirl the flask to mix.
4. Pipet the gel mix into a corner of the casting apparatus until the solution is approx one-and-a-half inches from the top of the gel plate (*see* **Note 3**).
5. Pipet approx 1 mL of N-Butanol on top of each lower gel and allow the lower gel to polymerize for at least 1 h.
6. Once polymerized, rinse the gel and the casting apparatus with distilled water and allow it to drain.

3.2.2. Preparation of Upper Gel

1. Combine the appropriate amounts (*see* **Table 2**) of the following ingredients in a 125-mL flask with vacuum extension: 30% Acrylamide/Bis solution, distilled water, 4X upper gel buffer, 69% glycerol, and 10% APS.

Table 2
SDS-PAGE Gel Calculations

	Reagents	1 Gel	2 Gels	3 Gels	4 Gels
Lower gel					
6% Gel	30% Acrylamide/Bis, 37:5:1 (2.6% C)	8 mL	16 mL	24 mL	32 mL
	H_2O	22 mL	44 mL	66 mL	88 mL
	4X Lower Gel Buffer	10 mL	20 mL	30 mL	40 mL
	10% APS	132 µL	264 µL	396 µL	528 µL
8% Gel	30% Acrylamide/Bis, 37:5:1 (2.6% C)	10.6 mL	21.2 mL	31.8 mL	42.4 mL
	H_2O	19.4 mL	38.8 mL	58.2 mL	77.6 mL
	4X Lower Gel Buffer	10 mL	20 mL	30 mL	40 mL
	10% APS	132 µL	264 µL	396 µL	528 µL
10% Gel	30% Acrylamide/Bis, 37:5:1 (2.6% C)	13.3 mL	26.6 mL	39.9 mL	53.2 mL
	H_2O	16.7 mL	33.4 mL	50.1 mL	66.8 mL
	4X Lower Gel Buffer	10 mL	20 mL	30 mL	40 mL
	10% APS	132 µL	264 µL	396 µL	528µL
12.5% Gel	30% Acrylamide/Bis, 37:5:1 (2.6% C)	16.7 mL	33.4 mL	50.1 mL	66.8 mL
	H_2O	13.3 mL	26.6 mL	39.9 mL	53.2 mL
	4X Lower Gel Buffer	10 mL	20 mL	30 mL	40 mL
	10% APS	132 µL	264 µL	396 µL	528 µL
Upper gel					
	30% Acrylamide/Bis, 37:5:1 (2.6% C)	1.5 mL	3.0 mL	4.5 mL	6.0 mL
	H_2O	5.3 mL	10.6 mL	15.9 mL	21.2 mL
	4X Lower Gel Buffer	2.5 mL	5.0 mL	7.5 mL	10.0 mL
	69% Glycerol	0.66 mL	1.32 mL	1.98 mL	2.64 mL
	10% APS	30 µL	60 µL	90 µL	120 µL

2. Again, de-gas flask for at least 1 min.
3. While waiting, place the combs into the gel apparatus, taking care to align the front and back combs when running multiple gels.
4. After de-gasing, add 10 µL of TEMED per gel and swirl the flask gently to mix.
5. Again, pipet the gel mix from a corner of the casting apparatus, taking care to gently remove any bubbles that form in or around the gel combs.
6. Allow the upper gel to polymerize for approx 45 min.
7. Once polymerized, both the gel and the casting apparatus can be either wrapped in cellophane and saved for the next day or loaded immediately.

3.2.3. Loading Samples

1. Remove the combs slowly, rinse the wells and the casting apparatus with distilled water, and allow them to drain.
2. Place the gel cassettes in the apparatus frame and remove any bubbles from the wells with a syringe (*see* **Notes 4** and **5**).
3. Sample buffer must be added to some of the samples before loading:
   a. Add 50 μL 2X sample buffer to a 50 μL aliquot of CM and the control specimen, if used.
   b. Add 20 μL 1X sample buffer to a 20 μL aliquot of each pre-stained molecular-weight marker.
   c. The cell pellet should have been collected in 1X sample buffer, making those samples ready to load.
4. Load the gel according to a prewritten gel plan (*see* **Notes 6–8**).
5. Use running buffer to top off all the wells and to fill the gel tank about one-third full.

3.2.4. Gel Assembly and Electrophoresis

1. Place the gel tank, with a stir bar, onto a stir pad.
2. Place the gel frame, with attached gel cassettes, into the gel tank.
3. Stir at low speed.
4. Use running buffer to fill the upper chamber of the gel tank to the top of the large gel plate.
5. Cover the gel tank and connect to a power supply.
6. Run the gel overnight at 50V.
7. Stop the run when the blue marker reaches the bottom of the gel plates.

3.3. Gel Transfer

1. In transfer buffer, soak pre-cut pieces of NC membrane and blotting paper and set aside the appropriate number of pre-cut pieces of porous cellophane (refer to **step 5** below).
2. Take the gel frame out of the tank and remove the gel cassettes from the frame.
3. Place the gels in transfer buffer for approx 5 min (*see* **Note 9**).
4. Coat the base of the semi-dry transfer cell with enough transfer buffer to sufficiently wet the surface.
5. Layer the transfer stack: 2 sheets blotting paper (presoaked), 1 NC membrane (pre-soaked), 1 gel (face-up), 1 piece porous cellophane (dip in Transfer Buffer to wet), 1 sheet blotting paper, 1 NC membrane, gel, and so on. Continue this pattern for all gels to be transferred, ending with 2 sheets of blotting paper on top of the last gel.
6. Gently roll a pasteur pipet over the top of the transfer stack to remove any bubbles, as they can affect the transfer efficiency of the proteins from the gel to the NC membrane.

7. Pour Transfer Buffer (remaining from **step 1** above) onto the transfer stack.
8. Place the top onto the semi-dry transfer machine, connect it to the power supply, and run at 170V for 2.5 h (*see* **Note 10**).
9. After 2.5 h, remove the layers of the transfer stack slowly, checking first to make sure the transfer was successful (i.e., that the prestained markers transferred to the NC membrane).
10. Using a needle, poke holes in a straight line across the middle of the molecular marker bands on the membrane. This will allow visualization of the molecular markers after film developing.
11. Trim the NC membrane (approx 3/4") on the top, long side (can also be done once the membrane is dry) to allow it to fit into shaker trays for future washes.
12. Hang the membranes and allow them to air dry.
13. Once dry, label and trim, if not already done.

3.4. Probing Blots

3.4.1. Western Ligand Blotting (WLB)

1. Wet the NC membranes in TBS for 1–2 min at 4°C, shaking at medium speed (*see* **Note 11**).
2. Wash the membranes in TBS/3% IGEPAL CA-630 for 30 min at 4°C.
3. Discard the TBS/3% IGEPAL CA-630 solution and wash each membrane in 20 mL TBS-T/1% BSA for at least 2 h at 4°C.
4. Add the radioisotopes at the appropriate dilutions and shake overnight at 4°C (*see* **Note 12**).
5. Remove and dispose of the radioactive waste according to institutional guidelines.
6. Shake the membranes briefly in TBS-T.
7. Hang the membranes up to air dry for at least 1 h.

3.4.2. Western Immunoblotting (IMB)

3.4.2.1. ANTIBODY LABELING

1. Place each dried NC membrane into a shaker tray with enough TBS to cover the membrane completely.
2. Stack the trays, cover and shake at medium speed for 5 min at room temperature (*see* **Note 13**).
3. Make a blocking solution of 5% nonfat dried milk in TBS. Once in solution, pour out the TBS from the shaker trays and add approx 50 mL of 5% dried milk/TBS to the tilted corner of each tray.
4. Shake for 1 h (*see* **Note 14**).
5. Make a solution of 2% nonfat dried milk in TBS-T for the primary and secondary antibody incubations. Manufacturer's protocols for antibody incubation solutions may vary.
6. After 1 h, pour out the 5% blocking solution and wash the NC membrane(s) in TBS-T for 5 min.

7. Pour out the TBS-T, add 20 mL of the 2% dried milk/TBS-T solution and the primary antibody, according to the manufacturer's specifications.
8. Shake the primary antibody solution for 2 h.
9. After 2 h, pour out the primary antibody solution and rinse each membrane with TBS-T solution 3 × 10 min.
10. Next, add 20 mL of 2% nonfat dried milk/TBS-T and the HRP-conjugated secondary antibody, according to the manufacturer's specifications (*see* **Note 15**).
11. Shake the secondary antibody solution for 1 h.
12. Following the secondary antibody incubation, wash the membranes: 4 × 5 min in TBS-T and then 2 × 5 min in TBS (*see* **Note 16**).
13. Proceed immediately to the ECL reaction.

3.4.2.2. ECL REACTION

1. With the Amersham ECL kit the reagents are combined in a 1 : 1 ratio. For four membranes: combine and mix 20 mL Reagent 1 and 20 mL Reagent 2.
2. Add 20 mL of the ECL reagent solution to each of two membranes and shake at medium high speed for 2 min.
3. Using the same 20-mL aliquots of ECL solution, repeat **step 2** for the last two membranes (*see* **Note 17**).
4. Wrap the NC membranes in cellophane (*see* **Notes 18–24**).

3.5. Visualization

1. Tape the corners of the face-up, cellophane-covered membranes (IMB) or the membrane itself (WLB) onto a piece of film paper. Film paper is included with some X-ray film.
2. Expose the film. For WLB membranes, expose for 4–14 d at –80°C. For IMB membranes, expose briefly for 10–30 s and alter the time as needed.
3. Develop film and label the lanes.

4. Notes

1. When resuspending the lyophilized pellet of CM in 1X PBS, pipet up and down the sides of the tube to assure all protein is resuspended. If not fully and evenly resuspended, this step may alter the concentrations of the proteins detected by the Western blots.
2. Once assembled, check the bottom of the gel sandwich for proper alignment of the gel spacers and glass plates in order to eliminate areas where leakage may occur. Quadruple folds of parafilm can be added to the base of the gel casting tray to help avoid leakage.
3. If pouring multiple gels (a maximum of four), pour the back gel first.
4. To minimize clean-up, use a sink when placing gel cassettes into apparatus frame. This also allows for better leverage in placing the cassettes securely into the frame.
5. To create a firm seal, pour running buffer over the apparatus frame before attaching the gel cassettes.

6. If loading multiple gels, load the back gel first. This allows for complete visualization of all wells as they are individually loaded.

7. Use an asymmetrical, prewritten gel plan to distinguish right-left orientation when working with multiple gels. Asymmetry can be achieved by loading molecular-weight markers in different lanes for each gel or by using markers with varied banding patterns. This will help to prevent confusion during the remaining steps, should a gel be flipped during transfer or a membrane be left unlabeled.

8. The corner of a kim-wipe can be used to remove bubbles from the tops of wells after sample loading.

9. When removing the gels from the gel plates, use the edge of a gel spacer (wet in transfer buffer first) to loosen one edge of the gel.

10. Alternatively, the gel transfer can be carried out at a lower voltage for a longer period of time.

11. All washes during the WLB are done at medium speed and at 4°C.

12. If desired, the radioisotope solution can be allowed to incubate longer than overnight at 4°C. Use the proper radioactive safety precautions, personal monitoring devices, and waste disposal for radioisotope work. Store the radioisotopes according to the manufacturer's specifications until ready to aliquot and use. Here, 5μCi of each radioisotope was resuspended in 1 mL of 1X PBS and then aliquots of 100 μL were used for each membrane. The exposure time may vary depending on the experiment.

13. During the IMB, all washes are done at a medium speed and room temperature (exception to temperature, *see* **Note 14** below)

14. The primary or secondary antibody solution can be left to shake at a medium speed overnight at 4°C.

15. The secondary antibody must be HRP-linked in order to be used in the ECL reaction, as it is the conjugated HRP that reacts with the chemiluminescent substrates to generate the light signal. It is this signal that is visualized when the exposed film is developed.

16. Prepare the reagents and utensils needed for the ECL reaction during the last 5-min wash with TBS. This saves time and optimizes the intensity of ECL, which is time-sensitive. Although it has preservative qualities, do not use Sodium Azide in TBS or TBS-T solutions, as it will largely inhibit the HRP-linked enzyme activity of the secondary antibody. Without Tween-II0 in the washing solutions, there may be more background upon developing of the films.

17. Re-using the ECL solution amongst membranes during the same IMB is advantageous financially, as the reagents are very expensive, and does not affect the quality of the exposure/developing.

18. Only the IMB membranes are wrapped in cellophane. The WLB membranes are taped directly to the film paper.

19. Cut several pieces of blotting paper into small strips (approx 1″ × 3″) and use the edge of them to push out any excess liquid when sealing a NC membrane in cellophane.

20. Wrapping the IMB membranes in cellophane is important, as it is essential that the membranes are not allowed to dry out after the ECL reaction.
21. Before exposing the film, nicks or cuts can be made in the membranes or film corners to distinguish the orientation of the membranes on the developed film.
22. Increase the exposure time if the band intensity is unsatisfactory, but keep in mind the ECL reaction has limited intensity (i.e. there is very little difference between a 2-h exposure and a film exposed overnight).
23. If high background occurs on the developed film, try one of the following: a) repeat the final series of 5-min washing steps and the ECL reaction, b) repeat both the Immunoblot and the ECL reaction, or c) repeat the IMB after using a blocking solution of 5% BSA in TBS.
24. The same membrane(s) can be probed several times using the same WLB/IMB procedure. Store the membranes at 4°C. Allow a few weeks between WLBs and a few days between IMBs.

Acknowledgments

This work was supported in part by the Lawson Wilkins Pediatric Endocrine Society Genentech Clinical Scholar Award (AG) and Molecular Approaches to Pediatric Science Child Health Research Center Program Award (AG). H460 cells were generously donated by Dr. Wafik El-Deiry. We are grateful to Dr. Pinchas Cohen, who first taught us the Western-blotting techniques for evaluating the IGFBPs.

References

1. Chin, E., Zhou, J., Dai, J., et al. (1994) Cellular localization of gene expression for components of the IGF ternary complex. *Endocrinol.* **134,** 2498–2504.
2. Baxter, R. C. (1994) Insulin-like growth factor binding proteins in the human circulation: a review. *Horm Res.* **42,** 140–144.
3. Guler, Z. S., Oh, Y., Kelley, K. M., and Rosenfield, R. G. (1989) Insulin-like growth factors I and II in healthy man: estimations of half-lives and production rates. *Acta Endocrinol.* **121,** 753–758.
4. Baxter, R. C. and Daughaday, W. H. (1991) Impaired formation of the ternary insulin-like growth factor binding protein complex in patients with hypoglycemia due to nonislet cell tumors. *J. Clin. Endocrinol. Metab.* **73,** 696–702.
5. Grimberg, A. and Cohen, P. (2000) Role of insulin-like growth factors and their binding proteins in growth control and carcinogenesis. *J. Cell Phys.* **183,** 1–9.
6. Underwood, L. E. (1996) Nutritional regulation of IGF-1 and IGFBPs. *J. Pediatr. Endocrinol. Metab.* **9(3 Suppl.),** 303–312.
7. Birnbacher, R., Amann, G., Breitschopf, H., et al. (1998) Cellular localization of insulin-like growth factor II mRNA in the human fetus and the placenta: detection with a digoxigenin-labeled cRNA probe and immounochemistry. *Pediatr Res.* **43,** 614–620.

8. Gerrard, D. E., Okamura, C. S., Ranalletta, M. A., and Grant, A. L. (1998) Developmental expression and location of IGF-1 and IGF-2 mRNA and protein in skeletal muscle. *J. Anim. Sci.* **76,** 1004–1011.

9. Ullrich, A., Gray, A., Tam, A. W., et al. (1986) Insulin-like growth factor I receptor primary structure: comparison with insulin receptor suggests structural determinants that define functional specificity. *EMBO J.* **5,** 2503–2512.

10. Treadway, J. L., Morrison, B. D., Goldfine, I. D., et al. (1989) Assembly of insulin-insulin-like growth factor-I hybrid receptors in vitro. *J. Biol. Chem.* **264,** 21450.

11. Ludwig, T., Eggenschwiler, J., Fisher, P., et al. (1996) Mouse mutants lacking the type 2 IGF receptor (IGF-2R) are rescued from perinatal lethality in Igf2 and Igf1r null backgrounds. *Dev. Biol.* **177,** 517–535.

12. Ellis, M. J., Leav, B. A., Yang, Z., et al. (1996) Affinity for the insulin-like growth factor-II (IGF-2) receptor inhibits autocrine IGF-2 activity in MCF-7 breast cancer cells. *Mol. Endocrinol.* **10,** 286–297.

13. Hwa, V., Youngman, O., and Rosenfeld, R. G. (1999) The insulin-like growth factor binding protein (IGFBP) superfamily. *Endocr. Rev.* **20,** 761–787.

14. Li, Y. M., Schacher, D. H., Liu, Q., et al. (1997) Regulation of myeloid growth and differentiation by the insulin-like growth factor-I receptor. *Endocrinol.* **138,** 362–368.

15. Oh, Y., Muller, H. L., Lamson, G. and Rosenfeld R. G. (1993) Insulin-like growth factor (IGF)-independent action of IGF-binding protein-3 in Hs578T human breast cancer cells. Cell surface binding and growth inhibition. *J. Biol. Chem.* **268,** 14964–14971.

16. Yamanaka, Y., Fowlkes, J. L., Wilson, E. M., et al. (1999) Characterization of insulin-like growth factor binding protein-3 (IGFBP-3) binding to human breast cancer cells: kinetics of IGFBP-3 binding and identification of receptor binding domain on the IGFBP-3 molecule. *Endocrinology* **140,** 1319–1328.

17. Mannhardt, B., Weinzimer, S.A., Wagner, M., et al. (2000) Human papillomavirus type 16 E7 oncoprotein binds and inactivates growth-inhibitory insulin-like growth factor binding protein 3. *Mol. Cell Biol.* **20,** 6483–6495.

18. Jaques, G., Noll, K., Wegmann, B., et al. (1997) Nuclear localization of insulin-like growth factor binding protein 3 in lung cancer cell line. *Endocrinol.* **138,** 1767–1770.

19. Schedlich, L. J., Young, T. F., Firth, S. M., and Baxter, R. C. (1998) Insulin-like growth factor-binding protein (IGFBP)-3 and IGFBP-5 share a common nuclear transport pathway in T47D human breast carcinoma cells. *J. Biol. Chem.* **273,** 18347–18352.

20. Wraight, C. J., Liepe, I. J., White, P. J., et al. (1998) Intranuclear localization of insulin-like growth factor binding protein-3 (IGFBP-3) during cell division in human keratinocytes. *J. Invest. Dermatol.* **111,** 239–242.

21. Liu, B., Lee, H. Y., Weinzimer, S. A., et al. (2000) Direct functional interactions between insulin-like growth factor-binding protein-3 and retinoid X receptor-alpha regulate transcriptional signaling and apoptosis. *J. Biol. Chem.* **275,** 33607–33613.

22. Miyakoshi, N., Richmann, C., Kasukawa, Y., et al. (2001) Evidence that IGF-binding protein-5 functions as a growth factor. *J. Clin. Invest.* **107**, 73–81.

23. Schedlich, L. J., Le Page, S. L., Firth, S. M., et al. (2000) Nuclear import of insulin-like growth factor-binding protein-3 and -5 is mediated by the importin beta subunit. *J. Biol. Chem.* **275**, 23462–23470.

24. Grimberg, A. (2000) p53 and IGFBP-3: apoptosis and cancer protection. *Mol. Genet. Metab.* **70**, 85–98.

25. Buckbinder, L., Talbott, R., Velasco-Miguel, S., et al. (1995) Induction of the growth inhibitor IGF-binding protein 3 by p53. *Nature* **377**, 646–649.

26. Bourdon, J. C., Deguin-Chambon, V., Lelong, J. C., et al. (1997) Further characterisation of the p53 responsive element-identification of new candidate genes for trans-activation by p53. *Oncogene* **14**, 85–94.

27. Dong, G., Rajah, R., Vu, T., et al. (1997) Decreased expression of Wilms' tumor gene WT-1 and elevated expression of insulin growth factor-II (IGF-II) and type 1 IGF receptor genes in prostatic stromal cells from patients with benign prostatic hyperplasia. *J. Clin. Endocrinol. Metab.* **82**, 2198–2203.

28. Shang, Y., Baumrucker, C. R., and Green, M. H. (1999) Signal relay by retinoic acid receptors alpha and beta in the retinoic acid-induced expression of insulin-like growth factor-binding protein-3 in breast cancer cells. *J. Biol. Chem.* **274**, 18005–18010.

29. Wang, D., Nagpal, M. L., Shimasaki, S., et al. (1995) Interleukin-I induces insulin-like growth factor binding protein-3 gene expression and protein production by Leydig cells. *Endocrinology* **136**, 4049–4055.

30. Grimberg, A., Bingrong, L., Bannerman, P., et al. (2002) IGFBP-3 mediates p53-induced apoptosis during serum starvation. *Int. J. Oncol.*, in press.

31. Doolittle, R. F. (1995) The multiplicity of domains in proteins. *Annu. Rev. Biochem.* **64**, 287–314.

32. Yu, H., Spitz, M. R., Mistry, J. et al. (1999) Plasma levels of insulin-like growth factor-I and lung cancer risk: a case-control analysis. *J. Natl. Cancer Inst.* **91**, 151–156.

33. Wu, X., Yu, H., Amos, C. I., Hong, W. K. and Spitz, M. R. (2000) Joint effect of insulin-like growth factors and mutagen sensitivity in lung cancer risk. *J. Natl. Cancer Inst.* **92**, 737–743.

34. Chan, J.M., Stampfer, M.J., Giovanucci, E., et al. (1998) Plasma insulin-like growth factor-I and prostate cancer risk: a prospective study. *Science* **279**, 563–566.

35. Wolk, A., Mantzoros, C.S., Andersson, O., et al. (1998) Insulin-like growth factor I and prostate cancer risk: a population-based, case-control study. *J. Natl. Cancer Inst.* **90**, 911–915.

36. Ma, J., Pollack, M. N., Giovanucci, E., et al. (1999) Prospective study of colorectal cancer risk in men and plasma levels of insulin-like growth factor (IGF)-I and IGF-binding protein-3. *J. Natl. Cancer Inst.* **91**, 620–625.

37. Petridou, E., Dessypris, N., Spanos, E., et al. (1999) Insulin-like growth factor-I and binding protein-3 in relation to childhood leukemia. *Intl. J. Cancer* **80**, 494–496.

38. Hankinson, S. E., Willett, W. C., Colditz, G. A., et al. (1998) Circulating concentrations of insulin-like growth factor-I and risk of breast cancer. *Lancet* **351**, 1393–1396.

39. Mantzoros, C. S., Tzonou, A., Signorello, L. B., et al. (1997) Insulin-like growth factor 1 in relation to prostate cancer and benign prostatic hyperplasia. *Br. J. Cancer* **76**, 1115–1118.

40. Cohen, P., Peehl, D. M., Stamey, T. A., et al. (1993) Elevated levels of insulin-like growth factor binding protein-2 in the serum of prostate cancer patients. *J. Clin. Endocrinol. Metab.* **76**, 1031–1035.

41. Grimberg, A. and Cohen, P. (1999) Growth hormone and prostate cancer: guilty by association? *J. Endocrinol. Invest.* **22(5 Suppl.)**, 64–73.

42. Quinn, K. A., Treston, A. M., Unsworth, E. J., et al. (1996) Insulin-like growth factor expression in human cancer cell lines. *J. Biol. Chem.* **271**, 11477–11483.

43. Favoni, R. E., de Cupis, A., Ravera, F., et al. (1994) Expression and function of the insulin-like growth factor I system in human non-small cell lung cancer and normal lung cell lines. *Intl. J. Cancer* **56**, 858–866.

44. Jiang, Y., Rom, W. N., Yie, T. A., et al. (1999) Induction of tumor suppression and glandular differentiation of A549 lung carcinoma cells by dominant-negative IGF-1 receptor. *Oncogene* **18**, 6071–6077.

45. Lee, C. T., Wu, S., Gabrilovich, D., et al. (1996) Antitumor effects of an adenovirus expressing antisense insulin-like growth factor I receptor on human lung cancer cell lines. *Cancer Res.* **56**, 3038–3041.

46. Long, L., Rubin, R., and Brodt, P. (1998) Enhanced invasion and liver colonization by lung carcinoma cells overexpressing the type 1 insulin-like growth factor receptor. *Exp. Cell Res.* **238**, 116–121.

47. Kiefer, P., Jaques, G., Schoneberger, J., et al. (1991) Insulin-like growth factor binding protein expression in human small cell lung cancer cell lines. *Exp. Cell Res.* **192**, 414–417.

48. Jaques, G., Kiefer, P., Schoneberger, H.J., et al. (1992) Differential expression of insulin-like growth factor binding proteins in human non-small cell lung cancer cell lines. *Eur. J. Cancer* **28A**, 1899–1904.

49. Wegmann, B. R., Schoneberger, H. J., Kiefer, P. E., et al. (1993) Molecular cloning of IGFBP-5 from SCLC cell lines and expression of IGFBP-4, IGFBP-5 and IGFBP-6 in lung cancer cell lines and primary tumours. *Eur. J. Cancer* **29A**, 1578–1584.

50. Noll, K., Wegmann, B. R., Havemann, K., and Jaques G. (1996) Insulin-like growth factors stimulate the release of insulin-like growth factor-binding protein-3 (IGFBP-3) and degradation of IGFBP-4 in non-small cell lung cancer cell lines. *J. Clin. Endocrinol. Metab.* **81**, 2653–2662.

51. Reeve, J. G., Brinkmann, A., Hughes, S., et al. (1992) Expression of insulin-like growth factor (IGF) and IGF-binding protein genes in human lung tumor cell lines. *J. Natl. Cancer Inst.* **84**, 628–634.

52. Reeve, J. G., Morgan, J., Schwander, J., and Bleehen, N. M. (1993) Role for membrane and secreted insulin-like growth factor-binding protein-2 in the regulation of insulin-like growth factor action in lung tumors. *Can. Res.* **53**, 4680–4685.

53. Hochscheid, R., Jaques, G., and Wegmann, B. (2000) Transfection of human insulin-like growth factor-binding protein 3 gene inhibits cell growth and tumorigenicity: a cell culture model for lung cancer. *J. Endocrinol.* **166,** 553–563.

54. Price, W. A., Moats-Staats, B. M., and Stiles, A. D. (1995) Insulin-like growth factor-I (IGF-1) regulates IGFBP-3 and IGFBP-4 by multiple mechanisms in A549 human adenocarcinoma cells. *Am. J. Respir. Cell Mol. Biol.* **13,** 466–476.

55. Sueoka, N., Lee, H. Y., Wiehle, S., et al. (2000) Insulin-like growth factor binding protein-6 activates programmed cell death in non-small cell lung cancer cells. *Oncogene* **19,** 4432–4436.

56. Hossenlopp, P., Seurin, D., Segovia-Quinson, B., et al. (1986) Analysis of serum insulin-like growth factor binding proteins using Western blotting: use of the method for titration of binding proteins and competitive bind studies. *Anal. Biochem.* **154,** 138–143.

57. Ferry, R. J., Jr., Katz, L. E. L., Grimberg, A., et al (1999) Cellular actions of insulin-like growth factor binding proteins. *Horm. Metab. Res.* **31,** 192–202.

58. Coverley, J.A. and Baxter, R.C. (1997) Phosphorylation of insulin-like growth factor binding proteins. *Mol. Cell Endocrinol.* **128,** 1–5.

59. Jones, J. I, D'Ercole, J. D., Camacho-Hubner, C., and Clemmons, D. R. (1991) Phosphorylation of insulin-like growth factor (IGF)-binding protein 1 in cell culture and in vivo: Effects on affinity for IGF-I. *Proc. Natl. Acad. Sci. USA* **88,** 7481–7485.

12

Screening of Mutations in the ras Family of Oncogenes by Polymerase Chain Reaction-Based Ligase Chain Reaction

Alfredo Martínez, Teresa A. Lehman, Rama Modali, and James L. Mulshine

1. Introduction

Lung cancer is the most common fatal type of cancer in the developed world. The overwhelming majority of cases of lung cancer are caused by tobacco products *(1)*, and even with the best therapeutic approaches, less than 15% of diagnosed cases survive 5 years *(2)*. It has been noted that even after smoking cessation, the risk of lung cancer remains elevated for over 15 years *(3)*. This observation clearly indicates that lung cancer has a protracted course developing over a 10–20-yr period, from the moment in which an epithelial cell becomes initiated by chronic exposure to chemical insults until a clinically evident cancer is detected. The long latency period generated by this biology provides an important window of opportunity to find transformed precancerous cells in high-risk populations and intervene in a timely manner.

The initiation of a malignant cell occurs through an accumulation of several somatic genetic alterations involving genes that have a critical role in normal cell growth regulation. Detection of the critical genetic events may provide biomarkers for early detection. Some molecular changes can lead to activation of a gene or gene product that enhances cell growth leading to cancer, whereas other changes can lead to loss of gene function of critical regulatory elements involved in the control of cell growth. These genes relevant to the formation of a cancer include oncogenes, tumor-suppressor genes, and growth factors and their receptors *(4,5)*. Oncogenes are dominant genes that can induce or maintain cellular transformation. They are related to normal cellular genes,

From: *Methods in Molecular Medicine, vol. 74: Lung Cancer, Vol. 1: Molecular Pathology Methods and Reviews*
Edited by: B. Driscoll © Humana Press Inc., Totowa, NJ

called proto-oncogenes, which have critical functions in cellular growth or differentiation. Proto-oncogenes are tightly regulated and are activated at specific spatio-temporal points during development or the cell cycle. When they escape these strict controls, the proto-oncogenes become oncogenes and the cell is continually stimulated towards proliferation. Oncogenes may be activated in various ways that include amplification, chromosome translocation, and point mutations, among others.

Substitutions in a single codon, affecting the proper genes, can also lead to gain-of-function resulting in cellular transformation. These point mutations produce a single amino acid substitution in the protein coded by the oncogene, enough to transform susceptible cells. The p53 tumor-suppressor gene and the ras family of proto-oncogenes are the best known examples of this mechanism. The ras family consists of three main members (K-ras, H-ras, and N-ras). Accumulating evidence indicates that mutation of K-ras may be an early event in several types of cancer, including lung, colon, and pancreatic cancers *(6)*. The K-ras proto-oncogene encodes a guanine nucleotide-binding protein that helps relay signals from receptor tyrosine kinases to the nucleus through the MAP-kinase pathway (*see* **Fig. 1**).

One of the main advantages of using K-ras as a biomarker for the early detection of lung cancer is that most of the mutations leading to cell transformation are restricted to codons 12, 13, and 61. Moreover, in non-small cell lung cancer (NSCLC) and in colorectal cancer, most of these mutations are in the first position of codon 12 *(7)*.

Several methods have been employed for detecting ras mutations. They include polymerase chain reaction (PCR) with single-strand conformation polymorphism analysis *(8)*, PCR amplification using mismatched primers to create a "designed restriction fragment length polymorphism" *(9)*, PCR-PIREMA (Primer-Introduced Restriction with Enrichment for Mutation Alleles) *(10)*, and PCR-based ligase chain reaction *(11,12)*. The first two methods provide a sensitivity ranging from 3–25% mutant alleles in a normal DNA background, whereas the other two have an apparent sensitivity of less than 1%. Assay sensitivity is critical in this analysis, since clinical samples usually available from a population-based screening application (bronchoalveolar lavage fluid, sputum smears, etc) contain only a small variable percentage of bronchial epithelial cells with the relevant point-mutation. In this report, we will focus on the technique known as PCR-based ligase chain reaction for the detection of point mutations in K-ras codon 12 in bronchoalveolar lavage (BAL) clinical specimens *(11,12)*.

The technique begins by collecting the specimens properly *(13)* and extracting the DNA from them. An initial PCR amplification increases the amount of template available for the analytical reaction, which is performed by ligase

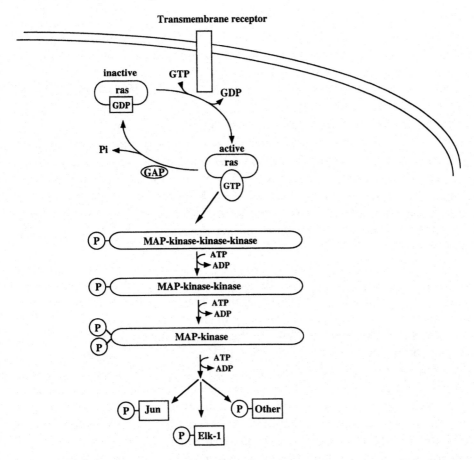

Fig. 1. Functional role of the ras proto-oncogene. When particular membrane receptor tyrosine kinases bind to their ligands in the cell surface, they activate ras by stimulating it to give up its GDP. As the concentration of GTP in the cytosol is 10 times greater than the concentration of GDP, ras will tend to bind GTP once GDP is ejected. In this state, ras will activate the cascade of MAP-kinases that ultimately will phosphorylate strategic proteins such as Jun and Elk-1, among others. The most common MAP-kinase-kinase-kinase that becomes activated by ras is a serine/threonine kinase called Raf. The whole system is deactivated by GTPase-activating proteins (GAP) that stimulate the hydrolysis of the ras bound GTP and keep the system in check. Mutations in codons 12, 13, or 61 result in amino acid changes, which in turn maintain ras in a permanently activated state.

chain reaction *(14)*. Finally, the reaction products are separated in a gel and exposed to X-ray film. The proper controls are provided by human tumor cell lines with known mutations in the first nucleotide of K-ras codon 12 *(15)*.

As an alternative to LCR, we (T.A.L., R.M.) have also developed a TaqMan-based assay to detect K-ras mutations at codon 12. TaqMan technology (ABI PRISM 7700 Sequence Detection System) has made significant advances in mutation detection and single nucleotide polymorphism (SNP) analysis. TaqMan analysis is a technique for the rapid real-time detection of specific DNA sequences using a closed-tube system *(16)*. This method utilizes fluorogenic oligonucleotide probes labeled with 5′ reporter and 3′ quencher dyes. A fluorescent signal is generated as the 5′ nuclease activity of Taq polymerase cleaves the reporter from the quencher during the amplification. The fluorescent emission is continuously monitored during the course of the reaction, and is represented as an amplification plot.

The frequency of detecting ras mutations in a clinical specimen is highly dependent on the sensitivity of the ras analysis assay. When using highly sensitive techniques such as those presented here, we can detect the presence of a particular mutation but the meaning of that mutation must be established with comprehensive clinical trials. In the reported studies *(11,12)*, 84% of the patients presented at least one mutation in K-ras codon 12, but the maximum expected rate of lung cancer development for this high-risk population is only 30% over the next 10 years. Therefore, the detection of a single point mutation does not necessarily mean the presence of an early lung cancer. Interestingly, the percentage of specimens with both a TGT and an AGT mutation (10/52, 19%) is closer to the cumulative expected percentage of cancer recurrences for this particular group. In addition, it has been reported that other events beyond an isolated ras mutation may be required to initiate a cancer *(17,18)*. Some of the cells carrying a single ras mutation may simply represent initiation events that do not become clonally expanded *(19)*.

It must be noted that the detection of ras mutations, though useful, must be put in perspective by analyzing other biomarkers and by developing a comprehensive protocol validated by pertinent clinical trials *(20–22)*. In addition, the clinical course for those individuals positive for a highly sensitive premalignant assay but without any actual evidence of a tumor must be determined. At the moment, the only possibility is to follow these individuals with more frequent check-ups, using such current technologies as chest X-rays, tomography, or even better the highly sensitive spiral computed tomography (CT) *(23)*. Nevertheless, we can envision a future in which these patients may receive treatment while tumor cells are still restricted to the respiratory epithelium. An important research effort is to define effective and minimally toxic chemopreventive agents to treat evolving lung cancer before that process develops invasive clinical behavior. These ongoing studies *(24–26)* will open the field of early intervention and chemoprevention in individuals of high-risk populations.

2. Materials

2.1. Positive Control Cell Lines

All can be purchased from the ATCC, Manassas, VA.

1. HeLa (K-ras codon 12 sequence GGT^{Gly}).
2. Calu 1 (K-ras codon 12 sequence TGT^{Cys}).
3. A549 (K-ras codon 12 sequence AGT^{Ser}).
4. H157 (K-ras codon 12 sequence CGT^{Arg}).
5. All of them grow on RPMI-1640 supplemented with 10% fetal calf serum (FCS).

2.2. Specimen Collection

1. Normal saline.
2. Protease inhibitors: aprotinin, EDTA, leupeptin, pepstatin, and phenylmethyl sulfonyl-fluoride (PMSF) (Sigma, St. Louis, MO).
3. Saccomanno's fixative: 50% ethanol plus 2% Carbowax 1540 (Union Carbide Corporation).

2.3. DNA Isolation

1. Proteinase K solution: 10 mM Tris-HCl, pH 7.8, 5 mM EDTA, 0.5% SDS, 200 µg/mL proteinase K (Boehringer Mannheim, Indianapolis, IN).
2. Phenol/chloroform (Insta-Mini-Prep kit, 5 Prime–3 Prime, Inc. Boulder, CO).
3. 100% ethanol.

2.4. PCR

All PCR reagents from Perkin Elmer, Boston, MA.
1. 1 M Tris-HCl, pH 8.4.
2. 1 M KCl.
3. 0.5 M MgCl$_2$.
4. Each dNTP, 40 mM stock.
5. Each primer (*see* **Table 1**).
6. Taq DNA polymerase.
7. 100 ng template DNA.

2.5. LCR

1. γ-AT-[^{32}P].
2. T4 polynucleotide kinase kit (Hoffmann-La Roche, Indianapolis, IN).
3. 1 M Tris-HCl, pH 7.6.
4. 0.5 M potassium acetate.

Table 1
**Sequence of the Primers Used for the PCR and LCR Phases
of the Technique**

Name	Bases	Sequence
PCR primers		
Sense	20	5′-CCT-GCT-GAA-AAT-GAC-TGA-AT-3′
Antisense	20	5′-TGT-TGG-ATC-ATA-TTC-GTC-CA-3′
LCR primers		
26 Ser	26	5′-GAT-ATT-TCT-TGT-GGT-AGT-TGG-AGC-TA-3′
23 Ser	23	5′-TTA-AAG-CTC-TTG-CCT-ACG-CCA-CT-3′
28 Cys	28	5′-ATG-ATA-TAA-CTT-GTG-GTA-GTT-GGA-GCT-T-3′
25 Cys	25	5′-AAT-TAA-AAC-TCT-TGC-CTA-CGC-CAC-A-3′
30 Arg	30	5′-AAA-TGA-TAT-AAC-TTG-TGG-TAG-TTG-GAG-CTC-3′
27 Arg	27	5′-AAA-ATT-AAA-ACT-CTT-GCC-TAC-GCC-ACG-3′
24 Gly	24	5′-TAA-AAC-TTG-TGG-TAG-TTG-GAG-CTG-3′
21 Gly	21	5′-AAC-ACT-CTT-GCC-TAC-GCC-ACC-3′
23 INV	23	5′-GTG-GCG-TAG-GCA-AGA-GTG-CGT-TG-3′
32 INV	32	5′-AGC-TCC-AAC-TAC-CAC-AAG-TTT-ATA-TTC-AGT-CA-3′

5. 3 M magnesium acetate.
6. 1 M DTT.
7. 0.1 M NAD⁺.

    7. 0.1 M NAD^+.
8. 10% Triton X-100.
9. 1 mg/mL salmon sperm DNA.
10. Taq DNA ligase (New England Biolabs, Beverly, MA).
11. Each diagnostic primer.
12. Each α-^{32}P-end-labeled invariant primer (at ≈ 4 × 10^5 cpm).
13. Template DNA from control cells and BAL samples.

2.6. Electrophoresis and Development

1. Gel loading buffer (Life Technologies, Gaithersburg, MD).
2. Precast 10% polyacrylamide gels containing 7 M urea (Novex, San Diego, CA).
3. X-OMAT AR film (Kodak, Rochester, NY).

2.7. TaqMan-Based Assay to Detect K-ras Mutations at Codon 12: Alternative to LCR

1. TaqMan probes, specific for wild-type plus each of 4 base pair changes in the K-ras 12 codon, fluorescent-labeled during synthesis. TaqMan probes are designed, synthesized and purified by BioServe Biotechnologies, Ltd. (Laurel, MD) using reagents from Applied Biosystems Division of Perkin Elmer (Foster City, CA).

2. 96-well reaction plates with optical grade caps (Applied Biosystems Division, Perkin Elmer).
3. 2X Universal Master Mix (Applied Biosystems Division, Perkin Elmer).
4. Primers (*see* **Subheading 3.7.1.**).
5. Template DNA from control cells and BAL samples.
6. ABI PRISM 7700 Sequence Detection System.

3. Methods

3.1. Positive Control Cell Lines

1. Cell lines are maintained in culture in RPMI-1640 supplemented with 10% FCS at 37°C in an atmosphere containing 5% CO_2 (*see* **Note 1**). DNA is extracted from 1×10^6 cells with Wizard Genomic DNA Purification Kit (Promega, Madison, WI), following manufacturer's guidelines.

3.2. Specimen Collection

1. Prepare normal saline for BAL collection and protease inhibitors for addition to collected material (*see* **Note 2**).
2. As part of an approved clinical protocol, following routine sedation of the patient, a flexible fiberoptic scope is inserted to examine the tracheal bronchial tree. The bronchoscope is wedged into one of the subsegments of the anterior segment of the right upper lobe for lavage. (In the event of right upper lobectomy, the anterior segment of the left upper lobe is lavaged.)
3. An aliquot of 60 mL sterile normal saline at room temperature is instilled through the bronchoscope. The fluid is immediately, but gently, hand-aspirated using the instilling syringe. The recovered fluid is placed in a sterile specimen cup, and a cocktail of protease inhibitors added at the following final concentrations: 7.8 μM aprotinin, 100 μM EDTA, 45 μM leupeptin, 1.0 μM pepstatin, 0.5 mM PMSF. Saline is instilled an additional three times for a total injected volume of 240 mL (*see* **Note 3**).
4. BAL fluid is divided in three portions and centrifuged at 200g for 10 min. In order to allow for multiple types of pathological analyses, supernatants are frozen in aliquots for further analysis (*see* **Note 4**).
5. Homogenize one of the pellets in a small volume of saline and freeze for future protein analysis.
6. Resuspended second pellet in normal saline, count cells, and aliquot into cell pellets containing about 1×10^6 cells each for future DNA extraction for Ligase chain reaction (LCR).
7. Fix remaining pellet in Saccomanno's fixative for morphological and immuno-cytochemical analysis *(13)*.

3.3. DNA Isolation

1. DNA is extracted from both cell lines and BAL specimens by incubating cell pellets of approximately 1×10^6 cells in proteinase K solution at 56°C overnight.

2. Cell lysate is subjected to phenol/chloroform extraction, and DNA is ethanol precipitated and pelleted.

3. DNA pellets are resuspended in 50 µL sterile water and quantitated by spectrophotometry: One µL of DNA solution is added to 500 µL H_2O and this solution read at a wavelength of 260 nm. The number obtained is multiplied by 25 and the result is expressed in µg/µL units.

3.4. PCR

1. PCR is required to amplify the region surrounding codon 12 of K-ras for further LCR analysis. Composition of a 50 µL reaction: 20 mM Tris-HCl, pH 8.4, 50 mM KCl, 2.5 mM MgCl$_2$, 0.2 mM each dNTP, 25 pmol each primer (*see* **Table 1**), 2.5 units Taq DNA polymerase, 100 ng template DNA. A typical analysis includes 20–30 BAL specimens plus the control cell lines.

2. The PCR primers (*see* **Table 1**) produce a 115 bp product. Samples are amplified for 35 cycles of 94°C for 1 min, 55°C for 1 min, and 72°C for 30 s (*see* **Note 5**).

3.5. LCR

1. Invariant primers (*see* **Table 1**) are end-labeled at the 5′ end with γ-AT-[^{32}P] using the T4 polynucleotide kinase kit from Hoffmann-La Roche (*see* **Note 6**).

2. Following PCR as described in **Subheading 3.4.**, 1 µL of each amplified DNA is added to a master mix of six mutated primers and two ^{32}P-labeled invariable primers (*see* **Table 1**) (*see* **Note 1**). Each 10 µL LCR reaction mixture contains: 20 mM Tris-HCl, pH 7.6, 25 mM potassium acetate, 10 mM magnesium acetate, 10 mM DTT, 1 mM NAD$^+$, 0.1% Triton X-100, 0.4 µg salmon sperm DNA, 15 nick closing units Taq DNA ligase, 40 fmol each diagnostic primer, 40 fmol each α-^{32}P-end-labeled invariant primer ($\approx 4 \times 10^5$ cpm), and approx 1 fmol template DNA.

3. A multiplex LCR is performed to determine the first base of codon 12 of the K-ras gene (*see* **Fig. 2**). Each 10 µL LCR reaction is overlaid with mineral oil and incubated at 94°C for 2.5 min, followed by 30 cycles of 94°C for 1 min and 65°C for 4 min (*see* **Note 5**).

3.6. Electrophoresis and Development for LCR

1. At the end of the LCR program, 2 µL of gel loading buffer and 4 µL of each reaction are heated together in a fresh tube at 94°C for 5 min, then chilled on ice.

2. Samples are loaded onto precast 10% polyacrylamide gels containing 7 M urea for polyacrylamide gel electrophoresis (PAGE).

3. Samples are subjected to PAGE at 150 V until the frontal dye reaches the bottom of the gel.

4. Gels are dried and exposed to X-ray film. An example of results is presented in **Fig. 3** (*see* **Notes 7,8**).

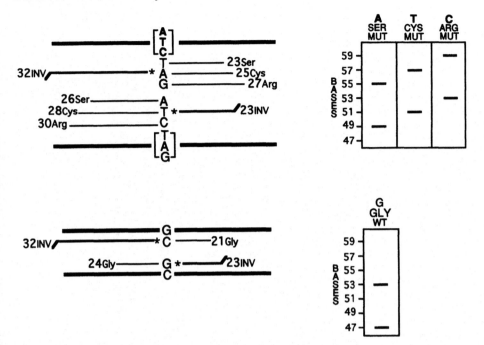

Fig. 2. Schematic representation of the PCR-based LCR assay strategy and primer design for determination of K-ras codon 12 mutations. (Upper diagram) A set of eight primers, including six diagnostic primers and two invariant labeled primers, are used in the LCR reaction mix for the determination of A, T, and/or C mutation (MUT) in the first base of K-ras codon 12. Diagnostic primer pairs are designated by their size and target base and represented schematically on the left panel. Gel analysis of LCR products of the reaction of each pair of diagnostic primers with the invariant primers 32INV and 23 INV (bold lines) results in the formation of the band patterns shown in the right panel. (Lower diagram) A schematic diagram illustrating the use of the wild-type primers 21 Gly and 24 Gly with the invariant primers 32INV and 23 INV in a separate LCR reaction. Gel analysis of the LCR products allows the detection of the presence of the wild-type base G in the first position of K-ras codon 12 as two bands of 47 and 53 bases shown in the right panel.

3.7. TaqMan-Based Assay to Detect K-ras Mutations at Codon 12: Alternative to LCR

1. Four TaqMan probes are prepared, one specific to the WT-G allele, and the other three specific to the A allele, C allele, and T allele (*see* **Note 9**).
   a. The WT probe is dual labeled with tetrachlorofluorescein (TET) and 6-carboxy-tetramethylrodhamine succinimidyl ester (TAMRA) during synthesis.

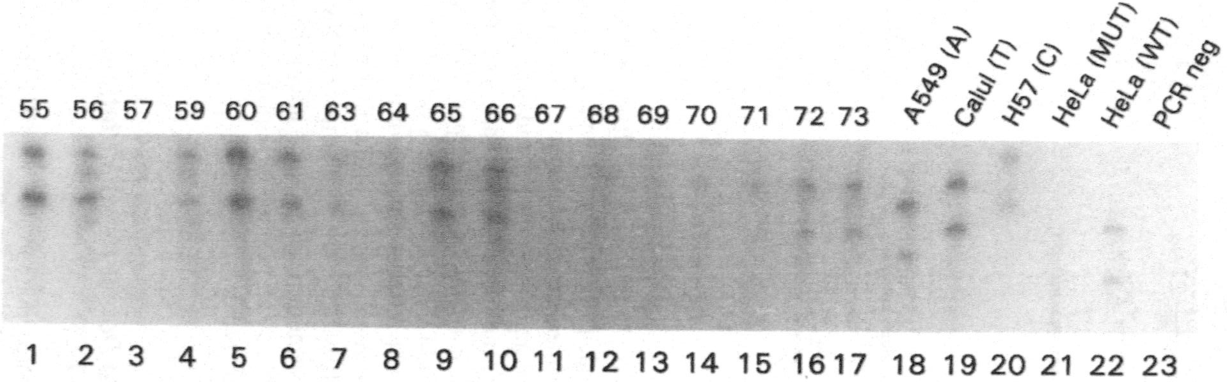

Fig. 3. PCR-based LCR analysis of BAL samples and positive and negative controls. DNA was isolated from a small fraction of each BAL sample, and PCR-based LCR was performed as indicated in the text. Lanes 1-17: LCR bands for 17 BAL specimens whose internal code is shown above the lanes. Lanes 18-20: results from mutant control DNA isolated from cell lines A549, Calu1, and H157, representing GGT → AGT, GGT → TGT, and GGT → CGT mutations, respectively. The results of HeLa DNA amplification by mutant or wild-type primers are shown in Lanes 21 and 22. Lane 23 is a PCR-negative control.

b. Each of the "mutant" probes is dual-labeled with 6-carboxyfluorescein (6-FAM) and TAMRA during synthesis.

2. TaqMan reactions are prepared in 25 μL volumes using 96-well reaction plates with optical grade caps. The PCR mixture contains 12.5 μL of 2X Universal Master Mix, 6.25 pmol of each primer, 3.125 pmol of each probe, and 10 ng of template DNA.

3. All amplifications are performed in "real time" using the 7700 Sequence Detection System. The amplification program consists of incubation at 50°C for 2 min (AmpErase UNG cleavage step), at 95°C for 10 min (activation of AmpliTaq Gold step), and then 40 cycles of 95°C for 15 s followed by 62°C for 1 min (*see* **Note 10**).

4. Notes

1. Many human tumor cell lines have been analyzed for the composition of their K-ras codon 12 sequence. For LCR we use four of them that cover all the possibilities. For the wild type control we use the HeLa cell line (GGT^{Gly}). For the mutants in the first position of codon 12 we use: Calu 1 (TGT^{Cys}), A549 (AGT^{Ser}), and H157 (CGT^{Arg}). The control cell lines guarantee that the experiment works properly and provide a clear comparison for the clinical specimens. For example, in a sample of 52 BAL specimens (a subset of which is shown in **Fig. 3**), 34 (65%) present the GGT→TGT mutation, 10 (19%) have the GGT→TGT plus the GGT→AGT, whereas the remaining 8 specimens are wild-type. The GGT→CGT mutation is not found in the clinical samples presented here, though the mutant control cell line H157 produces the expected result, indicating that the LCR analysis worked properly.

2. Protease inhibitors for BAL collection are designed to protect the specimens from all major types of proteases *(13)*. This precaution is not imperative for the preservation of DNA, but it is useful for other analyses that can be done on these specimens.

3. A potential limitation of every early detection technology arises from the way clinical specimens are collected. Even with the same team of experienced health specialists, the cellular representation in bronchoalveolar lavages from different patients may vary considerably. In addition, the number of precancerous cells collected, when compared to the number of normal components of the epithelium, is small, and more so the earlier the stage of the disease that is being evaluated. Therefore, the diagnostic tools must be highly sensitive and robust to overcome these potential problems.

4. All specimens are encoded so that the operator is blind to the source of the samples.

5. All experiments are repeated at least twice to avoid DNA polymerase and/or DNA ligase errors at the base of interest.

6. The primers are designed so that the respective lengths of the sense and antisense Gly^{GGT} ligated DNA are 47 and 53 bp, the Ser^{AGT} ligation products are 49 and 55 bp, the Cys^{TGT} products are 51 and 57 bp, and the Arg^{CGT} ligated DNAs

are 53 and 59 bp. In several primers, mismatched bases are incorporated to alter the T_ms.

7. The sensitivity of the diagnostic assay is paramount to provide meaningful results. This technique was tested by sequential dilutions of mutant DNA in a growing background of either wild-type DNA or water. Using such an approach, it was reported that this technique was able to detect less than 1% of the mutant allele *(11)*. In other words, we need to have at least 1% of all the cells in the sample carrying that particular mutation to be able to detect it. Anything below this threshold will be considered a wild-type specimen.

8. In several clinical samples we have observed combinations of the different mutations *(11,12)*. These results are seen as a collection of bands which represent the addition of the individual diagnostic bands. Evidently, the relative intensity of each pair of bands represents the frequency of each mutation in the sample. These results indicate the existence of polyclonal cell populations in the sample. Some examples can be seen in **Fig. 3**, Lanes 2, 4, 9, 10, and 17.

9. Since only two dyes can be utilized at once, only one specific mutant allele can be tested at a time. The wild type probe and each of the mutant allele probes are multiplexed, thus requiring a total of 3 individual TaqMan reactions to determine the genotype of the first base of K-ras codon 12.

10. The K-ras codon 12 TaqMan assay was validated using the same genomic DNA controls that were used to validate the PCR-based LCR method. Although the lower limit of sensitivity of mutation detection has not been tested for this TaqMan assay, the detection of mutations present at 1%, the limit of the PCR-based LCR assay, was easily accomplished. This method is faster than LCR and does not involve use of radioactivity. However, the two dye limit on probe labeling means only one specific mutant allele can be tested at a time. This is in contrast to the PCR-based LCR assay in which the multiplex analysis allows the determination of this genotype in a single reaction.

References

1. Peto, R., López, A. D., Boreham, J., Thun, M., and Heath, C. (1992) Mortality from tobacco in developed countries: indirect estimation from national vital statistics. *Lancet* **339**, 1268–1278.
2. Mulshine, J. L. (1998) Lung cancer: current progress, future promise. *Primary Care Cancer* **18**, 9–12.
3. Gaffney, M. and Altshuler, B. (1988) Examination of the role of cigarette smoke in lung carcinogenesis. *J. Natl. Cancer Inst.* **80**, 925–931.
4. Aunoble, B., Sanches, R., Didier, E., and Bignon, Y. (2000) Major oncogenes and tumor suppressor genes involved in epithelial ovarian cancer. *Int. J. Oncol.* **16**, 567–576.
5. Sakorafas, G. H., Tsiotou, A. G., and Tsiotos, G. G. (2000) Molecular biology of pancreatic cancer; oncogenes, tumor suppressor genes, growth factors, and their receptors from a clinical perspective. *Cancer Treat. Rev.* **26**, 29–52.

6. Minamoto, T., Mai, M., and Ronai, Z. (2000) K-ras mutation: early detection of molecular diagnosis and risk assessment of colorectal, pancreas, and lung cancers. *Cancer Detect. Prev.* **24**, 1–12.

7. Slebos, R. J. and Rodenhuis, S. (1992) The ras gene family in human non-small-cell lung cancer. *Monogr. Natl. Cancer Inst.* **13**, 23–29.

8. Suzuki, Y., Orita, M., Shiraishi, M., Hayashi, K., and Sekiya, T. (1990) Detection of ras gene mutations in human lung cancer by single-strand conformation polymorphism analysis of polymerase chain reaction products. *Oncogene* **5**, 1037–1043.

9. Kumar, R. and Dunn, L. L. (1989) Designed diagnostic restriction fragment length polymorphisms for the detection of point mutations in ras oncogenes. *Oncogene Res.* **1**, 235–241.

10. Jacobson, D. R. and Mills, N. E. (1994) A highly sensitive assay for mutant ras genes and its application to the study of presentation and relapse genotypes in acute leukemia. *Oncogene* **9**, 553–563.

11. Lehman, T. A., Scott, F., Seddon, M., Kelly, K., Dempsey, E. C., Wilson, V. L., et al. (1996) Detection of K-ras oncogene mutations by polymerase chain reaction-based ligase chain reaction. *Anal. Biochem.* **239**, 153–159.

12. Scott, F., Modali, R., Lehman, T. A., Seddon, M., Kelly, K., Dempsey, E. C., et al. (1997) High frequency of K-ras codon 12 mutations in bronchoalveolar lavage fluid of patients at high risk for second primary lung cancer. *Clin. Cancer Res.* **3**, 479–482.

13. Scott, F., Cuttitta, F., Treston, A. M., Avis, I., Gupta, P., Ruckdeschel, J., et al. (1993) Prospective trial evaluating immunocytochemical-based sputum techniques for early lung cancer detection: assays for promotion factors in the bronchial lavage. *J. Cell. Biochem. Suppl.* **17F**, 175–183.

14. Wiedmann, M., Wilson, W. J., Czajka, J., Luo, J., Barany, F., and Batt, C. A. (1994) Ligase chain reaction (LCR): overview and applications. *PCR Methods Appl.* **3**, S51–S64.

15. Mitsudomi, T., Viallet, J., Mulshine, J. L., Linnoila, R. I., Minna, J. D., and Gazdar, A. F. (1991) Mutations of ras genes distinguish a subset of non-small-cell lung cancer cell lines from small-cell lung cancer cell lines. *Oncogene* **6**, 1353–1362.

16. Livak, K. J., Flood, S. J., Marmaro, J., Giusti, W., and Deetz, K. (1995) Oligonucleotides with fluorescent dyes at opposite ends provide a quenched probe system useful for detecting PCR products and nucleic acid hybridization. *PCR Methods Appl.* **4**, 357–362.

17. Finney, R. E. and Bishop, J. M. (1993) Predisposition to neoplastic transformation caused by gene replacement of H-ras 1. *Science* **260**, 1524–1527.

18. Parada, L. F., Land, H., Weinberg, R. A., Wolf, D., and Rotter, V. (1984) Cooperation between gene encoding p53 tumour antigen and ras in cellular transformation. *Nature* **312**, 649–651.

19. Sidransky, D. (1994) Molecular screening; how long can we afford to wait? *J. Natl. Cancer Inst.* **87**, 955–956.

20. Tockman, M. S., Gupta, P. K., Myers, J. D., Frost, J. K., Baylin, S. B., Gold, E. B., et al. (1988) Sensitive and specific monoclonal antibody recognition of human lung cancer antigen on preserved sputum cells: A new approach to early lung cancer detection. *J. Clin. Oncol.* **6,** 1685–1693.
21. Tockman, M. S., Mulshine, J. L., Piantadosi, S., Erozan, Y. S., Gupta, P. K., Ruckdeschel, J. C., et al. (1997) Prospective detection of preclinical lung cancer: results from two studies of hnRNP expression. *Clin. Cancer Res.* **3,** 2237–2246.
22. Fielding, P. Turnbull, L., Prime, W., Walshaw, M., and Field, J. K. (1999) Heterogeneous nuclear ribonucleoprotein A2/B1 up-regulation in bronchial lavage specimens: a clinical marker of early lung cancer detection. *Clin. Cancer Res.* **5,** 4048–4052.
23. Mulshine, J. L. and Henschke, C. I. (2000) Prospects for lung-cancer screening. *Lancet* **355,** 592–593.
24. Wattenberg, L. W., Wiedmann, T. S., Estensen, R. D., Zimmerman, C. L., Galbraith, A. R., Steele, V. E., and Kelloff, G. J. (2000) Chemoprevention of pulmonary carcinogenesis by brief exposures to aerosolized budesonide or beclomethasone dipropionate and by the combination of aerosolized budesonide and dietary myo-inositol. *Carcinogenesis* **21,** 179–182.
25. Dahl, A. R., Grossi, I. M., Houchens, D. P., Scovell, L. J., Placke, M. E., Imondi, A. R., et al. (2000) Inhaled isotretinoin (13-cis retinoic acid) is an effective lung cancer chemopreventive agent in A/J mice at low doses: a pilot study. *Clin. Cancer Res.* **8,** 3015–3024.
26. Wang, D. L., Marko, M., Dahl, A. R., Engelke, K. S., Placke, M. E., Imondi, A. R., et al. (2000) Topical delivery of 13-cis retinoic acid by inhalation up-regulates expression of rodent lung but not liver retinoic acid receptors. *Clin. Cancer Res.* **9,** 3636–3645.

13

Assays for Raf-1 Kinase Phosphorylation and Activity in Human Small Cell Lung Cancer Cells

Rajani K. Ravi and Barry D. Nelkin

1. Introduction

Activation of the ras/raf signal transduction pathway has been shown to be involved in many proliferative and developmental signals as well as in transformation and tumorigenicity of many types of cancers *(1–4)*. However, small cell lung cancer (SCLC) cell lines, and SCLC in patients, rarely possess ras mutations *(5)*. In these cancers, ras mutations may not confer a growth advantage. In fact, in SCLC cell lines, introduction of an activated ras gene results in cell differentiation accompanied by slower cell growth *(6)*.

Ras-induced signaling often involves the activation of the c-raf-1 gene, a cytosolic serine/threonine protein kinase that is central to several intracellular signal-transduction pathways. Ras can translocate raf to the cell membrane where it is activated by a process possibly involving tyrosine phosphorylation. Upon activation, raf-1 phosphorylates mitogen- or extracellular-regulated-kinase (MEK) at Ser-217 and Ser-221, which in turn activates downstream mitogen-activated protein kinases (MAPKs) by phosphorylating Thr-183 and Tyr-185 *(3–4)*. This phosphorylation cascade leads to the activation of transcription factors involved in cell growth and differentiation *(1–4)*. In most immortalized cells, constitutive activation of this pathway results in the upregulation of cyclinD/cyclin-dependent kinase (CDK) activity or the downregulation of cdk inhibitors (CDKI) such as $p27^{KIP1}$ resulting in cellular proliferation *(7)*. However, in several cell types, the activation of the ras/raf-1 signal-transduction pathway, with resultant MAP kinase activation, can result in growth arrest and cell differentiation, which is mediated by the induction of CDKIs, either $p16^{INK4}$, $p21^{WAF1}$, or $p27^{KIP1}$, depending upon cell type *(7,18)*.

From: *Methods in Molecular Medicine, vol. 74: Lung Cancer, Vol. 1: Molecular Pathology Methods and Reviews*
Edited by: B. Driscoll © Humana Press Inc., Totowa, NJ

We have shown that activated raf-1 can induce growth arrest in SCLC cells via the induction of CDKIs. Thus, p27^{KIP1} is induced in Rb (retinoblastoma susceptibility protein) negative NCI-H209 and NCI-H510 cells, and p16^{INK4} is induced in Rb positive DMS53 cells *(9–10)*. Critical to the understanding of raf-1 signaling in cells are experimental methods to assess its activation. Because phosphorylation plays an intrinsic role in regulating raf-1 activity, it is important to assess raf-1 activation either by determining its phosphorylation state or by measuring its kinase activity on its downstream MAP kinases. Here we describe procedures for the assays of these kinases.

2. Materials
2.1. Preparation of Cell Lysates

1. Culture Medium: RPMI 1640 or medium depending on cell type.
2. Phosphate-buffered saline (PBS).
3. Lysis Buffer: 20 mM Tris-HCl, pH 8.0, 100 mM NaCl, 2 mM EGTA, 10 mM sodium fluoride (NaF), 40 mM β-glycerophosphate, 0.5% Triton X-100, 1 mM dithiothreitol (DTT), 10 μg/mL aprotinin, 10 μg/mL leupeptin, and 1 mM phenylmethylsulfonyl fluoride (PMSF). Cell lysis buffer is stored at 4°C without protease inhibitors and DTT, which are added from stock solutions stored at –20°C before use.
4. Bradford protein assay reagents: Bio-Rad protein assay dye reagent (Bio-Rad Laboratories, Hercules, CA) using bovine serum albumin (BSA) as the standard. (Bovine serum albumin [BSA, Fraction V] from Sigma, St. Louis, MO).

2.2. Immunoblotting

1. 2X sodium dodecyl sulfate (SDS) gel-loading buffer: 100 mM Tris-HCl, pH 6.8, 200 μM DTT, 4% SDS, 0.01% bromophenol blue and 20% glycerol. SDS gel-loading buffer lacking DTT can be stored at room temperature. DTT should then be added just before use.
2. Immobilon-P membrane (Millipore).
3. Wet transfer blotting apparatus (Bio-Rad Trans-blot Cell).
4. Tris-buffered saline (TBS): 10 mM Tris HCl, pH 7.6, and 150 mM NaCl.
5. TBST: TBS with 0.1% Tween 20.
6. Blocking buffer (1): 5% (w/v) nonfat dry milk in TBST.
7. Blocking buffer (2): 3% (w/v) BSA in TBST.
8. Polyclonal anti-raf-1 (C-12; an affinity purified rabbit antibody generated against carboxy-terminus of raf-1) (Santa Cruz Biotechnology, Santa Cruz, CA).
9. Anti-MEK-1 (C-18) (Santa Cruz Biotechnology).
10. Anti-MAPK/ERK1 (C-16) (Santa Cruz Biotechnology).
11. Anti-MAPK/ERK-2 (C-14) (Santa Cruz Biotechnology).
12. Monoclonal anti-c-raf-1 (generated against 162-378 residues of human raf-1) (BD Transduction Laboratories, San Diego, CA).
13. Anti-phospho MAPK (CellSignaling Technology, Inc., Beverly, MA).

14. Anti-phospho MEK-1. (CellSignaling Technology).
15. Antibody Diluent 1:5% (w/v) non fat dry milk in TBST.
16. Antibody Diluent 2:3% BSA in TBST.
17. Horseradish peroxidase-conjugated secondary antibodies (diluted from 1:3000 to 1:20,000) (Amersham, Arlington Heights, IL).
18. Enhanced chemiluminescent (ECL) reagents (Amersham).
19. Luminol reagents (Cell Signaling Technology).

2.3. Kinase Assays

2.3.1. Raf-1 Immunocomplex Assay

1. RIPA (Radio Immuno Precipitation Assay) lysis buffer: 1% (w/w) Nonidet-40 (NP-40), 1% (w/v) sodium deoxycholate, 0.1% (w/v) SDS, 0.15 M NaCl, 2 mM EDTA, 50 mM NaF, 0.2 mM sodium vanadate, 10 µg/mL aprotinin, and 1 mM PMSF (sodium vanadate, aprotinin, and PMSF are added fresh from stock solutions before use). Store buffer without vanadate at 4°C for up to 1 yr.
2. Whole-cell extraction (WCE) buffer: 50 mM Tris-HCl, pH 7.5, 137 mM NaCl, 5 mM MgCl$_2$, 1% TritonX-100, 50 mM β-glycerophosphate, 10 mM NaF, 0.1% (W/V) SDS, 2 mM EDTA, 10 mM EGTA, 1 mM DTT, 1 mM Na$_3$VO$_4$, 10 µg/mL aprotinin, 10 µg/mL leupeptin, 10 µg/mL pepstatin and 1 mM PMSF. Store WCE buffer at –20°C and add protease inhibitors just before use.

2.3.1.1. IMMUNOPRECITATION

1. Protein A-sepharose™ CLB (Pharmacia, Piscataway, NJ) (protein A-Sepharose is Protein A-agarose).
2. Protein A/G PLUS agarose (Santa Cruz Biotechnology).
3. Protein A slurry: Two hundred mg of protein A-sepharose or A/G PLUS agarose are dispersed in 5 mL of cold PBS and rocked on a slow rotator for 2 h at 4°C. The slurry is centrifuged at 1200g for 5 min at 4°C, and washed twice with cold PBS. The pelleted beads are then suspended in WCE buffer without protease inhibitors at a final concentration of 200 mg/mL and stored at 4°C. This Protein A-agarose slurry is good for 7–10 d at 4°C.
4. Wash Buffer: 10 mM HEPES (N-2-hydroxyethyl-piperazine-N′-Z-ethanesulfonic acid, pH 7.5), 100 mM NaCl, 0.5% (v/v) Nonidet P-40 (NP-40), 10 µg/mL leupeptin, and 10 µg/mL aprotinin. (Aprotinin and leupeptin should be added immediately before use.)
5. Kinase Reaction buffer: 20 mM HEPES, pH 7.5, 10 mM MgCl$_2$, 10 mM MnCl$_2$ (made fresh), 10 mM PNPP (p-Nitrophenyl phosphate, add fresh) and 10 mM EGTA. Store at 4°C.
6. Deoxy adenosine triphosphate (100 mM ATP).
7. [γ^{32}P]-ATP (3000Ci/mmol).
8. Recombinant MEK-1 (Santa Cruz Biotechnology).
9. Denaturing SDS-10% PAGE gels.
10. Gel fixative: 5% (v/v) methanol, 5% (v/v) glacial acetic acid.

2.3.2. MAP Kinase Assay

2.3.2.1. KINASE REACTION

1. Myelin basic protein (MBP) from Sigma, St. Louis, MO or Invitrogen Life Technologies, Gaithersburg, MD.
2. Kinase reaction buffer: 20 mM HEPES, pH 7.5, 10 mM MgCl$_2$, 1 mM EGTA, 1 mM DTT, 0.125 µCi/µL [γ-^{32}P] ATP and 0.5–1.0 µg MBP.
3. 12.5% SDS-PAGE gel.

3. Method

3.1. Preparation of Cell Lysates

The majority of the SCLC cells grow in suspension cultures. There are a few SCLC cell lines, including DMS 53, which grow as an adherent cell line. Such adherent cells must be dislodged from the tissue culture dish by scraping before assaying.

1. Harvest cells by centrifugation at 800g for 5 min at 4°C in a conical tube.
2. Gently resuspend the cell pellets in ice cold (4°C) PBS and wash twice with PBS.
3. Lyse the cell pellets in lysis buffer (100–150 µL of lysis buffer per 1 × 10^6 cells) for 20 min on ice.
4. Transfer cell lysates to 1.5-mL microfuge tubes and centrifuged at 12,000g for 10 min at 4°C to remove insoluble cell debris.
5. Collect supernatants and quantitate protein concentrations using the Bradford protein assay. These cell lysates can be used immediately for immunoblotting, or they may be snap-frozen and stored at –80°C for future use.

3.2. Immunoblotting

Western blotting is used to determine the level of specific protein expression.

1. 50–100 µg of lysates (prepared as described in **Subheading 3.1.**) are boiled with 2X SDS-gel loading buffer.
2. Subject proteins to SDS-PAGE. Any standard method can be used to make gel and to transfer proteins *(11–12)*.
3. Transfer proteins from SDS-PAGE gel to Immobilon-P membrane using a wet transfer blotting apparatus.
4. Rinse the membrane in TBS and block residual binding sites on the membrane in a solution containing either blocking buffer (1) or (2) for 1 h at room temperature (*see* **Note 1**).
5. Wash the membrane twice with TBST (5 min/wash), then incubate with the primary antibody (all listed in **Subheading 2.2.** at 1:1000 dilution or 0.1–0.5 µg/mL) for 2 h at RT (Diluent 1), or at 4°C overnight (Diluent 1), on a rocking platform.

6. Wash the membrane three times with TBST (5 min/wash) and incubated for one hour with horseradish peroxide-conjugated secondary antibody at RT.
7. Wash the membrane again at least three times with TBST (7 min/wash)
8. Detect immune reactions by enhanced chemiluminescence (ECL) following the supplier's instructions (*see* **Notes 2** and **3**).

3.3. Kinase Assays

3.3.1. Raf-1 Immunocomplex Assay

There are several assays for raf-1 activity *(13–15)*. Here we describe a basic method, based on the ability of activated raf-1 from cell lysates to phosphorylate its direct substrate, recombinant MEK-1, in the presence of [γ^{32}p] ATP in vitro (*see* **Notes 4** and **5**).

1. Harvest cells as described above in **Subheading 3.1.**
2. Resuspend the cell pellets in ice-cold (4°C) PBS and washed twice with PBS.
3. Lyse cell pellets either in WCE buffer or RIPA buffer (use either one of the lysis buffer that contain nonionic NP-40 or Triton X-100 as a detergent to solubilize nuclear and cytoplasmic proteins) (150–200 μL of lysis buffer per 1×10^6 cells) for 20 min on ice or on a slow rotator at 4°C.
4. Transfer whole-cell lysates to 1.5-mL microfuge tubes and centrifuge at 12,000g for 10 min at 4°C to remove insoluble cell debris.
5. Collect supernatants and determine protein concentrations. These whole-cell lysates can be used immediately for immunoprecipitation, or they may be snap-frozen and stored at –80°C for future use.

All the following steps are carried out in the cold.

3.3.1.1. IMMUNOPRECITATION

1. Pre-clear 100–250 μg of whole-cell lysates with 10–20 μL of Protein A-agarose slurry for at least 30 min to reduce nonspecific protein binding.
2. After this incubation, remove protein A-agarose by centrifugation for 2–3 min at 5000g, and collect supernatant into new microcentrifuge tubes.
3. Incubate supernatant with polyclonal or monoclonal anti-p74 raf-1 antibody (1 μg antibody/100–250 μg protein or 1:100 dilution; *see* **Note 6**) for at least 2 h at 4°C on a slow rotator.
4. Add 25–30 μL of 50:50 (v/v)) protein-A agarose slurry per sample (When using monoclonal anti-raf-1, use protein A+G Agarose). Incubate samples for an additional one hour on a rotator at 4°C (*see* **Note 7**).
5. Sediment the anti-raf-1 coated protein beads gently by centrifugation at 4000g for 2 min, and decant supernatant.
6. Wash the immunocomplexes two to three times in ice-cold lysis buffer, once in ice-cold wash buffer, and once in kinase reaction buffer supplemented with 0.5 μM DTT and 1 mM PMSF. The last wash with kinase buffer will equilibrate the immunocomplexes for the subsequent kinase reaction.

3.3.1.2. KINASE REACTIONS

1. To the immunoprecipitate, add a mixture of 20 μ*M* "cold" ATP, 0.125 μCi/1 μL [γ^{32}p] ATP (3000Ci/mmol), and 500 ng of recombinant MEK-1 in kinase reaction buffer (including 0.5 μ*M* DTT, 1 m*M* PMSF) in a total volume of 25–40 μL (*see* **Notes 8–10**).
2. Incubate reactions at 30°C for 20 min with gentle agitation to keep the immuno-precipitated Raf-1 protein bound beads in suspension (*see* **Note 11**).
3. Terminate the reaction by adding 2X SDS-gel loading buffer and heating to 100°C for 5–7 min in tightly capped tubes.
4. Centrifuge samples at 12,000*g* for 5 min. Resolve on denaturing SDS-10% PAGE gels until the free isotope is almost run off the gel (free isotope runs with the bromophenol blue dye).
5. Excise the free isotope region of the gel and discard. Fix the gel for 10 min, dry, and expose to autoradiographic film (*see* **Note 12**).
6. The radioactivity in the substrate bands can be quantitated on a phosphorimager (*see* **Note 13**).

3.3.2. MAP Kinase Assay

The procedure for measuring MAPK activity in immunoprecipitates is similar to the Raf-1 kinase assay.

3.3.2.1. IMMUNOPRECITATION

1. To immunoprecipitate p42/p44 MAPK/ERK, incubate 100 μg whole-cell lysates for 2 h at 4°C with 1 μg/mL anti-MAPK.
2. Incubate immune complexes with protein A-sepharose™ beads for 1 h. The immune complexes bound to the beads can then be washed with same lysis buffer and kinase buffer as described (*see* **Subheading 3.3.1.1.**).

3.3.2.2. KINASE REACTION

1. Incubate MAPK immunoprecipitates in 25–40 μL MAP kinase reaction buffer, containing myelin basic protein (MBP) as substrate, at 30°C for 20 min.
2. Stop the reactions by the addition of 2X SDS-gel loading buffer, boil for 5 min, separate the reaction products by electrophoresis on a 12.5% SDS-PAGE gel.
3. Visualize phosphorylated proteins are visualized by autoradiography and quanti-tate on a phosphorimager (Molecular Dynamics). **Figure 1** shows good correla-tion between MAPK activity as determined by the kinase assay, and p42/p44 phosphorylation as determined by Western blotting with an anti-phospho-MAPK antibody.

4. Notes

1. Although nonfat dried milk and BSA are compatible with nearly all detection systems, a careful choice is necessary to ensure compatibility with the detection system. Nonfat dried milk gives clean background but signal deteriorates rapidly.

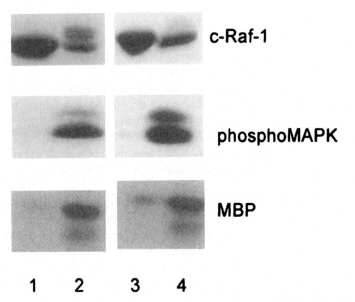

c-Raf-1

phosphoMAPK

MBP

1   2   3   4

Fig. 1. Whole cell lysates from SCLC cells NCI-H209 cells (lane 1), NCI-H209 cells with activated Raf-1 (lane 2), NCI-H510 cells (lane 3), and NCI-H510 cells with activated Raf-1 (lane 4) are immunoblotted with anti-Raf-1 and phospho-specific MAPK antibodies. The same cell lysates are immunoprecipitated with anti-MAPK antibody, and kinase activity is measured with myelin basic protein as substrate, as described in **Subheading 3.3.** Part of this figure is reproduced from Ravi et al. *(10)*, with permission from the American Society of Clinical Investigation.

Also biotin in dried milk may interfere with avidin-biotin reactions. In such situations, residual binding sites can be blocked using BSA which gives relatively good signal strength.

2. The activation of MEK and MAPK is usually correlated with their phosphorylation. Specific antibodies to assay MEK/MAPK phosphorylation in cells are commercially available (Cell Signaling Technology or Santa Cruz Biotechnology). These antibodies detect only the activated, phosphorylated forms of MEK and MAPK. The Western-blot protocol for these antibodies is exactly as specified by the manufacturer, and includes a blocking step with 5% (w/v) nonfat dry milk and the primary antibody incubations in 3% (w/v) BSA in TBS-T overnight at 4°C. The immune reactions are performed in Luminol or ECL reagents. Experiments using these phospho-specific antibodies should be accompanied by Western-blotting experiments using standard antibodies for MEK and MAPK, to determine whether the level of the protein remains constant.

3. Make sure the chemiluminescent reagents are evenly spread on the membrane and remove all the excess solutions before you expose to film.

4. Since MEK-1 is a kinase capable of autophosphorylation, kinase inactive MEK-1 must be used as a control in this assay. An alternative is use of FSBA (5'-P-flurosulfonyl benzoyladenosine) treated MEK-1 as a negative control. FSBA inactivates the autokinase activity of MEK.

5. This method assays the activity of immunoprecipitated raf-1 (p74[raf-1]). Either polyclonal or monoclonal raf-1 antibodies directed against human raf-1 can be used to immunoprecipitate raf-1 protein from cell lysates. Raf-1 antibodies for immunoprecipitation of raf-1 are available from a variety of commercial sources. An advantage of this assay is that immunoprecipitation of raf-1 removes the background kinase activity associated with other activated MAP kinases in cell lysates.

6. The concentration of Raf-1 antibody must be optimized for immunoprecipitation; the optimal concentration varies for different cell types and depends on the source of the antibody. The appropriate concentration is determined by immunoprecipitating c-raf-1 using increasing concentration of primary antibody, and assessing the efficiency of immunoprecipitation by Western blotting. At the optimized concentration of antibody, all of the c-raf-1 in the sample should be immunoprecipitated.

7. Alternatively, commercially available primary antibodies pre-bound to protein-A agarose beads may be incubated with the whole-cell lysate, allowing the immunoprecipitation to be done in a single 2-h incubation period.

8. To initiate the kinase reactions, defrost all stock solutions (which are stored at –20°C) before the last wash of immunoprecipitated samples, and keep them on ice.

9. Prepare the kinase reaction mix with all solutions including [γ^{32}P] ATP, and quickly add to tubes containing immunoprecipitated raf-1 on protein A- agarose beads. Quick spin for few seconds, and gently tap the tubes with your fingers, so that the beads can mix with kinase buffer mix.

10. If necessary, kinase reactions for the given system can be optimized by either increasing amounts of substrate with same incubation period, or by increasing incubation periods with constant amount of substrate.

11. If there is no shaker available at 30°C to incubate kinase reactions, reactions may be placed at 30°C and mixed two or three times during the incubation period.

12. Alternatively, gels may be transferred onto Immobilon-P membrane (Millipore, Bedford, MA) using a semi-dry transfer method. A semi-dry blotting method should be used to transfer kinase reaction products from SDS-PAGE gel to the Immobilon-P membrane, in order to reduce radioactive ^{32}P contamination. In this alternative, after the membrane is exposed to autoradiographic film, it can be incubated with a raf-1 specific antibody to ensure equal amount of raf-1 protein in different immunoprecipitates. A raf-1 antibody raised in different species should be used for incubating the membrane, so the secondary antibody used for developing the membrane does not cross react with the primary antibody used for immunoprecipitation.

13. Recently Bondzi et al. *(16)* described a single step non-radioactive kinase assay for Raf-1 using the activation-specific MEK antibody (Santa Cruz Biotechnology, Santa Cruz, CA,) that recognizes MEK-1 only when it is phosphorylated by raf-1. For this assay, the kinase reaction is performed as described above in the presence of "cold" ATP. The samples are resolved on SDS-PAGE gel, transferred to Immobilon-P membrane and Western blotted with the MEK-1 activation specific antibody.

References

1. Marshall, M. (1995) Interactions between ras and raf: Key regulatory proteins in cellular transformation. *Mol. Rep. Dev.* **42,** 493–499.
2. Williams, N. G. and Roberts, T. M. (1994) Signal transduction pathways involving the *Raf* proto-oncogene. *Cancer Metastasis Rev.* **13,** 105–116.
3. Morrison, D. K. and Cutler, Jr., R. E. (1997) The complexity of Raf-1 regulation. *Curr. Opin. Cell. Biol.* **9,** 174–179.
4. Seger, R. and Krebs, E. G. (1995) The MAPK signaling cascade. *FASEB J.* **9,** 726–735.
5. Mitsudomi, T., Viallet, J., Mulshine, R., Minna, J. D., and Gazdar, A. F. (1991) Mutations of ras genes distinguish a subset of non-small-cell lung cancer cell lines. *Oncogene* **6,** 1353–1362.
6. Mabry, M., Nakagawa, T., Baylin, S., Pettengill, O., Sorenson, G., and Nelkin, B. D. (1989) Insertion of the v-Ha-ras oncogene induces differentiation of calcitonin-producing human small cell lung cancer. *J. Clin. Invest.* **84,** 194–199.
7. Lloyd, A. C. (1998) Ras versus cyclin-dependent kinase inhibitors. *Curr. Opin. Genet. Dev.* **8,** 43–48.
8. Weintraub, S. J. (1999) Dormant tumor-suppressor pathways in tumors. *Am. J. Respir. Cell. Mol. Biol.* **20,** 540–542.
9. Ravi, R. K., Weber, E. McMahon, M., Williams, J. R., Baylin, S., Mal, A., et al. (1998) Activated Raf-1 causes growth arrest in human small cell lung cancer cells. *J. Clin. Invest.* **101,** 153–159.
10. Ravi, R. K., Thiagalingam, A., Weber, E., McMahon, M., Nelkin, B. D., and Mabry, M. (1999) Raf-1 causes growth suppression and alteration of neuroendocrine markers in DMS53 human small- cell lung cancer cells. *Am. J. Respir. Cell. Mol. Biol.* **20,** 543–549.
11. Sambrook, J., Fritsch, E. F., and Maniatis, T. (1989) *Molecular Cloning. A Laboratory Manual.* Cold Spring Harbor Laboratory Press, Cold Spring Harbor, NY.
12. Ausubel, F. A., Brent, R., Kingston, R. E., Moore, D. D., Seidman, J. G., Smith, J. A., and Struhl, K. (1995) *Current Protocols in Molecular Biology.* John Wiley & Sons, Inc., New York, NY.
13. Kyriakis, J. M., Force, I. L., Rapp, U. R., Bonventre, J. V., and Avruch, J. (1993) Mitogen regulation of c-Raf-1 protein kinase activity toward mitogen-activated protein kinase-kinase. *J. Biol. Chem.* **268,** 16009–16019.

14. Alessi, D. R., Cohen, P., Ashworth, A., Cowley, S., Leevers, S. J., and Marshall, C. J. (1995) Assay and expression of mitogen-activated protein kinase, MAP kinase kinase, and Raf. *Methods Enzymol.* **255,** 279–290.

15. Fabian, J. R., Daar, I. O., and Morrison, D. K. (1993) Critical tyrosine residues regulate the enzymatic and biological activity of Raf-1 kinase. *Mol. Cell. Biol.* **13,** 7170–7179.

16. Bondzi, C., Grant, S., and Krystal, G. W. (2000) A novel assay for the measurement of Raf-1 kinase activity. *Oncogene* **19,** 5030–5033.

14

γ-Glutamylcysteine Synthetase in Lung Cancer

Effect on Cell Viability

Kristiina Järvinen, Ylermi Soini, and Vuokko L. Kinnula

1. Introduction

Lung tissue is exposed to higher concentrations of oxygen than most other tissues. In addition, cigarette smoke and environmental toxic particles not only contain reactive oxygen species (ROS), but also enhance ROS production and activate various oxidant generating mechanisms in the cell. ROS include a number of highly reactive oxygen (superoxide radical $O_2^{\cdot-}$ hydrogen peroxide H_2O_2, hydroxyl radical $OH^{\cdot}$) and nitrogen (nitric oxide NO, peroxynitrite ONOO) metabolites *(1)*. At low concentrations, ROS may play a fundamental role in the regulation of signal transduction *(2)*, but persistent oxidant exposure can also cause injury to almost all cellular components, including membrane lipids and the genetic material of the cell. ROS also appear to play an important role in cancer biology, carcinogenesis, tumor growth, and drug therapy. Many aspects of ROS mechanisms in these pathways remain unsolved, but it has been hypothesized that antioxidant enzymes may play a role in the proliferation and apoptosis of cancer cells, and in the resistance of malignant cells to chemotherapeutic agents and radiation *(3–5)*.

Antioxidant enzymes (AOEs) and small molecular-weight antioxidants protect cells and tissues from free radical-related damage. So-called classical AOEs include superoxide dismutases (SOD), glutathione peroxidase (GPx), and catalase. SOD reduces superoxide radicals to H_2O_2. There are three SODs in mammalian cells and tissues: manganese SOD (MnSOD), copper zinc SOD (CuZnSOD), and extracellular SOD (ECSOD) *(1,6)*. Glutathione peroxidase and catalase reduce H_2O_2 into water and oxygen *(6)*. Other enzymes with

From: *Methods in Molecular Medicine, vol. 74: Lung Cancer, Vol. 1: Molecular Pathology Methods and Reviews*
Edited by: B. Driscoll © Humana Press Inc., Totowa, NJ

antioxidant capacity include thiol-containing proteins such as the families of thioredoxin, glutaredoxin, and peroxiredoxin *(7–9)*. One of the most important small molecular-weight antioxidants is glutathione (GSH), which is a thiol-containing tripeptide. GSH is oxidized to GSSG by GPx during the reduction of H_2O_2. Glutathione is synthesized from cysteine, glutamate, and glycine by glutathione synthase and gamma-glutamylcysteine synthetase (γGCS), the latter being the rate-limiting enzyme in glutathione synthesis. γGCS consists of two subunits: a heavy subunit with catalytic function (γGCSh) and a light subunit with a regulatory role (γGCSl). Both enzyme subunits contribute to enzyme activity, though the heavy subunit is considered more critical *(10)*. The complex mechanisms of AOEs include not only the synthesis of these enzymes, but also ATP-dependent transport of glutathione out of the cells, and function of several enzymes on the cell membrane as well. These glutathione-associated enzyme mechanisms have been investigated especially in the context of xenobiotic metabolism. They include γ-glutamyl transpeptidase (γGT), which participates in the degradation of extracellular glutathione, glutathione S-transferases (GST), and the family of multidrug resistance proteins (MRP) *(3)*. These mechanisms are described in **Fig. 1**.

Human bronchial epithelium contains detectable levels of SODs, catalase, GPx, γGT, and GSTs. The epithelial lining fluid of human lung has over 100 fold higher glutathione content than circulating blood *(11–14)*. Very few systematic studies have been conducted on malignant diseases as to the expression of antioxidant enzymes. Based on one study, MnSOD, GPx, and catalase were low in the 19 biopsies of human lung cancer when investigated by immunohistochemistry *(15)*. As to MnSOD, some studies have suggested that it is low *(16)* while others have suggested that it may be elevated, in malignant tumors *(17–19)*. In contrast, glutathione-dependent mechanisms have been shown to be associated both with carcinogenesis and with the drug resistance of malignant cells, since they may be induced by oxidant-generating cytotoxic drugs with consequent drug resistance *(3,4,10,20–24)*. The A549 cell line is a widely used, stable, and well-characterized human lung cancer cell line containing high glutathione content and detectable γGCS immunoreactivity *(25–27)*. This cell line is used here as a model to demonstrate the importance of glutathione-dependent mechanisms in these cells.

Buthionine sulphoximine (BSO) is a specific inhibitor of γGCS, and therefore it can be used to cause depletion of intracellular glutathione *(28)*.

In this chapter, we will describe an immunohistochemical staining method for γGCSh and γGCSl in both tumor biopsies and cell lines. We also describe the principles for investigating the importance of glutathione in malignant lung cells by modulation of glutathione levels by BSO in vitro. Cell-culture techniques and tests for cell viability and cytotoxicity are not included here, but

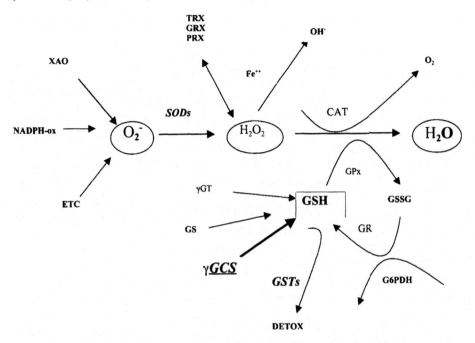

Fig. 1. The most important antioxidant mechanisms in cells. XAO, xanthine oxidase; NADPH-ox, NADPH-oxidase; ETC mitochondrial electron transport chain; TRX, thioredoxin; GRX, glutaredoxin; PRX, peroxiredoxin; SOD, superoxide dismutase; CAT, catalase; GPx, glutathione peroxidase; GR, glutathione reductase; GSH, glutathione; GSSG, oxidized glutathione; GST, glutathione S-transferase; γGCS, γ-glutamylcysteine synthetase; GS, glutathione synthase; γGT, γ-glutamyl traspeptidase; G6PDH, glucose-6-phosphate dehydrogenase.

have been exhaustively described elsewhere, including in this series, Methods in Molecular Medicine.

Several caveats must be emphasized when investigating AOEs and oxidant/antioxidant balance in malignant diseases. Some of those have been listed below.

- Only a fraction of intracellular compounds with antioxidant capacity have been characterized, and new enzymes are constantly being discovered.
- The relative importance of various AOEs in intact cells is unknown.
- The mRNA levels of thousands of genes can be simultaneously investigated (e.g., by micro-array), but they do not necessarily correlate with active protein in tumor biopsies in vivo. This would include analysis of mRNA expression of AOEs, which is why we emphasize protein expression and activity in this chapter.
- By immunohistochemistry, the location and expression of a protein can be detected; immunoreactivity does not necessarily correlate with enzyme activity,

especially in cancer tissues, which can produce proteins with altered conformation and activity.

- Though AOE immunohistochemistry is a valuable technique, only a few commercial high-quality antibodies for AOEs are available *(29)*.
- The measurement of enzyme activities from tumor tissues is not reliable, as tumor homogenates contain a mixture of multiple cell types and matrix proteins.
- The expression of the enzyme should be compared to healthy controls. Biopsies for those are, however, difficult to find. Additionally many "healthy" patients may smoke, which leads to chronic inflammation and induction of several AOEs.
- Cell cultures may be used to study antioxidants, but it must be noted that levels of AOEs usually decline in culture.
- The activity of enzymes such as γGCS in cultured cells may also be dependent on several factors, most importantly plating density, stage of cell growth, and constituents of the culture medium *(30)*.
- Specific inhibitors exist only for some AOEs (BSO for γGCS). Even if effective, it must be kept in mind that their application may be limited, as they may not be useful in clinical interventions.
- If cultured cells are induced by transfection to ectopically overexpress an AOE, the natural antioxidant/oxidant balance of the cell can be disturbed. Simultaneous induction of several AOEs has often been observed in vivo, and this situation may be quite difficult to duplicate by manipulation in vitro.
- The assessment of ROS production in intact cells is difficult, as radicals rapidly disintegrate, the methods are not particularly sensitive, and the determination of various oxidant metabolites, or their compartmentalization or quantification in the cell, is nearly impossible.

2. Materials

2.1. Preparation of Lung Biopsies for Immunohistochemistry of γGCS

2.1.1. Paraffin-Embedded Samples

1. Set up for paraffin embedding and sectioning.
2. 2% 3′-aminopropyltriethylsilane (A-3648, Sigma Chemicals, Cat. no. A-3648) in acetone.
3. Xylene.
4. Absolute ethanol.
5. 94% ethanol.
6. Phosphate-buffered saline (PBS).

2.1.2. Frozen Samples

1. Set up for frozen tissue sectioning.
2. Coated slides (Super Frost plus slides, Menzel-Gläzer, Germany).

2.2. Immunostaining

2.2.1. Preparation of Cultured Cells for Immohistochemistry

1. Human A549 lung adenocarcinoma cells (American Type Culture Collections, Rockville, MD).
2. Nutrient Mixture F-12 Ham growth medium with L-glutamine (Gibco, Paisley, UK) and 15% heat-inactivated fetal bovine serum (FBS; Gibco, Eggenstein, Germany), 100 U/mL penicillin and 100 µg/mL streptomycin (Gibco).
3. 0.05% Trypsin in PBS (Gibco, Paisley, UK).
4. 10% neutral formalin.
5. 2% agar in water.

2.2.2. Antigen Retrieval for Paraffin-Embedded Material

1. 10 mM citrate buffer, pH 6.0.

2.2.3. Incubation with the Antibodies

1. 2% nonfat milk powder in PBS.
2. Endogenous peroxidase block: 3% hydrogen peroxide in absolute methanol.
3. Primary (27) γGCS antibodies for γGCSh and γGCSl (dilution 1:1000) diluted in PBS.
4. Biotinylated secondary anti-rabbit antibody DAB method (Dakopatts, Glostrup, Denmark, Cat. no. E0353), dilution 1:200.
5. Biotinylated secondary anti-rabbit antibody AEC method (Zymed Laboratories Inc, San Francisco, CA, Cat. no. 85-9043, ready to use).
6. Rabbit primary antibody isotype control (Zymed Laboratories, Cat. no. 08-6199).

2.2.4. Chromogen Development

2.2.4.1. METHOD 1: DIAMINOBENZIDINE (DAB)

1. Streptavidin-biotin complex (ABC) (Histostain Plus Bulk kit, Zymed Laboratories, Cat. no. 85-9043).
2. DAB/hydrogen peroxide (Dakopatts).
3. Mayer hematoxylin (Oy Reagena Ab, Kuopio, Finland, Cat. no. 180210).
4. Immunomount (Shandon, Pittsburg, PA, Cat. no. 990402).
5. Aminoethylcarbaxole (Zymed Laboratories, Cat. no. 00-1111).

2.3. Inhibition of γ-Glutamylcysteine Synthetase

1. 0.1 mM to 1 mM BSO (L-Buthionine-[S,R]-Sulfoximine, Sigma Chemicals, Cat. no. B-2515).
2. Cisplatin, 0.5 mg/mL (Bristol-Myers Squibb AB).

3. Methods

3.1. Preparation of Lung Biopsies for Immunohistochemistry of γGCS

3.1.1. Paraffin-Embedded Samples

1. Prepare paraffin-embedded sections (*see* **Note 1**).
2. Cut 4-μm thick sections and place on 3′-aminopropyltriethylsilane-coated slides.
3. Deparaffinize through xylene 5 min × 3.
4. Dehydrate in absolute ethanol 3 min × 5, then 94 % ethanol 2 min × 2 and by double-distilled water 1 min × 1.
5. Rinse with PBS.

3.1.2. Frozen Samples

1. Cut 4-μm thick sections on Super Frost plus coated slides.
2. Air-dry for 15 min.
3. Wash with PBS.

3.2. Immunostaining

Representative staining reaction of γGCSh and γGCSl in the biopsies of lung carcinoma is shown in **Fig. 2**.

3.2.1. Preparation of Cultured Cells for Immunohistochemistry

1. Detach the A549 cells from culture with trypsin and centrifuge at 600*g* for 5 min.
2. Wash cell pellets with PBS.
3. Fix pellets in 10% neutral formalin for 24 h at 4°C.
4. Remove formalin and pour melted 2% agar in water over the pellets.
5. Embed the agar blocks in paraffin.
6. Cut 4-μm thick sections from the cell blocks and process further for immunohistochemistry as with paraffin blocks.

3.2.2. Antigen Retrieval for Paraffin-Embedded Material

1. Incubate the slides in 10 m*M* citrate buffer, pH 6.0, boil in a microwave oven for 2 min at 850 W (*see* **Note 2**), and after that for 10 min at 150 W.
2. Air-dry for 30 min.
3. Rinse in water and PBS.

3.2.3. Incubation with Antibodies

1. To block nonspecific binding, incubate slides in 2% nonfat milk powder for 15 min and rinse in tap water.
2. Block endogenous peroxidase by incubating the sections in 3% hydrogen peroxide in absolute methanol for 15 min.

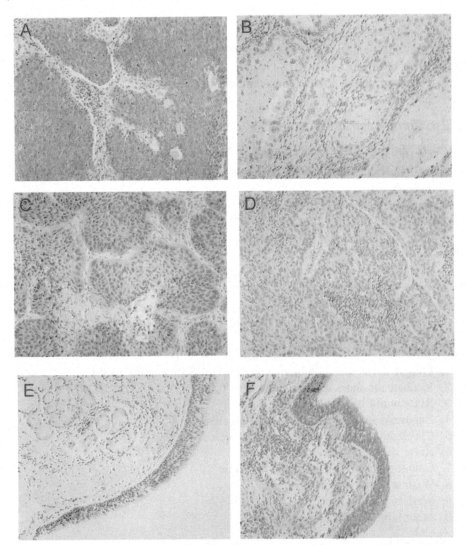

Fig. 2. Expression of γGCSh and γGCSl in the biopsies of human lung carcinoma and human nonmalignant bronchial epithelium. The panels display as follows: (**A**) Positive staining of γGCSh in lung squamous cell carcinoma; (**B**) Negative isotype control of γGCSh in lung carcinoma; (**C**) Positive staining of γGCSl in lung squamous cell carcinoma; (**D**) Negative isotype control of γGCSl in lung carcinoma; (**E**) Staining of γGCSh in bronchial epithelium; (**F**) Staining of γGCSl in bronchial epithelium.

3. Rinse in tap water 2 × 10 min and in PBS 3 × 10 min.
4. Incubate the slides in the primary (27) γGCS antibodies overnight at 4°C (*see* **Note 3**).

5. Wash three times in PBS.
6. Incubate in the biotinylated secondary anti-rabbit antibody appropriate for development using either DAB or AEC for 30 min at room temperature.
7. Rinse in PBS.
8. Negative control: Omit primary antibody and replace with PBS or rabbit primary antibody isotype control.

3.2.4. Chromogen Development

3.2.4.1. METHOD 1: DIAMINOBENZIDINE (DAB)

1. Prepare the streptavidin-biotin complex (ABC) according to manufacturer's instructions.
2. Incubate the slides in the avidin-biotin-peroxidase complex for 10 min.
3. Rinse with PBS.
4. Expose sample to DAB/hydrogen peroxide for 10 minutes.
5. Rinse with PBS 3 × 3 min.
6. Counterstain with hematoxylin for 5 min.
7. Wash with distilled water for 2 min.
8. Wash with tap water for 2 min.
9. Mount the slides with Immunomount.

3.2.4.2. METHOD 2: AMINOETHYLCARBAZOLE (AEC)

1. Prepare the streptavidin-biotin complex (*see* **Subheading 3.2.4.1.**).
2. Incubate the slides in ABC reagent for 10 min.
3. Rinse with PBS, 3 × 3 min.
4. Expose to aminoethylcarbaxole for 10 min.
5. Check development of color under a microscope.
6. Rinse slide in distilled water.
7. Counterstain with hematoxylin for 5 min.
8. Wash in distilled water for 2 min.
9. Wash in tap water for 2 min.
10. Mount the slides with Immunomount.

3.3. Inhibition of γ-Glutamylcysteine Synthetase

Effect of BSO on the cell survival of A549 lung adenocarcinoma cells is shown in **Fig. 3**.

1. Add BSO to subconfluent A549 lung adenocarcinoma for at least 16 h (*see* **Note 4**).
2. Remove the media and expose control and BSO- pretreated cells to cisplatin. To ensure the glutathione depletion during the whole incubation period, add the same concentration of BSO to the medium 24 h after starting the exposure, if the incubation time is over 24 h.
3. Determine intracellular GSH concentration (*28*).

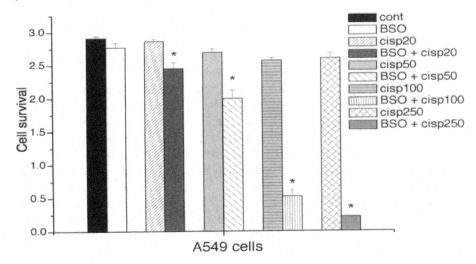

Fig. 3. The effect of glutathione depletion on the survival of cisplatin-treated A549 cells in culture. In this case the cell viability after 48 h exposure was examined using the XTT assay in a microplate reader.

4. Assess cell viability and/or cytotoxicity. In this particular case the microculture tetrazolium dye colorimetric assay (XTT) (Boehringer, Mannheim, Germany) was used according to the manufacturer's instructions. The results were analyzed using the Victor multilabel counter (1420 Wallac Inc., Turku, Finland) (*see* **Note 5**).

4. Notes

1. In order to achieve even tissue fixation and preserve morphology, pulmonary tissues can also be fixed intrabronchially with 10% buffered formalin
2. Microwave treatment was used to get optimal antigen retrieval. Retrieval times are not constant but should be standardized for each individual antibody.
3. Problems with the antibodies of antioxidant enzymes: The experience of our laboratory agrees with a recent investigation by Yan and coworkers, who found that many commercially available antibodies for antioxidant enzymes are of poor quality *(29)*. As stated by Yan et al. *(29)*, there are four catalase antibodies and one CuZnSOD antibody with sufficient specificity, but the MnSOD antibody detects only very high levels of the enzyme protein. Three glutathione peroxidases cannot detect the specific GPx band from cell lysates and have not been recommended for immunohistochemistry *(29)*. Rabbit antibodies to human γGCS, used here, are not commercially available. These antibodies were obtained from Dr. T. Kavanagh (University of Washington, Seattle, WA) and used here with his permission. A more detailed description of these particular antibodies has been given elsewhere *(27)*. Provided that the antibodies are available,

the immunohistochemical detection of other AOEs in human lung and lung malignancies are very similar to γGCS, with only slight modifications.

4. BSO should be made fresh every time. The appropriate concentration varies from 0.1 mM to 1 mM, depending on the GSH content of the cell. Determination of intracellular GSH concentration is recommended to test its depletion in the cell.

5. Either cell viability or cytotoxicity can be assessed. Most common assays for cytotoxicity include trypan blue exclusion, lactate dehydrogenase release, release of radioactive chromium, or thymidine incorporation. Most common methods for the assessment of cell survival include proliferation assays, such as the ability of the cell to form colonies. Cell cytotoxicity may also be investigated by assessing changes in the cellular energy state and apoptosis by numerous methodologies. Some of these methods have been described in detail in other volumes of this same book series (*see* for instance Methods in Molecular Medicine: *Cytotoxic Drug Resistance Mechanisms*, edited by R. Brown and U. Böger-Brown, Humana Press, 1999).

References

1. Halliwell, B. (1991) Reactive oxygen species in living systems: source, biochemistry, and role in human disease. *Am. J. Med.* **91,** 14S–22S.
2. Thannickal, V. J. and Fanburg, B. L. (2000) Reactive oxygen species in cell signaling. *Am. J. Physiol. Lung Cell Mol. Physiol.* **279,** L1005–L1028.
3. Tew, K. D. (1994) Glutathione-associated enzymes in anticancer drug resistance. *Cancer Res.* **54,** 4313–4320.
4. Zhang, K., Mack, P., and Wong, K. P. (1998) Glutathione-related mechanisms in cellular resistance to anticancer drugs. *Int. J. Oncol.* **12,** 871–882.
5. O'Brien, M. L. and Tew, K. D. (1996) Glutathione and related enzymes in multidrug resistance. *Eur. J. Cancer* **32A,** 967–978.
6. Halliwell, B. and Gutteridge, J. M. C. (1996) *Free Radicals in Biology and Medicine.* Oxford University Press, New York, NY.
7. Holmgren, A. (1985) Thioredoxin. *Annu. Rev. Biochem.* **54,** 237–271.
8. Powis, G., Mustacich, D., and Coon, A. (2000) The role of the redox protein thioredoxin in cell growth and cancer. *Free Radic. Biol. Med.* **29,** 312–322.
9. Rhee, S. G. (1999) Redox signaling: hydrogen peroxide as intracellular messenger. *Exp. Mol. Med.* **31,** 53–59.
10. Tipnis, S. R., Blake, D. G., Shepherd, A. G., and McLellan, L. I. (1999) Overexpression of the regulatory subumit of γ-glutamylcysteine synthetase in HeLa cells increases γ-glutamylcysteine synthetase activity and confers drug resistance. *Biochem. J.* **337,** 559–566.
11. Kinnula, V. L., Yankaskas, J. R., Chang, L., Virtanen, I., Linnala, A., Kang, B. H., and Crapo, J. D. (1994) Primary and immortalized (BEAS 2B) human bronchial epithelial cells have significant antioxidative capacity in vitro. *Am. J. Respir. Cell Mol. Biol.* **11,** 568–576.

12. Erzurum, S. C., Danel, C., Gillissen, A., Chu, C. S., Trapnell, B. C., and Crystal, R. G. (1993) In vivo antioxidant gene expression in human airway epithelium of normal individuals exposed to 100% O_2. *J. Appl. Physiol.* **75,** 1256–1262.

13. Cantin, A. M., North, S. L., Hubbard, R. C., and Crystal, R. G. (1987) Normal alveolar epithelial lining fluid contains high levels of glutathione. *J. Appl. Physiol.* **63,** 152–157.

14. Ingbar, D. H., Hepler, K., Dowin, R., Jacobsen, E., Dunitz, J. M., Nici, L., and Jamieson, J. D. (1995) gamma-Glutamyl transpeptidase is a polarized alveolar epithelial membrane protein. *Am. J. Physiol.* **269,** L261–L271.

15. Coursin, D. B., Cihla, H. P., Sempf, J., Oberley, T. D., and Oberley, L. W. (1996) An immunohistochemical analysis of antioxidant and glutathione S-transferase enzyme levels in normal and neoplastic human lung. *Histol. Histopathol.* **11,** 851–860.

16. Oberley, L. W. and Oberley, T. D. (1997) Role of antioxidant enzymes in the cancer phenotype. In: *Oxygen, Gene Expression, and Cellular Function.* Clerch, L. B. and Massano, D. J., eds. Lung Biology in Health and Disease. 105, Marcel Dekker, Inc., New York, 279–307.

17. Cobbs, C. S., Levi, D. S., Aldape, K., and Israel, M. A. (1996) Manganese superoxide dismutase expression in human central nervous system tumors. *Cancer Res.* **56,** 3192–3195.

18. Janssen, A. M., Bosman, C. B., Sier, C. F., Griffioen, G., Kubben, F. J., Lamers, C. B., et al. (1998) Superoxide dismutases in relation to the overall survival of colorectal cancer patients. *Br. J. Cancer* **78,** 1051–1057.

19. Kahlos, K., Anttila, S., Asikainen, T., Kinnula, K., Raivio, K. O., Mattson, K., et al. (1998) Manganese superoxide dismutase in healthy human pleural mesothelium and in malignant pleural mesothelioma. *Am. J. Respir. Cell Mol. Biol.* **18,** 570–580.

20. Cole, S. P., Downes, H. F., Mirski, S. E., and Clements, D. J. (1990) Alterations in glutathione and glutathione-related enzymes in a multidrug-resistant small cell lung cancer cell line. *Mol. Pharmacol.* **37,** 192–197.

21. Zaman, G. J., Lankelma, J., van Tellingen, O., Beijnen, J., Dekker, H., Paulusma, C., et al. (1995) Role of glutathione in the export of compounds from cells by the multidrug-resistance-associated protein. *Proc. Natl. Acad. Sci. USA* **92,** 7690–7694.

22. Rahman, I. and MacNee, W. (2000) Oxidative stress and regulation of glutathione in lung inflammation. *Eur. Respir. J.* **16(3),** 534–554.

23. Iida, T., Mori, E., Mori, K., Goto, S., Urata, Y., Oka, M., Kohno, S., and Kondo, T. (1999) Co-expression of gamma-glutamylcysteine synthetase sub-units in response to cisplatin and doxorubicin in human cancer cells. *Int. J. Cancer* **82,** 405–411.

24. Oguri, T., Fujiwara, Y., Isobe, T., Katoh, O., Watanabe, H., and Yamakido, M. (1998) Expression of γ-glutamylcysteine synthetase (γGCS) and multidrug resistance-associated protein (MRP), but not human canalicular multispecific organic anion transporter (cMOAT), genes correlates with exposure of human lung cancers to platinum drugs. *Br. J. Cancer* **77,** 1089–1096.

25. Hatcher, E. L., Alexander, J. M., and Kang, Y. J. (1997) Decreased sensitivity to adriamycin in cadmium-resistant human lung carcinoma A549 cells. *Biochem. Pharmacol.* **53,** 747–754.

26. al-Kabban, M., Stewart, M. J., Watson, I. D., and Reglinski, J. (1990) The effect of doxorubicin on the glutathione content and viability of cultured human lung cancer cell lines A549 and GLC4 210. *Clin. Chim. Acta.* **194,** 121–129.

27. Jarvinen, K., Pietarinen-Runtti, P., Linnainmaa, K., Raivio, K. O., Krejsa, C. M., Kavanagh, T., and Kinnula, V. L. (2000) Antioxidant defense mechanisms of human mesothelioma and lung adenocarcinoma cells. *Am. J. Physiol. Lung Cell Mol. Physiol.* **278,** L696–L702.

28. Buckley, B. J., Kent, R. S., and Whorton, A. R. (1991) Regulation of endothelial cell prostaglandin synthesis by glutathione. *J. Biol. Chem.* **266,** 16659–16666.

29. Yan, T., Jiang, X., Zhang, H. J., Li, S., and Oberley, L. W. (1998) Use of commercial antibodies for detection of the primary antioxidant enzymes. *Free Radic. Biol. Med.* **25(6),** 688–693.

30. Ray, S., Misso, N. L., Lenzo, J. C., Robinson, C., and Thompson, P. J. (1999) Gamma-glutamylcysteine synthetase activity in human lung epithelial (A549) cells: factors influencing its measurement. *Free Radic. Biol. Med.* **27,** 1346–1356.

15

Localization of Cyclooxygenase-2 Protein Expression in Lung Cancer Specimens by Immunohistochemical Analysis

Sarah A. Wardlaw and Thomas H. March

1. Introduction

Cyclooxygenase-2 (COX-2) inhibitors comprise a group of compounds that show promise as cancer preventives. COX-2 is an inducible enzyme that catalyzes the rate-limiting step in the synthesis of prostaglandins from arachidonic acid. The anti-inflammatory effects of aspirin and other non-steroidal antiinflammatory drugs (NSAIDs) are a result of their inhibition of this enzyme. A role for this enzyme in cancer development was first hypothesized when it was noted that people who ingest NSAIDs regularly for long periods of time have a significantly reduced risk of colon cancer *(1)*. Subsequently COX-2 was found to be expressed at high levels in about one-half of colorectal adenomas and most colorectal adenocarcinomas *(2)*. And more importantly, NSAIDs and other COX-2 inhibitors significantly reduced colon tumor number in both animal *(3,4)*, and clinical studies *(5)*.

Less is known about COX-2 expression in the lung and its role in lung tumorigenesis. NSAIDs and NS-398, a specific inhibitor of COX-2, repress in vitro and in vivo growth of murine and human lung cancer-derived cell lines *(6,7)*. These compounds also reduce the number of lung tumors that develop in mice exposed to a lung carcinogen *(6)*. COX-2 protein levels are low or undetectable in human small cell lung cancers *(8,9)*. However, COX-2 protein has been detected in all types of human non-small cell lung cancers (NSCLC), with the highest expression levels occuring in adenocarcinomas *(8–10)*. COX-2 is also expressed in the tumors that arise in several rodent models of lung adenocarcinoma *(11–13)*. In addition, in both murine and human lung COX-2

From: *Methods in Molecular Medicine, vol. 74: Lung Cancer, Vol. 1: Molecular Pathology Methods and Reviews*
Edited by: B. Driscoll © Humana Press Inc., Totowa, NJ

expression has been detected in premalignant/preinvasive lesions such as atypical adenomatous hyperplasia (AAH) and carcinoma *in situ (8,11–14)*.

The prognostic value of COX-2 expression levels in human lung adenocarcinomas has been examined in a small number of studies. One study found a correlation between COX-2 level and survival in a cohort of patients with Stage I disease *(15)*. However, in this study and two others *(8,14)*, no correlation was seen between COX-2 expression and overall survival or any clinical/pathological features such as tumor size, nodal involvement, or disease stage. What is not known at this time is whether COX-2 expression levels in tumor-progenitor cells, precursor lesions, or primary tumors will be indicative of the efficacy of the COX-2 inhibitor class of chemopreventive agents in repressing the incidence or recurrence of NSCLC.

This chapter describes the localization of COX-2 protein expression in lung cancer specimens by immunohistochemical analysis. The specimens are fixed and then incubated with an antibody that specifically recognizes COX-2. Bound antibody is then visualized by incubating the specimen with a biotinylated secondary antibody that recognizes the COX-2-specific antibody. Subsequent incubation with a mixture of avidin, biotin, and horseradish peroxidase (HRP), followed by the administration of a substrate of HRP, results in a colored reaction product localized to the areas of COX-2 protein expression. These results provide valuable information regarding the cellular and subcellular localization of COX-2 protein expression, as well as a semi-quantitative measure of expression levels. More quantitative results can be obtained by immunoblot analysis of tissue/tumor extracts. However, when analyzing tumors by immunoblotting, the results can vary significantly depending upon the region of the tumor from which the extract was prepared, or if the whole tumor is utilized, the ratio of tumor tissue to normal tissue present in the specimen. Similarly, COX-2 expression can be quantified on an mRNA level by means of Northern analysis, Ribonuclease Protection Assay (RPA), or quantitative reverse transcriptase polymerase chain reaction (RT-PCR), with the same limitations regarding the origin and composition of the specimen.

2. Materials

1. Formalin-fixed, 5-μm-thick tissue/tumor sections on positively charged glass slides (standard fixation/processing methods for human sections, *see* **Note 1** for mouse lung).
2. Dipping slide holder.
3. Histology-grade xylenes.
4. Ethanol.
5. Tris-buffered saline (TBS), pH 7.6.
6. Hydrogen peroxide.

7. Methanol.
8. Antigen Retrieval *Citra* Solution (BioGenex) (Optional).
9. Coplin jar(s) (Optional).
10. Humid chamber (*see* **Note 2**).
11. PAP pen.
12. VECTASTAIN®-Elite ABC Kit (Rabbit IgG specific) (Vector Laboratories).
13. Power Block™ blocking agent (BioGenex).
14. Primary Antibody Diluting Buffer™ (Biomeda).
15. Rabbit anti-COX-2 antibody (Cayman Chemical).
16. Rabbit IgG.
17. Aqueous Hematoxylin™ (Biomeda).
18. Xylene-based mounting medium (e.g., "Permount" from Fisher).
19. Cover slips.

3. Methods

1. Bake the tissue sections in a dry oven at 55–65°C for 1–3 h *if necessary* (*see* **Note 3**).
2. Place the tissue sections in a slide holder designed for liquid submersion of the slides. Deparaffinize the tissue sections by submerging them in xylene for 10 min. Repeat this two more times using clean xylene each time (*see* **Note 4**).
3. Rehydrate the tissue sections by submerging them in 100% ethanol for 5 min, followed by submersion in 95, 80, 70, 50, and 30% ethanol in water for 5 min each, ending with submersion in pure water for 5 min. *Once the tissue section is rehydrated it must not be allowed to dry out.*
4. Eliminate endogenous peroxidase activity in the tissue sections by submerging them in 0.1% hydrogen peroxide in methanol for 30 min. If antigen retrieval (**step 6**) will be performed, wash the tissue sections by submerging them three times in clean water for 5 min each time. If antigen retrieval will not be performed, wash the tissue sections by submerging them twice in clean water for 5 min each, followed by submersion in TBS for 5 min.
5. (Optional *see* **Note 5**). Enhance the antigenicity of the tissue sections by placing the slides in a Coplin jar and filling the jar with enough Antigen Retrieval *Citra* Solution to cover the tissue sections. Place the Coplin jar inside a larger container (e.g., a beaker) containing several inches of water. Microwave at high power until the antigen retrieval solution begins to boil. Reduce the power to 20–30% (just enough to maintain the boil) and microwave for an additional 15 min. *Cool to room temperature.* Wash the tissue sections by submerging them twice in clean water for 5 min each, followed by submersion in TBS for 5 min.
6. Air-dry the slides until the surface of the slide around the tissue section is dry, but the tissue section is still wet. Draw a circle around each tissue section with a PAP pen. Place the slides on a horizontal support inside of an uncovered humid chamber with the tissue sections facing up. Place some buffer on each tissue section until the entire area within the PAP circle is covered. (If you are analyzing more than 16–20 slides; *see* **Note 6**.)

7. Remove the buffer from each tissue section using a glass Pasteur pipet or plastic pipet tip inserted into the end of a flexible hose attached to a vacuum trap. Do not touch the tissue section with the pipet or tip. Point the pipet or tip away from the tissue section to prevent air from being pulled across the tissue section and drying it out.

8. Block nonspecific binding sites by applying Power Block blocking agent to each tissue section. Remove the Power Block after 5–10 min. Then apply a solution of 1.5% normal goat serum in TBS. (The serum is supplied in the VECTASTAIN Elite kit.) Cover/seal the humid chamber and place at 4°C overnight.

9. Remove the second blocking solution and apply the primary antibody (anti-COX-2) OR rabbit IgG (*see* **Note 7**) diluted in Primary Antibody Diluting Buffer (*see* **Note 8** for dilution information). Cover/seal the humid chamber and incubate at room temperature for at least 2 h.

10. Thoroughly wash away unbound primary antibody by applying and removing TBS three times or by holding each slide in a vertical orientation and gently directing a stream of TBS from a squeeze bottle to an area of the slide well above the tissue section.

11. Apply the secondary antibody (biotinylated anti-rabbit IgG, from VECTASTAIN Elite kit) in Primary Antibody Diluting Buffer at the dilution recommended in the kit instructions. Cover/seal the humid chamber and incubate at room temperature for 1 h.

12. Thoroughly wash away unbound secondary antibody as described in **step 10**.

13. Link the secondary antibody to horse radish peroxidase by preparing the ABC reagent as described in the VECTASTAIN Elite kit instructions and applying it to the tissue sections. Incubate at room temperature for 30 min. Wash the tissue sections with TBS.

14. Deliver substrate to the horse radish peroxidase by preparing the DAB solution as described in the VECTASTAIN Elite kit instructions and applying it to the tissue sections. Allow the enzymatic reaction and color development to proceed for 5–10 min (*see* **Note 9**). Stop the reaction by washing the tissue sections with *water*.

15. Dilute the Aqueous Hematoxylin 1:3 with water. Apply to the tissue sections for 2–5 min (*see* **Note 9**). Remove by washing the tissue sections with *water*. At this time the hematoxylin counterstain will appear purple. "Blue" the counterstain by applying TBS to the tissue sections for approx 5 min.

16. Return the slides to the dipping holder and dehydrate the tissue sections by submerging them for 5 min each in the same solutions used in **step 3**, but in reverse order, starting with water and ending with 100% ethanol.

17. Finish dehydrating the tissue sections by submerging them in xylene for 5 min. Repeat this two more times using clean xylene each time.

18. Air-dry the slides until the xylene has evaporated. Place a drop or two of mounting medium in the middle of each tissue section and gently place a coverslip on top

of the tissue section taking care not to trap any air bubbles. Leave the slides cover slip-up on a flat surface until the mounting medium has hardened.

19. Grade the expression of COX-2 in the immunohistochemically stained hyperplastic foci and neoplasms semi-quantitatively by light microscopic assessment (*see* **Note 10**).

4. Notes

1. To analyze mouse lungs, remove the lungs and cannulate the tracheas. Inflate the lungs with buffered 4% paraformaldehyde via the cannulas until the pleura is tense. Ligate the tracheas and further fix the lungs by immersion in fixative for 48–72 h. Trim the fixed lung lobes longitudinally along the axial airway before embedding and sectioning.

2. A humid chamber consists of an air-tight box that is open on top and contains elevated supports that hold slides horizontally above a small amount of water that is placed in the bottom of the box. Once sealed, the humid environment that develops inside of the box prevents the evaporation of reagents that have been applied to the tissue sections. Boxes can be bought that are made just for this purpose. Or one can simply use a shallow plastic container with a lid.

3. Baking increases the adherence of the tissue sections to the glass slides, but can also reduce their antigenicity. In general, lung tissue sections do not need to be baked. Bake them only if loss or folding of the tissue sections occurs during immunohistochemical analysis.

4. Three submersions in clean xylene ensure that all of the paraffin is removed. Tissue sections with paraffin residue will have a speckled appearance when the stained section is viewed with a light microscope.

5. Submerging and boiling tissue sections in any kind of "antigen retrieval" solution will often (but not always) increase the antigenicity of the tissue by making the antigen more accessible to the antibody. This allows the use of a higher dilution of antibody than would be used otherwise and is, therefore, of value when antibody is limited. Please note that antigen retrieval usually does not create antigen staining where none was seen before, will add 1–2 h to the entire procedure, and increases the likelihood that all or part of the tissue section will separate from the glass slide.

6. This method is cumbersome if one is working with more than 16–20 slides. Large numbers of slides can be processed easily using the MicroProbe Staining System (Fisher). The slides are placed in a special slide holder opposite clean Probe-On Plus glass slides (Fisher) (the tissue sections must also be on Probe-On Plus slides). Antibodies, substrate, and hematoxylin are then applied to and removed from all of the tissue sections at once through capillary action. A special detergent-containing buffer must be used in place of the TBS (10X Automation Buffer from Biomeda). Detergent (.075% Brij-35) must be added to the water used in **steps 14** and **15**. The slides are removed from the MicroProbe slide holder

and returned to the dipping slide holder prior to dehydration. The disadvantages of this method are that the tissue sections cannot be rinsed as thoroughly between reagent applications as with the "dropper method" described earlier, air bubbles can develop in the capillary space that will result in unstained areas of the tissue section, and parts of the tissue sections have a tendency to come loose when the slides are separated from their opposing clean glass slides.

7. For each section incubated with COX-2 antibody, a comparable section should be incubated with the "nonimmunized" equivalent of that antibody. In this way, nonspecific staining can be identified. Nonspecific staining occurs frequently; without a control slide for comparison, observed staining has little meaning. If the antibody is in the form of serum, serum from a nonimmunized animal should be applied to the control slides at the same dilution as the antibody. If the serum has been partially purified (as is the case with the rabbit polyclonal antibody from Cayman), purified IgG from a nonimmunized animal should be applied to the control slides. A second control that can further demonstrate the specificity of the staining is to pre-incubate the primary antibody solution with increasing amounts of the antigen used to immunize the host animal. (The peptide antigen used to create Cayman's polyclonal antibodies [PAbs] can be purchased from Cayman.) Exogenous antigen will block the binding of antibody to antigen in the tissue sections. Specific antigen staining should become fainter as the amount of exogenous antigen increases.

8. The best primary antibody dilution must be determined empirically, as results will vary depending upon species, fixation method, processing, antibody source, and so on. For the rabbit polyclonal antibody from Cayman, try dilutions in the range of 1:200 to 1:1000.

9. The brown color produced during application of the DAB can develop quickly. If the reaction is allowed to proceed for too long a background brown staining may begin to form. The blue hematoxylin counterstain can also be applied for too long or at too high of a concentration. This can obscure the brown DAB staining. The best time and dilution should be determined empirically.

10. COX-2 staining may be observed in normal lung tissue as well as in the neoplasms, particularly in the bronchial epithelium, vascular endothelium, and smooth muscle. The assessment of tumor staining can be subjectively graded in two parts consisting of distribution and intensity. First, the amount of the lesion containing positively stained cells is estimated on a percentage basis, and a score assigned to that percentage estimate. Thus, for <25% of the cells within the lesion staining positively, the score is 1. For 25–50%, the score is 2; for 50–75%, score = 3; and for 75–100%, score = 4. Simultaneously, the intensity of the DAB stain deposits within the positively stained cells is graded on a scale of 0 to 4+, with 4+ being the most intense (bronchiolar epithelium as a positive control). The product of the intensity and percentage distribution score give a subset of the total score. For example, within a single lesion, 25–50% of the cells stained with an intensity of 4+ (product = 8), while 25–50% of cells stained with a 3+ intensity (product = 6), and less than 25% of the cells within the lesion

stained with a 2+ intensity (product = 2). For the total score of the entire lesion, the subsets are summed (16 for the example given).

References

1. Thun, M. J., Namboodiri, M. M., and Heath, C. W. (1991) Aspirin use and reduced risk of fatal colon cancer. *N. Engl. J. Med.* **325,** 1593–1596.
2. Eberhart, C. E., Coffey, R. J., Radhika, A., Giardiello, F. M., Ferrenbach, S., and DuBois, R. N. (1994) Up-regulation of cyclooxygenase 2 gene expression in human colorectal adenomas and adenocarcinomas. *Gastroenterology* **107,** 1183–1188.
3. Pollard, M. and Luckert, P. H. (1982) Indomethacin treatment of rats with dimethylhydrazine-induced intestinal tumors. *Cancer Treat. Rep.* **64,** 1323–1327.
4. Jacoby, R. F., Marshall, D. J., Newton, M. A., Novakovic, K., Tutsch, K., Cole, C. E., et al. (1996) Chemoprevention of spontaneous intestinal adenomas in the *Apc*^Min mouse model by the nonsteroidal anti-inflammatory drug piroxicam. *Cancer Res.* **56,** 710–714.
5. Giardiello, F. M., Hamilton, S. R., Krush, A. J., Piantadosi, S., Hylind, L. M., Celano, P., et al. (1993) Treatment of colonic and rectal adenomas with sulindac in familial adenomatous polyposis. *N. Engl. J. Med.* **328,** 1313–1316.
6. Rioux, N. and Castonguay, A. (1998) Prevention of NNK-induced lung tumorigenesis in A/J mice by acetylsalicylic acid and NS-398. *Cancer Res.* **58,** 5354–5360.
7. Hida, T., Leyton, J., Makheja, A. N., Ben-Av, P., Hla, T., Martinez, A., et al. (1998) Non-small cell lung cancer cyclooxygenase activity and proliferation are inhibited by non-steroidal antiinflammatory drugs. *Anticancer Res.* **18,** 775–782.
8. Hida, T., Yatabe, Y., Achiwa, H., Muramatsu, H., Kozaki, K., Nakamura, S., et al. (1998) Increased expression of cyclooxygenase 2 occurs frequently in human lung cancers, specifically adenocarcinomas. *Cancer Res.* **58,** 3761–3764.
9. Wolff, H., Saukkonen, K., Anttila, S., Karjalainen, A., Vainio, H., and Ristimäki, A. (1998) Expression of cyclooxygenase-2 in human lung carcinoma. *Cancer Res.* **58,** 4997–5001.
10. Watkins, D. N., Lenzo, J. C., Segal, A., Garlepp, M. J., and Thompson, P. J. (1999) Expression and localization of cyclo-oxygenase isoforms in non-small cell lung cancer. *Eur. Respir. J.* **14,** 412–418.
11. Wardlaw, S. A., March, T. H., and Belinsky, S. A. (2000) Cyclooxygenase-2 expression is abundant in alveolar type II cells in lung cancer-sensitive mouse strains and in premalignant lesions. *Carcinogenesis* **21,** 1371–1377.
12. Bauer, A. K., Dwyer-Nield, L. D., and Malkinson, A. M. (2000) High cyclooxygenase 1 (COX-1) and cyclooxygenase 2 (COX-2) contents in mouse lung tumors. *Carcinogenesis* **21,** 543–550.
13. Kitayama, W., Denda, A., Yoshida, J., Sasaki, Y., Takahama, M., Murakawa, K., et al. (2000) Increased expression of cyclooxygenase-2 protein in rat lung tumors induced by *N*-nitrosobix(2-hydroxypropyl)amine. *Cancer Lett.* **148,** 145–152.
14. Hosomi, Y., Yokose, T., Hirose, Y., Nakajima, R., Nagai, K., Nishiwaki, Y., and Ochiai, A. (2000) Increased cyclooxygenase 2 (COX-2) expression occurs

frequently in precursor lesions of human adenocarcinoma of the lung. *Lung Cancer* **30**, 73–81.

15. Achiwa, H., Yatabe, Y., Hida, T., Kuroishi, T., Kozaki, K., Nakamura, S., et al. (1999) Prognostic significance of elevated cyclooxygenase 2 expression in primary, resected lung adenocarcinomas. *Clin. Cancer Res.* **5**, 1001–1005.

16

Non-RI Protocols for L-*myc* Allelotyping and Deletion Mapping of Chromosome 1p in Primary Lung Cancers

Keiko Hiyama, Ciro Mendoza, and Eiso Hiyama

1. Introduction

Deletion at a specific locus in a chromosome in cancer cells is assumed to imply the existence of a tumor-suppressor gene. As a result of multi-step carcinogenesis, there are several hotspots of allelic deletion in lung cancer *(1)*. The most frequent loci where allelic deletions occur in lung cancer tissues are the short arm of chromosome 3, which contains the *FHIT* gene at 3p14.2, the long arm of chromosome 13, which contains the *RB1* gene at 13q14, and the short arm of chromosome 17, which contains the *TP53* gene at 17p13. Deletions at these loci mean loss of the existing tumor-suppressor genes, resulting in carcinogenesis and/or tumorigenesis. Other loci, such as 5q, 9p, and 18q, are also frequently deleted in primary lesion of lung cancer, indicating the possible existence of other tumor-suppressor genes, which may also be responsible for carcinogenesis or early-stage development of lung cancer.

In contrast, the short arm of chromosome 1 is frequently deleted in metastatic lesions, but less often in primary lesions of the lung. Interestingly, the "S-allele" of the L-*myc* gene has been reported to be associated with metastasis, poor prognosis, and double cancer in patients with lung cancer *(2)*. These findings led to speculation of the existence of a tumor-suppressor gene associated with metastasis or late-stage development of lung cancer, and inactivation of this gene may have linkage disequilibrium with the L-*myc* "S-allele." To examine the propriety of this hypothesis, we determined the shortest regions of overlap (SROs) in 1p in lung cancer and found no association with the L-*myc* allelotype *(3)*. We demonstrated the three SROs from D1S2797 to pter, and proposed that

From: *Methods in Molecular Medicine, vol. 74: Lung Cancer, Vol. 1: Molecular Pathology Methods and Reviews*
Edited by: B. Driscoll © Humana Press Inc., Totowa, NJ

a tumor-suppressor gene, which might be involved in an inhibitory mechanism of cellular immortalization of lung cancer, may exist between D1S2797 and *MYCL1* at 1p34.3. Moreover, these non-RI techniques *(3,4)* are also applicable to other chromosomes for finding novel tumor-suppressor genes.

2. Materials

2.1. DNA Extraction

1. Medium buffer: 0.25 *M* sucrose, 0.1 *M* NaCl, 0.1 *M* Tris-HCl, pH 9.0. Autoclaved 100 mL 1 *M* Tris-HCl, pH 9.0, is added to the autoclaved 900 mL solution containing 85.56 g sucrose and 5.844 g NaCl. Store at room temperature. (Do not autoclave the mixture of Tris-HCl and sucrose.)
2. Extraction buffer: 10 m*M* EDTA, pH 8.0, 10 m*M* Tris-HCl, pH 8.0, 10 m*M* NaCl. Store at room temperature.
3. Proteinase K solution: Dissolved in the extraction buffer at 1 mg/mL. Stored at –20°C in small aliquots. Do not repeat freeze and thaw.
4. 10% SDS: Commercially available, or dissolve 10 g of SDS in 100 mL sterile distilled, deionized water (DDW). Store at room temperature.
5. Liquified phenol saturated with buffer: Ultra pure phenol saturated with buffer, pH > 7.8, is available from manufacturers (Nacalai Tesque, Kyoto, Japan). (Crystalline phenol must be melted at 68°C and saturated with buffer before use.) Never touch it without gloves and do not inhale (it causes severe burns). Store airtight and in the dark at 4°C. The upper layer is aqueous and use the lower layer (organic layer) in the experiments.
6. CIAA: chloroform containing 4% of isoamyl alcohol. Never touch it without gloves and do not inhale (chloroform is a carcinogen and irritating to the skin). To a 500-mL bottle of chloroform, add 20.8 mL of isoamyl alcohol. Store at room temperature.
7. 5 *M* NaCl: 146.1g NaCl in 500 mL DDW solution. Autoclave and store at room temperature.
8. 95% ethanol: commercially available. In the experiments using fluorescence, 95% ethanol is recommended rather than >99% ethanol. Store at room temperature.
9. TE buffer: 10 m*M* Tris-HCl, 1 m*M* EDTA, pH 8.0.

2.2. Primers for PCR

The sequences of the primers to be synthesized are listed below and other primers are available from Applied Biosystems (ABI Prism Linkage Mapping Set™, Foster City, CA) *(3–5)*. Primers are stored at –20°C in small aliquots and the fluorescent primers should be stored in dark.

1. Detection of L-*myc* amplification by fluorescent differential polymerase chain reaction (PCR).

    fluorescent L-*myc* sense primer: 5′-FAM-AGA GCT CAC CCA ATA GG-3′
    L-*myc* antisense primer: 5′-TGT GTG GAC AAT CGC AT-3′

β-globin sense primer: 5′-GTG TGC TGG CCC ATC ACT TT-3′

fluorescent β-globin antisense primer: 5′-HEX-CAA GAA AGC GAG CTT AG TGA-3′

2. Polymerase chain reaction-restriction fragment length polymorphism (PCR-RFLP) analysis of L-*myc* allelotype (nonlabeled).

L-*myc* sense: 5′-AGA GCT CAC CCA ATA GG-3′

L-*myc* antisense: 5′-TGT GTG GAC AAT CGC AT-3′

3. Deletion mapping for 1p by amplifying microsatellite markers with fluorescent primers (range of PCR product length).

D1S230 primer set (154–166 bp): ABI Prism Linkage Mapping Set™ (Applied Biosystems; HEX label)

D1S2890 primer set (214–238 bp): ABI Prism Linkage Mapping Set™ (HEX label)

D1S2797 primer set (102–138 bp): ABI Prism Linkage Mapping Set™ (FAM label)

fluorescent MYCL1 sense (140–209 bp): 5′-FAM-TGG CGA GAC TCC ATC AAA G-3′

MYCL1 antisense: 5′-CCT TTT AAG CTG CAA CAA TTT C-3′

fluorescent D1S168 sense (142–158 bp): 5′-NED-CTT TCC TCT CAC ACC AAG GC-3′

D1S168 antisense: 5′-CAA CGG TGA TGC CTT GAT C-3′

D1S255 primer set (91–111 bp): ABI Prism Linkage Mapping Set™ (HEX label)

fluorescent CRTM sense: 5′-NED-GAG AGC GTG TAA TGG CGT TT-3′

CRTM antisense (173–177 bp): 5′-AAA TGC AAA CGC AGT CCC TC-3′

fluorescent FGR sense (135–143 bp): 5′-FAM-TAT GTG GGT CCA TGT CAC CG-3′

FGR antisense: 5′-GCT AGC ATG CAC AAA TGC GG-3′

D1S234 primer set (268–288 bp): ABI Prism Linkage Mapping Set™ (FAM label)

4. Deletion mapping for 1p by amplifying minisatellite markers with nonfluorescent primers.

D1S80 sense: 5′-TGC GTG TGA ATG ACC CAG GAG CGT AT-3′

D1S80 antisense: 5′-TCT GGC TTG TTA TTT TGT CTT GTT GGA G-3′

D1S76 sense: 5′-GGG TCT CAG CGG ATG AAG GTT TTT G-3′

D1S76 antisense: 5′-GAA CGT GTC ACT GAT GTA GCG GTT G-3′

2.3. Materials for PCR, PCR-RFLP, and Deletion Mapping

1. Sterile distilled, deionized water (DDW).
2. Type I™ 10X PCR buffer: 500 mM KCl, 100 mM Tris-HCl, pH 9.0, 15 mM MgCl$_2$ (Applied Biosystems).
3. Type II™ 10X PCR buffer: 500 mM KCl, 100 mM Tris-HCl, pH 9.0 (Applied Biosystems).
4. dNTP mix: 0.2 mM each dNTP (Applied Biosystems).

5. Primer: High-performance liquid chromatography (HPLC)-purified oligonucle-otide primers are dissolved in TE (10 mM Tris-HCl, 1 mM EDTA, pH 8.0) at a concentration of 50 (nonlabeled PCR with Type I™ buffer) or 10 (fluorescent PCR with Type II™ buffer and MgCl$_2$ solution) pmol/μL.

6. 25 mM MgCl$_2$ solution (for Type II™ buffer).

7. AmpliTaq GOLD™ polymerase (Applied Biosystems).

8. Mineral oil.

9. Program Temp Control System PC-800™ (Astek, Fukuoka, Japan).

10. *Eco*RI (New England Biolabs, Beverly, MA).

11. 3% NuSieve™ 3:1 agarose gel (BioWhittaker Molecular Applications, Rockland, ME): 3 g NuSieve™ 3:1 agarose and 100 mL of TAE buffer (0.04 M Tris-acetate, 0.001 M EDTA), heated by microwave for 5 min.

12. Deionized formamide.

13. GeneScan-500 [ROX]™ (Applied Biosystems).

14. ABI Prism 310™ Genetic analyzer (Applied Biosystems).

15. GeneScan capillary (#401823™) with the Performance Optimized Polymer 4™ (POP-4, Applied Biosystems).

16. Dye: 0.05% xylene cyanol and 0.05% bromophenol blue in 50% glycerol.

17. 2% agarose gel (Type I™, Sigma, St. Louis, MO).

18. Charge-coupled device (CCD) imaging system (Densitograph AE-6900MF™, ATTO, Tokyo).

3. Methods

3.1. DNA Extraction

1. Cut a 0.5 g portion of frozen tissue into pieces using scissors. Homogenize 2–3 times in a Potter homogenizer™ with 10 mL medium buffer.

2. Transfer the homogenate to a 15-mL disposable tube, and centrifuge at 200g for 10 min at 4°C.

3. Suspend the pellet in medium buffer and centrifuge once again.

4. Re-suspend the pellet in 1 mL extraction buffer. Add 1 mL Proteinase K solution and 20 μL 10% sodium dodecyl sulfate (SDS) simultaneously. Mix gently by inversion.

5. Incubate the homogenate at 50°C for several hours.

6. Add 1 mL each of buffer-saturated phenol and CIAA and mix gently for 30 min.

7. Centrifuge at 1,400g for 20 min at room temperature.

8. Collect the upper phase and place in a new tube. Add 1 mL CIAA and mix gently for 15 min.

9. Centrifuge again, and collect the upper phase in a new tube. To this 2 mL solution, add 200 μL 5 M NaCl, mix, and add 5 mL 95% ethanol. Mix gently by inversion until whitish DNA strings appear.

10. Centrifuge at 1,400g for 20 min at 4°C. Gently remove the resultant supernatant, and rinse the pellet in the tube by adding 1 mL of 70–75% ethanol.

Table 1
PCR Conditions for L-*myc* Gene Analysis

	L-*myc* amplification	L-*myc* allelotype
Reaction mix		
Primers	L-*myc* & β-globin	L-*myc*
Conc. of each primer	10 pmol/μL	50 pmol/μL
Vol. of each primer	0.5 μL (× 4 primers)	0.5 μL (× 2 primers)
PCR buffer	Type II™, 1.5 μL	Type I™, 5 μL
dNTP mix	2 m*M*, 1.68 μL	2 m*M*, 5 μL
Genomic DNA (~50 ng/μL)	1.2 μL	1 μL
Additional MgCl₂	25 m*M* × 1.5 μL	–
H₂O (μL)	7 μL	38 μL
Ampli Taq Gold™	0.12 μL (0.6 u)	0.25 μL (1.25 u)
Total volume	15 μL	50 μL
PCR condition		
Initial denature (°C × min)	95 × 12	95 × 10
Cycle number	10 + 20	40
Denature (°C × s)	94 × 15; 89 × 15	95 × 60
Annealing (°C × s)	55 × 15; 55 × 15	52 × 60
Extension (°C × s)	72 × 30; 72 × 30	72 × 60
Final extension (°C × min)	72 × 10	72 × 3
Storage (°C)	4	4
Electrophoresis	ABI Prism 310™	3% NuSieve™3 : 1 agarose
Estimation	GeneScan™	CCD system

11. Transfer the DNA to a 2-mL microcentrifuge tube and centrifuge at 10,000*g* for 10 min at 4°C. Remove the supernatant, dry at 50°C briefly, and dissolve the wet pellet in 500–1000 μL TE buffer. Store at 4°C (*see* **Notes 1–3**).

3.2. Detection of L-myc Amplification by Differential PCR

1. Add ~50 ng genomic DNA to a PCR mixture containing 5 pmol each of fluorescent L-*myc* sense and β-globin antisense primers and nonlabeled L-*myc* antisense and β-globin sense primers, 224 μ*M* each dNTP, 0.6 units Ampli Taq GOLD™, Type II™ PCR buffer, and 2.5 m*M* MgCl₂ in a total volume of 15 μL.
2. Top the mixture with one drop of mineral oil and subject to PCR amplification using conditions listed in **Table 1**.
3. Amplification of L-*myc* is diagnosed when the observed L-*myc* peak area in one allele is more than 150% expected from the corresponding β-globin peak area (*see* **Fig. 1**). This value is equivalent to ≥fivefold amplification, as determined by Southern-blot analysis.

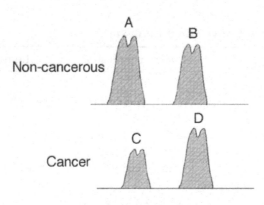

Expected peak area of "C" = A x D/B
Expected peak area of "D" = B x C/A

Fig. 1. Fragment analysis using ABI Prism 310™ Genetic Analyzer and GeneScan™ software. In detecting L-*myc* amplification by differential PCR, peaks A and C represent the β-globin gene, while peaks B and D represent the L-*myc* gene. When (peak area of D) > (peak area of B) × (peak area of C)/(peak area of A) × 1.5, the cancer sample is diagnosed as having L-*myc* amplification. In detecting allelic loss for deletion mapping, when (peak area of C) < (peak area of A) × (peak area of D)/(peak area of B) × 0.7, the cancer sample is diagnosed as having loss of allele C.

3.3. L-myc *Allelotype Determined by PCR-RFLP*

1. Add ~50 ng genomic DNA to a PCR mixture containing 25 pmol of each primer, 200 μ*M* each dNTP, 1.25 units Ampli Taq GOLD, and Type I PCR buffer (containing 1.5 m*M* MgCl₂) in a volume of 50 μL, and subjected to PCR amplification (*see* **Table 1**).
2. Add 1 μL each of 20 m*M* DTT, 170 m*M* MgCl₂, and restriction enzyme *Eco*RI to a 17 μL aliquot of the unpurified PCR product and incubate at 37°C for 1–2 h.
3. Electrophorese the digested samples on a 3% NuSieve™ 3:1 agarose gel. Stain with ethidium bromide and photograph under UV light. The undigested "L-allele" appears as a 138-bp fragment and the digested "S-allele" appears as 100-bp and 38-bp fragments (*see* **Note 4**).

3.4. Deletion Mapping

Analyze microsatellite markers (repeat of 2–4 bp) by fragment analysis using the ABI Prism 310™ Genetic Analyzer, and minisatellite markers (repeat of several dozen bp) by agarose gel electrophoresis.

1. For detecting microsatellite markers (D1S230, D1S2890, D1S2797, MYCL1, D1S168, D1S255, CRTM, FGR, and D1S234), mix 1 μL of the PCR product

Table 2
PCR Conditions for Microsatellite Markers in Deletion Mapping

Reaction mix			
Primers	One fluorescent and one nonfluorescent		
Conc. of each primer	10 pmol/μL		
Vol. of each primer	0.5 μL (× 2 primers)		
PCR buffer	Type II™, 1.5 μL		
dNTP mix	2 mM, 1.68 μL		
Genomic DNA (~50 ng/μL)	1.2 μL		
Additional MgCl$_2$	25 mM × 1.5 μL		
H$_2$O (μL)	7 μL		
Ampli Taq Gold™	0.12 μL (0.6 u)		
Total volume	15 μL		
PCR condition	Condition A[a]	Condition B[a]	Condition C[a]
Initial denature (°C × min)	95 × 12	95 × 10	95 × 10
Cycle number	10 + 20	30	10 + 20
Denature (°C × s)	94 × 15; 89 × 15	95 × 60	94 × 15; 89 × 15
Annealing (°C × s)	55 × 15; 55 × 15	58 × 60	61 × 15; 58 × 15
Extension (°C × s)	72 × 30; 72 × 30	72 × 60	72 × 30; 72 × 30
Final extension (°C × min)	72 × 10	72 × 3	72 × 3
Storage (°C)	4	4	4
Electrophoresis	ABI Prism 310™		
Estimation	GeneScan™		

[a]Microsatellite markers for condition A, D1S230, D1S2890, D1S2797, D1S255, D1S234, MYCL1; condition B, D1S168, CRTM; condition C, FGR.

    amplified using conditions listed in **Table 2** with 12 μL of deionized formamide and 0.5 μL of GeneScan-500 [ROX]™.

2. Heat the mixture at 95°C for 5 min, chill on ice, and load into the ABI Prism 310™ Genetic analyzer. It will take approx 40 min per sample for capillary electrophoresis (*see* **Note 5**).

3. For detecting minisatellite markers, mix 5 μL each of the PCR product amplified using conditions listed in **Table 3** with 3-μL dye.

4. Electrophorese samples on a 2% agarose gel, stain with ethidium bromide, and analyze using a charge-coupled device.

5. For both microsatellite and minisatellite markers, loss of heterozygosity (LOH) is diagnosed when the peak area of one allele is less than 70% expected from the corresponding noncancerous tissue (*see* **Fig. 1**).

4. Notes

1. Cancer and corresponding noncancerous tissue samples are stored at –80°C as soon as possible after surgery. For PCR analysis using genomic DNA, tissue

Table 3
PCR Conditions for Minisatellite Markers in Deletion Mapping

Reaction mix		
Primers	nonfluorescent primers	
Conc. of each primer	50 pmol/µL	
Vol. of each primer	0.5 µL (× 2 primers)	
PCR buffer	Type 1™, 5 µL	
dNTP mix	2 mM, 5 µL	
Genomic DNA (~50 ng/µL)	1 µL	
Additional MgCl$_2$	–	
H$_2$O (µL)	38 µL	
Ampli Taq Gold™	0.25 µL (1.25 u)	
Total volume	50 µL	
PCR condition	D1S76	D1S80
Initial denature (°C × min)	95 × 10	95 × 10
Cycle number	30	35
Denature (°C × s)	95 × 60	95 × 60
Annealing (°C × s)	63 × 70	57 × 70
Extension (°C × s)	72 × 180	72 × 180
Final extension (°C × min)	72 × 10	72 × 10
Storage (°C)	4	4
Electrophoresis	2% agarose	
Estimation	CCD system	

samples kept for several hours at room temperature could be used, although they are unsuitable for RNA or telomerase analysis.

2. If the sample DNA will be used only for PCR, easier and faster protocols of extracting DNA are applicable, using commercial kits, such as DNA Extractor WB Kit™ (Wako, Osaka, Japan). However, with the protocol listed in **Subheading 3.3.1.**, larger amounts of high molecular-weight DNA sufficient for Southern-blot analysis of large fragments (e.g., analysis for telomere) can be obtained.

3. If genomic DNA will be used also for Southern-blot analysis of large fragments, storage at 4°C is recommended to avoid mechanical breakage during freeze-thaw repetition. However, because fungi may contaminate the sample DNA at 4°C resulting in DNA degradation, it is recommended that an aliquot be stored at −20°C. If the DNA sample is used only for PCR, freeze-thaw repetition causes no problem.

4. Unlike a type I agarose gel of 2% or less, which can be used for 1 wk as long as it is kept wet, the 3% gel should be used within a day.

5. It is possible to mix PCR products (up to half volume of formamide) for several markers labeled with different kinds of fluorescence or PCR products without overlapping in the range of the lengths, subject to the capillary electrophoresis

as a mix, and analyze separately. Detail protocol of fragment analysis using ABI Prism 310™ Genetic Analyzer with the Performance Optimized Polymer 4™ (Applied Biosystems) is according to the manufacturers' manuals for GeneScan™ Chemistry Guide Update and ABI PRISM 310™.

References

1. Rom, W. N., Hay, J. G., Lee, T. C., Jiang, Y., and Tchou-Wong, K. M. (2000) Molecular and genetic aspects of lung cancer. *Am. J. Respir. Crit. Care Med.* **161,** 1355–1367.
2. Kawashima, K., Nomura, S., Hirai, H., Fukushi, S., Karube, T., et al. (1992) Correlation of L-myc RFLP with metastasis, prognosis and multiple cancer in lung-cancer patients. *Int. J. Cancer* **50,** 557–561.
3. Mendoza, C., Sato, H., Hiyama, K., Ishioka, S., Isobe, T., Maeda, H., et al. (2000) Allelotype and loss of heterozygosity around the L-myc gene locus in primary lung cancers. *Lung Cancer* **28,** 117–125.
4. Hiyama, E., Hiyama, K., Ohtsu, K., Yamaoka, H., Fukuba, I., Matsuura, Y., and Yokoyama, T. (2001) Biological characteristics of neuroblastoma with partial deletion in the short arm of chromosome 1. *Med. Ped. Oncol.* **36,** 67–74.
5. Ohtsu, K., Hiyama, E., Ichikawa, T., Matsuura, Y., and Yokoyama, T. (1997) Clinical investigation of neuroblastoma with partial deletion in the short arm of chromosome 1. *Clin. Cancer Res.* **3,** 1221–1228.

III

Molecular Abnormalities in Lung Cancer

C. Detection of Altered Cell Surface Markers

17

Intercellular Adhesion Molecules (ICAM-1, VCAM-1, and LFA-1) in Adenocarcinoma of Lung

Technical Aspects

Armando E. Fraire, Bruce A. Woda, Louis Savas, and Zhong Jiang

1. Introduction

Cell adhesion molecules (CAMs) such as intercellular adhesion molecule (ICAM-1), vascular adhesion molecule (VCAM-1), and lymphocyte function-associated antigen (LFA-1) facilitate interaction among cells of various lineages and are therefore crucial in the complex processes of inflammation and tumor growth *(1,2)*. This chapter discusses the mechanisms of action of CAMs and offers methodologic information for their detection and identification in fresh-frozen lung tissue. In particular, this chapter describes our experience with these CAM's in pulmonary non-small cell carcinoma and also in non-neoplastic tissue compartments of the lung such as endothelial cells, lymphocytes, fibroblasts, alveolar epithelial cells, and bronchial epithelial cells.

Among nine patients with pulmonary adenocarcinoma, three had acinar (gland forming, nonbronchioloalveolar) adenocarcinomas, five had bronchoalveolar carcinomas, and one had an adenocarcinoma metastatic from the colon. **Table 1** shows our findings on the expression of cell-adhesion molecules in the various components of the adenocarcinomas, including tumor cells proper, tumor endothelial cells, tumor stromal cells, and lymphocytes infiltrating the tumor substance. **Table 2** contains data pertaining to expression of the cell adhesion molecules in normal non-neoplastic cellular compartments of the lung, which included capillary endothelial cells (pulmonary circulation), lymphocytes, interstitial fibroblastic cells, alveolar epithelial cells, and bronchial epithelial cells. An example of positive immunostaining for

From: *Methods in Molecular Medicine, vol. 74: Lung Cancer, Vol. 1: Molecular Pathology Methods and Reviews*
Edited by: B. Driscoll © Humana Press Inc., Totowa, NJ

Table 1
Expression of Cell-Adhesion Molecules in Lung Tumors

Tumor histologic type (n)	ICAM-1 TC TEC TSC	VCAM-1 TC TEC TSC	LFA-1 TIL
BAC(5)	5/5 5/5 5/5	0/5 5/5 5/5	5/5
AAD (3)	3/3 3/3 3/3	0/3 3/3 3/3	3/3
MCC (1)	1/1 1/1 1/1	0/1 1/1 1/1	1/1

ICAM, intercellular adhesion molecule; VCAM, vascular cell-adhesion molecule; LFA, lymphocyte function-associated antigens; TC, Tumor cells; AAD, Acinar Adenocarcinoma; TEC, Tumor Endothelial cells; MCC, Metastatic Colon Cancer; TSC, Tumor stromal cells; TEC,Tumor Endothelial Cells; BAC, Bronchoalveolar carcinoma; TIL, Tumor Infiltrating Lymphocytes. (Reproduced with permission from **ref. 3**).

Table 2
Expression of Cellular-Adhesion Molecules in Normal Lung Tissue Compartments

CAM	LEC	PL	IFC	AEC	BEC
ICAM-1	+	+	+	+	+
VCAM-1	±	+	+	–	–
LFA-1	–	+	+	–	–

CAM, Cellular Adhesion Molecules; AEC, Alveolar Epithelial Cells; LEC, Lung Endothelial Cells; BEC, Bronchial Epithelial Cells; PL, Pulmonary Lymphocytes; +/–, Positive/Negative CAM Expression; IFC, Interstitial Fibroblastic Cells; ICAM, intercellular adhesion molecule; VCAM, vascular cell adhesion molecule; LFA, lymphocyte function-associated antigen. Reproduced with permission from **ref. 3**.

ICAM-1 in a frozen section of primary pulmonary adenocarcinomas is shown in **Fig. 1**.

Adhesion molecules such as ICAM-1, VCAM-1, and LFA-1 play important roles in the complex process of airway inflammation and tumor growth. Among these three adhesion molecules, ICAM-1 in particular has been the subject of considerable interest and research. While the expression of soluble circulating ICAM-1 in non-small cell carcinoma of lung has been extensively studied its expression in fresh-frozen tissues is less well-understood. Using immuno-histochemical staining of non-small cell lung cancers (NSCLC), Passlick et al. assessed the expression pattern of molecules mediating efficient cellular immune response *(4)*. Among 91 patients with NSCLC, the tumor cells of 27 (29.7%) patients expressed ICAM-1 in their tumor cells *(4)*. Vascular adhesion molecules such as VCAM-1, which belong to the immunoglobulin super gene

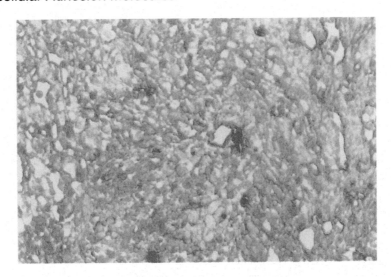

Fig. 1. ICAM-1 immunostain, note positive signal in tumor cells, endothelial cells, tumor stromal cells and tumor infiltrating lymphocytes. Original magnification ×100. Reproduced with permission from **ref. 3**.

family, are involved in the process of strong adhesion of mononuclear cells to endothelial cells. VCAM-1 is expressed in several nonvascular cell types including dendritic cells, bone marrow, and synovial cells among others (5). Furthermore, VCAM-1 is known to mediate adhesion of tumor cells such as melanoma cells to endothelial cells and may be involved in the complex process of metastatic spread of tumors. Integrins are a family of transmembrane glycoproteins that function in both cell-cell and cell-substratum adhesion (6). Integrins are ubiquitous, with at least one heterodimer present on all nucleated cells (6). LFA-1, a member of the integrin family of CAMs is present in neutrophils, monocytes, and lymphocytes as well as platelets. LFA-1 acts as a ligand for ICAM-1 and also ICAM-2.

In a previous study, we demonstrated the expression of ICAM-1 in all (100%) of the nine examined adenocarcinomas. This expression was strongest in the tumor cells proper, but it was also seen in tumor endothelial cells and tumor stromal (nonepithelial) cells. Previous studies of lung tumors also demonstrated expression of ICAM-1 in nonsmall cell carcinoma of the lung (4) but not at the level that we have shown. Passlick et al. (4) reported ICAM-1 expression in 19 (42.2%) of 45 adenocarcinomas and also in 5 (13.5%) of 37 squamous cell carcinomas. The reason for the higher rate of expression of ICAM-1 in our hands, as compared with that of Passlick et al. (4), is unclear, but it might be the result of differences in methodology such as differences in antibody strength.

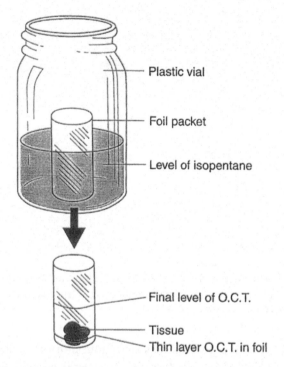

Fig. 2. Apparatus used for slow freezing of specimens.

2. Materials

2.1. Tissue Preparation

1. Neoplastic and non-neoplastic lung tissue, obtained from patients with adeno-carcinoma accessioned at the University of Massachusetts Medical Center, Worcester, MA *(3)*.
2. Hematoxylin and eosin stain.
3. Isopentane.
4. Aluminum foil.
5. Plastic vial (about 2 inches tall and 1 inch wide).
6. Dram bottle.
7. Wide-mouthed thermo-flask.
8. Applicator sticks (wooden).
9. O.C.T. (Optimum Cutting Temperature) medium.
10. Long forceps to hold the foil pocket and plastic vial.
11. Liquid nitrogen.
12. Razor blade.
13. Permanent marker pen (to label the foil pocket).

2.2. Manual Immunoperoxidase Staining

1. Acetone.
2. Vaseline.
3. Phosphate-buffered saline (PBS), pH 7.4.
4. 5 mL PBS with Goat Serum (PBS/GS): Goat serum (heat-inactivated). Store at 4°C.
5. Hydrogen peroxide (3%) (Commercial sources) store at room temperature.
6. Primary monoclonal antibodies (MAbs): anti-ICAM-1 (1:8000 dilution Becton-Dickinson, San Jose, CA), anti-VCAM-1 (1:4000 dilution Becton-Dickinson), and anti-LFA-1 (dilution 1:2000 Becton-Dickinson).
7. Biotinylated horse anti-mouse IgG (Vector BA-2001) 1:40 dilution (12.5 µg/mL) in 1% PBS/GS. Store at 4°C.
8. Horseradish peroxidase avidin D (HRP/AD) (Vector A-2004) 1:50 dilution (100 µg/mL) in 1% PBS/GS. Store at 4°C.
9. Stock diaminobenzidine: While working under the hood wearing gloves and a labcoat, carefully add the entire contents of a 25 g. bottle of 3,3′ diaminobenzidine tetrahydrochloride (Sigma D5637) to 450 mL of PBS. With the aid of a stir bar, mix the solution until dissolved (several hours) then bring the volume up to 500 mL. While still working under the hood, divide into 2-mL aliquots, store at –20°C.
10. Working DAB Solution: 0.1 mg/mL diaminobenzidine (DAB), with 0.2% hydrogen peroxide. Combine stock DAB (2 mL), working PBS (98 mL) and hydrogen peroxide (666 mL).
11. Ethanol.
12. Synthetic resin: Polymount (Poly Scientific, Bay Shore, NY).

3. Methods

3.1. Tissue Preparation

3.1.1. Histological Examination

1. Hematoxylin and eosin stained sections of surgically resected lung tumors were reviewed by one of us to evaluate the histologic classifications of the tumors and to ascertain the grade of differentiation, according to standard criteria *(3)* (*see* **Note 1**).

3.1.2. Freezing Tissue (see **Note 2**)

1. Use the dram bottle as a mold to make a foil pocket. Make sure the pocket is labeled.
2. Place a thin layer of O.C.T. at the bottom of the foil pocket.
3. Quickly place tissue in the O.C.T., tapping quickly with applicator if necessary to center and orient the specimen.

4. Place the foil pocket in the plastic vial containing isopentane. The foil pocket should not float, but the isopentane should reach a level higher than the level of O.C.T. (**Fig. 2**) (*see* **Note 3**).
5. Set the vial with the aluminum pocket in liquid nitrogen. The O.C.T. will freeze from outside in. The tissue is completely frozen when a small peak forms in center of the O.C.T.
6. Place the frozen block in a –20°C or –70°C.

3.2. Manual Immunoperoxidase Staining

1. Cut 4-μm frozen sections and allow to air dry for 10–15 min.
2. Fix frozen sections in room temperature acetone for 10 min and allow to air dry.
3. Circle section with a thin outline of vaseline.
4. Place slides in PBS/GS buffer. Subsequent incubations are carried out at room temperature in a chamber by first shaking off excess buffer and then flooding the slide with the appropriate reagents. Upon completion of the incubations shake off excess reagent before placing in buffer.
5. Block endogenous peroxidase activity by incubating for 8–10 min in hydrogen peroxide solution followed by two changes of PBS/GS for 3 min each.
6. Apply appropriate primary antibody to each slide and incubate in a room temperature moist chamber for 30–45 min.
7. Shake off excess antibody and wash in 2 changes of PBS/GS for 3 min each.
8. Apply biotinylated secondary antibody to each slide and incubate in a room temperature moist chamber for 30 min.
9. Shake off excess antibody and wash in 2 changes of PBS/GS for 3 min each.
10. Apply avidin/peroxidase complex to each slide and incubate in a room temperature wet chamber for 30 min.
11. Shake off excess avidin/peroxidase complex and wash in 2 changes of PBS without GS for 3 min each.
12. With the slides arranged in a rack, incubate in DAB solution for 10 min. At the end of the incubation, transfer the rack of slides to PBS and check for appropriate staining under the microscope.
13. Counterstain the slides for 30–60 s in hematoxylin. Rinse the slides in several changes of tap water. Check under the microscope for adequate contrast.
14. Dehydrate, clear in xylene, and mount in polymount.

4. Notes

1. Neoplastic and non-neoplastic lung tissue was obtained from nine patients with adenocarcinoma (eight women and one man; age range, 60–77) accessioned at the University of Massachusetts Medical Center, Worcester, MA, from 1994 to 1996 (*3*). Non-neoplastic tissue was obtained from lung tissue sampled at least 5 cm from the primary tumors. The nine tumor cases included eight primary pulmonary adenocarcinomas and one adenocarcinoma metastatic from the colon. Five of the eight primary pulmonary adenocarcinomas were bronchioloalveolar carcinomas, and three were acinar adenocarcinomas (*3*).

2. In our experience freezing the tissue is the most important step needed to obtain adequate morphology and optimum staining.

3. Directly freezing the tissue in liquid nitrogen causes ice crystal formation and freezing artifact due to the formation of a nitrogen gas envelope insulating the tissue (Leidenfrost effect). Freezing at −20°C in a cryostat is too slow and will also cause ice-crystal formation. Isopentane chilled with liquid nitrogen helps to avoid these problems.

References

1. Polverine, P. J. (1996) Cellular adhesion molecules: Newly identified mediators of angiogenesis. *Am. J. Pathol.* **148,** 1023–1029.
2. Ree, H. J., Khan, A. A., Elasakr, M., Liau, S., and Teplitz, C. (1993) Intercellular adhesion molecule-1 (ICAM-1) staining of reactive and neoplastic follicles. *Cancer* **71,** 2817–2822.
3. Jiang, Z., Woda, B. A., Savas, L., and Fraire, A. E. (1998) Expression of ICAM-1, VCAM-1 and LFA-1 in adenocarcinoma of lung with observations on the expression of these adhesion molecules in non neoplastic lung tissue. *Mod. Pathol.* **11(12),** 1189–1192.
4. Passlick, B., Izbicks, J. R., Simmel. S., Kuboschok, B., Karg, O., Habekost, M., et al. (1994) Expression of major histocompatibility Class I and Class II antigen and intercellular adhesion molecule-1 on operable non small cell lung carcinomas: frequency and prognostic significance. *Eur. J. Cancer* **30A,** 376–381.
5. Brekel, A. J. S.-van den, Thunnissen, F. B. J. M., Buurman, W. A., and Wouters, E. F. M. (1996) Expression of E-selectin, intercellular adhesion molecule (ICAM-1) and vascular cell adhesion molecule (VCAM)-1 in non-small-cell lung carcinoma. *Virchows Arch.* **428,** 21–27.
6. Pilewski, J. M. and Abelda, S. M. (1993) Adhesion molecules in the lung. An overview. *Am. Rev. Respir. Dis.* **148,** 31–37.

18

MUC1 Expression in Lung Cancer

Eva Szabo

1. Introduction

Abnormalities in mucin-type glycoprotein expression have been documented in a variety of cancers, identifying these molecules as targets for immunologically based therapies and prognostic/diagnostic assays. Epithelial mucin proteins are synthesized by cells lining the ducts and lumens of various epithelial surfaces and contribute to the protective and lubricating functions of mammalian mucus (1). These proteins are characterized by a variable number of amino acid tandem repeats and extensive O-glycosylation at serine and threonine residues, resulting in a composition of 50–80% carbohydrate by weight. To date, at least 9 mucin genes, encoding the protein backbone of these glycoproteins, have been identified and at least partially sequenced.

Several different mucins are expressed in normal and neoplastic human respiratory epithelium. Depending on the sensitivity of assays employed (e.g., reverse transcriptase polymerase chain reaction [RT-PCR] vs immunohisto-chemistry), a variety of cells within the normal bronchial epithelium have been shown to express MUC1, MUC2, MUC4, MUC5AC, MUC5B, and MUC8 (2,3). MUC 3 and MUC6 are generally not expressed. MUC1 has also been shown to be highly expressed in type II pneumocytes of the alveolar epithelium (4). In corresponding non-small cell lung cancers (NSCLC), frequent expression of MUC1, MUC2, MUC4, and MUC8 has been observed, while MUC5AC is infrequently expressed (2–4). The significance of decreased MUC5AC expression is not known; it may reflect the cell of origin for NSCLC or it may have functional importance. Small cell lung cancers (SCLC) express only MUC1 with any significant frequency (3). MUC1 expression has also been correlated with poor prognosis in NSCLC (5).

From: *Methods in Molecular Medicine, vol. 74: Lung Cancer, Vol. 1: Molecular Pathology Methods and Reviews*
Edited by: B. Driscoll © Humana Press Inc., Totowa, NJ

Several studies have suggested that MUC1 may facilitate epithelial carcinogenesis by a variety of mechanisms. Immunohistochemical expression of MUC1 has been shown to correlate with increased invasiveness, migration, and angiogenesis in ovarian and lung cancer *(5,6)*. Cell lines transfected with *MUC1* cDNA have reduced cell-matrix and cell-cell adhesion, which may account for greater metastatic ability *(7–9)*. *MUC1*-transfected melanoma cells are not able to form conjugates with lymphokine-activated killer cells and cytotoxic T lymphocytes *(8)* and purified MUC1 protein reversibly inhibits proliferation of cultured T cells *(10)*. MUC1 has also been shown to form complexes with Grb2 and Sos through its cytoplasmic tail, suggesting a potential role in signal transduction *(11)*. Thus MUC1 may contribute to carcinogenic progression through modulation of cell adhesion, the immune system, and cell signaling.

Upregulated expression of MUC1 in carcinomas has pointed to possible uses in prognosis, immunotherapy, and gene therapy. Assays for CA 15-3, which recognize MUC1, have been used to monitor early breast cancer *(12–14)*, and given the aberrant expression of MUC1 in many cancers, several recent studies have focused on MUC1 as a target for vaccine development *(15–17)*. Data from Mensdorff-Pouilly et al. suggest that a humoral immune response to MUC1 protects against disease progression in mammary carcinogenesis *(15)*. In addition, Chen et al. have used the *MUC1* promoter for adenoviral delivery of therapeutic genes to cancer cells *(18)*.

We have previously shown that MUC1 expression is tightly linked with the type II pneumocyte lineage in normal and neoplastic lung, being highly expressed in normal type II pneumocytes as well as in atypical and neoplastic lesions derived thereof *(4)*. The type II pneumocytes, along with other lung cell lineages, function as progenitor cells for normal and neoplastic epithelium during the repair of injury and during carcinogenesis. In cell lines, modulation of the differentiation status through pharmacologic manipulation leads to downregulation of MUC1 *(4,19)*. Immunohistochemical analysis using well characterized monoclonal MUC1 antibodies *(4)* offers a powerful tool to study MUC1 expression and the type II pneumocyte lineage during the process of carcinogenesis.

2. Materials

Immunohistochemistry for MUC1 can be performed on paraffin-embedded sections (4–8 microns thick), cryostat-cut frozen sections, or cell line cytospins.

2.1. Preparation of Tissue Sections or Cytospins

1. Xylene.
2. 95% ethanol.

3. 100% ethanol.
4. Acetone, −4°C (for frozen sections or cytospins).
5. Peroxidase quenching buffer: 0.3% hydrogen peroxide in absolute methanol.
6. 0.01 M Phosphate-buffered saline (PBS), pH 7.4 (PBS pH 7.4 dry powder is commercially available from Sigma, St, Louis, MO; dissolve contents of 1 packet in 1 L of dH$_2$O).
7. Slide staining set, including slide holder with detachable handle (hold 25 slides) and staining dishes (Tissue-Tek; Sakura, Torrance, CA).
8. Timer.

2.2. Citrate-Microwave Antigen Retrieval

1. 0.01 M citric acid, pH 6.0 (adjust pH with 2 M NaOH).
2. Microwave with adjustable power settings.

2.3. Immunoperoxidase Technique

2.3.1. Incubation with Primary Anti-serum

1. Vectastain ABC peroxidase mouse kit (Vector Laboratories, Burlingame, CA); Blocking serum: Add 4 drops of stock solution (yellow bottle) to 10 mL PBS, can be prepared ahead of time.
2. Humidity chamber (Shandon, Pittsburgh, PA).
3. 1% Normal rabbit serum (NRS) in PBS, 0.1% sodium azide, as diluent for antibodies.
4. NCL-MUC1-CORE antibody (clone Ma552, recognizes a hexapeptide in the tandem repeat region of the MUC1 protein core, Novocastra, Burlingame, CA) 1 : 100 dilution in NRS.
5. NCL-MUC1 antibody (clone Ma695, recognizes a carbohydrate epitope of the MUC1 glycoprotein, Novocastra, Burlingame, CA) 1 : 100 dilution in NRS.

2.3.2. Incubation with Secondary Antibody and ABC Reagent

1. Secondary antibody (from Vectastain ABC peroxidase mouse kit, *see* **Subheading 2.3.1.**): Add 1 drop of stock solution (from blue bottle) to 10 mL PBS, should be prepared fresh on the day of use.
2. ABC reagent (from Vectastain ABC peroxidase mouse kit, *see* **Subheading 2.3.1.**): Add 2 drops of A stock (orange bottle) and 2 drops of B stock (brown bottle) to 10 ml PBS (make up fresh on day of use, at least 30 min before using).

2.3.3. DAB Incubation and Counterstaining

1. 3,3′-Diaminobenzidine tetrahydrochloride (DAB) stock solution: Add 7.5 g DAB powder to 200 mL dH$_2$O, cover with aluminum foil and stir for 20 min. Aliquot 4-mL portions and keep frozen at −20°C until use.
2. 0.05 M Tris-HCl, pH 7.5: Trizma, pH 7.5, reagent (Sigma), 6.024 g/800 mL dH$_2$O).

3. DAB working solution: Prepare fresh just prior to each use (i.e., during last 15 min of incubation in ABC reagent). Add 150 mg DAB (4 mL of thawed stock solution, protected from light) to 200 mL 0.05 M Tris. Add 15 µL of 30% hydrogen peroxide. Keep away from light.

4. 2% osmium (dilute 4% osmium solution in dH$_2$O; Polysciences, Inc., Warrington, PA).

5. Light Green SF Yellowish (Sigma, St. Louis, MO) or other green counterstain. Prepare stock solution by dissolving 0.8 g Light Green and 0.8 mL glacial acetic acid in 400 mL dH$_2$O. Prepare working solution by dissolving 40 mL stock solution in 200 mL dH$_2$O.

2.3.4. Slide Preparation for Storage

1. Cover slips.
2. Permount.

3. Methods

3.1. Preparation of Tissue Sections or Cell Line Cytospins

Formalin-fixed, paraffin-embedded tissues must be deparaffinized with xylene and rehydrated prior to immunostaining. Tissues that are not fixed in formalin (frozen sections and cell line cytospins) need to be fixed prior to immunostaining. With the exception of antigen retrieval, all subsequent procedures are the same for both types of specimens (from **step 3** onward) and are performed at room temperature except where specified otherwise. Once tissue sections are hydrated, they must not be allowed to dry out at any point during the procedure (*see* **Note 1**).

1. For formalin-fixed tissues: Deparaffinize by soaking for 3 changes of xylene for 3 min each. Hydrate through graded ethanol solutions by soaking in 100% EtOH twice (3 min each), 95% EtOH twice (3 min each), and rinsing in distilled water.

2. For frozen sections or cell line cytospins: Fix in cold acetone (–4°C) for 10 min, keeping refrigerated the entire time. Rinse in PBS.

3. Quench endogenous peroxidase activity by soaking for 15 min in quenching buffer, then rinse in PBS.

3.2. Citrate-Microwave Antigen Retrieval (for Formalin-Fixed Paraffin Embedded Sections Only)

Antigen retrieval by heating slides in a citrate buffer optimizes access of antibodies used in immunostaining to the antigenic epitopes that may become masked during formalin cross-linking. The tissue sections must not dry out at any time.

1. Place slides in plastic container filled to brim with 0.01 M citrate buffer, pH 6.0, and loosely cover. Microwave at full strength for 5 min, check and add buffer if

necessary, repeat for 5 additional min. Check and add buffer if necessary, repeat for 5 min at reduced microwave setting of "8."

2. Cool slides in the citrate buffer for 15 min at room temperature, rinse in three changes of fresh PBS for 2 min each. Proceed to immunostaining.

3.3. Immunoperoxidase Technique

3.3.1. Incubation with Primary Antiserum

Either MUC1 antibody listed in **Subheading 2.** can be used. Commercially available immunostaining kits facilitate the technique. The following technique is based on the Vectastain ABC peroxidase mouse kit (Vector Laboratories). Three drops, or 75 µL of liquid, are usually sufficient to cover the tissue sections (*see* **Note 2**).

1. Apply blocking serum for 10 min (3 drops).
2. Apply primary antibody with pipet (75 µL) directly to blocking serum and place slides overnight in humidity chamber at 4°C.

3.3.2. Incubation with Secondary Antibody and ABC Reagent

1. Remove slides from incubation racks and place in PBS for 3 min.
2. Apply blocking serum for 3 min (3 drops).
3. Apply secondary (biotinylated) antibody (3 drops) and incubate in humidity chamber at room temp for 45 min.
4. Remove from incubation racks and place in PBS for 3 min.
5. Apply ABC reagent (3 drops) and incubate in humidity chamber racks at room temp for 45 min.
6. Remove slides from incubation racks and place in PBS for 3 min.

3.3.3. DAB Incubation and Counterstaining

1. Prepare fresh DAB working solution. Immerse slides in DAB solution for 10 min, with constant stirring. Keep away from light.
2. Rinse slides in 200 mL Tris buffer for 3 min, followed by PBS for 3 min.
3. Optional: Place slides in osmium vapor chamber for 10 min (3 drops of 2% osmium in dH$_2$O on wet paper towel in chamber, use parafilm on chamber top to keep airtight and moist).
4. Rinse in PBS for 5 min.
5. Counterstain with light green for 2 min; dip in H$_2$O.

3.3.4. Slide Preparation for Storage

1. Dehydrate in two changes of 95% EtOH (2 min each); two changes of 100% EtOH (2 min each); and three changes of xylene for a minimum of 15 min (3 min, 3 min, then 9 min). Slides can be left in xylene for several hours.
2. Cover slip in Permount (*see* **Note 3**).

3.6. Interpretation of Results

Three distinct staining patterns of MUC1 immunoreactivity can be seen in human NSCLC tissue sections. Membranous staining (*see* **Fig. 1A**), along the lumen, showing the apical polarity described for MUC1 expression in normal tissues, is expressed primarily in papillary adenocarcinomas. Diffuse cytoplasmic staining demonstrating a loss of normal apical polarity (*see* **Fig. 1B**) is also frequently seen, while an intense focal globular staining pattern (*see* **Fig. 1C**) occurs occasionally. More than one staining pattern can occur in different areas of the same tumor sample.

Immunohistochemical results can be scored using the following scale: 0, no positive cells; 1, <1% tumor cells positive; 2, ≥1% and <10% tumor cells positive; 3, ≥10% and <50% tumor cells positive; 4, ≥50% and <75% tumor cells positive; and 5, ≥75% tumor cells positive. Intensity of the staining can be scored on a scale of 0 to + (weak) to +++ (strong). In our studies, tumor specimens containing ≥10% cells with MUC1 immunoreactivity, regardless of intensity (score 3–5), were considered positive for use in clinicopathological correlation. Atypical regions containing 4 or more contiguous positively staining cells were also considered positive.

4. Notes

1. Positive and negative control tissue sections or cell line cytospins should be included with every immunohistochemical assay batch. Normal type II pneumocytes strongly express MUC1 and thus can serve as an internal control in tissue sections where they are present. Tissues that could serve as positive controls include MUC1 expressing lung or breast tumors or normal lung, while nonexpressing tumors or lymph node can serve as a negative control.

2. It is essential that once tissue slides are hydrated, that they remain moist and do not dry out at any point during the procedure. Slides that dry out are not interpretable. When small amounts of liquid are to be added to a slide (e.g., blocking serum or primary antibody), a Kimwipe can be used to first wipe off all extra liquid from around the tissue section, keeping the tissue section itself moist. Care should be taken to not wipe off small, hard-to-see tissue sections or cytospins. Liquid can then be added to the tissue section, and surface tension will generally keep the small volume from flowing throughout the slide. In some cases it may be useful (but is not usually necessary) to use a hydrophobic slide marking pen such as the PAP Pen (Zymed, San Francisco, CA) to outline the tissue section to keep the small amounts of liquid concentrated over the tissue.

3. Troubleshooting: Omitting any one of several crucial steps during the immunohistochemical procedure (e.g., primary antibody, secondary antibody, hydrogen peroxide from DAB solution) will lead to negative results. A positive control slide should help identify this problem. As long as the slides have been kept moist at all times, one can return to the antibody blocking step and repeat the

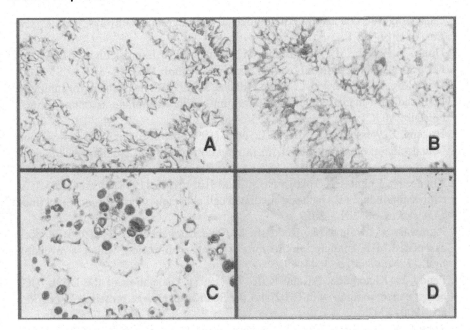

Fig. 1. Photomicrograph of MUC1 expression in NSCLC. (**A**) Positive membranous staining (immunoperoxidase, ×75). (**B**) Diffuse cytoplasmic staining (immunoperoxidase, ×75). (**C**) Intense focal globular staining (immunoperoxidase, ×75). (**D**) Lack of MUC1 expression in a primary adenocarcinoma (immunoperoxidase, ×75).

immunoperoxidase procedure. Even if the slides have been dehydrated, mounted in Permount, and coverslipped, they can be soaked in xylene to gently remove the cover slip, rehydrated through graded alcohols, and immunostained again.

References

1. Gendler, S. and Spicer, A. (1996) Epithelial mucin genes. *Ann. Rev. Physiol.* **57,** 607–634.
2. Copin, M.-C., Devisme, L., Buisine, M.-P., et al. (2000) From normal respiratory mucosa to epidermoid carcinoma: expression of human mucin genes. *Int. J. Cancer* **86,** 162–168.
3. Lopez-Ferrer, A., Curull, V., Barranco, C., et al. (2001) Mucins as differentiation markers in bronchial epithelium: squamous cell carcinoma and adenocarcinoma display similar expression patterns. *Am. J. Respir. Cell Mol. Biol.* **24,** 22–29.
4. Jarrard, J. A., Linnoila, R. I., Lee, H., et al. (1998) MUC1 is a novel marker for the type II pneumocyte lineage during lung carcinogenesis. *Cancer Res.* **58,** 5582–5589.
5. Giatromanolaki, A., Koukourakis, M. I., Sivridis, E., et al. (2000) Coexpression of MUC1 glycoprotein with multiple angiogenic factors in non-small cell lung

cancer suggests coactivation of angiogenic and migration pathways. *Clin. Cancer Res.* **6,** 1917–1921.

6. Dong, Y., Walsh, M., Cummings, M., et al. (1997) Expression of MUC1 and MUC2 mucins in epithelial ovarian tumors. *J. Pathol.* **183,** 311–317.

7. Wesseling, J., van der Valk, S., and Hilkens, J. (1996) A mechanism for inhibition of E-cadherin-mediated cell-cell adhesion by the membrane-associated mucin episialin/MUC1. *Mol. Biol. Cell* **7,** 565–577.

8. Hilkens, J., Wesseling, J., Vos, H. L., et al. (1995) Involvement of the cell surface-bound mucin, episialin/MUC1, in progression of human carcinomas. *Biochem. Soc. Transact.* **23,** 822–826.

9. Kondo, K., Kohno, N., Yokoyama, A., and Hiwada, K. (1998) Decreased MUC1 expression induces E-Cadherin-mediated cell adhesion of breast cancer cell lines. *Cancer Res.* **58,** 2014–2019.

10. Agrawal, B., Krantz, M., Reddish, M., and Longenecker, B. (1998) Cancer-associated MUC1 mucin inhibits human T-cell proliferation, which is reversible by IL-2. *Nature Med.* **4,** 43–49.

11. Pandy, P., Kharbanda, S., and Kufe, D. (1995) Association of the DF3/MUC1 breast cancer antigen with Grb2 and the Sos/Ras exchange protein. *Cancer Res.* **55,** 4000–4003.

12. Romero, S., Fernandez, C., Arriero, J., et al. (1996) CEA, CA 15-3 and CYFRA 21-1 in serum and pleural fluid of patients with pleural effusions. *Eur. Respir. J.* **9,** 17–23.

13. Vizcarra, E., Lluch, A., Cibrian, R., et al. (1996) Value of CA 15.3 in breast cancer and comparison with CEA and TPA: A study of specificity in disease-free follow-up patients and sensitivity in patients at diagnosis of the first metastasis. *Breast Cancer Res. Treat.* **37,** 209–216.

14. Pectasides, D., Pavlidis, N., Gogou, L., et al. (1996) Clinical value of CA 15-3, mucin-like carcinoma-associated antigen, tumor polypeptide antigen, and carcinoembryonic antigen in monitoring early breast cancer patients. *Am. J. Clin. Oncol.* **19,** 459–464.

15. von Mensdorff-Pouilly, S., Gourevitch, M. M., Kenemans, P., et al. (1996) Humoral immune response to polymorphic epithelial mucin (MUC-1) in patients with benign and malignant breast tumors. *Eur. J. Cancer* **32A,** 1325–1331.

16. Katayose, Y., Kudo, T., Suzuki, M., et al. (1996) MUC1-specific targeting immunotherapy with bispecific antibodies: inhibition of xenografted human bile duct carcinoma growth. *Cancer Res.* **56,** 4205–4212.

17. Apostolopoulos, V., Osinski, C., and McKenzie, I. (1998) MUC1 cross-reactive Galα(1,3)Gal antibodies in humans switch immune responses from cellular to humoral. *Nature Med.* **3,** 315–320.

18. Chen, L., Chen, D., Manome, Y., et al. (1995) Breast cancer selective gene expression and therapy mediated by recombinant adenovirus containing the DF3/MUC1 promoter. *J. Clin. Invest.* **96,** 2775–2782.

19. Chang, T.-H. and Szabo, E. (2000) Induction of differentiation and apoptosis by ligands of peroxisome proliferator-activated receptor γ in non-small cell lung cancer. *Cancer Res.* **60,** 1129–1138.

19

Altered Surface Markers in Lung Cancer

Lack of Cell-Surface Fas/APO-1 Expression in Pulmonary Adenocarcinoma May Allow Escape from Immune Surveillance

Yoshihiro Nambu and David G. Beer

1. Introduction

Bronchogenic carcinoma is the leading cause of cancer-related mortality, with the prognosis of pulmonary adenocarcinoma remaining poor in advanced-staged tumors despite improved efforts in earlier diagnosis and combination chemotherapy and radiation therapy. Understanding the potential mechanisms underlying the poor survival of these cancers will potentially lead to better therapeutics. One important area that has received significant attention, and with it a greater understanding is the role of apoptosis, or genetically encoded programmed cell death. Apoptosis is defined by distinct characteristic morphological and biochemical changes *(1)*. In malignant cells, these physiological apoptotic pathways are often altered, resulting in a significant survival advantage for these cells *(2)*. Tumors with developed resistance to apoptosis can survive despite an active immune system. The Fas receptor (APO-1 or CD95) and its ligand play a key role in the initiation of one apoptotic pathway in malignant tumor *(3–5)*. Loss of the Fas protein has been reported to induce resistance to apoptosis, however, apoptotic resistance in some Fas-expressing malignant cells has also been reported *(4,5)*. The Fas receptor is located in the cell surface of tumor cells, and loss of cell-surface Fas protein expression by dislocation of Fas protein is one of the essential mechanisms for tumor immune resistance *(6,7)*. Because of the central roles of FACScan analysis and confocal microscopy in the evaluation of the cell surface Fas protein

From: *Methods in Molecular Medicine, vol. 74: Lung Cancer, Vol. 1: Molecular Pathology Methods and Reviews*
Edited by: B. Driscoll © Humana Press Inc., Totowa, NJ

expression, this chapter focuses on the utilization of these tools in assessment of Fas in lung adenocarcinomas.

2. Materials

2.1. FACScan Analysis for Cell-Surface Fas Protein Expression

1. Cell lines: A549 (human lung adenocarcinoma cells) and BJAB (human B-cell lymphoma cells), which serve as a positive control for cell-surface Fas protein expression, were obtained from The American Type Culture Collection (Rockville, MD).
2. Culture Medium: DMEM containing 10% FBS and 1% penicillin/streptomycin was used for the culture of A549 cells, and RPMI 1640 medium (Sigma Chemical, St. Louis, MO) containing 10% FBS and 1% penicillin/streptomycin was used for BJAB cells. All cells were cultured at 37°C with 5% CO_2.
3. Flow cytometry buffer: PBS with 0.5% rabbit serum and 10^{-3} mM NaN$_3$. Note: toxicity hazard for NaN$_3$. (Save at 4°C, light protection by aluminum foil is needed, stable for 1 mo).
4. 10 mM EDTA, pH 8.0, at 4°C.
5. Phosphate-buffered saline (PBS): 10 mM sodium phosphate, 0.9% NaCl, pH 7.5, with 10^{-3} mM NaN$_3$ (without rabbit serum) if maintained at 4°C it is stable without rabbit serum.
6. Antibodies for FACScan analysis: primary antibody: DX-2 (PharMingen, San Diego, CA), secondary antibody: FITC-conjugated anti-mouse antibody (Biosource International, Camarillo, CA).
7. FACScan® (Becton Dickinson, San Jose, CA).

2.2. Anti-Fas Antibody-Mediated Apoptosis

1. 96-well plates.
2. Antibody: DX-2 without NaN$_3$ (should be utilized for biological assays, because NaN$_3$ has significant toxicity for cells).
3. Recombinant protein G (Sigma, St. Louis, MO) 20 µg/mL.
4. 0.25% trypsin-1 mM EDTA.
5. Propidium iodide-containing cell lysis buffer: 0.1% sodium citrate, 0.1% Triton X-100, and 10 µg/mL propidium iodide.

2.3. Transfection and Confocal Microscopy

1. MCF-7 (human breast cancer cells) used as positive control for cell surface Fas protein expression (American Tissue Culture Collection).
2. Chambered microscope slides.
3. pcDNA3 vector containing the 1.0-kb human Fas-FLAG (FLAG epitope NH2-terminal) fusion protein cDNA (kindly provided by Dr. V.M. Dixit).
4. Lipofectin (Life Technologies, Rockville, MD) used according to manufacturer's instructions.
5. Acetone.

6. Blocking solution: 1:20 dilution of goat serum in PBS.
7. Anti-FLAG antibody (clone M2; Eastman Kodak, Rochester, NY). 1:500 dilution in PBS with 1% rabbit serum and 10^{-3} mM NaN$_3$.
8. FITC-conjugated anti-mouse antibody (Biosource International, Camarillo, CA).
9. Fluoromount-G (Southern Biotechnology Associates, Birmingham, AL). This medium will not quench fluorescence.
10. Confocal microscope (Bio-Rad, Hercules, CA).

3. Methods

3.1. FACScan Analysis for Cell-Surface Fas Protein Expression

1. Rinse adherent A549 adenocarcinoma cells in PBS, and then incubate in 10 mM EDTA for 20 min at 4°C, and harvest by gentle pipetting (*see* **Note 1**). Incubation with 10 mM EDTA is not needed for BJAB cells, because they grow in suspension.
2. Wash cells three times in PBS, and then suspend A549 and BJAB cells (10^6 cells/ 200 µL) in flow cytometry buffer. Label for 30 min at 4°C with anti-Fas primary antibody (clone DX-2; PharMingen) diluted with 200 µL flow cytometry buffer to 1.25 µg/mL.
3. After three washes with flow cytometry buffer, label the cells with FITC-conjugated anti-mouse secondary antibody diluted to 1:1,000 in flow cytometry buffer (protect from light by wrapping bottle in aluminum foil).
4. Perform flow cytometric analysis using a FACScan® gated to exclude fractured cells and small cellular debris. Examine approx 10,000 cells for each determination. The size of cells differ for each of the malignant cell lines, so an adequate plotting area (gate) should be determined for each (*see* **Note 2**). Prior to FACScan analysis, the samples should always be kept protected from light using aluminum foil.
5. **Figure 1** represents a typical result of the analysis of cell surface Fas protein expression in A549 and BJAB cells. In A549 cells, the cell populations are those containing the FITC-conjugated secondary antibody alone (gray fill) and with anti-Fas antibody (no fill). Most of BJAB cells express Fas protein. Approximately 48% of A549 cells express Fas protein. The levels of cell-surface expression of Fas protein are significantly lower than in BJAB cells.

3.2. Anti-Fas Antibody-Mediated Apoptosis

1. Plate A549 and BAJB cells in 96-well plates at 4×10^4 cells/well and incubate overnight (*see* **Note 3**).
2. After replacing the media, incubate cells with 12.5 µg/mL DX-2 anti-Fas antibody (without NaN$_3$) (*see* **Note 4**) and recombinant protein G for 20 h. Wells containing no treatment (recombinant protein G alone) serve as control.
3. Harvest adherent A549 using trypsin and also collect and non-adherent cells (*see* **Note 5**). Wash in PBS, and then incubate at 4°C for 12 h in propidium iodide-containing cell lysis buffer. Cell nuclei will remain intact but must be protected from light.

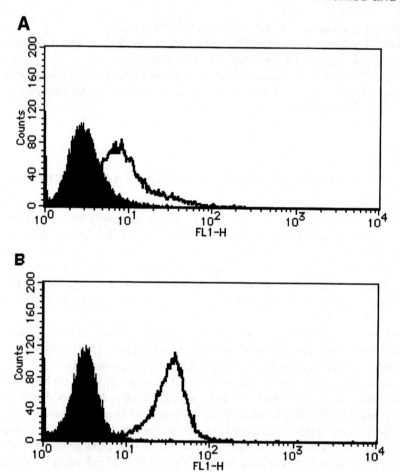

Fig. 1. Analysis of cell-surface Fas protein expression in A549 and BJAB cells. (**A**) A549 cells, or (**B**) BJAB cells incubated with the FITC-conjugated secondary antibody alone (dark fill), or with anti-Fas antibody (no fill). A greater percentage of the BJAB cells express the Fas protein.

4. Use the FACScan flow cytometer to quantify the percentage of cells undergoing apoptosis *(8,9)*.
5. Plot the fluorescence of propidium iodide in each nucleus graphically. Nuclei demonstrating fluorescence below the peak which represents a G1 DNA content are counted as apoptotic (*see* **Note 6** and **Fig. 2**). These cells are reported as a percentage of the total number of nuclei counted (5,000 gated events) (*see* **Note 7**).

3.3. Transfection and Confocal Microscopy

Ectopic expression of FLAG-tagged fas protein can be achieved by transient transfection of A549 and MCF-7 cells. The location of protein expression

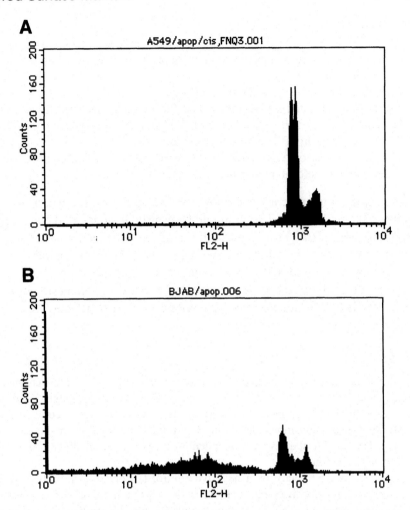

Fig. 2. Histograms of the analysis of apoptotic cells using flow cytometry. The percent of A549 (**A**) or BJAB (**B**) cells undergoing apoptosis 20 h after treatment with anti-Fas antibody and cross-linked with protein G. The large number of BJAB cells located below the G1 peak represent apoptotic cells.

can then be analyzed using an anti-FLAG monoclonal antibody (MAb) and confocal microscopy.

1. Grow cells (A549 and MCF-7: 3×10^6 per each cell line) on chambered slides.
2. Transiently transfect with the FLAG-tagged Fas expression vector for 48 h. Efficiency should be approx 10%, non-transfected cells serve as a control for staining specificity (*see* **Note 8**). For all transient transfections, use Lipofectin.
3. Fix cells for 10 min in 100% acetone kept cold at –20°C.

4. Wash in PBS at room temperature.
5. Block nonspecific binding using blocking solution for 30 min at room temperature.
6. Remove blocking solution and add monoclonal anti-FLAG antibody for 30 min at room temperature.
7. Wash three times in PBS at room temperature.
8. Use FITC-conjugated secondary antibody to detect immunoreactivity of Fas. Incubate with cells for thirty minutes at room temperature.
9. Wash three times in PBS at room temperature.
10. Mount cover slips onto the stained and washed slides using Fluoromount-G.
11. Image using a confocal microscope (*see* **Note 9**).

Using confocal microscopy and an anti-FLAG antibody, the Fas-protein on the cell surface in the MCF-7 cells should be clearly demonstrated (*see* **Fig. 3**). However, the Fas-FLAG protein, though it may be visualized within the cytoplasm of A549 cells, should not be observed on the cell-surface membrane (*6*). These findings suggested that in A549 cells, both the expression of the native Fas protein, as well as the transfected and expressed Fas protein, do not result in sufficient levels of surface Fas protein expression to render these cells sensitive to Fas-mediated apoptosis.

4. Notes

1. If A549 fail to detach, the incubation time in 10 mM EDTA at 4°C may need to be increased, or temperature can be shifted to 37°C. However, longer incubation damages cells, and precise cell-surface protein evaluation can become difficult. Minimal incubation times should be determined empirically for the cell lines used. Trypan blue stain is recommended for assessing cell viability after 10 mM EDTA incubation.
2. In each FACScan analysis, a negative control (secondary antibody alone) is essential, and a positive control (BJAB cells) is preferred. For each primary and secondary labeling step, the labeling conditions may be modified depending on the incubation time and temperature. FITC-conjugated primary antibody is also recommended as a negative control for FACScan analysis. In this case the step for labeling using a secondary antibody is omitted.
3. For a positive control of cells undergoing apoptosis, Jurkat cells (human T-cell lymphoma cell lines) is often reported. Jurkat cells, however, are sometimes not extremely susceptible to the anti-Fas antibody. Before experimentation an analysis of the susceptibility BJAB and/or Jurkat cells to DX-2 treatment should be evaluated as positive control.
4. The primary antibody (DX-2), which was used for FACScan and immuno-histochemistry, contains NaN$_3$. For the anti-Fas mediated apoptosis assay, the DX-2 antibody without containing NaN$_3$ should be used to avoid cell damage.
5. Adherent and nonadherent cells should be collected since apoptotic cells become nonadherent easily. For harvesting adherent A549 cells, trypsinization with

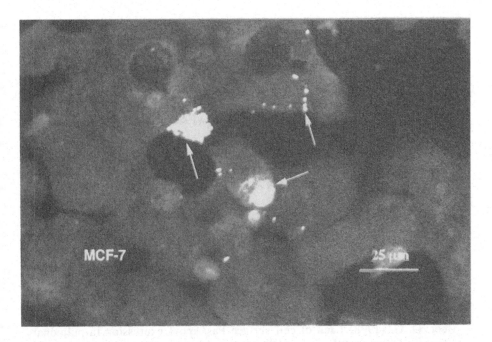

Fig. 3. Confocal microscopy with an anti-FLAG antibody. The Fas-protein on the cell surface in the MCF-7 cell transfected with FLAG-tagged Fas cDNA and expressing Fas is clearly visible (arrow) (**Fig. 3**). Most of the nontransfected cells do not show any immunoreactivity.

standard 0.25% trypsin-EDTA for only 2–3 min is often all that is required. Longer tripsinization should be avoided, as it severely damages cells and may cause cells go undergo necrosis rather than apoptosis.

6. The fluorescent peak lower than the G1 peak does represent nuclei which are apoptotic, however, a very low peak may also indicate necrotic cells. Precise gating may be needed for analysis, in order to avoid necrotic cells and debris.

7. **Figure 2** shows typical histograms for analysis of apoptosis in A549 and BJAB cells. The percent of cells undergoing apoptosis 20 h after treatment with anti-Fas antibody and cross-linked with protein G, or the control treated of protein G alone are analyzed. The size of the cell can differ depending upon each type of malignant cell line used, thus adequate plotting area (gate) should be determined for each. A549 cells are resistant to Fas-mediated apoptosis, however most of BJAB cells are observed to undergo apoptosis (*see* **Fig. 2**). It is established that BAJB cells express cell surface Fas and are susceptible to anti-Fas antibody treatment. A549 cells, however, lack cell-surface Fas protein and are resistant to anti-Fas antibody.

8. The efficacy of transient transfection is often low, usually less than 10%. For confocal microscopical analysis, careful attention to well-stained FLAG-labeled cells should be evaluated.

9. For confocal microscopical analysis, cells are not as easily focused upon as in thin sections of cells or tissues and it may be difficult to evaluate the whole-cell structures. For these analyses, the surface areas of the cells may be focused upon to detect the tranfected Fas protein.

References

1. Wyllie, A. H., Kerr, J. F. R., and Currie, A. R. (1980) Cell death: significance of apoptosis. *Int. Rev. Cytol.* **68,** 251–306.
2. Thompson, C. B. (1995) Apoptosis in pathogenesis and genes and treatment of disease. *Science* **267,** 1456–1461.
3. Nagata, S. and Goldstein, P. (1995) The Fas death factor. *Science* **267,** 1449–1456.
4. Cheng, J., Zhou, T., Liu, C., Shapiro, J. P., Brauer, M. J., Keifer, M. C., et al. (1994) Protection from Fas-mediated apoptosis by a soluble form of the Fas molecule. *Science* **263,** 1759–1762.
5. Cascino, I., Fiucci, G., Papoff, G., and Ruberti, G. (1995) Three functional soluble forms of the human apoptosis-inducing Fas molecule are produced by alternative splicing. *J. Immunol.* **154,** 1157–1164.
6. Nambu, Y., Hughes, S. J., Rehemtulla, A., Hamstra, D., Orringer, M. B., and Beer, D. G. (1998) Lack of cell surface Fas/Apo-1 expression in pulmonary adenocarcinoma. *J. Clin. Invest.* **101,** 1102–1110.
7. Hughes, S. J., Nambu, Y., Soldes, O. S., Hamstra, D., Rehemtulla, A., et al. (1997) Fas/APO-1 (CD95) is not translocated to the cell membrane in esophageal adenocarcinoma. *Cancer Res.* **57,** 5571–5578.
8. Nicoletti, I., Mgliorati, G., Pagliacci, M. C., Grignani, F., and Riccadi, C. (1991) A rapid and simple method for measuring thymocyte apoptosis by propidium iodide staining and flow cytometry. *J. Immunol. Methods* **139,** 271–279.
9. Darzynkiewicz, Z., Bruno, S., Del Bino, G., Gorczyca, W., Hotz, M. A., Lassota, P., and Traganos, F. (1992) Features of apoptotic cells measured by flow cytometry. *Cytometry* **13,** 795–808.
10. Weller, M., Frei, K., Groscurth, P., Krammer, P. H., Yonekawa, Y., and Fontana, A. (1994) Anti-Fas/APO-1 antibody-mediated apoptosis of cultured human glioma cells. Induction and modulation of sensitivity by cytokines. *J. Clin. Invest.* **94,** 954–964.
11. Chinnaiyan, A. M., O'Rourke, K., Tewari, M., and Dixit, V. M. (1995) FADD, a novel death domain-containing protein, interacts with the death domain of Fas and initiates apoptosis. *Cell* **81,** 505–512.

III

MOLECULAR ABNORMALITIES IN LUNG CANCER

D. DETECTION OF ALTERATIONS IN THE APOPTOTIC PATHWAY

20

Prognostic Relevance of Angiogenic, Proliferative, and Apoptotic Factors in Lung Carcinomas

A Case Review

Manfred Volm and Reet Koomägi

1. Introduction
1.1. Angiogenic and Anti-angiogenic Factors

Angiogenesis—the development and formation of new blood vessels—is important in a variety of processes such as growth and differentiation, wound healing, and the formation of neoplasms. An avascular tumor grows to a size of 2–3 mm and only rapidly expands when it becomes vascularized. Many cells, including tumor cells, affect the formation of new vessels by secreting angiogenic and anti-angiogenic factors (1). The balance of positive and negative angiogenic factors determines whether cells remain in a state of vascular homeostasis, or whether they proceed to the stage of neovascularization. These factors may include a combination of vascular endothelial growth factor (VEGF), basic fibroblast growth factor (bFGF), platelet-derived endothelial cell growth factor (PD-ECGF), and/or angiostatin.

The role played by VEGF in tumor-associated angiogenesis has been clearly demonstrated in many solid tumors, This suggests that VEGF upregulation may be a general property of highly vascularized neoplasms. bFGF was the first endothelial growth factor to be identified and is similar to VEGF, a directly acting angiogenic molecule. PD-ECGF has been characterized as a major mitogen for a variety of normal mesenchymal and related tumor cells. It plays an important role in angiogenesis and endothelial cell chemotaxis. An analysis of cultured lung cancer cells detected the frequent expression of PD-ECGF in all histological types of lung cancer. O'Reilly et al. (2) reported the identifica-

From: *Methods in Molecular Medicine, vol. 74: Lung Cancer, Vol. 1: Molecular Pathology Methods and Reviews*
Edited by: B. Driscoll © Humana Press Inc., Totowa, NJ

tion and purification of a human plasminogen fragment with endothelial inhibitory activity. They named this fragment angiostatin. They demonstrated that a primary mouse tumor can generate angiostatin, which almost completely suppresses the growth of primary tumor metastases. Additionally, they inhibited the growth of three human and three murine primary carcinomas in mice by systematically administering human angiostatin. In order to determine a possible prognostic role for these factors, in the study described herein we examine the effect of the pro-angiogenic factors VEGF, bFGF, PD-ECGF, and the anti-angiogenic factor angiostatin on the survival of patients with non-small cell lung cancers (NSCLC).

1.2. Apoptotic Factors

Programmed cell death is one of the most important regulatory mechanisms of cellular homeostasis in organisms. This process has acquired a number of names and has been well-known for more than 100 years. The term finally adopted for it in recent years is "apoptosis" *(3)*. Most of the morphological changes observed in apoptosis are caused by a set of cysteine proteases named caspases. Apoptosis involves the activation of death-inducing ligand/receptor systems, the cleavage of caspases, and the perturbation of mitochondrial functions. Another component of apoptosis includes the induction of Fas-ligand and the upregulation of Fas by external factors, which has been observed in tumor cells. Mitochondrial function during apoptosis seems to be controlled by the Bcl-2 family, which may inhibit apoptosis. In this study we analyzed Fas ligand, Fas, caspase 3, and Bcl-2.

1.3. Proliferative Factors

Cyclins and cyclin-dependent kinases are universal regulators of cellular proliferation in eukaryotic cells. Regulatory mechanisms include varying the abundance of cyclin, the phosphorylation of the kinase subunit that may yield either positive or negative effects and the actions of cyclin-kinase inhibitory proteins. Several classes of mammalian cyclins that are synthesized in different ways and degraded at specific points during the cell cycle have been described *(4)*. The complex formed by cyclin D1 and cdk4 governs the G1 progression, while cyclin A together with cdk2 regulates entry into and progression through the S phase. The proliferating cell nuclear antigen (PCNA) is essential for cellular DNA synthesis. Therefore, in the present study we analyzed the significance of changes in cyclin A, cdk2, and PCNA expression as measured by immunohistochemistry, and of alterations in cell-cycle phases, as measured by flow cytometry, on patient survival.

The main purpose of the current study was to ascertain the most critical prognostic factors and then to evaluate whether a combination of angiogenic, proliferative, and/or apoptotic factors can provide improved prognostic information for the overall survival of patients with NSCLC.

2. Results

2.1. Patient Population Statistics

One hundred and fifty patients (135 men, 15 women) with previously untreated non-small cell lung carcinomas were admitted into this study. The morphological classification of the carcinomas was conducted according to the World Health Organization (WHO) specifications. Of the carcinomas, 85 (56.6%) were squamous carcinomas, 40 (26.7%) were adenocarcinomas, and 25 (16.7%) were large cell carcinomas. The patients were staged according to the guidelines of the UICC. Eight patients had stage IA (5.3%), 23 (15.3%) stage 1B, 4 (2.7%) patients had stage IIA and 39 (26.0%) stage IIB tumors. Seventy-six patients (50.7%) had stage IIIA tumors. The average age of the patients was 58 (25–76) yr. Sixty-three patients (42%) did not exhibit lymph node involvement while 87 did (58%). One hundred nine patients were given only surgical treatment. Fifteen patients were also given cytotoxic drugs and 25 patients (mainly squamous cell lung carcinomas) were treated with palliative irradiation. The additional radiation treatment and chemotherapy had no significant effect on overall patient survival time ($p > 0.1$).

2.2. Combined Methods for Analysis

Follow-up data were obtained from hospital charts and by corresponding with the referring physicians. Patient survival was determined from the date of surgery until the last follow-up visit or reported death and was evaluated by using a life table analysis according to the method of Kaplan and Meier. Immunohistochemistry (biotin-streptavidin method) was used to determine the angiogenic, proliferative, and apoptotic factors in the formalin-fixed, paraffin-embedded, tumor specimens. Cell cycle analysis was conducted by flow cytometry.

2.3. Cellular Prognostic Factor Analysis

The overall prognosis of patients with lung carcinomas is mainly determined by tumor size, lymph node involvement, and the stage. This holds true for our group of patients. To discover new cellular prognostic factors in addition to the clinical factors, we analyzed the expressions of angiogenic, proliferative, and apoptotic factors (*see* **Table 1**).

2.3.1. Correlation of Survival with Altered Expression of Angiogenic and Antiangiogenic Factors

The median survival time was shorter for patients with VEGF-positive carcinomas than for those with VEGF-negative carcinomas (69 vs 141 wk)

Table 1
Median Survival Times (MST) and Relative Risk of Patients with NSCLC According to Angiogenic, Proliferative, and Apoptotic Factors

	Patients/ death	MST (wk)	Log rank test p-value	Relative risk
Angiogenic factors				
VEGF				
Negative	53/33	141		1.0
Positive	80/60	69	0.17	1.3
bFGF				
Negative	50/35	68		1.0
Positive	93/67	80	0.73	1.0
PD-ECGF				
Negative	67/45	79		1.0
Positive	63/51	69	0.27	1.2
Angiostatin				
Negative	87/63	65		1.6
Positive	25/16	146	0.10	1.0
Proliferative factors				
Cyclin A				
Negative	65/41	92		1.0
Positive	75/58	64	0.09	1.4
CDK2				
Negative	39/26	89		1.0
Positive	105/76	76	0.36	1.2
PCNA				
Negative	99/67	89		1.0
Positive	43/34	51	0.05	1.5
SG2M				
>23	40/24	108		1.0
<23	35/28	85	0.10	1.6
Apoptotic factors				
Fas ligand				
Negative	37/31	41		1.6
Positive	90/62	87	0.05	1.0
Fas/CD95				
Negative	71/58	69		1.5
Positive	78/48	86	0.02	1.0
Caspase 3				
Negative	26/20	34		1.5
Positive	69/49	87	0.16	1.0
Bcl-2				
Negative	98/72	78		1.1
Positive	43/28	102	0.58	1.0

(**Table 1, Fig. 1**). The relative risk estimate for these patients was increased by a factor of 1.3. The expression of the angiogenic factors bFGF and PD-ECGF did not exhibit a significant correlation with survival. The angiogenesis inhibitor, angiostatin, exhibited an inverse correlation with survival time. Patients with angiostatin-positive carcinomas survived longer than patients with angiostatin-negative carcinomas (**Table 1, Fig. 1**). The median survival of patients with angiostatin-positive carcinomas was 146 wk while that of patients with angiostatin-negative carcinomas was only 65 wk. The relative risk of patients with angiostatin-negative carcinomas was 1.6 when compared with patients who had angiostatin-positive carcinomas.

2.3.2. Correlation of Survival with Altered Expression of Proliferative Factors and Altered Cell-Cycle Phases

We then determined the expression of different proliferative factors and detected a relationship between patient survival and these factors. In this analysis, the survival times were shorter when the proliferative factors were upregulated (**Table 1**). For patients with cyclin A-negative carcinomas the median survival was 92 wk and for patients with cyclin A-positive carcinomas only 64 wk. The corresponding values for cdk2 and PCNA were 89 vs. 76 wk and 89 vs 51 wk (**Table 1, Fig. 1**). Consistent with the data obtained by immuno-histochemistry, we found that the survival times were shorter for cancer patients with a higher proportion of S, G2, and M phase cells than for patients with a lower proportion of these cell-cycle cells.

2.3.3. Correlation of Survival with Altered Expression of Apoptotic Factors

Additionally, we analyzed expression of the pro-apoptotic factors Fas ligand, Fas, and caspase 3 and discovered an inverse relationship between the pro-apoptotic factors and patient survival time. Patients with a greater expression of the apoptotic factors had a more favorable prognosis (**Table 1**). The median survival times of lung cancer patients with Fas ligand expression was 87 wk and of those without such expression only 41 wk. The relative risk estimate for patients with Fas ligand-negative carcinomas was 1.6 compared to patients with Fas ligand-positive carcinomas. Corresponding results were obtained with Fas. Additionally, we analyzed the relationship between caspase 3 and patient survival (**Fig. 1**). Analogous to the findings with Fas and Fas ligand, we discovered that patients who expressed caspase 3 had a favorable outcome.

2.3.4. Prognostic Value for Cellular Factors Analysis at a Particular Tumor Stage and Lymph Node Involvement

The overall prognosis of patients with lung cancer is mainly determined by tumor size, lymph node involvement, and stage. This holds true for our group

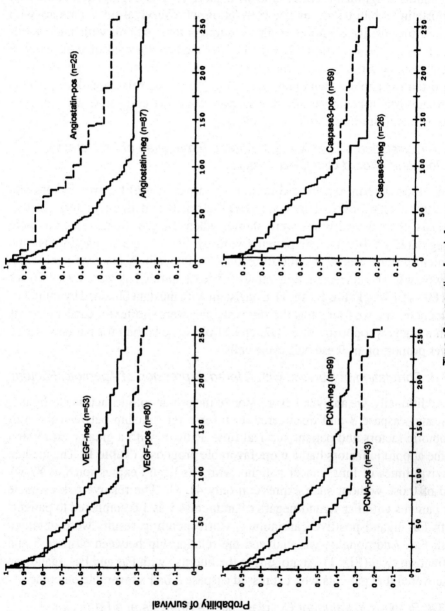

of patients. To exclude the effect or the possible introduction of a bias into the current analysis, we further evaluated the cellular factors according to patients with stage IIIA tumors and those with lymph node involvement. The analysis of these more homogeneous groups of patients can be found in **Table 2** (stage IIIA) and **Table 3** (patients with lymph node involvement). Limiting the survival time analysis to patients with stage IIIA tumors and to patients with lymph node involvement shows that the prognostic power of the angiogenic, proliferative, and apoptotic factors remains. **Figures 2** and **3** show the homogeneous groups of patients grouped according to the cellular factors. It is obvious that the prognostic power of the angiogenic, proliferative, and apoptotic factors remains in the homogeneous patient groups.

2.3.5. Combined Analysis of Cellular Factors

In order to determine whether a combination of factors can yield improved prognostic information, we investigated all possible combinations of the angiogenic, proliferative and apoptotic factors. **Table 4** shows the results of six combinations. It can clearly be seen that the differences between the patient groups are both greater and statistically significant. The patient group with VEGF-negative and FAS-positive carcinomas had a median survival time of 184 wk while the patient group with VEGF-positive and Fas-negative carcinomas had a medium survival time of only 68 wk. The relative risk of patients with VEGF-positive/Fas-negative carcinomas was 1.8. Patients with angiostatin-positive/Fas-positive carcinomas had a median survival time of > 260 wk. In contrast, the survival time of the patients with angiostatin-negative and Fas-negative carcinomas was only 80 wk. The relative risk for patients with angiostatin- negative and Fas-negative tumors was 3.4. Patients with carcinomas having a high proliferative activity (high proportion of S/G2/M phase cells, PCNA-positive, and cyclin A-positive tumors), but which did not express apoptotic factors (Fas, caspase 3) or angiostatin had the shortest survival times, while patients with carcinomas having a low proliferative activity and a high expression of apoptotic factors or angiostatin exhibited the most favorable outcome (**Table 4, Fig. 4**). The median survival time of patients with tumors containing a high proportion of S/G2/M phase cells and with tumors that were Fas-negative was only 38 wk while the median survival time of patients with Fas-positive carcinomas and a low proportion of S/G2/M

Fig. 1. (*opposite page*) Survival curves (Kaplan-Meier estimates) of patients with NSCLC grouped according to the expression of VEGF, angiostatin, PCNA, and caspase 3.

Table 2
Median Survival Times (MST) and Relative Risk of Stage IIIA Patients According to Angiogenic, Proliferative, and Apoptotic Factors

Stage IIIA	Patients/ death	MST (wk)	Log rank test p-value	Relative risk
Angiostatin				
Negative	42/35	33		1.2
Positive	11/10	76	0.60	1.0
Cyclin A				
Negative	30/22	68		1.0
Positive	38/34	26	0.17	1.4
PCNA				
Negative	48/38	47		1.0
Positive	21/20	21	0.047	1.7
SG2M				
<23%	20/12	68		1.0
>23%	16/12	21	0.016	2.4
Caspase 3				
Negative	19/17	16		1.5
Positive	26/23	69	0.16	1.0
Fas ligand				
Negative	25/22	21		1.3
Positive	36/30	47	0.30	1.0

phase cells was > 260 wk. Corresponding results were obtained with the other combinations (**Table 4**).

To summarize, the results confirmed that VEGF, cyclin A, PCNA, and a high proportion of S/G2/M phase cells are unfavorable prognostic factors while angiostatin, Fas ligand, Fas, and caspase 3 are favorable prognostic factors for the survival times of patients with NSCLC. Furthermore, an inverse relationship exists between angiogenic, proliferative, and apoptotic factors.

3. Discussion

Prognostic factors can serve many purposes. They can be used to understand the natural history of cancer, to identify homogeneous patient populations, to characterize subsets of patients with a favorable or unfavorable outcome, to predict the success of therapy, or to plan follow-up strategies. In this context, the balance between angiogenic, proliferative, and apoptotic factors within a tissue is important in controlling its overall growth. Therefore, the factors

Table 3
Median Survival Times (MST) and Relative Risk of Patients
with Lymph Node Involvement According to Angiogenic,
Proliferative, and Apoptotic Factors

Lymph node involvement	Patients/ death	MST (wk)	Log rank test p-value	Relative risk
Angiostatin				
Negative	50/39	43		1.1
Positive	13/11	76	0.83	1.0
Cyclin A				
Negative	39/27	69		1.0
Positive	41/36	28	0.07	1.6
PCNA				
Negative	56/41	57		1.0
Positive	24/23	21	0.002	2.1
SG2M				
<23%	25/14	129		1.0
>23%	17/16	21	0.005	2.6
Caspase 3				
Negative	20/17	22		1.4
Positive	32/26	69	0.23	1.0
Fas ligand				
Negative	26/23	21		1.4
Positive	45/35	68	0.06	1.0

mentioned earlier prove useful in assessing a patient's prognosis. In our analysis, we demonstrated that a combination of angiogenic, proliferative, and apoptotic factors can provide improved prognostic information of overall patient survival. This analysis also discovered direct and indirect correlations between angiogenesis, apoptosis, and proliferation in lung cancer. Several studies provide some indications of a causal relationship between angiogenic, proliferative, and apoptotic factors. For instance, VEGF withdrawal in xenografts of glioma cells in mice results in apoptosis; angiostatin, which inhibits angiogenesis and tumor growth in mice, induces endothelial cell apoptosis *(5)*. Likewise, 2-methoxyestradiol, which inhibits angiogenesis and tumor growth, induces apoptosis *(6)*. These observations suggest that endothelial cell apoptosis may be responsible for inhibiting angiogenesis and preventing the growth of tumors.

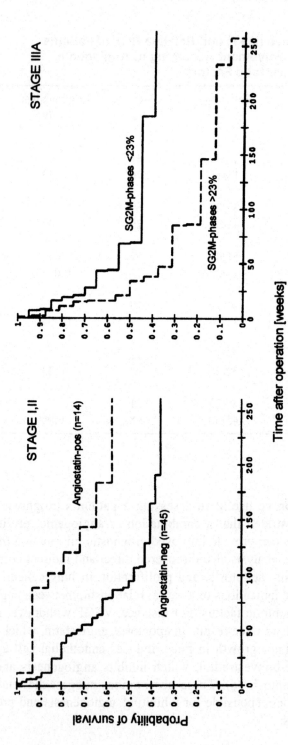

Fig. 2. Survival curves of stage I and II patients grouped according to angiostatin expression (left) and of stage IIIA patients grouped according to the proportion of SG2M phase cells (right).

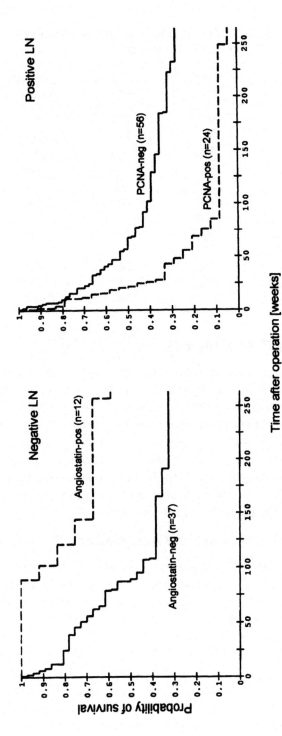

Fig. 3. Survival curves of patients without lymph node involvement grouped according to the expression of angiostatin (left) and of patients with lymph node involvement grouped according to the expression of PCNA (right).

Table 4
Median Survival Times (MST) and Relative Risk of Patients
with NSCLC According to Two Cellular Factors

Combinations	Patients/ death	MST (wk)	Log rank test p-value	Relative risk
VEGF-pos/Fas-neg	40/33	68		1.8
VEGF-neg/Fas-pos	29/16	184	0.047	1.0
Angiostatin-neg/Fas-neg	43/35	80		3.4
Angiostatin-pos/Fas-pos	11/5	>260	0.004	1.0
SG2M-pos/Fas-neg	18/16	38		3.0
SG2M-neg/Fas-pos	23/10	>260	0.004	1.0
PCNA-pos/Fas-neg	18/16	19		2.6
PCNA-neg/Fas-pos	49/27	146	0.002	1.0
Cyclin A-pos/Casp-neg	10/9	16		2.3
Cyclin A-neg/Casp-pos	32/21	107	0.024	1.0
PCNA-pos/Angio-neg	19/16	25		2.6
PCNA-neg/Angio-pos	19/12	146	0.007	1.0

3.1. The Possible Role of Hypoxia

Hypoxia may be the link between angiogenesis, apoptosis, and proliferation. Hypoxia can exert a selective pressure for the expansion of transformed cell populations with a reduced apoptotic potential. This process is modulated by p53 (7). Gene-inactivation studies have shown that angiogenesis is also regulated by hypoxia. Normal cells and cancer cells both produce VEGF under hypoxic stress (8). Hypoxia also affects the proliferation. The increased genetic instability of tumor cells may result in the generation of a greater number of genetic variants, which can be the source of more aggressive cell populations within the process of malignant progression (9).

3.2. The Importance of Combined Analyses and Future Directions

It is evident that a variety of angiogenic, proliferative, and apoptotic factors are important for a patient's clinical outcome. All of these and other factors must be considered when a systematic analysis of gene and protein changes in tumors is undertaken in order to provide prognostic information. Morphological analysis still forms the basis of diagnostic pathology. Additional information is obtained by immunohistochemistry, Western blotting, Northern blotting, and reverse transcription polymerase chain reaction (RT-PCR). Some of these techniques are relatively complex and time-consuming. This drawback can be overcome by using the recently developed microarray technique. It facilitates the simultaneous analysis of thousands of genes in a single experiment. Using

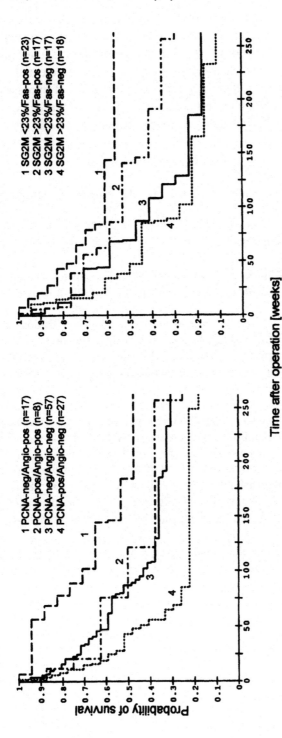

Fig. 4. Survival curves of patients with NSCLC grouped according to the expression of PCNA and angiostatin (left) and grouped according to the proportion of SG2M phase cells and Fas expression (right).

this technique, RNA is converted into cDNA (or cRNA) probes in a reverse transcription reaction that incorporates labeled nucleotides. The cDNA (cRNA) probes are then hybridized to arrays. After hybridization, the quantity of the probe hybridizing to each gene (spot) on the array is detected. The relative intensity of each spot on the array represents the level of expression for each individual gene. A corresponding analysis of proteins can be conducted with peptide arrays. Employing these analyses, investigators can then generate a prognostic test.

References

1. Folkman, J. (1995) Clinical applications of research on angiogenesis. *N. Eng. J. Med.* **333,** 1757–1763.
2. O'Reilly, M. S., Holmgren, L., Chen, C., and Folkman, J. (1996) Angiostatin induces and sustains dormancy of human primary tumors in mice. *Nat. Med.* **2,** 689–692.
3. Kerr, J. F. R., Wyllie, A. H., and Currie, A. R. (1972) Apoptosis: a basic biological phenomenon with wide-ranging implications in tissue kinetics. *Br. J. Cancer* **26,** 239–257.
4. Cordon-Cardo, C. (1995) Mutation of cell cycle regulators. Biological and clinical implications for human neoplasia. *Am. J. Path.* **147,** 545–560.
5. Lucas, R., Holmgren, L., Garcia, I., Jimenez, B., Mandriota, J., Borlat, F., et al. (1998) Multiple forms of angiostatin induce apoptosis in endothelial cells. *Blood* **92,** 4730–4741.
6. Yue, T. L., Wang, X., Louden, C. S., Gupta, S., Pillarisetti, K., Gu, J., et al. (1997) 2-methoxyestradiol, an endogenous estrogen metabolite, induces apoptosis in endothelial cells and inhibits angiogenesis: possible role for stress-activated protein kinase signaling pathway and Fas expression. *Mol. Pharmacol.* **51,** 951–957.
7. Brown, J. M., and Giaccia, A. J. (1998) The unique physiology of solid tumors: Opportunities (and problems) for cancer therapy. *Cancer Res.* **58,** 1408–1416.
8. Shweiki, D., Itin, A., Soffer, D., and Kashet, E. (1992) Vascular endothelial growth factor induced by hypoxia may mediate hypoxia-initiated angiogenesis. *Nature* **359,** 843–845.
9. Reynolds, T. Y., Rockwell, S., and Glazer, P. M. (1996) Genetic instability induced by the tumor's microenvironment. *Cancer Res.* **56,** 5754–5757.

21

Morphological Assessment of Apoptosis in Human Lung Cells

Lori D. Dwyer-Nield, David Dinsdale, J. John Cohen,
Margaret K. T. Squier, and Alvin M. Malkinson

1. Introduction

Apoptosis, a unique mode of cell death that occurs physiologically as part of a "program" to eliminate unwanted cells, was first described in 1972 (1) and is now one of the most active areas of biologic research. This process occurs during development, as a defense mechanism when cells are damaged by disease or toxins, and as a major constituent of normal homeostatic maintenance. Many biochemical assays have been developed to detect and quanitify apoptosis, but altered nuclear morphology is the most reliable feature.

1.1. Apoptosis vs Necrosis

Oncosis (2) is the prelytic cytoplasmic swelling and karyolysis (nuclear breakdown) that precedes necrosis. Necrosis comprises the postmortem changes that follow apoptosis or oncosis and consists of a loss of plasma membrane integrity; other characteristics of necrosis are secondary. A classic model of necrosis is the lysis of antibody-coated cells by complement proteins. These cells are "dead" because membrane barriers are lost as shown by the uptake of trypan blue, eosin Y, propidium iodide, ethidium bromide, and other vital dyes. Nuclear morphology remains intact until lysosomal enzymes are released, after which DNA is degraded and nuclear disintegration begins. In a cell undergoing apoptosis, a series of morphological changes occur that are distinct from oncosis or necrosis. Cells degrade chromatin early during apoptosis, and damaged DNA and nuclear collapse are visible even though cytoplasmic

From: *Methods in Molecular Medicine, vol. 74: Lung Cancer, Vol. 1: Molecular Pathology Methods and Reviews*
Edited by: B. Driscoll © Humana Press Inc., Totowa, NJ

organelles and the plasma membrane remain intact. Assays that simultaneously measure membrane integrity and nuclear condensation are thus highly desirable. Other hallmarks of apoptosis include cellular shrinkage, fragmentation of DNA, "flipping" of phosphatidylserine from the inner to the outer leaflet of the plasma membrane, zeiosis (a "boiling" action or blebbing of the plasma membrane), break-up of the cell into apoptotic bodies (*see* **Fig. 1A**), and phagocytosis of apoptotic cells and vesicles by a nearby phagocytic cell. Phagocytosis rarely occurs in vitro, and thus "secondary" or "apoptotic necrosis" often ensues. Most of these changes can be observed by transmission electron microscopy (TEM), but it is often useful to correlate these observations with complementary methods.

1.2. Assays of Apoptosis

These simple methods based on nuclear morphology are useful for detecting, confirming, and/or quantitating apoptosis in most experimental systems and particularly in pulmonary samples. We recommend beginning with a simple morphological assay that is rapid, highly-informative, makes no a priori assumptions, and uses inexpensive materials and readily available blue-light fluorescence microscopy (*see* **Subheading 3.1.**). More complex or advanced methods have been described in detail elsewhere *(5)*. An optimal combination of techniques for demonstrating apoptosis utilizes morphology plus an assay of DNA damage or membrane alterations.

DNA laddering, the separation of inter-nucleosomal DNA cleavage products on an agarose gel that produces a ladder-like appearance of DNA bands in multiples of 200 base pairs, is indisputable evidence of apoptosis. Unfortu-

---

Fig. 1. *(facing page)* **(A)** Spontaneous apoptosis in a freshly isolated (using a tissue-slice method) human type II cell showing the characteristic condensation of chromatin (*) towards one pole of the fragmented nucleus. Condensed chromatin and nucleolar remnants (arrowheads) are also evident in a smaller nuclear fragment and in a separate, apoptotic body. The nuclear envelope and endoplasmic reticulum of the apoptotic cell are swollen, resulting in zeiosis (Z), but the mitochondria show no signs of swelling. The vesicular nature of the Golgi apparatus (G) is also characteristic of apoptotic (and mitotic) cells. **(B)** TUNEL/TEM of an A549 cell, 3 h after treatment with 1 μM Tumor Necrosis Factor-Related Apoptosis Inducing Ligand (TRAIL), processed for routine electron microscopy. TUNEL labeling is evident over the partially condensed chromatin (*) but not over euchromatin, the nucleolus (n) or the cytoplasmic inclusion (arrow). **(C)** Detail of the area indicated in "B". **(D)** Cell similar to that shown in (B), processed in acrylic resin and incubated with the "CytoDeath" antibody. Caspase-cleaved cytokeratin is present in the cytoplasmic inclusion (arrow) but not in the adjacent nucleus (N). All bars = 1 μm.

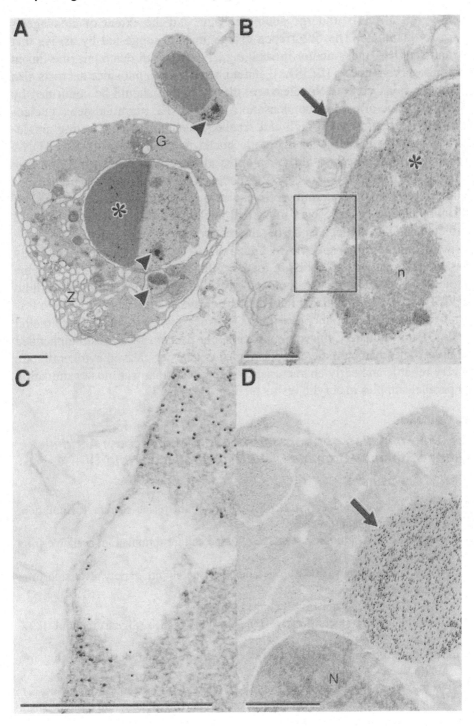

nately, not all cells undergo such cleavage, and the extent of cleavage is hard to quantitate. The occurrence of apoptosis is suggested by assays that quantitate DNA nicks and/or breaks (e.g., TUNEL, cell death enzyme-linked immunosorbent assays [ELISAs], and diphenylamine), but since necrosis also results in nonspecific DNA cleavage, these methods should be confirmed by TEM evidence of nuclear condensation. The TUNEL (terminal deoxynucleo-tidyltransferase-mediated nick-end labeling) technique for detecting single-strand nicks in the DNA of apoptotic nuclei is widely used to detect DNA damage and can be applied to samples already processed for TEM (*see* **Fig. 1B,C**). Interpretation of TUNEL specimens is not straightforward because nuclear remnants of necrotic cells can also label intensely. A low level of TUNEL labeling even occurs in normal nuclei, possibly as a result of nicks inflicted on DNA molecules during the sectioning process.

A technique more specific to apoptosis is the "CytoDEATH" antibody assay, which utilizes an antibody that specifically detects a caspase (cysteine protease family involved in apoptosis) cleavage site in cytokeratin 18 at amino acids DALD^{397}↓S (the arrow indicates the cleavage site). This provides a less ambiguous indicator of apoptosis than DNA cleavage, particularly in epithelial cells *(3)*; unfortunately, this antibody cannot be used on epoxy resin-embedded samples. The characteristic cytoplasmic aggregates of cleaved cytokeratin are a very reliable and early characteristic of apoptosis that warrants examination of parallel samples in acrylic resin (*see* **Fig. 1D**; *4*).

2. Materials

2.1. Determination of Apoptosis by Light Microscopy: Acridine Orange/Ethidium Bromide (AO/EB) Method (see Note 1)

2.1.1. Cell Culture

1. Phosphate-buffered saline (PBS): use standard tissue-culture formulation, available from many vendors.
2. Trypsin/EDTA solution: use standard tissue culture formulation, available from many vendors.
3. Fetal bovine serum (FBS): use standard tissue culture variety, available from many vendors.
4. 1.5-mL microfuge and 15-mL conical tubes.
5. Acridine orange stock: dissolve 1 mg acridine orange (Sigma) in 1 mL 0.9% saline.
6. Ethidium bromide stock: dissolve 1 mg ethidium bromide (Sigma) in 1 mL 0.9% saline.
7. Acridine orange/ethidium bromide (AO/EB) working solution (*see* **Note 2**): combine 100 µL acridine orange stock solution, 100 µL ethidium bromide stock

solution, and 800 μL 0.9% saline. Working solution and dye stocks are stable for >1 yr when stored, protected from light, at 4°C.

2.1.2. Preparation of Slides

1. Microscope slides, 10 × 10 mm coverslip (no. 1 thickness; VWR Scientific).
2. Fluorescence microscope (Zeiss or equivalent equipped with a fluorescein filter set).
3. Five-channel counter (Fisher Scientific).

2.2. Electron Microscopy

The materials needed for most of these procedures are available from several specialist suppliers [e.g., Agar Scientific (Stansted, CM24 8DA, UK); Electron Microscopy Sciences (Ft. Washington, PA); Ernest F. Fullam, Inc. (Latham, NY); Ted Pella Inc. (Redding, CA); Polysciences (Warrington, PA); or TAAB Laboratories (Aldermaston, RG7 8NA, UK)]. Suppliers of specific reagents are indicated in the text.

2.2.1. Morphology

1. Primary fixative: Mix 8 mL glutaraldehyde (use a 25% solution, EM grade) with 50 mL 0.2 M sodium cacodylate (*see* **Notes 3** and **4**). Adjust to pH 7.3 with 0.1 M HCl and bring to a final volume of 100 mL with distilled water. Check pH before use. Make fresh on the day of the experiment.
2. Wash buffer: 0.1 M sodium cacodylate buffer, pH 7.3.
3. Secondary fixative: Add a stock solution of 0.2 M sodium cacodylate containing 2% potassium ferrocyanide [$K_4Fe(CN)_6$] to an equal volume of 2% osmium tetroxide (*see* **Note 5**) in distilled water (*see* **Note 6**). Make fresh on the day of the experiment.
4. 5% Aqueous uranyl acetate (*see* **Note 7**).
5. Series of aqueous ethanol solutions: 70, 90, 95, 100%.
6. 100% propylene oxide.
7. TAAB resin (TAAB Laboratories, Aldermaston, UK): Mix 53 g TAAB embedding resin with 43 g dodecanyl succinic anhydride (DDSA), 6 g methyl nadic anhydride (MNA), and 2 mL 2,4,6-tridimethylamino methyl phenol (DMP-30) on a roller-mixer for several hours before use. Many other suitable epoxy resins (*see* **Note 8**) are available, including Agar 100, Araldite and Epon.
8. Resin working reagents: 50% solution in propylene oxide and 100% resin.
9. Coffin mold.
10. Lead citrate stain (*see* **Note 9**): Add 30 mL 8.86% lead nitrate to an equal volume of 11.53% tri-sodium citrate ($C_6H_5Na_3O_7$•$2H_2O$). Mix vigorously for 1 min, and then intermittently for 30 min. Add 16 mL 1 M sodium hydroxide (freshly made and filtered) to clear. Add 24 mL water and mix by inversion (*see* **Note 10**).

2.2.2. TUNEL/TEM

Reagents for this technique are available from several suppliers but we have found the "ApopTag" kit (Intergen Company, Purchase, NY) effective and convenient.

1. 300 Mesh nickel grids.
2. Sterile 90-mm diameter polystyrene petri dishes.
3. Normal sheep serum (British Biocell International, Cardiff, UK).
4. PBSSAT: PBS containing 1% normal sheep serum, 1% bovine serum albumin (BSA), and 1% Tween 20.
5. Secondary antibody: sheep anti-digoxigenin antibody conjugated with 10 nm colloidal gold particles (British Biocell International, Cardiff, UK).
6. Aliquot the "Apotag" components into micro-centrifuge tubes in the volumes listed below to avoid repeated freeze/thaw cycles. Store in freezer.
   a. Equilibration Buffer: 200 µL
   b. TdT Enzyme Solution: 50 µL
   c. Reaction Buffer: 100 µL
   d. Stop Wash Buffer: 50 µL

2.2.3. Immunocytochemistry

1. 4% paraformaldehyde: Heat 75 mL 1.78% dibasic sodium phosphate ($Na_2HPO_4 \cdot 2H_2O$) for 1 min at a setting of 1000W in a microwave oven (almost boiling). Add 4 g paraformaldehyde and shake until dissolved. Add 0.89 g sodium chloride and 25 mL of 1.56% monobasic sodium phosphate ($NaH_2PO_4 \cdot 2H_2O$). Cool to room temperature.
2. Primary fixative: Combine 4% paraformaldehyde with 0.1% glutaraldehyde (*see* **Note 3**) in PBS. Check pH (*see* **Note 11**).
3. Unicryl resin (British Biocell International).
4. Polymerization rack and refrigerated chamber with UV lamps.
5. Epoxy resin adhesive.
6. Normal goat serum (British Biocell International).
7. Primary antibody: mouse monoclonal antibody (MAb) M30 "CytoDEATH" (Roche Diagnostics, Mannheim, Germany).
8. PBSGAT: PBS containing 1% normal goat serum, 1% BSA, and 1% Tween 20.
9. Secondary antibody: goat anti-mouse IgG conjugated with10 nm gold (British Biocell).

3. Methods

3.1. Determination of Apoptosis by Light Microscopy: Acridine Orange/Ethidium Bromide (AO/EB) Method

3.1.1. Cell Culture

Treat cells with putative apoptotic inducers to determine dose-response curves and time courses. The purpose of this step is to elucidate conditions for optimal apoptosis while maintaining cell integrity (*see* **Note 12**). The AO/EB technique also works well with primary cell isolates, but is not suited for tissues. Tissue sections can be stained with a single DNA intercalating fluorescent dye such as DAPI (4,6-diamidino-2-phenylindole) or Hoechst 33342 (Sigma, St. Louis, MO) to examine nuclear morphology, but membrane integrity cannot be readily examined on tissue slices.

1. Following the treatment, harvest 10,000–50,000 cells in 15 mL conical tubes (*see* **Note 13**).
   a. Cells that grow in suspension are readily harvested by drawing the media from cell culture plates or bottles, rinsing with PBS, and centrifuging the pooled cells at 200*g* for 5–10 min. Aspirate the supernatant, leaving about 25 µL of media on the pellet.
   b. Adherent cells are harvested with trypsin. It is important to pool media, cell washes, and trypsinized cells, as apoptotic cells may be floating in the media or only loosely adherent. Following detachment of cells from tissue-culture surface, FBS should be added to the trypsinized cells to neutralize trypsin.
2. Following pelleting, resuspend the cells in the remaining supernatant.
3. Place twenty-five µL of cell suspension into a microcentrifuge tube and add 2 µL of the AO/EB mixture (*see* **Note 14**). Mix very gently by hand. Leave the pipet tip in the tube for later use.
4. If a series of samples is to be examined, store the cells on ice until nearly ready for evaluation, and then add the dye mixture.

3.1.2. Preparation of Slides

1. Place 10 µL of the cell/dye mixture onto a microscope slide and cover with a 10 × 10 mm No. 1 cover slip (*see* **Note 15**).
2. Examine with a 40–60X dry objective, using epi-illumination and filters appropriate for detecting fluorescein fluorescence. An inexpensive quartz halogen bulb provides ideal light. Filters should provide illumination at 488 nm and emission at 520 nm.

3.1.2.1. SCORING LIVE VS DEAD CELLS

Both acridine orange and ethidium bromide intercalate into DNA to preferentially stain cell nuclei (*see* **Note 16**). Acridine orange is cell-permeant, allowing visualization of the nuclear structure in living cells. Nuclei stained with acridine orange appear yellow-green; red fluorescence may also be seen in the cytoplasm of normal cells (e.g., from RNA, mitochondrial DNA, or various types of granules). As is true for trypan blue or eosin, ethidium bromide does not penetrate intact cell membranes; when plasma membranes rupture, ethidium bromide reaches the nucleus and, overwhelming the contribution of acridine to fluorescence emission, stains the nucleus orange-red.

3.1.2.2. Scoring Apoptotic vs Nonapoptotic Cells by Nuclear Morphology

Normal cell nuclei have "structure" or a lacy appearance caused by variations in intensity reflecting the distribution of euchromatin and heterochromatin (*see* **Fig. 2A**). Apoptotic nuclei, in contrast, have very condensed chromatin that appear as crescents around the nuclear periphery, or the entire nucleus can present as one or more featureless, bright, spherical beads (**Fig. 2**; *see* **Notes 17** and **18**). In advanced apoptosis, a cell may lose DNA, so the overall brightness may be less than that of a normal cell.

3.1.2.3. Differential Cell Quantitation

Score 100 cells (minimum) into one of four categories: live nonapoptotic (green nuclei, normal distribution of chromatin), live apoptotic (green nuclei, condensed chromatin), dead nonapoptotic (orange nuclei, normal distribution of chromatin), or dead apoptotic (orange nuclei, condensed chromatin; *see* **Notes 19–22**).

3.2. Electron microscopy

3.2.1. Morphology

1. Harvest cells.
   a. Harvest suspension cultures by centrifugation at 3000*g* for 10 min in 1.5-mL microcentrifuge tubes using a swing-out rotor (*see* **Note 23**).
   b. Harvest adherent cultures of cells so as to enrich the proportion of apoptotic cells. Apoptotic cells can be dislodged from underlying cells by vigorously swirling the medium and immediately decanting and centrifuging as above (*see* **Note 24**).
2. Replace the supernatant on the cells with primary fixative and fix the pellet overnight at 4°C (*see* **Note 25**).
3. Wash pellet 3 × 15 min in buffer. At this point the cells can be stored at 4°C if necessary.
4. Incubate pellet in the secondary fixative for 1 h at room temperature.
5. Wash 3 × at 2 h/wash in distilled water.
6. Incubate pellet in 5% aqueous uranyl acetate (*see* **Note 27**) overnight at 4°C.
7. Wash in distilled water, 3 × at 20 min/wash.
8. Dehydrate in a series of ethanol solutions: 70% (2 × 15 min), 90% (1 × 15 min), 95% (1 × 15 min), 100% (3 × 15 min) followed by 100% propylene oxide (2 × 15 min) (*see* **Notes 26** and **27**).
9. Infiltrate the fixed tissue bloc with a 50% solution of resin in propylene oxide for 2 h, and then in 100% resin for 4 changes/d for 3 d (*see* **Note 28**).
10. Polymerize for 48 h at 60°C.
11. Reorient pellet by sawing the tip from the tube (2–3 mm from the tip) and inverting it, cut-surface down, into a "coffin" mold.

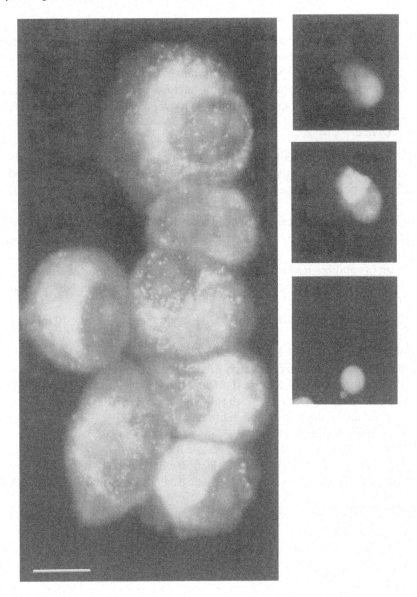

Fig. 2. Human adenosquamous carcinoma H125 cells were treated with 20 μ*M* Calpain Inhibitor 1 for 24 h. Cells were harvested by trypsinization as described, pelleted, and treated with AO/EB. Cells were then visualized and photographed using a Nikon Optiphot fitted with a Nikon HFX-II camera. The large panel shows the AO/EB staining of several nonapoptotic H125 nuclei. Note the heterogeneous staining. The small panels represent 3 separate examples of apoptotic H125 nuclei in the same sample. Note the differences in size and the lack of detail in the apoptotic nuclei. Bar = 10 μm.

12. Fill the mold with fresh resin and polymerize for 48 h at 60°C.
13. Cut semithin (1 μm) sections through all layers of the pellet and then cut ultrathin (70 nm) sections from selected areas, collect them on 300 mesh copper or nickel grids, and stain with lead citrate for 10 min (*see* **Note 29**).
14. Examine grids in a transmission electron microscope. **Figure 1A** shows an example of an electron micrograph generated from a cell prepared using this protocol.

3.2.2. TUNEL/TEM

1. Use sections (unstained) prepared as described in **Subheading 3.2.1.**, collected on 300 mesh nickel grids. Arrange the reagents as 35 μL droplets in sterile 90-mm diameter polystyrene petri dishes Completely immerse the grids face-up for all stages (*see* **Note 30**).
2. Block nonspecific binding by incubating in serum from the species in which the secondary antibody has been raised (sheep) for 4 h at room temperature (*see* **Note 31**).
3. Wash in equilibration buffer 1 × 10 min at room temperature.
4. Incubate in TdT Enzyme solution diluted 30:70 in reaction buffer, overnight at 4°C.
5. Block in stop/wash Buffer, diluted 1:34 in ultrapure water, 1 × 10 min at room temperature.
6. Wash in PBSSAT 3 × 1 h and then 2 × 2 h at room temperature.
7. Incubate in the secondary antibody diluted 1:50 in PBSSAT, overnight at 4°C.
8. Blot and then *plunge*-wash grid (hold grid firmly with the tips of the forceps and plunge it, edge-first, into the wash solution) into PBSSAT (*see* **Note 32**).
9. Blot and then *plunge*-wash grid in ultrapure water.
10. Allow grid to air dry.
11. Stain grid with 5% aqueous uranyl acetate for 1 min.
12. Examine grid in a transmission electron microscope. **Figure 1B, C** show TUNEL/TEM micrographs of an apoptotic A549 cell prepared using this method.

3.2.3. Immunocytochemistry

1. Harvest cells as described in **Subheading 3.1.1.**
2. Gently replace the supernatant with primary fixative and fix the pellet for 1 h at room temperature.
3. Wash pellet in PBS 2 × 15 min.
4. Store overnight in a fresh change of PBS at 4°C.
5. Wash pellet in distilled water 3 × 15 min.
6. Dehydrate in a series of ethanol solutions: 70% (3 × 15 min), 90% (1 × 15 min), 95% (1 × 15 min), 100% (3 × 15 min) (*see* **Note 27**).
7. Infiltrate pellet with a 50% solution of Unicryl resin in ethanol (2 h), 100% resin (1 h) and then overnight. This is followed by 4 changes/d for the following 5 d (hold samples in 100% resin during any intervening weekend; *see* **Note 33**).
8. Insert micro-centrifuge tubes into the polymerization rack and equilibrate for 6 h at 4°C (*see* **Note 34**).

9. Polymerize resin for 5 d with UV radiation ($\lambda = 360$ nm) at 4°C (*see* **Note 35**).
10. Reorient pellet by sawing the tip from the tube and mounting it, transversely, onto a blank stub using epoxy resin adhesive. ('Araldite Rapid' sets within 1 h.)
11. Cut semi-thin (1-μm) sections axially through all layers of each pellet to select areas for ultramicrotomy.
12. Cut ultrathin sections from selected areas and collect on 300 mesh nickel grids (*see* **Notes 30** and **36**).
13. Block nonspecific binding by incubating in serum of the species in which the secondary antibody has been raised (e.g., goat) for 4 h at room temperature (*see* **Note 36**).
14. Incubate with the primary antibody, diluted 1:5 in PBSGAT, overnight at 4°C.
15. Blot grid, wash in PBSGAT for 3 × 1 h, and then again 2 × 2h.
16. Incubate grid in secondary antibody, diluted 1:50 in PBSGAT, overnight at 4°C.
17. Blot grid, then *plunge*-wash in PBSGAT (*see* **Note 32**).
18. Blot, then *plunge*-wash in ultrapure water.
19. Allow grid to air dry.
20. Stain with 5% aqueous uranyl acetate for 1 min.
21. Examine grid in a transmission electron microscope. **Figure 1D** shows an electron micrograph of caspase-cleaved cytokeratin (Cyto-Death antibody) antibody.

4. Notes

1. Nuclear morphology has been the universal standard for detection of apoptosis for 30 years. This can be detected and quantitated by assays such as the AO/EB method. For final confirmation with any new cell type, light microscopy should not stand alone; the definitive identification of apoptosis is by TEM.
2. Acridine orange and ethidium bromide are DNA intercalating dyes and are mutagens by the Ames test. Avoid all skin contact, wear gloves, lab coat, and eye protection.
3. Glutaraldehyde and formaldehyde are toxic by ingestion and harmful by skin absorption and inhalation. They are skin, eye, and respiratory irritants and may cause long term sensitization. Always wear gloves, lab coat, face mask, and eye-protection and use in a fume hood where possible or in a well-ventilated area.
4. Sodium cacodylate is an arsenical compound; it is a very toxic, cumulative poison and confirmed carcinogen. Avoid all skin contact, use in a fume hood, and always wear gloves, lab coat, and eye protection.
5. Osmium tetroxide is very toxic and highly volatile. Always wear gloves and a lab coat and work in a fume hood.
6. The potassium ferrocyanide solution should be adjusted to pH 7.3 and aged, at 4°C, for at least 7 d before use. It is yellow in color and turns dark brown upon addition to osmium tetroxide.
7. Uranyl acetate is very toxic and radioactive. Always wear gloves and a lab coat. When handling powder, wear a face mask. Any spills should be cleaned

immediately and thoroughly. Store urany lacetate solution at 4°C, protect it from strong light during use, and discard if cloudy.

8. Epoxy resins and their components are harmful by inhalation and are skin, eye, and respiratory irritants. A lab coat and gloves should be worn at all times and all work carried out in a fume hood where possible. Otherwise, a face mask and gloves should be worn, and the experiments performed in a well-ventilated area. Epoxy resin dust is harmful by inhalation. A face mask and eye protection should be worn at all times and the dust should be contained during and after trimming.

9. Lead nitrate is toxic by ingestion and absorption. It is also an eye irritant. Always wear gloves, lab coat, and face mask when handling powder.

10. Boiled, ultra-pure water (>18.2MΩ) should be used throughout. Aliquot the final solution into 1.5-mL micro-centrifuge tubes, each one filled to the brim to exclude carbon dioxide, and discard after use.

11. The fixative should be made up fresh on the day of use; if final pH is not 7.3 (± 0.05), then check components and repeat procedure.

12. The power of the AO/EB combination lies in the ability, with a single filter set, to examine both nuclear morphology and viability simultaneously on any given cell. This prevents common errors in data interpretation. For example, treating cells with distilled water might be seen as preventing apoptosis if nuclear morphology was the only variable assessed (since a lysed cell cannot commit suicide), whereas it would be interpreted as causing apoptosis if cell death was the only variable assessed.

13. Troubleshooting: excessive debris is observed. Common causes include cell lysis and damage to cells during harvest. Harvesting at earlier time points may help. Careful handling of cells, such as avoiding cytospinning, scraping, or vigorous pipetting, also reduces debris.

14. Alternative dyes: other stains can be used to differentially visualize nuclear morphology (e.g., Hoechst 33342, DAPI) and viability (e.g., trypan blue, eosin). Hoechst 33342 staining is particularly useful for visualizing nuclei in tissue sections. One millimolar (in water) Hoechst dye stock is mixed with cells or placed over a tissue section at 10 µ*M* final concentration. Hoechst dyes require ultraviolet illumination, and filters that pass excitation light at 360 nm and emit light at 460 nm.

15. Classification into cell-staining categories must be performed immediately after placing the cells on the slide so that the cells do not dry out. If the coverslip is dropped too hard on the cells, they may lyse or develop globular processes that can cause errors in counting. Three samples fit on each slide.

16. A color photograph of cells stained by this technique with all four categories demonstrated can be seen in Dwyer-Nield et al. (*6*).

17. Distinguishing apoptotic lung cells from nonapoptotic lung cells is cell type-specific. A nonapoptotic nucleus generally has a heterogeneous appearance. Some cell types have prominent nucleoli that appear as densely staining circles inside the nucleus, and these should not be confused with the condensed chromatin beads often seen in an apoptotic nucleus. Apoptotic cells with intact membranes

are easily distinguished from their normal counterparts. Membrane-compromised cells, however, sometimes shrink, and this diminishes the size difference between the apoptotic and nonapoptotic nuclei. Carefully observe the appearance of the chromatin and determine if there is any structure or definition, being careful not to count individual apoptotic bodies produced from the same cell as separate apoptotic events.

18. Different cell types tend to have distinct nuclear characteristics. Thymocytes, for example, have little cytoplasm and are very small. Mouse lung epithelial cells have larger nuclei with large nucleoli, while human lung cancer cells run the gamut. Human lung H125 cells of adenosquamous tumor origin (*see* **Fig. 2**) are large with prominent nucleoli. Human small cell lung carcinoma variants, H82 and H446, have smaller nuclei and are harder to score. Positive and negative controls for nuclear morphology are necessary in each experiment; untreated cells should be examined to familiarize the eye with normal cellular architecture. To recognize apoptotic nuclei, it is helpful to observe cells tested with an agent known to induce apoptosis in that cell type. If no such agent has been yet delineated, serum starvation (growing cells in serum-free medium overnight) often induces apoptosis.

19. Unlike other apoptosis detection methods in which the sample is subjected to an automated analysis, the assays described here take time. To obtain meaningful statistics, one should count 100 cells/sample and at least 3 samples/condition. When examining multiple slides, prepare only one or two at a time since drying of the slide distorts cellular architecture. A hemocytometer may be used instead of a slide, but nuclear morphology is more distinct on a slide because of the moderate compression provided by the No. 1 cover slip. A cover slip thicker than No.1 causes too much compression, resulting cell blebbing and lysis. The cells should be prepared fresh and counted immediately. The time required for counting depends on cell density, amount of debris, and the cell type.

20. Cells do not always appear unambiguously apoptotic or normal. Thus, judgement calls have to be made on cells in early stages of apoptosis or that have been otherwise compromised. Counting at least 100 cells/sample helps to eliminate effects of questionable judgements. It is also advisable to count fields from different parts of each coverslip to ensure an unbiased count.

21. Troubleshooting: If nuclei are difficult to detect, try adding more dye. Other DNA intercalating agents in the experimental system may interfere with AO/EB determinations.

22. Troubleshooting: bleaching—check that filters are intact and provide only blue light to the sample. Unfiltered UV light produces rapid bleaching with these dyes.

23. An ideal pellet for preparing sections for TEM is 1 mm at its thickest point and usually consists of about 3×10^6 cells.

24. The underlying cells may then be fixed and processed through to stage 7 *in situ* before being removed using a cell-scraper, pelleted and embedded in resin.

25. Addition and removal of the fixative and wash solutions is performed gently to avoid disturbing the pellet.

26. Propylene oxide is harmful by ingestion, inhalation, and absorption; it is irritating to the skin, eyes, and respiratory systems; is carcinogenic and teratogenic; and is highly flammable and explosive. Gloves and a lab coat should be worn and all procedures carried out in a fume hood away from sources of ignition.

27. One hundred percent ethyl alcohol is stored over a molecular sieve (to maintain dehydration) and filtered with a 0.2-μm syringe filter before use.

28. Lids should be removed during all stages involving 100% resin to allow release of any traces of propylene oxide. If most of the resin has been removed with a pasteur pipet, the remainder can be eliminated by inverting the tube over absorbent tissue for 1 h.

29. The intensity of lead staining can be enhanced by pretreating the grids with 5% uranyl acetate for 10 min.

30. To minimize loss of sections during subsequent procedures, the grids should be etched with concentrated nitric acid and then dipped into an adhesive solution. This adhesive solution is prepared by dipping 20-mm Scotch® cellulose adhesive tape in 10 mL chloroform to remove adhesive. Sections should be "baked" onto these grids overnight at 37°C before use.

31. The blocking serum is diluted 1:50 in PBS containing both 1% BSA and 1% Tween 20.

32. If sections are dislodged during *plunge*-washing the grids may be washed on droplets of PBSSAT and ultrapure water instead.

33. The timing of the holding stage (weekend) has no discernible effect. Shorter infiltration times can result in the formation of creases in sections of apoptotic nuclei.

34. The rack suspends the tubes over the mid-line between two Philips TL 8w/05 fluorescent lamps mounted 140 mm apart, the tip of each tube being 150 mm from both lamps. This is placed in a chest freezer (–20°C) modified to provide precise temperature control (± 0.5°C).

35. Unlike many other acrylic resins, oxygen need not be excluded but the temperature should be closely monitored.

36. All steps are carried out in 35-μL droplets in sterile 90-mm diameter plastic petri dishes. Grids should be fully immersed, face-up, for all stages.

Acknowledgments

We are grateful to Judy McWilliam and Tim Smith for their help in refining these techniques and in the preparation of this chapter and to Dr. Pamela Rice for photographing the H125 cells. This work was supported by USPHS Grant CA33497.

References

1. Kerr, J. F., Wyllie, A. H., and Currie, A. R. (1972) Apoptosis: a basic biological phenomenon with wide-ranging implications in tissue kinetics. *Br. J. Cancer* **26,** 239–257.

2. Levin, S., Bucci, T. J., Cohen, S. M., Fix, A. S., Hardisty , J. F., LeGrand, E. K., et al. (1999) The nomenclature of cell death: recommendations of an *ad hoc* Committee of the Society of Toxicologic Pathologists. *Toxicol. Pathol.* **27**, 484–490.
3. MacFarlane, M., Merrison, W., Dinsdale, D., and Cohen, G.M. (2000) Active caspases and cleaved cytokeratins are sequestered into cytoplasmic inclusions in TRAIL-induced apoptosis. *J. Cell Biol.* **148**, 1239–1254.
4. Leers, M. P., Kolgen, W., Bjorklund, V., Bergman, T., Tribbick, G., Persson, B., et al. (1999) Immunocytochemical detection and mapping of a cytokeratin 18 neo-epitope exposed during early apoptosis. *J. Pathol.* **187**, 567–572.
5. Squier, M. K. and Cohen, J. J. (2000) Assays of apoptosis. *Methods Mol. Biol.* **144**, 327–337.
6. Dwyer-Nield, L. D., Thompson, J. A., Peljak, G., Squier, M. K., Barker, T. D., Parkinson, A., et al. (1998) Selective induction of apoptosis in mouse and human lung epithelial cell lines by the *tert*-butyl hydroxylated metabolite of butylated hydroxytoluene: a proposed role in tumor promotion. *Toxicology* **130**, 115–127.

22

[D-Arg^6, D-Trp^{7,9}, N^{me}Phe^8]-Substance P (6-11) Activates JNK and Induces Apoptosis in Small Cell Lung Cancer Cells via an Oxidant-Dependent Mechanism

Alison MacKinnon and Tariq Sethi

1. Introduction

[D-Arg^6, D-Trp^{7,9}, N^{me}Phe^8]-substance P (6-11) (antagonist G) is a novel class of anti-cancer agent that inhibits small cell lung cancer (SCLC) cell growth in vitro and in vivo and is entering Phase II clinical investigation for the treatment of SCLC *(1,2)*. Although antagonist G blocks SCLC cell growth (IC$_{50}$ = 24.5 ± 1.5 and 38.5 ± 1.5 µM for the H69 and H510 cell lines, respectively), its exact mechanism of action is unclear. Factors affecting the balance between SCLC cell proliferation and apoptosis will have a profound effect on tumor growth. However, the mechanisms which regulate apoptosis remain poorly understood. The p46/p54 c-jun N-terminal kinases (JNKs) are members of the MAPK family that activate the transcription factors c-jun and ATF2 and are stimulated by environmental stress (e.g., heat shock, UV, TNF-α), receptor tyrosine kinases and G-protein-linked receptors *(3–5)*. Activation of JNK1 has been shown to be important for UV-induced apoptosis in SCLC cells *(6)*. Reactive oxygen species (ROS) are involved in signaling events leading to apoptosis in many cell types *(7)*. ROS have been shown to activate JNK *(8)*, c-jun expression, and AP-1 activity *(9,10)*. The role of ROS in pathways leading to programmed cell death is particularly pertinent in cancers where the oxygen tension at the center of tumors may be particularly low *(11)*.

Our studies have shown that antagonist G activates JNK via free radical oxygen generation, which may be important for antagonist G-induced apoptosis of SCLC cells in vitro. We suggest that both of these effects are likely to be

From: *Methods in Molecular Medicine, vol. 74: Lung Cancer, Vol. 1: Molecular Pathology Methods and Reviews*
Edited by: B. Driscoll © Humana Press Inc., Totowa, NJ

crucial for antagonist G's maximal anti-tumor effect in vivo. In the present chapter we describe the procedures that are commonly used to assay for apoptosis and for the activity of JNK.

2. Materials

All reagents should be of the purest grade available.

The SCLC cell line NCI-H69 was purchased from the American Type Tissue Culture Collection (Rockville, MD); RPMI-1640 was obtained from Sigma (Poole, UK); antagonist G ([D-Arg^6, D-Trp^{7,9}, N^{me}Phe^8]-substance P (6-11)) was a kind gift from Peptec (Copenhagen, Denmark); [γ^{32}P]-ATP (3000 Ci/mmol) was purchased from Amersham PLC (Amersham, UK); JNK1-FL, p42^{MAPK} polyclonal antibodies (PAbs), GST c-jun (79), myelin basic protein and protein A/G agarose were purchased from Santa Cruz Biotechnology.

2.1. Cell Culture

1. MK3 anaerobic incubator with 0% oxygen (Don Whitely Scientific Ltd., Yorkshire, UK).

2.2. SCLC Proliferation Assay

1. NCI-H69 SCLC cells.
2. Culture medium: RPMI 1640 medium with 25 mM HEPES supplemented with 10% (v/v) fetal calf serum (PCS), 50 U/mL penicillin, 50 µg/mL streptomycin, and 5 µg/mL L-glutamine.
3. SITA medium: RPMI 1640 medium supplemented with 30 nM selenium, 5 µg/mL insulin, 10 µg/mL transferrin, and 0.25% (w/v) bovine serum albumin (BSA).
4. 21-gauge sterile needle.
5. Coulter counter (Coulter Electronics).
6. 24-well tissue-culture plates.

2.3. Measurement of Apoptosis

1. Serum-free medium: RPMI 1640 medium containing 0.25% (w/v) BSA.
2. Antagonist G, 25 µM (Kind gift from the Imperial Cancer Research Fund, Edinburgh).
3. N-acetyl cysteine (10 mM n-AC) (Sigma).
4. Cytospin set up.
5. Methanol.
6. May-Grünwald-Giemsa stain.

2.4. Measurement of JNK/MAPK Activity

1. Phosphate-buffered saline (PBS), pH 7.4 (Sigma).
2. PBS containing CaCl$_2$ and MgCl$_2$ (Sigma).

3. Lysis buffer: 25 mM HEPES (sodium salt), pH 7.4, 0.3 M NaCl, 1.5 mM MgCl$_2$, 0.2 mM EDTA (store at 4°C). On the day of use, add 0.1% (v/v) Triton X-100, 1 protease inhibitor tablet/50 mL (Boehringer), 20 mM β-glycerophosphate, 0.5 mM dithiothreitol (DTT), 1 mM orthovanadate (0.25 mL of 200 mM stock). Lysis buffer is stable for approx 1 d on ice.
4. 200 mM sodium orthovanadate stock: Prepare in distilled H$_2$O. Boil and allow to cool. Adjust to pH 10.0. Repeat boiling and adjusting pH until pH is stable. Aliquot and store at –20°C.
5. Rotary mixer

2.4.1. JNK1-Immune-Complex Kinase Assay

1. PAb to JNK1 (Santa Cruz C-15 FL).
2. Protein A/G agarose beads.
3. Wash buffer: 20 mM HEPES (sodium salt), pH 7.4, 50 mM NaCl, 2.5 mM MgCl$_2$, 0.1 mM EDTA. Store at 4°C.
4. Kinase buffer: 20 mM HEPES (sodium salt), pH 7.4, 0.5 mM NaF, 7.5 mM MgCl$_2$, 0.2 mM EGTA (store at 4°C). On the day of use add 2 mM DTT, 10 mM β-glycerophosphate, 0.5 mM orthovanadate. Store kinase buffer on ice for 1 d.
5. Adenosine triphosphate (ATP).
6. [γ³²P]-ATP (3000 Ci/mmol).
7. GST-c-jun substrate (Santa Cruz Biotechnologies).
8. Eppendorf thermomixer.
9. Sodium dodecyl sulfate polycrylamide gel electrophoresis (SDS-PAGE) sample buffer (4X): Tris (2 mL of a 1 M stock), pH 6.8, 4 mL glycerol, 0.8 g SDS, 40 mg bromophenol blue, 4 mL mercaptoethanol. Store at room temperature.
10. 12% SDS-PAGE gel.
11. SDS-PAGE gel fixative: 10% acetic acid, 30% methanol
12. Coomassie Blue (Sigma).
13. Phosphorimager (Storm Molecular Dynamics).

2.4.2. P42^{MAPK}-Immune-Complex Kinase Assay

1. P42^{MAPK} specific lysis buffer: 25 mM HEPES (sodium salt), pH 7.4, 0.3 M NaCl, 1.5 mM MgCl$_2$, 0.2 mM EDTA (store at 4°C). On the day of use, add 0.5% (v/v) Triton X-100, 1 protease inhibitor tablet/50 mL (Boehringer), 20 mM β-glycerophosphate, 0.5 mM DTT, 1 mM orthovanadate.
2. Polyclonal p42^{MAPK} antibody, (Santa Cruz Biotechnologies).
3. Myelin basic protein (Sigma).
4. 2.5 cm^2 pieces of P81 phosphocellulose paper (Sigma).
5. 0.5% phosphoric acid.
6. Acetone.

3. Methods

3.1. Cell Culture

1. For experimental purposes, the cells were transferred to SITA medium consisting of RPMI 1640 medium supplemented with 30 nM selenium, 5 µg/mL insulin, 10 µg/mL transferrin and 0.25% (w/v) BSA. Cells were quiesced in serum-free RPMI 1640 medium containing 0.25% (w/v) BSA. In anoxic studies, cells were incubated at 37°C in a MK3 anaerobic incubator with 0% oxygen (Don Whitely Scientific Ltd.).

3.2. SCLC Proliferation Assay

Standard culture conditions for NCI-H69 SCLC are maintenance in culture medium at a density of 1–2 × 10^6/mL in a humidified atmosphere of 5% CO_2/95% air at 37°C.

1. Transfer SCLC cells to SITA medium and culture for 2–3 d prior to experiment, to a density of 1–2 × 10^6/mL.
2. Pellet cells from one 75 cm^3 flask at 200g for 4 min and resuspend in approx 5 mL SITA medium.
3. Disaggregate cells by passing though a 21-gauge sterile needle. Take an aliquot for counting.
4. Determine cell density using a Coulter counter (Coulter Electronics). Adjust cell number to 5 × 10^4 cells/mL.
5. Plate cells in 1-mL aliquots in 24-well tissue-culture plates and leave in incubator for 1–4 h. Set up six plates for a full time-course.
6. Add test drugs or control diluent (at 100X concentration) in a 10 µL volume, wrap plates in foil, and place in an incubator at 37°C.
7. Determine cell number at d 1, 3, 5, 7, 9, and 12.

3.3. Measurement of Apoptosis

1. Culture SCLC cells in SITA medium and then place in a quiescent state by overnight incubation in serum-free medium.
2. Incubate SCLC cells (10^6 cells/mL in 24-well plates) in the presence or absence of test agents (example antagonist G, 25 µM, plus or minus ROS scavenger N-acetyl cysteine (10 mM n-AC)) for 24 h.
3. Collect cells and gently disaggregate by pipetting (×3) through a p1000 plastic pipet tip.
4. Cytocentrifuge cells (150 µL) onto glass slides, fix with methanol, stain with May-Grünwald-Giemsa stain, and examine using an Olympus BH-2 microscope, at a magnification of ×400.
5. Apoptotic SCLC cells are identified as displaying typical morphological features, including cell shrinkage and chromatin condensation as previously detailed (*12*); (**Fig. 1**). Estimate the percentage of apoptotic cells from >500 cells counted from 4–5 random fields (*see* **Note 1**). An alternative method for assessing apoptosis morphologically is available and is briefly outlined in **Note 2**.

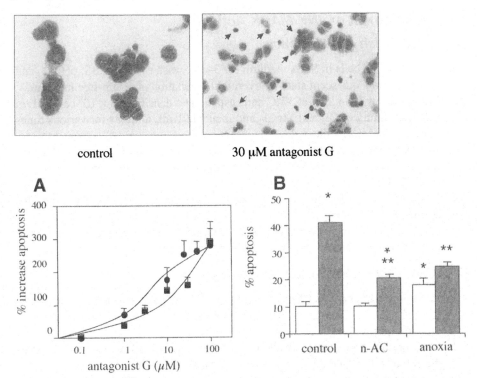

Fig. 1. Effect of antagonist G on SCLC cell apoptosis. (**A**) SCLC cells H69 (●) and
H510 (■) were washed and incubated in serum free quiescent medium with antagonist
G or diluent (H_2O) for 24 h at 37°C. Apoptosis was assessed morphologically using
May-Grünwald-Giemsa stain as described in Methods. The data is expressed as %
increase in apoptosis and represents the mean ± SEM of 4 independent experiments
performed in triplicate. Representative photomicrographs (upper panel) of histologically stained H69 cells treated with diluent (left) or 30 μM antagonist G (right) for
24 h, showing the presence of apoptotic bodies. (**B**) Antagonist G-induced apoptosis
is inhibited by anoxia and n-acetyl cysteine. H69 cells cultured in SITA medium were
quiesced overnight in serum-free medium, washed, and incubated (1×10^6 cells/mL)
in the absence (open bars) or presence (closed bars) of 25 μM antagonist G with or
without 10 mM n-acetyl cysteine (n-AC) for 24 h at 37°C. H69 cells were made anoxic
by incubation in a MK3 anaerobic incubator (0% O_2) at 37°C for 24 h. Apoptosis was
assessed morphologically using May-Grünwald-Giemsa stain as described in Methods.
The results are expressed as % apoptotic cells and represent the mean ± SEM of
3–4 separate experiments performed in duplicate. *statistically different from control;
**statistically different from corresponding antagonist G control; $p < 0.05$ ANOVA).

3.4. Measurement of JNK/MAPK Activity

3.4.1. Preparation of Cell Extracts

1. Culture SCLC cells in SITA medium for 3–4 d, wash twice in PBS, pH 7.4, and then place in a quiescent state by overnight incubation in serum-free medium.
2. Wash cells twice in PBS at 37°C and suspend at a density of 5×10^6 cells/mL in PBS containing $CaCl_2$ and $MgCl_2$ and incubate 1 mL aliquots for various times with test agents as indicated.
3. After appropriate treatments, cells are rapidy sedimented at 4°C and the resulting pellets washed in ice-cold PBS. From this point all procedures until electrophoresis should be carried out at 4°C.
4. Suspend cells in 0.5 mL lysis buffer at 4°C and mix on a rotary mixer for 30 min at 4°C.
5. Clarify extracts by centrifugation at 13,000g for 10 min (*see* **Note 2**). Estimate protein concentration using Pierce BCA protein assay reagent (*see* **Note 3**).

3.4.2. JNK1-Immune-Complex Kinase Assay

1. Immunoprecipitate JNK1 from cell lysates (500 µg protein) using 3 µg antibody to JNK1 (Santa Cruz C-15 FL). Incubate for 2 h at 4°C or overnight at 4°C on a rotating shaker.
2. Wash protein A/G agarose beads twice in PBS and add 50 µL (50:50 slurry) to the extracts. Incubate 2 h at 4°C on a rotating shaker.
3. Wash the beads three times by repeated centrifugation (13,000g for 1 min at 4°C) and resuspension in ice-cold wash buffer, and then once in ice-cold kinase buffer. Extreme care should be taken at this stage to avoid aspiration of the beads. After the final wash carefully remove all the kinase buffer to the top of the beads.
4. Suspend the beads in 20 µL kinase buffer containing 20 µ*M* ATP, 1 µCi [γ^{32}P]-ATP (3000 Ci/mmol) and 1 µg GST-c-jun (a 1-79) substrate. Incubate at 30°C for 20 min in an Eppendorf thermomixer.
5. Stop the reaction by adding 7 µL 4X SDS-PAGE sample buffer and heat to 95°C for 10 min.
6. Load samples onto a 12% SDS-PAGE gel and electrophorese until the sample front reaches the bottom of the gel.
7. Fix the gel for 10 min and stain in Coomassie Blue for 2 h at room temperature. Destain by washing in fixing solution with repeated changes for 5 h.
8. Identify phosphorylated c-jun by autoradiography of the dried gels, or by phosphorimager (Storm Molecular Dynamics) (*see* **Note 4**).

3.4.3. P42^{MAPK}-Immune-Complex Kinase Assay

Assay p42^{MAPK} activity exactly as described for JNK1, with the noted exceptions.

1. Lyse cells in P42^{MAPK} specific lysis buffer.
2. Immunoprecipitate P42^{MAPK} using 2 µg polyclonal p42^{MAPK} antibody.

3. Incubate washed immunoprecipitates in kinase buffer containing 100 μM ATP, 1 μCi $[\gamma^{32}P]$-ATP (3000 Ci/mmol), and 10 μg myelin basic protein and incubate at 30°C for 20 min in an Eppindorf thermomixer.

4. Spot 20 μL of supernatant onto phosphocellulose paper and wash paper 3 times in 0.5% phosphoric acid.

5. Dip filters in acetone and air dry before counting for $[^{32}P]$ in a beta-scintillation counter (*see* **Note 5**).

4. Notes

1. **Figure 1** shows a typical experiment where SCLC cells are treated with antagonist G for 24 h. Antagonist G stimulated apoptosis in SCLC cells as judged morphologically. In the SCLC cell line H69, antagonist G (25 μM) increased basal apoptosis from 10.5 ± 4.2% to 37.1 ± 5.4% ($n=4$), with an EC$_{50}$ of 5.9 ± 0.1 μM, ($n=4$; **Fig. 1A**). Antagonist G also induced apoptosis in the SCLC cell line H510 with an EC$_{50}$ value of 15.2 ± 2.7 μM (**Fig. 1A**). Antagonist G-induced apoptosis was blocked by co-incubation with the ROS scavenger N-acetyl cysteine (10 mM n-AC) and by incubation under anoxic conditions (**Fig. 1B**). This suggests that antagonist G-induced apoptosis occurs via an oxidant-dependent mechanism in SCLC cells.

2. Cells can be stained with acridine orange and ethidium bromide to detect necrotic vs apoptotic cells. Quiesced SCLC cells suspended in 96-well plates (2×10^5 cells/mL) are treated with test agents. Following a desired incubation period, 1 μL of a mixture of acridine orange (100 μg/mL) and ethidium bromide (100 μg/mL) are added. This mixture is protected from light and stored at 4°C. NB. Extreme caution should be used when handling and disposing of ethidium bromide. After a 2 min incubation at room temperature cells are viewed under fluorescence microscopy. Viable cells have a bright green nucleus with intact structure. Apoptotic cells have a bright green or orange nucleus showing condensation of chromatin as dense areas. Necrotic cells have an orange nucleus with intact structure.

3. An additional clearing step can be included by adding 50 μL (50:50 slurry in lysis buffer) of albumin agarose and mixing at 4°C for 30 min. The resultant supernatant is assayed for protein.

3. 20 μL aliquots of lysate are diluted 1:5 with PBS prior to protein determination. This is necessary to bring the protein concentration within the sensitivity of the assay and to dilute out the reducing agent (DTT) in the lysis buffer that interferes with the colorimetric assay.

4. Antagonist G (25 μM), caused a marked and sustained activation of JNK activity in H69 cells. This effect was maximal at 2 h, and sustained for at least 6 h (**Fig. 2A**). The activation of JNK by antagonist G was concentration-dependent (**Fig. 2B**), with an EC$_{50}$ value of 3.2 ± 0.1 μM ($n=3$).

5. Antagonist G caused a modest increase in p42^{MAPK} activity in H69 cells, which was not evident at concentrations lower than 25 μM (**Fig. 2B** inset). Therefore, antagonist G causes a selective stimulation of JNK over MAPK which may be instrumental in its ability to induce apoptosis in SCLC cells.

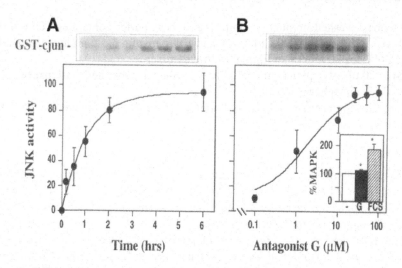

Fig. 2. Effect of antagonist G on MAPK and JNK activity in SCLC cells. (A) Time course of JNK activation. H69 cells (5×10^6 cells/mL) were incubated with 25 μM antagonist G at 37°C for the times indicated. JNK activity was assessed by immunoprecipitation of the cell lysates with a polyclonal anti-JNK1 antibody and phosphorylation of GST-cjun as described in Materials and Methods. The data are expressed as % maximal response and represent the mean ± SEM of 3 experiments performed in duplicate. The basal JNK activity did not change significantly during the incubation (data not shown). A representative autoradiograph is shown. (B) Concentration dependence of JNK activation. H69 cells were incubated with antagonist G at the concentrations indicated for 60 min at 37°C. The results are expressed as % maximal response and represent the mean ± SEM of 2–4 experiments performed in duplicate. A representative autoradiograph is shown. Inset, MAPK activity. H69 cells were incubated with 50 μM antagonist G (G) for 20 min or 10% (v/v) FCS for 10 min at 37°C. p42^{MAPK} was immunoprecipitated from cell lysates and activity was measured as described in Materials and Methods. The data are expressed as % control and represent the mean ± SEM of 3 experiments performed in duplicate.

References

1. MacKinnon, A. C., Armstrong, R. A., Waters, C., Cummings, J., Smyth, J. F., Haslett, C., and Sethi, T. (1999) [Arg^6, D-Trp^{7,9}, N^{me}Phe^8]-substance P (6-11) activates JNK and induces apoptosis in small cell lung cancer cells via an oxidant dependent mechanism. *Br. J. Cancer* **80,** 1026–1034.

2. MacKinnon, A. C., Waters, C. M., Rahman, I., Harani, N., Rintoul, R., Haslett, C., and Sethi, T. (2000) [Arg^6, D-Trp^{7,9}, N^{me}Phe^8]-substance p (6-11) (antagonist G) induces induces AP-1 transcription and sensitises cells to chemotherapy. *Br. J. Cancer* **83,** 941–948.

3. Chen, Y., Meyer, C. F., and Tan, T. (1996) Persistant activation of c-jun N-terminal Kinase 1 (JNK1) in γ radiation-induced apoptosis. *J. Biol. Chem.* **271,** 631–634.

4. Verheij, M., Bose, R., Lin, X. H., Yao, B., Jarvis, W. D., Grant, S., et al. (1996) Requirement for ceramide-initiated SAPK/JNK signalling in stress-induced apoptosis. *Nature* **380,** 75–79.
5. Coso, O. A., Chiariello, M., Kalinec, G., Kyriakis, J. M., Woodgett, J., and Gutkind, J. S. (1995) Transforming G protein coupled receptors potently activate JNK (SAPK). *J. Biol. Chem.* **270,** 5620–5624.
6. Butterfield, L., Storey, B., Maas, L., and Heasley, L. E. (1997) c-jun NH2-terminal kinase regulation of the apoptotic response of small cell lung cancer cells to ultraviolet radiation. *J. Biol. Chem.* **272,** 10110–10116.
7. Buttke, T. M. and Sandstrom, P. A. (1994) Oxidative stress as a mediator of apoptosis. *Immunol. Today* **15,** 7–11.
8. Laderoute, K. R. and Webster, K. A. (1997) Hypoxia/reoxygenation stimulates jun kinase activity through redox signalling in cardiac myocytes. *Circ. Res.* **80,** 337–344.
9. Janssen, Y. M. W., Matalon, S., and Mossman, B. T. (1997) Differential induction of c-*fos*, c-*jun* and apoptosis in lung epithelial cells exposed to ROS or RNS. *Am. J. Physiol.* **273,** L789–L796.
10. Xu, Y., Bradham, C., Brenner, D. A., and Czaja, M. J. (1997) Hydrogen peroxide-induced liver cell necrosis is dependent on AP-1 activation. *Am. J. Physiol.* **273,** G795–G803.
11. Bush, R. S., Jenkin, R. D. T., Allt, W. E. C., Beale, F. A., Bean, H., Dembo, A. J., and Pringle, J. F. (1978) Definitive evidence for hypoxic cells influencing cure in cancer therapy. *Br. J. Cancer* **37,** 302–306.
12. Tallet, A., Chilvers, E. R., Hannah, S., Dransfield, I., Lawson, M. F., Haslett, C., and Sethi, T. (1996) Inhibition of neuropeptide-stimulated tyrosine phosphorylation and tyrosine kinase activity stimulates apoptosis in small cell lung cancer cells. *Cancer Res.* **56,** 4255–4263.

23

Isolation of Cells Entering Different Programmed Cell Death Pathways Using a Discontinuous Percoll Gradient

Patrick P. Koty, Haifan Zhang, Wendong Lei, and Mark L. Levitt

1. Introduction

Cancer is a disease of altered cellular homeostasis. Therefore, pathways for induction of differentiation and programmed cell death are being considered as targets for therapeutic approaches (1,2). Data indicate that those lung cancer patients whose tumors demonstrate squamous differentiation tend to survive longer (3,4). Because lung tumors appear to be metaplastic to an extent (5,6), attainment of the squamous state of differentiation may be feasible for all lung tumors, resulting in control of malignancy through terminal differentiation or programmed cell death (7,8).

Keratinocyte transglutaminase (kTG), a membrane-associated enzyme, is induced during irreversible terminal squamous differentiation of keratinocytes and normal human bronchial epithelial cells (9–11). Tissue transglutaminase (tTG), a cytosolic enzyme, is downregulated during squamous differentiation in these cell types (12), but upregulated during programmed cell death in several cell types (13–17). During differentiation, kTG catalyzes the formation of the cornified cross-linked envelope (CLE) (18). Similarly, during programmed cell death in squamous lung cancer cell lines, tTG catalyzes protein cross-linking, a variant type of CLE referred to as the apoptotic envelope (14,16,19–22). This raises the possibility of alternative terminal programs in lung cancer, under control of the squamous phenotype, based on either differentiation or programmed cell death pathways. Interferon-β (IFN-β) is capable of affecting growth, terminal squamous differentiation, and programmed cell death in non-small cell lung cancer (NSCLC) cell lines (23,24). Interestingly, IFN-β

From: *Methods in Molecular Medicine, vol. 74: Lung Cancer, Vol. 1: Molecular Pathology Methods and Reviews*
Edited by: B. Driscoll © Humana Press Inc., Totowa, NJ

Table 1
Density Fractionated Cells Using a Discontinuous
Percoll Gradient

Density	Untreated	IFN-β treated
1.04 g/mL		19.6 ± 2.9%
1.05 g/mL		17.0 ± 2.8%
1.06 g/mL		12.7 ± 6.7%
1.07 g/mL	99% ± 0.5%	70.8 ± 4.7%

induces envelope competence only in NSCLC cells with squamous features *(25)*, suggesting that in NSCLC there is a relationship between the squamous phenotype and envelope competence. It has also been demonstrated that tTG is cleaved by caspase 3 during late stages of programmed cell death *(26)*. tTG cleavage causes loss of cross-linking function but is accompanied by DNA fragmentation.

Differentiation and programmed cell death are often accompanied by a change in cellular density. It has been shown that terminal differentiation in keratinocytes is associated with increasing cell size *(27)* and with decreasing density *(28)*. Furthermore, in the human promyelocytic cell line HL-60, a change in cellular density occurs during differentiation and subsequent apoptosis *(29)*. We have previously investigated the effect of IFN-β on cellular density *(30)*. IFN-β treated cells were subject to fractionation on a discontinuous Percoll density gradient, which revealed a shift in cell density (*see* **Table 1**). This study also included analyzing the fractionated cells for growth, kTG and tTG expression and activity, programmed cell death (as measured by DNA fragmentation and PARP cleavage *[31]*), and CLE competence (summarized in **Table 2**).

These studies indicate the existence of subpopulations of squamous NSCLC cells that respond differently to IFN-β treatment by entering distinct squamous differentiation-related cell death pathways. Growth response to IFN-β may be a driving force for the pathway selection. Cells retaining a higher growth rate and density have increased tTG protein and enzymatic activity and an increase in envelope competence (only seen in squamous NSCLC cell lines, as stated earlier). On the other hand, cells exhibiting a significant decrease in growth rate and density undergo DNA fragmentation and have higher levels of kTG, a sign of terminal squamous differentiation. The choice of which pathway a particular cell enters may reflect an attempt to maintain cellular homeostasis under different growth conditions. In rapidly growing cells, programmed cell death may occur via a tTG-mediated pathway without evidence of squamous

Table 2
Summary of Growth, Programmed Cell Death, and Differentiation Assays

	Density	Growth	DNA fragmentation	kTG expression	tTG expression	PARP cleavage	CLE competent
IFN-β treated							
	1.04 g/mL	+	+++	++	+	++	+
	1.05 g.mL	+	++	+++	+	++	++
	1.06 g/mL	+	+	+	+++	+++	++
	1.07 g/mL	++	+/–	+	++	+++	+++
Untreated							
	1.07 g/mL	++	+/–	–	++	+	++

None detected, +/– very low, + low, ++ moderate, +++ high.

differentiation, whereas in cells whose growth rate has been diminished by IFN-β treatment, cell death may be the result of terminal squamous differentiation. Possibly, parallels can be drawn to the maintenance of homeostasis during epidermal squamous differentiation. In this situation, the rapidly proliferating basal cells demonstrate elevated levels of tTG with no evidence of DNA fragmentation *(32)*. Programmed cell death under these circumstances would serve to regulate the rapid proliferation of these precursor cells. The growth rate slows as the cells become increasingly differentiated and migrate towards the alveolar surface, at which point kTG is the preferentially expressed transglutaminase and DNA fragmentation can be detected *(32)*. Under these circumstances, we speculate that programmed cell death may be causally related to terminal squamous differentiation. Although programmed cell death occurs in each case, the pathways are different (as represented by DNA fragmentation or CLE formation) and the choice of cell death pathway may be driven by the growth rate of the cell population.

Alternatively, the subpopulations of fractionated cells after exposure to IFN-β may be representative of cells in different stages of programmed cell death. DNA fragmentation is generally considered a late event in the apoptotic cascade while cleavage of PARP is thought to occur much earlier. The distribution of PARP cleavage suggests that this event precedes the shift in density. As stated earlier, tTG is cleaved by caspase 3 during late-stage programmed cell death resulting in a loss of cross-linking function but accompanied by DNA fragmentation *(26)*. While there are several possible interpretations of this data, it may explain why low density cells have decreased expression and activity of tTG and lack CLE competence but exhibit DNA fragmentation. What it fails to explain, however, is the relation, if any, that PARP cleavage may have to the upregulation of kTG and DNA fragmentation associated with a loss of cell density.

Clearly, these initial findings need further characterization. Thus, the approach and protocols provided in this chapter can be very useful tools to further investigate selected subpopulations of cells exposed to IFN-β or any other agent that affects growth, terminal squamous differentiation, or programmed cell death.

2. Materials

2.1. Tissue Culturing-Adherent Lung Cancer Cells

1. RPMI-1640 media supplemented with 0.3 µg/mL L-glutamine, 10% (v/v) heat-inactivated fetal bovine serum (FBS), 50 U/mL penicillin, 50 µg/mL streptomycin, 0.5 µg/mL fungizone (Gibco/BRL). Store at 4°C.
2. 25 mm^2 tissue-culture flasks or 24-well tissue culture plates.

2.2. Density Gradient Fractionation

1. Interferon-β (Berlex Laboratories, Inc.). Use at 180 IU/mL. Store at 4°C.
2. 1X PBS buffer, pH 7.4: 137 mM NaCl, 2.7 mM KCl, 10 mM Na$_2$HPO$_4$, 2 mM KH$_2$PO$_4$.
3. 0.05% trypsin-EDTA. Store at 4°C.
4. Stock solution of Percoll/NaCl: Add Percoll (1.13 g/mL) at a ratio of 9:1 to 1.5 M NaCl.
5. Sterile 15-mL conical tubes.

2.3. Cell Growth Assay

1. [^{3}H]thymidine. Store at 4°C. **Caution:** Radioactive, use proper safety procedures.
2. 10% trichloroacetic acid (TCA). **Caution:** Highly corrosive and toxic; wear gloves and a mask when handling.
3. 0.25 N NaOH.
4. Scintillation vials, fluid, and counter.

2.4. Analysis of DNA Fragmentation by Flow Cytometric Analysis

1. 70% Ethanol.
2. DNase-free RNase A (Sigma) solution: 1 mg/mL diluted in 10 mM Tris-HCl, pH 7.5, 15 mM NaCl.

3. Propidium iodide (PI) solution: 100 µg/mL diluted in PBS. Light sensitive, store in dark. **Caution:** PI is a mutagen, wear gloves and a mask.
4. Fluorescein isothiocyanate (FITC): 10 µg/mL diluted in ethanol. Light sensitive, store in dark at –20°C.
5. Flow cytometer (Becton Dickerson FACscan).
6. Lysis II flow cytometry data analysis software.

2.5. Analysis of DNA Fragmentation by TUNEL Staining

1. 10% neutral buffered formalin in PBS, pH 7.4.
2. Peroxidase quenching buffer: 0.3% hydrogen peroxide in methanol.
3. TdT buffer, pH 7.2: 30 mM Tris-HCl, 140 mM sodium cacodylate. Store at 4°C.
4. TdT labeling mixture: digoxigenin-conjugated dUTP (0.5 nmoles) and TdT enzyme (5 units). Store components TdT enzyme and digoxigenin-conjugated dUTP at –20°C. Prepare TdT labeling mixture just before use.
5. Humidity chamber.
6. Peroxidase conjugated anti-digoxigenin antibody (Dako) diluted 1 : 1000 in PBS. Store at 4°C.
7. 3-amino-9-ethyl carbazole (AEC) solution (Biomeda Corp). Store at 4°C. **Caution:** AEC is a suspected carcinogen, wear gloves.
8. Mayer's hematoxylin (Sigma).
9. Aqueous-based slide mounting medium (Biomeda Corp).
10. Coplin jars.
11. Microscope slides.
12. Light microscope with photographic capabilities.

2.6. Western Blot Analysis for tTG and kTG Proteins and PARP Cleavage

2.6.1. Total Protein Isolation

1. tTG and kTG lysis buffer: 50 mM Tris-HCl, pH 7.4, 150 mM NaCl, 0.02% NaN$_3$, 1% Triton X-100. Add proteinase inhibitors prior to use: 2 µg/mL aprotinin, 2 µg/mL leupeptin, 1 µg/mL pepstatin A, 100 µg/mL PMSF. Store at 4°C. **Caution:** PMSF is toxic and may be fatal if inhaled, swallowed, or absorbed through the skin. Wear gloves and a mask when using PMSF and flush eyes or skin with copious amounts of water in case of contact.
2. Poly (ADP-ribose) polymerase (PARP) lysis buffer: 6.25 mM Tris base, pH 6.8, 6 M urea, 2% (w/v) SDS, 5% (v/v) β-mercaptoethanol (**add β-mercaptoethanol just before use**). Store at –20°C.
3. Sterile 1.5-mL tubes.
4. 96-well plates.
5. DC Protein Assay (Bio-Rad Laboratories).
6. Microtiter plate reader (wavelength 650–750 nm).

2.6.2. Gel Electrophoresis

1. Vertical gel electrophoresis unit.
2. 30% (w/v) polyacrylamide (29.2 g/100 mL)/Bis (0.8 g/100 mL) stock solution. Store at 4°C. Light sensitive, store in dark. **Caution:** Acrylamide is a potent cumulative neurotoxin that is absorbed through the skin; wear gloves and a mask when handling.
3. Resolving gel buffer: 1.5 *M* Tris-HCl, pH 8.8.
4. Stacking gel buffer: 0.5 *M* Tris-HCl, pH 6.8.
5. 10% (w/v) ammonium persulfate (APS). Make fresh.
6. TEMED. Store at 4°C.
7. 10% sodium dodecyl sulfate (SDS) (electrophoresis grade).
8. 10% SDS-polyacrylamide gel electrophoresis (PAGE) gel. For every 10 mL of either resolving or stacking gel solution: 4 mL 30% acrylamide/Bis solution, 2.5 mL of either resolving or stacking gel buffer, 0.1 mL 10% SDS, 3.4 mL deionized H_2O.
9. 2X SDS gel-loading buffer: 100 m*M* Tris-HCl, pH 6.8, 4% (w/v) SDS, 0.2% (w/v) bromophenol blue, 20% (v/v) glycerol, 200 m*M* β-mercaptoethanol (**add β-mercaptoethanol just before use**).
10. Prestained molecular-weight markers (Bio-Rad Laboratories). Store at –20°C.
11. 1X electrode buffer, pH 8.3: 25 m*M* Tris-HCl, 250 m*M* glycine, 0.1% SDS.

2.6.3. Western Blot Transfer

1. Electrophoretic transfer unit.
2. Nitrocellulose membrane.
3. Whatman 3MM filter paper.
4. Transfer buffer, pH 8.3: 25 m*M* Tris, 192 m*M* glycine, 20% (v/v) methanol, 0.5% SDS.

2.6.4. Probing Western Blot with kTG, tTG, or anti-PARP Antibody

1. Blocking buffer: 2% horse serum in TBS. Store at 4°C.
2. Tris-buffered saline (TBS): 10 m*M* Tris-HCl, pH 7.4, 150 m*M* NaCl. Store at 4°C.
3. Wash buffer: 0.1% Tween 20 in TBS.
4. Anti-kTG antibody (B.C1, a gift from Dr. Scott Thacher) diluted 1:100 in TBS. Store at –20°C.
5. Anti-tTG antibody (CUB74.1, a gift from Dr. Paul Birchbickler) (*see* **Note 1**) diluted 1:200 in TBS. Store at –20°C.
6. Anti-PARP antibody (Transduction Lab). Use at a 1:2000 dilution in TBS. Store at –20°C.
7. HRP-conjugated secondary antibody (Amersham Pharmacia Biotech) diluted 1:1000 in TBS. Store at 4°C.
8. ECL Western Blotting Detection Kit (Amersham Pharmacia Biotech).
9. Autoradiographic film.

10. Autoradiograph developer.
11. Densitometer with the capability of scanning autoradiographs.

2.7. Transglutaminase Activity Assay

2.7.1. Preparation of tTG Containing Fraction

1. Cytosolic lysis buffer: 10 mM Tris-HCl, pH7.4, 2 mM EDTA. Add proteinase inhibitors prior to use: 2 µg/mL aprotinin, 2 µg/mL leupeptin, 1 µg/mL pepstatin A, 100 µg/mL PMSF. Store at 4°C. **Caution:** PMSF is toxic and may be fatal if inhaled, swallowed, or absorbed through the skin. Wear gloves and a mask when using PMSF and flush eyes or skin with copious amounts of water in case of contact.
2. Sterile cell scraper.
3. Sterile 1.5-mL microcentrifuge tube.
4. Glycerol.

2.7.2. Preparation of kTG Containing Fraction

1. Pellet lysis buffer: 10 mM Tris-HCl, pH 7.4, 2 mM EDTA, 0.2 mM DTT, 0.3% (v/v) Triton X-100. Add proteinase inhibitors prior to use: 2 µg/mL aprotinin, 2 µg/mL leupeptin, 1 µg/mL pepstatin A, 100 µg/mL PMSF. Store at 4°C.

2.7.3. tTG and kTG Activity Assay

1. Transglutaminase activity assay buffer: 0.125 M Tris-HCl, pH 8.3, 1.5 mg/mL dimethylated casein, 5 mM CaCl, 1.25 mM EDTA, 2.5 mM dithiothreitol (DTT), 25 µCi/ml ^{3}H-putrescine. Store at 4°C. **Caution:** ^{3}H-putrescine is radioactive, use proper safety procedures.
2. Scintillation vials (Scatron Inc.), fluid, and counter.
3. 20% trichloroacetic acid (TCA).

2.8. Dual Parameter Flow Cytometry for DNA Fragmentation and kTG or tTG Protein Expression

1. 1% (v/v) formaldehyde in PBS, pH 7.4
2. Methanol.
3. Blocking buffer: 2% horse serum in TBS. Store at 4°C.
4. Anti-kTG antibody (**Subheading 2.6.4.**).
5. Anti-tTG antibody (**Subheading 2.6.4.**).
6. Biotinylated anti-mouse secondary antibody (Vector Laboratories). Use diluted at 1:1000 in PBS. Store at 4°C.
7. FITC-conjugated anti-digoxigenin antibody (Roche). Use diluted at 1:1000 in PBS. Store at 4°C. Light sensitive, store in dark.
8. Phycoerythrin (PE)-conjugated streptavidin (Vector Laboratories). Use diluted at 1:1000 in PBS. Store at 4°C. Light sensitive, store in dark.

2.9. Immunohistochemical Dual Analysis for DNA Fragmentation and kTG or tTG Protein Expression

2.9.1. TUNEL Assay for DNA Fragmentation

1. Acetone.

2.9.2. Immunohistochemical Staining for kTG or tTG Protein

1. Blocking buffer: 10% horse serum in PBS. Store at 4°C.
2. Anti-kTG antibody (B.C1, gift from Dr. Scott Thacher) diluted at 1:10 in PBS. Store at 4°C.
3. Anti-tTG antibody (CUB74.1, gift from Dr. Paul Birchbickler) (*see* **Note 1**) diluted at 1:10 in PBS. Store at 4°C.
4. Biotin conjugated anti-mouse antibody (Vector Laboratories). Use diluted at 1:250 in PBS. Store at 4°C.
5. Streptavidin-conjugated alkaline phosphatase (Vector Laboratories). Use diluted at 1:250 in PBS. Store at 4°C.
6. Alkaline phosphatase substrate III (Vector Laboratories). Store at 4°C.

2.10. Cross-linked Envelope Competence Assay

1. Dulbecco's Modified Eagle Medium (DMEM) (Gibco/BRL). Store at 4°C.
2. Calcium ionophore A23187 (Sigma): stock solution 50 mg/mL in dimethyl sulfoxide (DMSO). Store at 4°C.
3. DTT (molecular-biology grade): 1 *M* stock concentration.
4. 10% (w/v) SDS (molecular-biology grade).
5. Hemocytometer.
6. Phase contrast microscope.

3. Methods

3.1. Tissue Culturing Adherent Lung Cancer Cells

1. Seed adherent lung cancer cell lines into either 25 mm^2 tissue-culture flasks or 24-well tissue-culture plates.
2. Grow cells to confluence in serum supplemented RPMI-1640 media at 37°C in an atmosphere of 5% CO_2.

3.2. Density Gradient Fractionation

1. After cells have grown to confluence, starve in serum-free RPMI-1640 medium for 48 h (*see* **Note 2**).
2. Remove media and incubate cells in freshly supplemented RPMI-1640 medium containing IFN-β for 24 h.
3. Remove medium and rinse cells with PBS.
4. Add 1 mL trypsin to cells for 5–10 min (*see* **Note 3**).
5. Stop trypsinization with 1 mL supplemented RPMI-1640 media.
6. Remove cells and centrifuge at 100*g* for 10 min.

7. Remove supernatant and discard. Resuspend cells in 1 mL PBS.
8. Dilute the stock solution of Percoll:NaCl with 0.15 M NaCl into 1.07, 1.06, 1.05, and 1.04 g/mL solutions using the formulas:
   X + Y = 100 mL
   and
   1.1258X + 1.0088Y = Z × 100 mL
   Solve for X, then determine Y where:
   X = mL Percoll:NaCl stock
   Y = mL 0.15 M NaCl
   Z = final density
   A gradient is obtained by placing 1 mL of each Percoll solution (starting from 1.07 to 1.04 g/mL) carefully into a 15-mL conical tube before addition of the cells.
9. Place cells on the discontinuous Percoll gradient and centrifuge at 500g for 20 min at room temperature.
10. Remove and fractionate cell subpopulations according to their position within the surface bands by pipetting aliquots from the top band down.
11. Wash cells once in PBS and centrifuge at 500g for 20 min at room temperature.
12. Remove supernatant and resuspend cell pellet in appropriate solution for each assay.

3.3. Cell Growth Assay

1. Resuspend the density fractionated cells (1×10^5) in 2 mL supplemented RPMI-1640 media and seed onto 24-well plates. Incubate overnight to achieve cell adherence (*see* **Note 4**).
2. Incubated cells with [^{3}H]thymidine, at a final concentration of 0.4 Ci/mL diluted in prewarmed unsupplemented RPMI-1640 medium, for 1.5 h at 37°C in an atmosphere of 5% CO_2.
3. Remove medium and wash twice with PBS to remove residual radioactive material.
4. Remove PBS and add 0.5 mL of cold 10% TCA for 10 s.
5. Remove TCA (*see* **Note 5**) and add 0.8 mL 0.25 N NaOH to solubilize the cells.
6. Gently shake plate for 20 min.
7. Place 0.6 mL each sample into scintillation vials containing 3 mL scintillation fluid and vortex.
8. [^{3}H]thymidine incorporation is determined by liquid-scintillation spectrometry.

3.4. Analysis of DNA Fragmentation by Flow Cytometric Analysis

1. Fix density fractionated cells (1×10^6) in 70% cold ethanol overnight at 4°C (*see* **Note 6**).
2. Wash with PBS and centrifuge at 100g for 10 min.
3. Repeat **step 2**.
4. Resuspend cells in 450 μL PBS and add 50 μL RNase A solution to digest cellular RNA at 37°C for 1 h.

5. Add 0.5 mL propidium iodide stock solution and incubate the cells in the dark for 30 min (*see* **Note 7**).
6. Stain cells with 5 μL fluorescein isothiocyanate for 5 min in the dark.
7. Determine cell protein and DNA content simultaneously by flow cytometry.
8. Analyze data using Lysis II flow cytometry software.

3.5. Analysis of DNA Fragmentation by TUNEL Staining

1. Fix density fractionated cells in formalin solution for 10 min to maintain cell morphology.
2. Drop cells (1×10^5) onto microscope slides and dry at room temperature overnight.
3. Wash slides for three times 2 min each in PBS in Coplin jars. Use forceps to handle slides.
4. Quench endogenous peroxidase in quenching buffer for 30 min.
5. Wash three times for 2 min each in PBS.
6. Wash once with TdT buffer for 2 min.
7. Incubate in TdT labeling mixture containing TdT and digoxigenin-conjugated dUTP at 37°C in a high humidity chamber for 90 min.
8. Wash three times for 2 min each in PBS.
9. Incubate in diluted peroxidase conjugated anti-digoxigenin antibody for 60 min in a high humidity chamber at room temperature.
10. Visualize bound peroxidase by incubating in 3-amino-9-ethyl carbazole (AEC) solution for 2–10 min.
11. Wash in distilled water and counterstain with Mayer's hematoxylin for 2 min.
12. Wash in tap water and incubate in PBS for 2 min.
13. Wash in distilled water, apply aqueous-based mounting medium, and dry at room temperature.
14. Analyze cells for DNA fragmentation by counting 200 cells per field, from a minimum of three fields, using a 10× eyepiece and 20× objective.

3.6. Western Blot Analysis for tTG and kTG Proteins and PARP Cleavage

3.6.1. Total Protein Isolation

1. Lyse density fractionated cells in wells with 500 μL of either tTG and kTG lysis buffer or PARP lysis buffer for 15 min at room temperature.
2. Scrape and remove cell lysate and place into sterile 1.5-mL microcentrifuge tubes.
3. Freeze lysate at –80°C for 10 min, thaw, and vortex.
4. Repeat **step 3**.
5. Centrifuge (12,000*g*) lysate for 10 min at 4°C.
6. Take supernatant and transfer to a sterile 1.5-mL microcentrifuge tube. Add 50 μL glycerol to 500 μL clarified lysate, mix thoroughly, and store at –80°C.
7. Determine protein concentration using commercially available assay.

3.6.2. Gel Electrophoresis

1. Prepare 10% SDS-PAGE resolving gel solution by adding 50 μL 10% APS and 10 μL TEMED per 10 mL resolving gel solution, cast, overlay with water, and allow to polymerize for 1 h.
2. Remove water and gently dry top of resolving gel with Whatman 3MM filter paper.
3. Prepare SDS-PAGE stacking gel solution by adding 50 μL 10% APS and 10 μL TEMED per 10 mL stacking gel solution, cast on top of polymerized resolving gel, insert comb, and allow to polymerize for 45 min.
4. Remove comb and rinse wells of stacking gel with distilled water then add 1X electrode buffer to reservoirs.
5. Aliquot equal quantities of protein extracts (80 μg/lane). Mix extracts 1:1 with 2X SDS gel-loading buffer. Be sure each gel includes a lane for molecular-weight markers.
6. Denature samples at 95°C for 4 min, place on ice, and load samples into wells.
7. Separate proteins by gel electrophoresis at 200V for 30–60 min.

3.6.3. Western Blot Transfer

1. Cut nitrocellulose membrane and Whatman 3MM filter paper to fit gel size (*see* **Note 8**).
2. Remove gel from electrophoresis unit and soak gel, membrane, and filter paper in transfer buffer for 1 h.
3. Prepare gel sandwich consisting of transfer cassette, fiber pad, filter paper, SDS-PAGE gel, membrane, filter paper, and fiber pad (*see* **Note 9**).
4. Assemble transfer unit (*see* **Note 10**).
5. Transfer overnight at 30V and 90mA.

3.6.4. Probing Western Blot with anti-kTG, anti-tTG, or anti-PARP Antibody

1. Block membrane for 20 min at room temperature with gentle agitation (*see* **Note 11**).
2. Wash membrane three times for 10 min each at room temperature.
3. Incubate membrane with diluted primary antibodies to kTG, tTG, or PARP overnight at 4°C with gentle agitation.
4. Wash membrane three times for 10 min each at room temperature.
5. Incubate membrane in diluted HRP-conjugated secondary antibody for 1 h at room temperature with gentle agitation (*see* **Note 12**).
6. Visualize the antigens bound to the membranes using ECL reagents.
7. Expose blot to autoradiographic film for 1–5 min, then develop and fix film.
8. Quantify protein expression using a densitometer capable of analyzing autoradiographs.

3.7. Transglutaminase Activity Assay

3.7.1. Preparation of tTG Containing Fraction

1. Lyse density fractionated cells using 500 µL cytosolic lysis buffer for each well for 15 min.
2. Scrape cells and transfer to a sterile 1.5-mL microcentifuge tube.
3. Freeze cells at –80°C for 10 min, thaw, then vortex.
4. Repeat **step 3**.
5. Centrifuge at 12,000g for 15 min at 4°C.
6. Take supernatant (cytosolic fraction contains tTG) and transfer to a sterile 1.5 mL microcentrifuge tube. Add 50 µL glycerol to 500 µL cytosolic fraction, mix thoroughly, and store at –80°C. Reserve pellet fraction on ice.

3.7.2. Preparation of kTG Containing Fraction

1. Resuspend pellet fraction (**Subheading 3.7.1.**) in cytosolic lysis buffer and centrifuge at 12,000g at 4°C for 5 min.
2. Repeat **step 1**.
3. Resuspend pellet in 0.5 mL pellet lysis buffer.
5. Freeze the pellet at –80°C for 10 min, thaw, then vortex.
6. Repeat **step 5**.
7. Centrifuge at 12,000g at 4°C for 30 min.
8. Take supernatant (membrane fraction contains kTG) and transfer to a sterile 1.5-mL microcentrifuge tube. Add 50 µL glycerol to 500 µL membrane fraction, and store at –80°C.

3.7.3. tTG and kTG Activity Assay

1. Determine protein concentration of cytosolic and membrane fractions using a commercially available assay (*see* **Subheading 2.6.1.**).
2. Incubate 20 µg total cytosolic (containing tTG) or membrane fraction (containing kTG) protein with 200 µL transglutaminase activity assay buffer in a 4 mL scintillation vial for 30 min with agitation at 37°C.
3. Quench reaction by adding 2 mL 20% cold TCA.
4. Centrifuge at 2,000g for 20 min at 4°C.
5. Aspirate and discard supernatant, then wash pellet with 2 mL 10% TCA.
6. Centrifuge at 2,000g for 20 min at 4°C.
7. Aspirate and discard the supernatant.
8. Add 3 mL scintillation fluid to the vial.
9. Determine [^{3}H]putrescine incorporation by liquid scintillation spectrometry.

3.8. Dual Parameter Flow Cytometry for DNA Fragmentation and kTG or tTG Protein Expression

3.8.1. TUNEL Staining for DNA Fragmentation

1. Fix density fractionated cells in formaldehyde solution (*see* **Note 13**).
2. Centrifuge at 500g for 5 min, then remove and discard supernatant.

3. Fix cells in cold methanol overnight at 4°C.
4. Centrifuge at 500*g* for 5 min, then discard supernatant.
5. Wash cells for 2 min with PBS, then centrifuge at 500*g* for 5 min. Discard supernatant.
6. Repeat **step 5** twice.
8. Wash cells once with 1 mL TdT buffer (*see* **Subheading 2.5.**) for 2 min.
9. Centrifuge at 500*g* for 5 min, then discard supernatant.
10. Incubate in 1 mL TdT labeling mixture (*see* **Subheading 2.5.**) at 37°C for 90 min.
11. Wash cells three times for 2 min each in 1 mL PBS. Use these same samples for co-analysis of kTG and tTG protein expression.

3.8.2. Immunofluorescent Staining for kTG or tTG Protein

1. Incubate slides from previous step in blocking buffer for 20 min.
2. Centrifuge at 500*g* for 5 min, then discard supernatant.
3. Incubate cells in diluted primary antibody, either anti-kTG or anti-tTG (**Subheading 2.6.4.**), for 1 h.
4. Centrifuge at 500*g* for 5 min, then discard supernatant.
5. Wash once for 2 min in 1 mL PBS, centrifuge at 500*g* for 5 min, then discard supernatant.
6. Incubate cells in diluted biotin conjugated anti-mouse antibody for 1 h.
7. Wash once for 2 min in 1 mL PBS, centrifuge at 500*g* for 5 min, then discard supernatant.
8. Incubate cells in diluted anti-digoxigenin-FITC and streptavidin-phycoerythrin (PE) for 2 h in the dark.
9. Wash once for 2 min in 1 mL PBS, centrifuge at 500*g* for 5 min, then discard supernatant.
10. Resuspend cells in 1 mL PBS.
11. Determine DNA fragmentation (by analyzing FITC fluorescence) and kTG or tTG expression (by analyzing PE fluorescence) simultaneously by flow cytometry (*see* **Note 14**).
12. Analyze data using flow cytometry software (Lysis II software).

3.9. Immunohistochemical Dual Analysis for DNA Fragmentation and kTG or tTG Protein Expression

3.9.1. TUNEL Staining for DNA Fragmentation (see **Note 15**)

1. Fix density fractionated cells in formaldehyde solution (*see* **Subheading 2.8.**) for 10 min.
2. Drop cells (1 × 10^5) onto microscope slides and dry at room temperature overnight.
3. Fix cells in cold acetone for 10 min.
4. Wash three times for 2 min each in PBS.
5. Quench endogenous peroxidase activity by incubating in quenching buffer (*see* **Subheading 2.5.**) for 30 min.

6. Wash three times for 2 min each in PBS.
7. Wash once with TdT buffer (*see* **Subheading 2.5.**) for 2 min.
8. Incubate in TdT labeling mixture (*see* **Subheading 2.5.**) containing TdT and digoxigenin-conjugated dUTP at 37°C in a high humidity chamber for 90 min.
9. Wash three times for 2 min each in PBS.
10. Incubate in diluted peroxidase conjugated anti-digoxigenin antibody (*see* **Subheading 2.5.**) for 60 min in a high humidity chamber at room temperature.
11. Visualize bound peroxidase by incubating in 3-amino-9-ethyl carbazole (AEC) solution (*see* **Subheading 2.5.**) for 2–10 min.
12. Wash in distilled water. Use these same samples for analysis of kTG and tTG protein expression.

3.9.2. Immunohistochemical Staining for kTG or tTG Protein

1. Wash slides three times for 2 min each in PBS.
2. Incubate in blocking buffer proteins for 20 min in a high humidity chamber at room temperature.
3. Incubate in diluted primary antibody (anti-kTG or anti-tTG diluted 1:10 in PBS) overnight at 4°C.
4. Wash slides three times for 2 min each in PBS.
5. Incubate in diluted biotin conjugated anti-mouse antibody for 1 h at room temperature in a high humidity chamber.
6. Wash slides three times with PBS for 2 min each wash.
7. Incubate in diluted streptavidin-conjugated alkaline phosphatase for 1 h at room temperature in a high-humidity chamber.
8. Wash slides three times in PBS for 2 min each wash.
9. Visualize bound alkaline phosphatase using an alkaline phosphatase substrate III.
10. Wash in distilled water and counterstain with Mayer's hematoxylin (*see* **Subheading 2.5.**) for 2 min.
11. Wash in tap water, then incubate in PBS for 2 min.
12. Wash in distilled water, apply aqueous-based mounting medium (*see* **Subheading 2.5.**), and dry at room temperature.
13. Analyze cells for DNA fragmentation and kTG or tTG protein by counting 200 cells per field, from a minimum of three fields, using a 10× eyepiece and 20× objective.

3.10. Cross-linked Envelope (CLE) Competence Assay (see Note 16)

1. Incubate density fractionated cells (1×10^6) in 1 mL DMEM with 2 µg/mL calcium ionophore A23187 (*see* **Note 17**) for 4 h at 37°C, with agitation (*see* **Note 18**).
2. Quench reaction on ice with 2% (v/v) SDS and 10 mM DTT.
3. Incubate cells in a drybath at 100°C for 5 min.
4. CLEs are counted under a phase contrast microscope using a hemocytometer (*see* **Note 19**).

4. Notes

1. A commercially produced tTG antibody (Transglutaminase II) is now available through Upstate Biotechnology.
2. Use serum starvation to optimize the cells for differentiation potential.
3. When isolating subpopulations of cells using a Percoll gradient, it is critical that the cells are in a single cell suspension. Therefore, trypsinize and gently agitate flasks or plates until all cells are in single cell suspension. In addition, Percoll, PBS, and RPMI-1640 media need to be warmed to room temperature prior to use to prevent cells from clumping in a cold solution.
4. It is necessary to select those cells that are viable by allowing them to adhere after isolation from the Percoll gradients. If this is not done and total cells (viable and nonviable) are used after fractionation, the growth assay may be incorrectly influenced by the presence of this nonviable cell population (which may vary between fractions).
5. Cells may detach from the bottom of the wells when precipitated with TCA. Therefore, attention should be paid to avoid cell loss when discarding TCA.
6. Fixation with 70% cold ethanol is recommended because it allows FITC and PI to enter the plasma membrane easier, thus resulting in better protein and DNA staining. Overnight ethanol fixation is recommended; however, variations in time will influence the binding of PI to DNA and the fragility of the cells.
7. Warm the PBS prior to use at 37°C for 30 min. This will aide in the loss of small DNA fragments from the cell.
8. Wear gloves at all times when handling nitrocellulose membranes and use flat forceps to hold membranes.
9. Remove all bubbles between the gel and the nitrocellulose membrane by smoothing them out with a sterile glass Pasteur pipet.
10. Some transfer units utilize an ice block or a cold water circulator to cool the transfer unit. Otherwise, if necessary, transfer units can be run in a cold room. Also, place a magnetic stir bar in the buffer tank and place unit on a magnetic stirrer.
11. If it is necessary to decrease nonspecific background on the nitrocellulose membrane, use 1% (w/v) dry nonfat milk in the reaction buffer for the primary and secondary antibodies, and for the conjugated biotin and avidin-HRP solutions, if used.
12. If not using a conjugated HRP secondary antibody, it is important to dilute the concentration of avidin conjugated HRP to 1:5000 or 1:10000.
13. For dual parameter staining flow cytometry, use 1% formaldehyde in PBS, pH 7.4, to fix cells. The formaldehyde solution will maintain the integrity of cell surface proteins.
14. The samples should be subject to flow cytometry as soon as possible, to minimize the effect of the fluorescence extinction over time.
15. The TUNEL protocol should always precede immunohistochemical staining.
16. The term "envelope competence" indicates the presence of all cellular components necessary for CLE formation, but that the envelope forms only when it is

induced by any of several methods, usually incubation with a calcium ionophore. While normal human bronchial epithelia and epidermal keratinocytes are capable of spontaneous envelope formation, lung cancer cell lines are only envelope competent.

17. Calcium ionophore may precipitate at 4°C. If so, it needs to be warmed and resuspended in solution.
18. Use a 6-mL tube for this step to allow cells to maximally interact with calcium ionophore.
19. After cells are boiled in 2% SDS and 10 mM DTT, the only remaining structures are CLEs. CLEs appear as ghost-like structures under microscopy and are difficult to see.

References

1. Seifter, E. J., Levitt, M. L., and Kramer, B. S. (1987) An outlier theory of cancer curability. Tumor cell differentiation as a therapeutic goal. *Am. J. Med.* **83,** 757–760.
2. Thompson, H. J., Strange, R., and Schedin, P. J. (1992) Apoptosis in the genesis and prevention of cancer. *Cancer Epidemiol. Biomarkers. Prev.* **1,** 597–602.
3. Minna, J. D., Pass, H., Gladstein, E. J., and Ihde, D. C. (1989) Cancer of the lung, in *Cancer: Principals and Practice of Oncology* (DeVita, V. T., Hellman, S., and Rosenberg, S. A., eds.), J. B. Lippincott Co., Philadelphia, pp. 591–705.
4. Mountain, C. F. (1988) Prognostic implications of the International Staging System for lung cancer. *Semin. Oncol.* **15,** 236–245.
5. Steele, V. E. and Nettesheim, P. (1981) Unstable cellular differentiation in adenosquamous cell carcinoma. *J. Natl. Cancer Inst.* **67,** 149–154.
6. Terasaki, T., Shinosato, Y., Nakajima, T., Tsumuraya, M., Ichinose, H., Nagatsu, T., and Kato, K. (1987) Reversible squamous cell characteristics induced by vitamin A deficiency in a small cell lung cancer cell line. *Cancer Res.* **47,** 3533–3537.
7. Ohashi, K., Nemoto, T., Eishi, Y., Matsuno, A., Nakamura, K., and Hirokawa, K. (1997) Expression of the cyclin dependent kinase inhibitor p21WAF1/CIP1 in oesophageal squamous cell carcinomas. *Virchows Arch.* **430,** 389–395.
8. Modjtahedi, H., Eccles, S., Sandle, J., Box, G., Titley, J., and Dean, C. (1994) Differentiation or immune destruction: two pathways for therapy of squamous cell carcinomas with antibodies to the epidermal growth factor receptor. *Cancer Res.* **54,** 1695–1701.
9. Greenberg, C. S., Birckbichler, P. J., and Rice, R. H. (1991). Transglutaminases: multifunctional cross-linking enzymes that stabilize tissues. *FASEB J.* **5,** 3071–3077.
10. Jetten, A. M. (1989) Multistep process of squamous differentiation in tracheo-bronchial epithelial cell in vitro: Analogy with epidermal differentiation. *Environ. Health Perspect.* **80,** 149–160.
11. Green, H. (1980) The keratinocyte as differentiated cell type. *Harvey. Lect.* **74,** 101–139.

12. Vollberg, T. M., George, M. D., Nervi, C., and Jetten, A. M. (1992) Regulation of type I and type II transglutaminase in normal human bronchial epithelial and lung carcinoma cells. *Am. J. Respir. Cell Mol. Biol.* **7(1)**, 10–18.

13. Fesus, L., Thomazy, V., Autuori, F., Ceru, M. P., Tarcsa, E., and Piacentini, M. (1989) Apoptotic hepatocytes become insoluble in detergents and chaotropic agents as a result of transglutaminase action. *FEBS Lett.* **245,** 150–154.

14. Piacentini, M., Fesus, L., Farrace, M. G., Ghibelli, L., et al. (1991) The expression of "tissue" transglutaminase in two human cancer cell lines is related with the programmed cell death (apoptosis). *Eur. J. Cell Biol.* **54,** 246–254.

15. Piacentini, M., Annicchiarico-Petruzzelli, M., Oliverio, S., Piredda, L., Biedler, J. L., and Melino, E. (1992) Phenotype-specific "tissue" transglutaminase regulation in human neuroblastoma cells in response to retinoic acid: correlation with cell death by apoptosis. *Int. J. Cancer* **52,** 271–278.

16. el Alaoui, S., Mian, S., Lawry, J., Quash, G., and Griffin, M. (1992) Cell cycle kinetics, tissue transglutaminase and programmed cell death (apoptosis). *FEBS Lett.* **311(2),** 174–178.

17. Fesus, L., Madi, A., Balajthy, Z., Nemes, Z., and Szondy, Z. (1996) Transglutaminase induction by various cell death and apoptosis pathways. *Experientia* **52,** 942–949.

18. Thacher, S. M. and Rice, R. H. (1985) Keratinocyte-specific transglutaminase of cultured human epidermal cells: Relation to cross-linked envelope formation and terminal differentiation. *Cell* **40,** 685–695.

19. Fesus, L., Thomazy, V., Autuori, F., Ceru, M. P., Tarcsa, E., and Piacentini, M. (1989) Apoptotic hepatocytes become insoluble in detergents and chaotropic agents as a result of transglutaminase action. *FEBS Lett.* **245,** 150–154.

20. Fesus, L. (1993) Biochemical events in naturally occurring forms of cell death. *FEBS Lett.* **328,** 1–5.

21. Piacentini, M., Ceru, M. P., Dini, L., and Di Rao, M. (1992) In vivo and in vitro induction of "tissue" transglutaminase in rat hepatocytes by retinoic acid. *Biochim. Biophys. Acta* **1135(2),** 171–179.

22. Piacentini, M., Fesus, L., and Melino, G. (1993) Multiple cell cycle access to the apoptotic death programme in human neuroblastoma cells. *Eur. J. Biochem.* **320(2),** 150–154.

23. Nair, S., Mayotte, J., Lokshin, A., and Levitt, M. (1994) Induction of squamous differentiation by interferon β in a human non-small-cell lung cancer cell line. *J. Natl. Cancer Inst.* **86,** 378–383.

24. Lokshin, A., Mayotte, J. E., and Levitt, M. L. (1995) Mechanism of interferon beta-induced squamous differentiation and programmed cell death in human non-small-cell lung cancer cell lines. *J. Natl. Cancer Inst.* **87,** 206–212.

25. Levitt, M. L., Gazdar, A. F., Oie, H. K., Schuller, H., and Thacher, S. M. (1990) Cross-linked envelope-related markers for squamous differentiation in human lung cancer cell lines. *Cancer Res.* **50,** 120–128.

26. Fabbi, M., Marimpietri, D., Martini, S., Brancolini, C., Amoresano, A., Scaloni, A., et al. (1999) Tissue transglutaminase is a caspase substrate during apoptosis.

Cleavage causes loss of transamidating function and is a biochemical marker of caspase 3 activation. *Cell Death Differ.* **6,** 992–1001.

27. Bergstresser, P. R., Pariser, R. J., and Taylor, J. R. (1978) Counting and sizing of epidermal cells in normal human skin. *J. Invest. Dermatol.* **70,** 280–284.

28. Simon, M. and Green, H. (1984) Participation of membrane-associated proteins in the formation of the cross-linked envelope of the keratinocyte. *Cell* **36,** 827–834.

29. Martin, S. J., Bradley, J. G., and Cotter, T. G. (1990) HL-60 cells induced to differentiate towards neutrophils subsequently die via apoptosis. *Clin. Exp. Immunol.* **79,** 448–453.

30. Zhang, H., Koty, P.P., Mayotte, J., and Levitt, M.L. (1999) Induction of multiple programmed cell death pathways by IFN-γ in human non-small-cell lung cancer cell lines. *Exper. Cell Res.* **247,** 133–141.

31. Kaufmann, S.H., Desnoyers, S., Ottaviano, Y., Davidson, N. E., and Poirier, G. G. (1993) Specific proteolytic cleavage of poly(ADP-ribose) polymerase: an early marker of chemotherapy-induced apoptosis. *Cancer Res.* **53,** 3976–3985.

32. Polakowska, R. R., Piacentini, M., Bartlett, R., Goldsmith, L. A., and Haake, A. R. (1994) Apoptosis in human skin development: morphogenesis, periderm, and stem cells. *Dev. Dyn.* **199,** 176–188.

III

MOLECULAR ABNORMALITIES IN LUNG CANCER

E. DETECTION OF ALTERATIONS IN LUNG CELL-DIRECTED ANGIOGENESIS

24

Angiogenesis, Metastasis, and Lung Cancer

An Overview

Amir Onn and Roy S. Herbst

1. Introduction

Tumor angiogenesis enables a pre-existing tumor to grow and metastasize. The term angiogenesis designates development of new blood vessels from preexisting vasculature. Goldman *(1)*, in 1907, was the first to describe the formation of new blood vessels, i.e., angiogenesis, around tumors. Growth and survival of normal cells, as well as tumors, are dependent on an adequate blood supply. Folkman *(2)* suggested in 1971 that tumors, like any other tissue, can only receive oxygen and nutrients by diffusion if the tumors are smaller than 1–2 mm in diameter. Further growth necessitates the formation of new blood vessels. Without a blood supply, tumors cannot grow beyond this critical size, or metastasize. However, at the time of their initial treatment, most patients with cancer have clinically or microscopically detectable metastases *(3)*. In addition, most deaths from cancer result from metastases resistant to conventional therapy *(3)*. Understanding these fundamental principles of cancer biology has been the main drive for comprehensive research in that field. Kerbel *(4)* recently discussed the history of angiogenesis research and the striking increase in interest in tumor angiogenesis and development of anti-angiogenesis drugs in the 1990s. This research resulted in the discovery of a growing number of genes and molecules that regulate the physiology of angiogenesis and metastasis. The balance between positive and negative regulatory molecules released by both tumors and host cells mediates the induction of angiogenesis. How this occurs, and the known pro- and anti-angiogenic molecules were recently reviewed in detail *(3,5–7)*. The accumulated data

From: *Methods in Molecular Medicine, vol. 74: Lung Cancer, Vol. 1: Molecular Pathology Methods and Reviews*
Edited by: B. Driscoll © Humana Press Inc., Totowa, NJ

support the evaluation of tumor angiogenesis as a prognostic factor, in cancer in general, and in lung cancer in particular. In this chapter we describe the principles of the biology of cancer angiogenesis and metastasis, the methods used to evaluate these processes, and the current therapeutic modalities for intervening in angiogenesis and metastasis, with special emphasis on the studies of lung cancer. Our discussion focuses only on studies involving human tumors and/or human cell lines.

2. Tumor Angiogenesis and Metastasis

2.1. Principal Regulators in Angiogenesis and Metastasis

A list of the known endogenous factors attributing to the homeostasis of angiogenesis is presented in **Table 1**. During the past two decades, more than 20 growth factors, cytokines, and other substances have been found to have pro-angiogenic activity *(7)*. Some of these, as well as some anti-angiogenic factors, are described below. Altering their functions by using specific drugs may affect other necessary and sometimes vital physiological mechanisms.

1. Vascular Endothelial Growth Factor (VEGF)/Vascular Permeability Factor (/VPF). VEGF/VPF is the best-studied pro-angiogenic factor. It was first identified by Dvorak and colleagues *(8)* by its ability to induce vascular leaking and permeability in ascites, and so was called VPF. VEGF/VPF plays a central role in the regulation of angiogenesis: it induces proliferation of endothelial cells, increases vascular permeability, and induces promotion of urokinase plasminogen activator by endothelial cells *(7)*. In addition to its pivotal role as an angiogenic factor, VEGF/VPF was shown recently to function as a survival factor for endothelial cells and to prevent endothelial cell apoptosis *(9)*. Currently, five members of the VEGF family are known. They are named according to their amino-acid lengths: VEGF-206, -189, -165, -145, and -121. VEGF-121 and VEGF-165 are the most common and are produced by tumor cells *(7,10)*. These isoforms bind to the tyrosine-kinase VEGF receptors (VEGFR-1, previously known as flt-1), which may have negative role of action, and VEGFR-2 (previously known as KDR or flk-1), which mediates the major permeability, growth, and endothelial cell survival actions of VEGF. Both receptors are expressed almost exclusively on endothelial cells. A third receptor, VEGFR-3 (previously known as flt-3), seems to play a particular role in formation of lymphatic vessels *(11)*. VEGF expression is controlled by hypoxia, activation of oncogenes such as *ras*, inactivation of tumor-suppressor genes such as *p53*, and the action of other cytokines, such as transforming growth factor (TGF)-β and nitric oxide (NO) *(7)*.

2. Basic Fibroblast Growth Factor (bFGF). bFGF was the first pro-angiogenic factor discovered. It also has a mitogenic effect on endothelial cells. However, unlike the activity of VEGF, the mitogenic activity of bFGF activity is not specific, as it enhances the proliferation of a wide variety of ectoderm and mesoderm-derived

Table 1
Endogenous Pro- and Anti-Angiogenic Molecules

	References
Pro-angiogenic molecules	
Angiopoietin 1	*(30)*
bFGF	*(61)*
E-cadherin	*(62)*
EGF	*(63)*
Ephrins	*(30)*
HGF/SF	*(64)*
IL-8	*(65)*
Integrins	*(66)*
NOS, COX-2	*(50)*
PD-ECGF	*(10)*
PDGF	*(7)*
Plasminogen activator, MMP	*(10)*
TGF-α, -β	*(10)*
TNF-α	*(64)*
VEGF/VPF	*(7)*
Anti-angiogenic molecules	
Angiopoietin 2	*(30)*
Angiostatin	*(13)*
Endostatin	*(14)*
IFN-α, -β, -γ	*(61)*
IL-12	*(67)*
Thrombospondin	*(7)*

cells, such as epithelial cells and fibroblasts. Endothelial cells produce bFGF in an autocrine fashion *(7)*. In addition, bFGF stimulates endothelial cells to migrate, to increase production of proteases, and to undergo morphogenesis *(10)*.

3. Platelet-Derived Endothelial Cell Growth Factor (PD-ECGF). PD-ECGF was first isolated from platelets, but is now known to be produced by malignant tumors as well as by macrophages, stromal cells, and glial cells. It is a less potent endothelial cell mitogen than bFGF and VEGF. It stimulates endothelial cell DNA synthesis and chemotaxis and induces production of bFGFs *(7,10)*.

4. Transforming Growth Factor (TGF). TGF-α and TGF-β stimulate endothelial cell proliferation. TGF-β is also involved in the regulation of cellular replication and synthesis of many components of the extracellular matrix (ECM) *(7)*.

5. Epidermal Growth Factor Receptor (EGFR). EGFR belongs to a family of four receptors: EGFR (HER1 or ErbB1), ErbB2 (HER2/neu), ErbB3 (HER3), and ErbB4 (HER4). EGFR has an intrinsic tyrosine kinase activity. Many human cancers of epithelial origin express high numbers of EGFRs, and are stimulated

by activation of the receptor via a TGF-α/EGFR autocrine loop, thus contributing to angiogenesis *(12)*.

6. Angiogenin. Angiogenin is a peptide that induces angiogenesis, not by increasing endothelial cell proliferation, but through an indirect effect, probably through interactions with other molecules *(7)*.

7. Interleukin-8 (IL-8). IL-8 is a chemoattractant cytokine. It is angiogenic and is produced by a variety of tissue and blood cells that attract and activate neutrophils in inflamed regions *(10)*.

8. Platelet-Derived Growth Factor (PDGF). PDGF belongs to a family of heterodimeric or homodimeric isoforms of A and B chains. They act as potent nonspecific growth factors for mesenchymal and glial cells *(10)*.

9. Thrombospondin. Thrombospondin is a potent inhibitor of endothelial proliferation and migration. It is downregulated during tumorigenesis *(7)*.

10. Interferon (IFN). The IFNs include IFN-α, IFN-β, and IFN-γ. In addition to their natural antiviral activity, they regulate multiple biological activities such as cell growth, differentiation, oncogene expression, host immunity, and tumorigenicity. They have antiproliferative actions, especially on tumor cells and on endothelial cells in vitro. Systemic therapy using recombinant IFNs produces antiangiogenic effects in vascular tumors, including hemangioma, Kaposi's sarcoma, melanoma, basal cell and squamous cell carcinoma, and bladder carcinoma *(10)*.

11. Angiostatin. Angiostatin is a 38-kDa fragment of plasminogen. O'Reilly et al. *(13)*, who purified this compound, suggested that certain primary mouse tumors can inhibit their own metastases. This activity may be mediated, at least in part, by angiostatin.

12. Endostatin. Endostatin is an angiogenesis inhibitor produced by hemangioendotheliomas and was, like angiostatin, first described by O'Reilly et al. *(14)*. Endostatin is a 20-kDa C-terminal fragment of collagen XVIII that specifically inhibits endothelial proliferation and potently inhibits angiogenesis and tumor growth.

2.2. Principles of Metastasis

In 1889, Paget *(15)* noted that patients with breast cancer had a disproportionate incidence of metastasis to the ovaries and that the incidence of skeletal metastasis was different for different tumors. Based on these observations, Paget proposed that metastasis occurs only when certain favored tumor cells (the "seed") have a special affinity for the growth milieu provided by certain specific organs (the "soil"). That formation of metastasis required the interaction of the right cells with the compatible organ environment is not incidental. Fidler *(3)* summarized the modern definition of the "seed and soil" hypothesis in three principles. First, tumors may be regarded as small organs, consisting of multiple cell populations having heterogeneous biological properties. These cells differ in their ability to undergo angiogenesis, invasion, and metastasis, and in their sensitivity to various cytotoxic agents. Second, metastasis strongly selects for cells that succeed in completing the sequential and interrelated

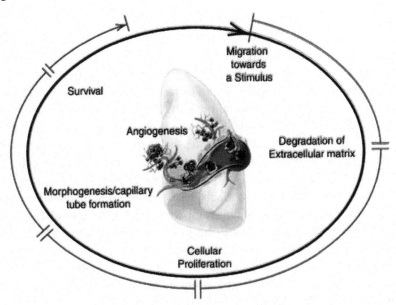

Fig. 1. The metastasis cascade. For metastasis to occur, cells from the primary tumor have to complete a meticulous multistep process. Each step is a balance between aiding and opposing factors. Only when the balance tilts forward, can the cells proceed to the next step. First, the cells detach from the primary tumor and overcome local anchoring forces, and then they invade and travel along the blood vessels or lymphatics. Next they penetrate the target organ connective tissue, reproduce and survive the local immune system. Newly formed blood vessels supply the growing metastatic tumor.

steps of this process. To produce clinically relevant lesions, metastatic cells must complete all steps in the process: invasion, embolization, survival in the circulation, arrest in a distant capillary bed, and extravasation into and multiplication within the organ parenchyma *(16)*. Although some of the steps in the process occur randomly, as a whole, metastasis favors the survival and growth of only a few subpopulations of cells within the parent neoplasm. Thus, metastases can have a clonal origin, and different metastases can originate from the proliferation of different single cells. Third, once a metastasis is established, its outcome, growth, and survival depend on many interactions with homeostatic factors and mechanisms *(3)*. The steps in metastasis are shown in **Fig. 1**.

2.3. Details of Model of Metastasis

Following the initial transformation and growth of cells, vascularization must occur for tumors to grow to more than 2 mm in diameter *(17)*. The synthesis and secretion of several angiogenic factors by the tumor and the host cells play a key role in establishing a capillary network from the surrounding host tissue *(18)*. Local invasion of the host stroma occurs next as a consequence of the enhanced expression of a series of enzymes (e.g., matrix metalloproteinases [MMPs]) *(19)*. Tumor cells can penetrate lymphatic channels and venules, because their thin walls offer little resistance, thus providing easy entry to the circulation. Detachment and embolization of small tumor cell aggregates occurs next. However, most of these circulating tumor emboli are rapidly destroyed *(17)*. The few tumor cells that survive in the circulation come to rest in the capillary beds of organs. Tumor cells adhere to the walls of blood vessels and extravagate into the organ parenchyma. Proliferation within the organ parenchyma completes the metastatic process, at which point the lesion must again develop a new vascular network (i.e., undergo angiogenesis) while also evading the host immune system. The metastatic potential of a tumor is the result of a balance between positive and negative regulatory factors controlled by a multitude of genetic processes. For instance, growth is controlled by EGFR, angiogenesis by VEGF/VPF, bFGF, and IL-8, invasion by MMP-2 and MMP-9, and cell-to-cell adhesion by E-cadherin. The expression of these factors has been assessed in several kinds of neoplasms, including colon *(20)*, gastric *(21)*, pancreatic *(22)*, prostate *(23)*, renal *(24)*, and lung cancers *(25)*, and found to correlate with prognosis.

2.4. Control of Neovascularization

As mentioned earlier, angiogenesis is a crucial step in the transformation of a small, local, and noninvasive tumor (which is benign in this respect) to a growing, spreading tumor *(10)*. To survive, mammalian cells must be within 100–200 µm of blood vessels, the diffusion limit for oxygen. For multicellular organisms to grow beyond this size, they must recruit new blood vessels by vasculogenesis (assembly of vessels from endothelial precursors, as in the embryo) or by angiogenesis (sprouting of an existing vessel network, as in wound healing and tumor growth) *(5)*. It is now widely accepted that under normal conditions, the "angiogenic switch" is in the "off" position because of the balance between pro-angiogenic and anti-angiogenic molecules. The switch is turned to "on" when the net balance is tipped in favor of angiogenesis *(5)*. Various signals that trigger the switch have been discovered. These include metabolic stress (e.g., low PO_2, low pH, or hypoglycemia), mechanical stress (e.g., pressure generated by proliferating cells), immune or inflammatory responses, and genetic mutations (e.g., activation of oncogenes or deletion of tumor-suppressor genes that control angiogenesis regulators). It has been suggested that decreases in the negative inhibition (i.e., regression of the anti-angiogenesis arm of the seesaw) accelerate the angiogenic process *(10)*. This hypothesis is based on the observation that IFN-β, a known anti-angiogenic factor, is found in high levels in epithelial cells and fibroblasts surrounding kidney tumor implanted subcutaneously in nude mice whereas bFGF expression by the tumor is low. In contrast, the IFN-β is not found in or around the same tumors implanted in the kidneys of nude mice, and bFGF expression by the tumor is 10–20 times higher *(10)*.

2.5. Mechanisms of Tumor-Vessel Formation

Tumor vessels develop mainly by angiogenesis, i.e., they sprout from pre-existing vessels. Other contributing mechanisms are intussusception, in which tumor tissue columns insert into the lumen of preexisting vessels and divide into several vessels *(5)*, recruitment of circulating endothelial cell precursors shed from blood vessel walls or mobilized from the bone marrow *(26)*, and/or vessel co-optation, in which tumors metastasizing into vascularized tissue initially grow by co-opting existing host vessels. The co-opted host vasculature then regresses, and the cells that survive the process are rescued by robust angiogenesis at the tumor margins *(27)*.

2.6. The Process of Angiogenesis

This process consists of multiple, sequential, interdependent steps *(10)*. It begins with local proteolytic activity that degrades the basement membrane surrounding capillaries. The enzymes most widely implicated in this process are MMPs, such as interstitial collagenase (MMP-1) and the gelatinases (MMP-2 and MMP-9), serine protease, and plasminogen activator. After degradation, the underlying endothelial cells invade the surrounding stroma and head toward the angiogenic stimulus. The endothelial cells proliferate as they migrate and are then organized into three-dimensional structures to form new capillary tubes *(28)*.

Kumar et al. *(29)* examined the relative activity of several factors on different phases of angiogenesis in vitro by treating human umbilical vein endothelial cells (HUVEC) with varying concentrations of bFGF, VEGF/VPF, PDGF, PD-ECGF, hepatocyte growth factor (HGF), and IL-8. Degradation of the extracellular matrix and morphogenesis endothelial cell division, migration, and survival were examined. The main finding was that VEGF/VPF and bFGF ensure survival of the cells in serum-free medium (endothelial cells cannot survive in culture without serum). Other important findings were that bFGF is the most potent mitogen, while VEGF/VPF and PD-ECGF are the next most potent. bFGF is the only factor able to upregulate the expression of the degradation enzymes plasminigen activator and interstitial collagenase (MMP-1). VEGF/VPF, bFGF, and HGF all induce chemotactic migration of the endothelial cells, but more specifically, bFGF and VEGF/VPF are chemotactic for endothelial cells, while HGF enhances their random migration, consistent with its property as a scatter factor *(10)*. Finally, IL-8, VEGF/VPF, and bFGF all induce the organization of HUVEC into an extensive network that resembles a capillary mesh *(28)*.

Recently, Yancopoulos et al. *(30)* concluded that the vascular endothelium-specific growth factors needed for angiogenesis include the five known members of the VEGF family. Also required are four members of the angiopoietin family, and at least one member of the large ephrin family. In addition, many other growth factors that are not specific for vascular endothelium are required for blood vessel formation, such as bFGF and members of the PDGF and TGF-β families. VEGF is regarded as the most critical driver of vascular formation, as it is required to initiate the formation of immature vessels. Angiopoietin (Ang)-1 and ephrin-B2 are subsequently required for further remodeling and maturation of this initially immature vasculature. Ephrin-B2 is particularly important in distinguishing developing arterial and venous vessels. After vessel maturation, Ang-1 seems to continue to be important in maintaining the quiescence and stability of the mature vasculature. Destabilization of the vasculature occurs at the beginning of vascular remodeling and involves in autocrine induction by the endothelium of a natural antagonist of Ang-1, most probably Ang-2 *(30)*. In a contrasting study, Ahmad et al. *(31)* transfected colon cancer cells with Ang-1 and Ang-2, injected the cells into nude mice, and assessed tumor growth to examine the balance between Ang-1 and Ang-2. The tumors produced by the Ang-2-transfected cells were larger and had more vessels than did the Ang-1 cells, suggesting that increases in Ang-2 activity enhance tumor angiogenesis and growth.

2.7. Macrostructure and Microstructure of Tumor Vessels

Although most solid tumors are highly vascular, their vessels are structurally and functionally abnormal. They are disorganized, tortuous, and dilated with an uneven diameter and excessive branches and shunts. Consequently, tumor blood flow is chaotic and leads to hypoxic and acidic regions in tumors *(5)*. In addition, tumor vessels differ from normal blood vessels in their cellular composition, permeability, stability, and slower growth *(3)*. Chang et al. *(32)* reported the presence of "mosaic" vessels with both endothelial cells and tumor cells form the luminal surface of tumor vessels. They also showed that 15% of perfused vessels of colon carcinoma xenografts in mice are mosaic, having focal regions where no endothelial cells can be detected and tumor cells appeared to contact the vessel lumen, and found similar numbers of mosaic vessels in human colon carcinoma biopsy samples *(32)*. In light of these data, it is especially interesting, that endothelial cells from different and apparently normal regions of human lung differ in the expression of the cell antigen thrombomodulin and von Willebrand factor *(33)*. This endothelial cell heterogeneity extends also to function, such as response to anti-angiogenic molecules *(34)*. Taken together, these observations suggest that strategies for targeting endothelial cells must take into account their molecular diversity and the organ specificity of the vasculature *(35)*.

2.8. Tumor Heterogeneity and Interactions with the Microenvironment

As discussed earlier, the tumor has to be regarded as an organ, composed of different cells with different biological activities. Giatromanolaki et al. *(35)* compared the peripheral and the inner patterns of vascularization in 178 surgical specimens of primary lung cancer and found that VEGF could induce blood vessel formation in the inner, hypoxic area, but not the periphery. Fidler et al. *(10)* showed that the decrease in IFN expression surrounding human kidney tumors implanted in kidney and nude mice correlates with an elevation in bFGF expression at the periphery of the tumor, and vice versa, when the tumor was implanted subcutaneously. Kuniyasu et al. *(39)* examined the expression of angiogenic factors by hyperplastic colonic mucosa adjacent to 40 Dukes' stage B and 34 Dukes' stage C surgical colon cancer specimens. They found higher expression of EGFR and TGF-α in the Dukes' C specimens, whilst the expression of IFN-β was inversely correlated with the level of pro-angiogenic molecules. They also showed that injection of colon cells into the cecal wall of mice induces hyperplastic changes in the adjacent mucosa, which expressed higher levels of pro-angiogenic molecules and lower levels of IFN-β than did the control mucosa. These data suggest that certain cancers, such as those of the colon, can induce hyperplasia in adjacent mucosa, which in turn produces angiogenic molecules that contribute to neoplastic angiogenesis *(37)*.

3. Pulmonary Implications of Angiogenesis

3.1. Noncancerous Conditions

VEGF and its receptors, VEGFR-1 and VEGFR-2, are essential facilitators of vessel formation in the embryo. Lung embryonic morphogenesis is further mediated by many other factors, including fibroblast growth factor (FGF), epidermal growth factor (EGF), TGF-β, and PDGF *(37)*. Recently, overexpression of lung VEGF was shown to correlate with induction of acute pulmonary edema, a process involving high vascular permeability, in mice *(39)*. Because angiogenesis is a prerequisite for airway remodeling in bronchial asthma, Hoshino et al. *(40)* examined the expression of VEGF, bFGF, and angiogenin in bronchial biopsy specimens from asthmatic and healthy control subjects.

Asthmatic subjects have more cells expressing VEGF, bFGF, and angiogenin in the airways and more blood vessels in the submucosa than do control subjects. The imbalance between IL-8 and IFN-γ-inducible protein is widely accepted as the key mechanism in the pathological process of idiopathic pulmonary fibrosis *(41)*.

3.2. Lung Cancer

Weidner et al. *(42)* were the first to report that, as the degree of angiogenesis detected in a primary tumor correlates with the prognosis. Their work established a direct relationship between metastasis and angiogenesis. The number of microvessels predicts the probability of metastatic disease and survival in non-small cell lung cancer (NSCLC), as it does in other solid tumors *(43,44)*. Formerly, anti-Factor VIII (von Willibrand factor) vessel immunostaining was used for detection of angiogenesis in cancer. Recently, several new antibodies have shown a higher sensitivity, and anti-CD34 and anti-CD31 antibody staining has been proposed as the standard for microvessel studies *(7)*. Dewhirst et al. *(44)* recently reviewed the methods to study oxygen transport at the microcirculatory level and proposed usage of some modern technology for further assessment of the degree of angiogenesis for prognostic purposes.

Poon et al. *(7)* recently reviewed the clinical implications of circulating angiogenic factors in cancer patients and reported that VEGF as well as bFGF correlate with poor prognosis in lung cancer. In extensive research of animal models of lung cancer, Yano et al. *(46)* found that VEGF is actually the cause of pleural effusion. However, it is necessary but not sufficient for the production and growth of brain metastasis *(47)*. IL-8 was also assessed in NSCLC and was found to correlate with tumor progression, tumor angiogenesis, patient survival, and timing of relapse *(48)*. Herbst et al. *(25)* have shown that the ratio of MMP (which is related to invasion) to E-cadherin (which is related to cell adhesion) is significantly higher in patients with recurrent lung cancer than in lung cancer patients in remission. They examined 60 surgical specimens of clinically stage 1 lung cancer for a battery of metastasis-related factors by using a rapid colorimetric mRNA *in situ* hybridization technique developed in the Fidler laboratory at M. D. Anderson for detecting the activity of different steps of angiogenesis and metastasis *(20)*. This technique is readily applicable to tissue-culture cells and frozen or formalin-fixed, paraffin-embedded tissues (archival specimens) and allows the measurement of the specific mRNA levels of particular genes. The technique is relatively quick (it can be completed in less than 5 h) and uses oligonucleotide probes synthesized with six biotin molecules at their 3′ ends, which affords a higher signal than with internally labeled fragments. These oligonucleotide probes are more specific and because they are not radioactive, they preserve tissue morphology, allowing the identifica-

Table 2
Angiogenesis Inhibitors in US Clinical Trials

Drug	Sponsor	Phase	Mechanism
Thalidomide	Celgene	I, I/II, II, III	Unknown
Carboxyamidotriazole	National Cancer Institute	I, II	Inhibitor of calcium influx
Col-3	Collagenex Pharmaceuticals	I, I/II, II	A tetracycline analog, selectively inhibits expression and production of MMP-2 and MMP-9
Endostatin	EntreMed	I	Direct inhibition of endothelial cells
Suramin	Parke-Davis	I, II	Nonspecific multisite effects
SU5416	Sugen Inc.	I, I/II, II, III	Blocks VEGF receptor signaling
(Pegalated) IFN-α 2b	Schering Plough	I, II, III	Inhibits bFGF and VEGF production
Interleukin-12	Genetics Institute	I/II, II	Upregulates IFN-γ and IP-10
EMD121974	Merck KCgaA	I/II	Small molecule blocker of integrin present on endothelial cell surface
RhuMabVEGF (recombinant human monoclonal antibody); Bevacizumab	National Cancer Institute; Genentech	I, II, II/III, III	Monoclonal antibody to VEGF
IM862	Cytran	II	Unknown mechanism
Squalamine	Geneara Pharmaceuticals	II	Extract from dogfish shark liver; inhibits sodium-hydrogen exchanger, NHE
RPI 4610	Ribozyme Pharmaceuticals, Inc.	II	Chemically synthesized anti-VEGF receptor ribozyme
BMS 275291	Bristol-Myers Squibb	II/III	An MMP inhibitor
AE-941/Neovastat	Aeterna Laboratories Inc.	III	A shark cartilage extract, Naturally occurring MMP inhibitor
Marimastat	British Biotech	III	Synthetic inhibitor (MMP)

Adapted from http://cancertrials.nci.nih.gov/news/angio/table.html, July 2001.

tion of subtle differences in staining intensity between the nucleus and cytoplasm and between the center and periphery of a tumor *(20)*.

As shown by Kuniyasu et al. *(22)*, different factors are expressed in different areas of a tumor: EGF, MMP, and bFGF in the periphery and VEGF in the center. Herbst et al. *(25)* also examined bFGF, VEGF, and IL-8 on these specimens, but did not find correlation with clinical parameters. Volm et al. *(49)* reported a similar finding for the relationship of several factors in assessing patients' survival: the individual levels of PD-ECGF, bFGF, and VEGF are not prognostic for NSCLC, but when the factors were combined in multivariate analysis, only 43% of patients expressing none of the factors had metastatic disease, whereas 77% expressing all factors had metastasis *(49)*. Recently, Marrogi et al. *(50)* investigated the correlation of several vasodilators with angiogenesis in 106 surgical specimens of NSCLC. They reported that nitric oxide synthase (NOS), cyclooxygenase-2 (COX-2), VEGF, and CD31 are differentially expressed in approx 50% of cases and that the expression of nitric oxide synthase 2 (NOS-2) and COX-2 correlates positively with VEGF status as well as CD31 staining (microvessel density) in tumors. Interestingly, NOS-2 overexpression was higher in adenocarcinoma and large cell carcinoma specimens than in squamous cell carcinoma samples, suggesting heterogeneous expression in different cell types. While the expression of NOS-2, COX-2, and microvessel density correlates with disease stage, it does not predict nor correlate with survival *(50)*. Cox et al. *(51)* performed immunohistochemical analysis of paraffin-embedded surgical sections from 167 lung cancer patients staining for the microvessel markers CD34, MMP-2, and MMP-9 and the erb/HER type (tyrosine kinase receptor. Patients with many microvessels and high tumor MMP-9 expression had a worse outcome than cases with only one or neither of these markers. Immunoreactivity for both erb/HER and MMP-9 expression was associated with poor prognosis. The authors suggested using this biological staging in addition to the conventional TNM staging system for the evaluation of lung cancer patients *(51)*.

4. Cancer Treatment Targeting Metastasis And Angiogenesis
4.1. Principles

Anti-angiogenic therapy was made possible by the development of mono-clonal antibodies (MAbs) targeting proteins active at specific phases in metastasis or angiogenesis. By the time of diagnosis, most tumors are biologi-cally heterogeneous and contain multiple subpopulations of cells with different properties *(52)*. Because not all cells in a neoplasm are likely to metastasize, it is important to identify the more malignant populations of cells, which confer an adverse prognosis. Therefore, to improve the survival rate of patients with early-stage NSCLC and to better stratify patients with advanced disease, novel methods must be developed to identify individuals at increased risk who might benefit from more aggressive treatment. Although chemotherapy for lung cancer has improved in the last decade, it is still only marginally effective (and often toxic), and routine adjuvant or neoadjuvant therapy for lung cancer is most often not performed. The development of new therapeutic agents with novel targets of action (i.e., antiangiogenic agents and MMP inhibitors) must be based on a better understanding of the processes of metastasis and angiogenesis in human lung tumors *(52)*.

Carter *(53)* discussed the design of clinical studies using angiogenesis inhibitors and concluded that since angiogenesis inhibitors target normal cells, the traditional strategy used in clinical development of cytotoxic agents may not be appropriate for these novel agents. Thus, the criterion used in many of the early clinical studies is the time to progression *(53)*. It may not be easy to assess response to therapy with anti-angiogenic agents (e.g., treatment of fatal infantile hemangiomas using IFN-α requires daily administration of nontoxic, relatively low doses for many months *[54]*). In addition, it is difficult to measure the serum levels of many of the factors *(7)*. Thus, surrogate markers are needed for each molecule. Also, it has been suggested that cancer should be regarded as a chronic disease and should be treated like other chronic conditions, with continuous low-dose therapy *(55)*.

4.2. Preclinical and Clinical Studies

Dozens of compounds are currently in preclinical or clinical studies (**Table 2**). It is of special interest to find anti-angiogenic mechanisms in the function of conventional chemotherapy or COX-2 inhibitors *(4,6)*. We will focus on those drugs whose main mechanism of action is attributed to blocking of angiogenesis.

4.2.1. Anti-VEGF Studies

Two modes to block the action of VEGF have been developed: selective inhibition of the VEGFR and inhibition of VEGFR tyrosine kinase phosphorylation. Many studies of in vitro models and animal models have shown significant tumor regression or tumor arrest in response to therapy *(56)*. Yano et al. *(57)* were the first to demonstrate a reduction in pleural effusion formation, but not the number of lung lesions, in an animal model. They used PTK 787, an oral tyrosine kinase phosphorylation inhibitor that affects the VEGF and PDGF receptors *(57)*. Verheul et al. *(58)* showed that treatment with ascetic and pleural effusion samples incubated with SU5416, a VEGFR-2 inhibitor, reduces endothelial cell proliferation.

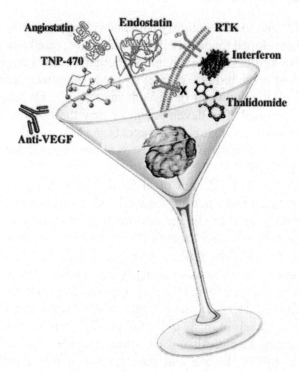

Fig. 2. Patient-tailored therapeutic cocktail. Patients will be treated with small molecules targeted to specific proteins manifested by their tumors. RTK, receptor tyrosine kinase.

4.2.2. Anti EGFR Studies

Liu et al. *(12)* treated human colon cancer cells with anti-EGFR MAb to produce apoptosis in vitro. Bruns et al. *(59)* implanted human pancreatic carcinoma into the pancreases of nude mice and treated the animals with PKI166, an oral EGFR tyrosine kinase inhibitor, which decreased growth and metastasis and increased survival as a result of increased apoptosis of tumor-associated endothelial cells. Acquired resistance to EGFR was described by Viloria-Petit et al. *(60)*, who found that the most resistant tumors express increased levels of VEGF. (These results were in an animal model, using a cell line that expresses high levels of EGFR.)

4.2.3. MMP Inhibitors

Several synthetic MMP inhibitors, that in preclinical studies had shown an effect on tumor growth, are in clinical trials. They are not expected to interfere with cell proliferation and therefore are not intended to eliminate tumor cells but rather to inhibit cell functions associated with the malignant process.

However, some clinical trials of MMP inhibitors were recently halted because of undesirable side effects *(57)*.

5. Conclusions

Lung cancer is a major health problem in the United States and in many other countries. Prevention methods, i.e., anti-smoking campaigns, have not proved entirely effective. The early detection of lung cancer by computerized tomography and sputum analysis is regarded as controversial. The state-of-the-art for chemotherapy is not beneficial for most patients. We therefore believe that this is the time for the addition of anti-angiogenesis therapy to the current arsenal of chemotherapy. These compounds should target specific tumors in specific organs, according to the gene expression of the specific tumor by the influence of the surrounding organ (*see* **Fig. 2**). It is likely that a cocktail of inhibitors will be required based on the specific phenotype of a given tumor. The optimal timing of this therapy in relation to conventional chemotherapy, as well as optimal dosages, are yet to be determined. In our experience, cancer must be regarded as a chronic disease and should be treated as such with these agents at all stages including maintenance therapy.

References

1. Goldman, E. (1907) The growth of malignant disease in man and the lower animals with special reference to the vascular system. *Lancet* **2**, 1236–1240.
2. Folkman, J. (1971) Tumor angiogenesis: therapeutic implications. *N. Engl. J. Med.* **285**, 1182–1186.
3. Fidler, I. J. (2000) Angiogenesis and cancer metastasis. *Cancer J. Sci. Am.* **6**, S134–S141.
4. Kerbel, R. S. (2000) Tumor angiogenesis: past, present and the near future. *Carcinogenesis* **21**, 505–515.
5. Carmeliet, P. and Jain, R. K. (2000) Angiogenesis in cancer and other diseases. *Nature* **407**, 249–257.
6. Miller, K. D., Sweeney, C. J., Sledge, G. W., Jr. (2001) Redefining the target: chemotherapeutics as antiangiogenics. *J. Clin. Oncol.* **19**, 1195–1206.
7. Poon, R. T., Fan, S. T., and Wong, J. (2001) Clinical implications of circulating angiogenic factors in cancer patients. *J. Clin. Oncol.* **19**, 1207–1225.
8. Senger, D. R., Galli, S. J., Dvorak, A. M., Perruzzi, C. A., Harvey, V. S., and Dvorak, H. F. (1983) Tumor cells secrete a vascular permeability factor that promotes accumulation of ascites fluid. *Science* **219**, 983–985.
9. Bruns, C. J., Liu, W., Davis, D. W., Shaheen, R. M., McConkey, D. J., Wilson, M. R., et al. (2000) Vascular endothelial growth factor is an in vivo survival factor for tumor endothelium in a murine model of colorectal carcinoma liver metastases. *Cancer* **89**, 488–499.
10. Fidler, I. J., Singh, R. K., Yoneda, J., Kumar, R., Xu, L., Dong, Z., et al. (2000) Critical determinants of neoplastic angiogenesis. *Cancer J. Sci. Am.* **6**, S225–S236.

11. Joukov, V., Pajusola, K., Kaipainen, A., Chilov, D., Lahtinen, I., Kukk, E., et al. (1996) A novel vascular endothelial growth factor, VEGF-C, is a ligand for the Flt4 (VEGFR-3) and KDR (VEGFR-2) receptor tyrosine kinases. *EMBO J* **15(2)**, 290–298.

12. Liu, B., Fang, M., Schmidt, M., Lu, Y., Mendelsohn, J., and Fan, Z. (2000) Induction of apoptosis and activation of the caspase cascade by anti-EGF receptor monoclonal antibodies in DiFi human colon cancer cells do not involve the c-jun N-terminal kinase activity. *Br. J. Cancer* **82,** 1991–1999.

13. O'Reilly, M. S., Holmgren, L., Shing, Y., Chen, C., Rosenthal, R. A., Moses, M., et al. (1994) Angiostatin: a novel angiogenesis inhibitor that mediates the suppression of metastases by a Lewis lung carcinoma. *Cell* **79,** 315–328.

14. O'Reilly, M. S., Boehm, T., Shing, Y., Fukai, N., Vasios, G., Lane, W. S., et al. (1997) Endostatin: an endogenous inhibitor of angiogenesis and tumor growth. *Cell* **88,** 277–285.

15. Paget, S. (1889) The distribution of secondary growths in cancer of the breast. *Lancet* **1,** 571–573.

16. Price, J. E., Aukerman, S. L., and Fidler, I. J. (1986) Evidence that the process of murine melanoma metastasis is sequential and selective and contains stochastic elements. *Cancer Res.* **46,** 5172–5178.

17. Fidler, I. J. (1997) Molecular biology of cancer: invasion and metastasis (De Vita, V. T., Jr., Hellman, S., and Rosenberg, S. A., eds.), in *Cancer: Principles and Practice of Oncology*, 5th ed., JB Lippincott Co., pp. 135–152.

18. Folkman, J. (1995) Angiogenesis in cancer, vascular, rheumatoid and other disease. *Nature Med.* **1,** 27–31.

19. Liotta, L. A. and Stetler-Stevenson, W. G. (1990) Metalloproteinases and cancer invasion. *Semin. Cancer Biol.* **1,** 99–106.

20. Kitadai, Y., Ellis, L. M., Takahashi, Y., Bucana, C. D., Anzai, H., Tahara, E., and Fidler, I. J. (1995) Multiparametric in situ messenger RNA hybridization analysis to detect metastasis-related genes in surgical specimens of human colon carcinomas. *Clin. Cancer Res.* **1,** 1095–1102.

21. Anzai, H., Kitadai, Y., Bucana, C. D., Sanchez, R., Omoto, R., and Fidler, I. J. (1998) Expression of metastasis-related genes in surgical specimens of human gastric cancer can predict disease recurrence. *Euro. J. Cancer* **34,** 558–565.

22. Kuniyasu, H., Ellis, L. M., Evans, D. B., Abbruzzese, J. L., Fenoglio, C. J., Bucana, C. D., et al. (1999) Relative expression of E-cadherin and type IV collagenase genes predicts disease outcome in patients with resectable pancreatic carcinoma. *Clin. Cancer Res.* **5,** 25–33.

23. Kuniyasu, H., Troncoso, P., Johnston, D., Bucana, C. D., Tahara, E., Fidler, I. J., and Pettaway, C. A. (2000) Relative expression of type IV collagenase, E-cadherin, and vascular endothelial growth factor/vascular permeability factor in prostatectomy specimens distinguishes organ-confined from pathologically advanced prostate cancers. *Clin. Cancer Res.* **6,** 2295–2308.

24. Slaton, J. W., Inoue, K., Perrotte, P., El-Naggar, A. K., Swanson, D. A., Fidler, I. J., and Dinney, C. P. (2001) Expression levels of genes that regulate metastasis and

angiogenesis correlate with advanced pathological stage of renal cell carcinoma. *Am. J. Pathol.* **158,** 735–743.

25. Herbst, R. S., Yano, S., Kuniyasu, H., Khuri, F. R., Bucana, C. D., Guo, F., et al. (2000) Differential expression of E-cadherin and type IV collagenase genes predicts outcome in patients with stage I non-small cell lung carcinoma. *Clin. Cancer Res.* **6,** 790–797.

26. Raffi, S. (2000) Circulating endothelial precursors: mystery, reality, and promise. *J. Clin. Invest.* **105,** 17–19.

27. Holash, J., Maisonpierre, P. C., Compton, D., Boland, P., Alexander, C. R., Zagzag, D., et al. (1999) Vessel cooption, regression, and growth in tumors mediated by angiopoietins and VEGF. *Science* **284,** 1994–1998.

28. Auerbach, W. and Auerbach, R. (1994) Angiogenesis inhibition: a review. *Pharmacol. Therapeut.* **63,** 265–311.

29. Kumar, R., Yoneda, J., Bucana, C. D., and Fidler, I. J. (1998) Regulation of distinct steps of angiogenesis by different angiogenic molecules. *Intl. J. Oncol.* **12,** 749–757.

30. Yancopoulos, G. D., Davis, S., Gale, N. W., Rudge, J. S., Wiegand, S. J., and Holash, J. (2000) Vascular-specific growth factors and blood vessel formation. *Nature* **407,** 242–248.

31. Ahmad, S. A., Liu, W., Jung, Y. D., Fan, F., Wilson, M., Reinmuth, N., et al. (2001) The effects of angiopoietin-1 and -2 on tumor growth and angiogenesis in human colon cancer. *Cancer Res.* **61,** 1255–1259.

32. Chang, Y. S., di Tomaso, E., McDonald, D. M., Jones, R., Jain, R. K., and Munn, L. L. (2000) Mosaic blood vessels in tumors: frequency of cancer cells in contact with flowing blood. *Proc. Natl. Acad. Sci. USA* **97,** 14608–14613.

33. Kawanami, O., Jin, E., Ghazizadeh, M., Fujiwara, M., Jiang, L., Ohaki, Y., et al. (2000) Mosaic-like distribution of endothelial cell antigens in capillaries and juxta-alveolar microvessels in the normal human lung. *Pathol. Intl.* **50,** 136–141.

34. Baker, C. H., Bruns, C. J., Fan, D., Killion, J.J., and Fidler, I.J. (2000) Different effects of angiostatin (K1-4) and K5 on cultured endothelial cells of different origin. *Proc. Am. Assoc. Cancer Res.* **41,** 308.

35. Pasqualini, R., McDonald, D. M., and Arap, W. (2001) Vascular targeting and antigen presentation. *Nature Immunol.* **2,** 567–568.

36. Giatromanolaki, A., Koukourakis, M. I., Sivridis, E., O'Byrne, K., Gatter, K. C., and Harris, A. L. (2000) 'Invading edge vs. inner' (edvin) patterns of vascularization: an interplay between angiogenic and vascular survival factors defines the clinical behaviour of non-small cell lung cancer. *J. Pathol.* **192,** 140–149.

37. Kuniyasu, H., Yasui, W., Shinohara, H., Yano, S., Ellis, L. M., Wilson, M. R., et al. (2000) Induction of angiogenesis by hyperplastic colonic mucosa adjacent to colon cancer. *Am. J. Pathol.* **157,** 1523–1535.

38. Warburton, D., Schwarz, M., Tefft, D., Flores-Delgado, G., Anderson, K. D., and Cardoso, W. V. (2000) The molecular basis of lung morphogenesis. *Mechan. Dev.* **92,** 55–81.

39. Kaner, R. J., Ladetto, J. V., Singh, R., Fukuda, N., Matthay, M. A., and Crystal, R. G. (2000) Lung overexpression of the vascular endothelial growth factor gene induces pulmonary edema. *Am. J. Respir. Cell Mol. Biol.* **22,** 657–664.

40. Hoshino, M., Takahashi, M., and Aoike, N. (2001) Expression of vascular endothelial growth factor, basic fibroblast growth factor, and angiogenin immunoreactivity in asthmatic airways and its relationship to angiogenesis. *J. Allergy Clin. Immunol.* **107,** 295–301.

41. Belperio, J. A., Keane, M. P., Arenberg, D. A., Addison, C. L., Ehlert, J. E., Burdick, M. D., and Strieter, R. M. (2000) CXC chemokines in angiogenesis. *J. Leukocyte Biol.* **68,** 1–8.

42. Weidner, N., Semple, J. P., Welch, W. R., and Folkman, J. (1991) Tumor angiogenesis and metastasis—correlation in invasive breast carcinoma. *N. Engl. J. Med.* **324,** 1–8.

43. Fontanini, G., Lucchi, M., Vignati, S., Mussi, A., Ciardiello, F., De Laurentiis, M., et al. (1997) Angiogenesis as a prognostic indicator of survival in non-small-cell lung carcinoma: a prospective study. *J. Natl. Cancer Instit.* **89,** 881–886.

44. Fontanini, G., Vignati, S., Lucchi, M., Mussi, A., Calcinai, A., Boldrini, L., et al. (1997) Neoangiogenesis and p53 protein in lung cancer: their prognostic role and their relation with vascular endothelial growth factor (VEGF) expression. *Br. J. Cancer* **75,** 1295–1301.

45. Dewhirst, M. W., Klitzman, B., Braun, R. D., Brizel, D. M., Haroon, Z. A., and Secomb, T. W. (2000) Review of methods used to study oxygen transport at the microcirculatory level. *Intl. J. Cancer* **90,** 237–255.

46. Yano, S., Shinohara, H., Herbst, R. S., Kuniyasu, H., Bucana, C. D., Ellis, L. M., and Fidler, I. J. (2000) Production of experimental malignant pleural effusions is dependent on invasion of the pleura and expression of vascular endothelial growth factor/vascular permeability factor by human lung cancer cells. *Am. J. Pathol.* **157,** 1893–1903.

47. Yano, S., Shinohara, H., Herbst, R. S., Kuniyasu, H., Bucana, C. D., Ellis, L. M., et al. (2000) Expression of vascular endothelial growth factor is necessary but not sufficient for production and growth of brain metastasis. *Cancer Res.* **60,** 4959–4967.

48. Yuan, A., Yang, P. C., Yu, C. J., Chen, W. J., Lin, F. Y., Kuo, S. H., and Luh, K.T. (2000) Interleukin-8 messenger ribonucleic acid expression correlates with tumor progression, tumor angiogenesis, patient survival, and timing of relapse in non-small-cell lung cancer. *Am. J. Respir. Crit. Care Med.* **162,** 1957–1963.

49. Volm, M., Koomagi, R., and Mattern, J. (1999) PD-ECGF, bFGF, and VEGF expression in non-small cell lung carcinomas and their association with lymph node metastasis. *Anticancer Res.* **19,** 651–655.

50. Marrogi, A. J., Travis, W. D., Welsh, J. A., Khan, M. A., Rahim, H., Tazelaar, H., et al. (2000) Nitric oxide synthase, cyclooxygenase 2, and vascular endothelial growth factor in the angiogenesis of non-small cell lung carcinoma. *Clin. Cancer Res.* **6,** 4739–4744.

51. Cox, G., Jones, J. L., Andi, A., Waller, D. A., and O'Byrne, K. J. (2001) A biological staging model for operable non-small cell lung cancer. *Thorax* **56**, 561–566.
52. Herbst, R. S. and Fidler, I. J. (2000) Angiogenesis and lung cancer: potential for therapy. *Clin. Cancer Res.* **6**, 4604–4606.
53. Carter, S. K. (2000) Clinical strategy for the development of angiogenesis inhibitors. *Oncologist* **5**, 51–54.
54. Ezekowitz, R. A., Mulliken, J. B., and Folkman, J. (1992) Interferon alpha-2a therapy for life-threatening hemangiomas of infancy. *N. Engl. J. Med.* **326**, 1456–1463.
55. Fidler, I. J. and Ellis, L. M. (2000) Chemotherapeutic drugs: more really is not better. *Nature Med.* **6**, 500–502.
56. Brekken, R. A., Overholser, J. P., Stastny, V. A., Waltenberger, J., Minna, J. D., and Thorpe, P.E. (2000) Selective inhibition of vascular endothelial growth factor (VEGF) receptor 2 (KDR/Flk-1) activity by a monoclonal anti-VEGF antibody blocks tumor growth in mice. *Cancer Res.* **60**, 5117–5124.
57. Yano, S., Herbst, R. S., Shinohara, H., Knighton, B., Bucana, C. D., Killion, J. J., et al. (2000) Treatment for malignant pleural effusion of human lung adenocarcinoma by inhibition of vascular endothelial growth factor receptor tyrosine kinase phosphorylation. *Clin. Cancer Res.* **6**, 957–965.
58. Verheul, H. M., Hoekman, K., Jorna, A. S., Smit, E. F., and Pinedo, H. M. (2000) Targeting vascular endothelial growth factor blockade: ascites and pleural effusion formation. *Oncologist* **5**, 45–50.
59. Bruns, C. J., Solorzano, C. C., Harbison, M. T., Ozawa, S., Tsan, R., Fan, D., et al. (2000) Blockade of the epidermal growth factor receptor signaling by a novel tyrosine kinase inhibitor leads to apoptosis of endothelial cells and therapy of human pancreatic carcinoma. *Cancer Res.* **60**, 2926–2935.
60. Viloria-Petit, A., Crombet, T., Jothy, S., Hicklin, D., Bohlen, P., Schlaeppi, J. M., et al. (2001) Acquired resistance to the antitumor effect of epidermal growth factor receptor-blocking antibodies in vivo: a role for altered tumor angiogenesis. *Cancer Res.* **61**, 5090–5101.
61. Singh, R. K., Gutman, M., Bucana, C. D., Sanchez, R., Llansa, N., and Fidler, I. J. (1995) Interferons alpha and beta down-regulate the expression of basic fibroblast growth factor in human carcinomas. *Proc. Natl. Acad. Sci. USA* **92**, 4562–4566.
62. Frixen, U. H., Behrens, J., Sachs, M., Eberle, G., Voss, B., Warda, A., et al. (1991) E-cadherin-mediated cell-cell adhesion prevents invasiveness of human carcinoma cells. *J. Cell Biol.* **113**, 173–185.
63. Mendelsohn, J. (1990) The epidermal growth factor receptor as a target for therapy with antireceptor monoclonal antibodies. *Semin. Cancer Biol.* **1**, 339–344.
64. Rosen, E. M., Zitnik, R. J., Elias, J. A., Bhargava, M. M., Wines, J., and Goldberg, I. D. (1993) The interaction of HGF-SF with other cytokines in tumor invasion and angiogenesis. *Exs* **65**, 301–310.

65. Singh, R. K., Gutman, M., Radinsky, R., Bucana, C. D., and Fidler, I. J. (1994) Expression of interleukin 8 correlates with the metastatic potential of human melanoma cells in nude mice. *Cancer Res.* **54,** 3242–3247.
66. Bauer, J., Margolis, M., Schreiner, C., Edgell, C. J., Azizkhan, J., Lazarowski, E., and Juliano, R. L. (1992) In vitro model of angiogenesis using a human endothelium-derived permanent cell line: contributions of induced gene expression, G-proteins, and integrins. *J. Cell. Physiol.* **153,** 437–449.
67. Voest, E. E., Kenyon, B. M., O'Reilly, M. S., Truitt, G., D'Amato, R. J., and Folkman, J. (1995) Inhibition of angiogenesis in vivo by interleukin 12. *J. Natl. Cancer Inst.* **87,** 581–586.
68. Giavazzi, R. and Taraboletti, G. (2001) Preclinical development of metalloproteasis inhibitors in cancer therapy. *Crit. Rev. Oncol. Hematol.* **37,** 53–60.

25

Matrix Metalloproteinase Expression in Lung Cancer

Melissa Lim and David M. Jablons

1. Introduction

The importance of matrix metalloproteinases (MMPs) in the growth and spread of solid tumors has been known for over a decade *(1,2)*. However, the molecular mechanisms that regulate their expression and the elucidation of their role in angiogenesis are subjects of extensive, ongoing investigation. The MMPs are a family of extracellular, zinc-dependent proteinases that control tumor growth via tumor promotion *(3)* and angiogenesis *(2,4)*. They are secreted as latent proenzymes and become activated after cleavage of their propeptide domain. MMPs are regulated on several levels including transcription, protein activation, and the interaction with endogenous inhibitors such as the tissue inhibitors of metalloproteinases (TIMPs) *(5)*. Over 20 MMPs have been described to date *(6; see* **Table 1**). Although traditionally subclassified according to substrate specificity (e.g., collagenases, gelatinases, stromelysins), collectively they are capable of breaking down all of the components of the extracellular matrix (ECM), including components of basement membranes (BMs) and submucosa *(1,5,6)*. MMP-2 and MMP-9, gelatinase A and B, respectively, are of particular interest because they degrade type IV collagen, the major component of basement membranes. Recently, Fang et al. *(7)* demonstrated in an animal model of chondrosarcoma that MMP-2 shifts the "proteolytic balance" towards an angiogenic phenotype, and is required for new blood vessel formation.

Our goal here is to examine the expression of metalloproteinases in lung cancer, and outline the development and application of synthetic metalloproteinase inhibitors in preclinical and early clinical trials.

From: *Methods in Molecular Medicine, vol. 74: Lung Cancer, Vol. 1: Molecular Pathology Methods and Reviews*
Edited by: B. Driscoll © Humana Press Inc., Totowa, NJ

Table 1
Matrix Metalloproteinase Classification

MMP family	MMP number	Common name
Collagenases	1	Interstitial collagenase
	8	Neutrophil collagenase
	13	Collagenase-3
	18	Xenopus collagenase
Gelatinases	2	Gelatinase A
	9	Gelatinase B
Stromelysins	3	Stromelysin-1
	10	Stromelysin-2
	11	Stromelysin-3
	7	Matrilysin
Elastase	12	Metalloelastase
Membrane-type	14	MT-MMP-1
	15	MT-MMP-2
	16	MT-MMP-3
	17	MT-MMP-4
	21	MT-MMP-5
Unclassified	20	Enamelysin
	19	
	23	
	24	

Adapted from **ref.** *6*.

1.1. MMPs and Lung Cancer

Several years ago MMPs were suspected to be related to the level of invasiveness of lung and head and neck and cancers. Muller et al. *(8)* found high levels of stromelysin-2 (MMP-10), collagenase-1 (MMP-1), and pump-1 (matrilysin, or MMP-7) messenger RNA in human non-small cell lung cancer (NSCLC) tissues compared to normal bronchial mucosa. MMPs-2 and -9, the gelatinases, are also upregulated in squamous cell cancer of the lung, although a correlation with clinical staging was not confirmed *(9)*. However, the prognostic significance of MMPs has been explored *(10,11)*, and serum MMP-2 levels (as determined by enzyme-linked immunosorbent assays) correlated with the stage of NSCLC and decreased with a response to chemotherapy *(10)*. A correlation with stage of disease was also found by Nawrocki et al. *(12)*, who surveyed the tissues of 88 patients with NSCLC (plus 13 samples of non-neoplastic lung tissue) and studied the expression of MMPs-1, -2, -3, -7, -9, -11, and -14, in addition to TIMPs-1, -2, and -3. In this study, gelatinase

A (MMP-2) was the most commonly overexpressed MMP (66% of tumor samples), although it was also detected in 31% of normal tissues. Stromelysin-3 (MMP-11), collagenase-1 (MMP-1), gelatinase B (MMP-9), and matrilysin (MMP-7) were significantly higher in tumor vs normal tissue, but only gelatinase A, gelatinase B, and collagenase-1 mRNA levels correlated with TNM stage of disease.

1.1.1. The Role of MMPs in Varying Stages of Cancer

More recently, attention has turned toward defining the roles of specific metalloproteinases during different stages of disease. The progression from squamous dysplasia to carcinoma *in situ* is best described for squamous cell lung cancer *(13)*. In studies comparing MMP expression within different tissue compartments, Bolon et al. *(14)* demonstrated MMP mRNA expression (MMPs 1, -3, -11, and -7) within epithelial cells of early intraepithelial lesions, whereas MMP-1, -3, and -11 expression shifted to stromal fibroblasts within microinvasive and invasive lesions. This shift in expression suggests an active role by tumor-associated connective tissue cells in regulating the proteolysis required for invasion. The role tumor cells play in stimulating fibroblast production of metalloproteinases is currently under investigation. Both membrane-bound and soluble tumor cell factors have been implicated in the regulation of tumor cell-associated fibroblast MMP expression *(15,16)*. Biswas et al. isolated EMMPRIN (extracellular matrix metalloproteinase inducer) from human non-small cell lung carcinoma cell membranes *(15)*. Purified EMMPRIN upregulates the steady-state mRNA expression of MMPs-1, -2, and -3 *(17)*. We reported previously that EMMPRIN upregulation of human lung fibroblast MMP-1 (16-Lu cells) is through the p38 signal transduction pathway *(18)*. Recently, we discovered that purified EMMPRIN also increases the expression of MMP-9 in vitro (unpublished data; *see* **Fig. 1**). Gelatinase expression is demonstrated by substrate (gelatin)-impregnated acrylamide gel electrophoresis, as shown below. White zones of lysis indicate gelatinase activity.

MMP overexpression is also found in small cell lung cancer, although the profile and pattern of expression are distinct from non-small cell. For instance, Bolon et al. *(19)* found strong expression of stromelysin-3 (MMP-11), but no expression of stromelysin-1 (MMP-3) or matrilysin (MMP-7), by *in situ* hybridization. This difference in MMP expression may reflect unique cell type-specific molecular regulation of MMPs.

1.2. Metalloproteinase Inhibitors

Numerous studies in animals have found that MMP inhibition retards tumor growth and extends survival *(4,20,21,22)*. The relative importance of each MMP family member in contributing to tumor progression has not been

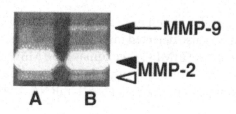

Fig. 1. Gelatin zymography of 3T3 fibroblasts stimulated with vehicle alone (**A**) and with purified EMMPRIN (**B**). Arrow points to MMP-9 expression, black and white arrowheads the latent and active isoforms of MMP-2, respectively.

determined, however, synthetic MMP inhibitors target multiple MMPs in order to achieve an optimal cytostatic effect *(23,24)*. The first generation of broad-spectrum synthetic MMP inhibitors was led by batimastat (*Mr* 477), or BB-94, which was designed to mimic the peptide residues of the cleavage site of the main substrate of MMPs, collagen. Its inhibitory profile, in order of increasing IC_{50}s is MMP-1 (3 n*M*), MMPs-2 and -9 (4 n*M*), MMP-7 (6 n*M*), and MMP-3 (20 n*M*) *(23)*. Although batimastat is insoluble and shows poor oral bioavailability, sustained plasma concentrations may be achieved with intraperitoneal *(25)* and intrapleural *(26)* injections. A Phase I dose-escalation study in patients with malignant pleural effusions who received intrapleural batimastat showed that plasma concentrations peaked within hours of administration and could be detected up to 12 wk post-injection (in the highest dose group) *(26)*. Three patients at each dose level (15, 30, 60, 105, 135, and 300 mg/m^2) were enrolled in the study. Seven of eighteen patients experienced low-grade fever within 24–48 h after drug administration, eight experienced elevated liver enzymes, six had nausea, six malaise, and five pleural pain. Only elevated liver enzymes were found to be associated with the higher drug doses (60 mg/m^2 and above), although there was no correlation with plasma drug levels. The repeat aspiration rate in the month after batimastat was significantly lower than in the month before administration (10 aspirations vs 42, $p = 0.0004$).

Marimastat (BB2516) is a second-generation broad spectrum MMP that shows greater oral bioavailability than batimastat. It contains a zinc-chelating hydroxamate structure as well as a collagen-like core *(27)*. A Phase I study in patients with advanced lung cancer (10/12 cases were non-small cell) was conducted to determine the maximum tolerated dose of marimastat *(28)*. Patients were assigned one of three dose levels, 25 mg, 50 mg, or 100 mg twice daily for up to 12 wk. During the first 8 wk of treatment the patients receiving the highest dose experienced a diffuse polyarthritis, fatigue, and joint swelling. With prolonged treatment, similar but less severe symptoms were seen in the lower dose groups. Nonsteroidal anti-inflammatory agents and prednisone did not appear to prevent these side effects. No complete or partial responses to MMP therapy were observed. This and other Phase I studies helped to define the current dose of marimastat used in clinical studies, 10 mg twice daily *(27)*. Marimastat has advanced to Phase III clinical studies in patients with advanced gastric and pancreatic cancer *(29–31)*. No survival benefit of marimastat alone or in combination with gemcitabine has been found with advanced pancreatic cancer *(29,30)*. Patients with inoperable gastric cancer receiving marimastat vs placebo had no statistically significant improved survival at the primary endpoint of 85% mortality in one study arm; however, the patients that received marimastat have shown statistically significant longer progression-free survival, a secondary endpoint *(31)*.

Using X-ray crystallography of recombinant MMPs that demonstrates the active site pocket, Agouron Pharmaceuticals developed a somewhat more selective synthetic MMP inhibitor *(32)*. AG3340, or prinomastat, is a small (MW 423), orally available, nonpeptidic, hydroxamate inhibitor with an inhibitory profile substantially favoring MMP-13 and MMP-2 *(32)*. MMPs inhibited, in order of increasing 50% inhibitory concentrations, are MMP-13 (0.03 nM), MMP-2 (0.05 nM), MMP-9 (0.26 nM), MMP-3 (0.30 nM), MMP-14 (0.33 nM), MMP-1 (8.3 nM), and MMP-7 (54 nM). Numerous preclinical models using human tumor cells implanted into immunocompromised mice, showed that prinomastat given both orally and intraperitoneally inhibited tumor growth in a dose-dependent manner *(33,34)*. This promising agent moved to Phase III clinical trials in patients with advanced prostate and non-small cell lung cancer. Patients received standard chemotherapy with or without prinomastat. Although prinomastat appeared to be well-tolerated, the preliminary data did not indicate any beneficial effects of the agent and the trials were discontinued in the fall of 2000 *(35)*. A separate study with patients with stage IIIB disease is ongoing.

1.3. Summary and Future Directions

Matrix metalloproteinases play a key role in both the local growth and distant spread of solid tumors. Several MMPs are upregulated in lung cancer, especially the gelatinases (MMPs-2 and -9), interstitial collagenase (MMP-1), and stromelysin-3 (MMP-11). Synthetic metalloproteinase inhibitors are designed to mimic MMP substrate and block the enzyme active site. Several inhibitors have been developed to date, with increasing oral bioavailability and improved selectivity. Despite great promise in preclinical studies, the results of Phase III trials have been disappointing. These agents are cytostatic instead of cytotoxic, and the clinical endpoint of disease stabilization has not been statistically demonstrated. However, this lack of efficacy in advanced disease only serves to underscore the importance of evaluating MMP inhibitors earlier, when the MMP-dependent proteolytic switch of angiogenesis may be interrupted.

References

1. Mignatti, P. and Rifkin, D. B. (1993) Biology and biochemistry of proteinases in tumor invasion. *Physiolog. Rev.* **73**, 161–195.
2. Liotta, L. A., Steeg, P. S., and Stetler-Stevenson, W. G. (1991) Cancer metastasis and angiogenesis: an imbalance of positive and negative regulation. *Cell* **64**, 327–336.
3. Matrisian, L. (1999) Cancer biology: extracellular proteinases in malignancy. *Curr. Biol.* **9**, R776–R778.
4. Bergers, G., Javaherian, K., Lo, K-M., Folkman, J., and Hanahan, D. (1999) Effects of angiogenesis inhibitors on multistage carcinogenesis in mice. *Science* **284**, 808–812.
5. Kleiner, D. E. and Stetler-Stevenson, W. G. (1999) Matrix metalloproteinases and metastasis. *Cancer Chemother. Pharmacol.* **43(Suppl.)**, S42–S51.
6. Nelson, A. R., Fingleton, B., Rothenberg, M. L., and Matrisian, L. M. (2000) Matrix metalloproteinases: biologic activity and clinical implications. *J. Clin. Oncol.* **18(5)**, 1135–1149.
7. Fang, J., Shing, Y., Wiederschain, D., Yan, L., Butterfield, C., Jackson, G., et al. (2000) Matrix metalloproteinase-2 is required for the switch to the angiogenic phenotype in a tumor model. *Proc. Natl. Acad. Sci. USA* **97(8)**, 3884–3889.
8. Muller, D., Breathnach, R., Engelmann, A., Millon, R., Bronner, G., Flesch, H., et al. (1991) Expression of collagenase-related metalloproteinase genes in human lung or head and neck tumours. *Int. J. Cancer* **48**, 550–556.
9. Nakagawa, H. and Yagihashi, S. (1994) Expression of type IV collagen and its degrading enzymes in squamous carcinoma of the lung. *Japn. J. Cancer Res.* **85**, 934–938.
10. Garbisa, S., Scagliotti, G., Masiero, L., DiFrancesco, C., Caenazzo, C., Onisto, M., et al. (1992) Correlation of serum metalloproteinase levels with lung cancer metastasis and response to therapy. *Cancer Res.* **52**, 4548–4549.
11. Delebecq, T. J., Porte, H., Zerimach, F., Copin, M. C., Gouyer, V., Dacquembronne, E., et al. (2000) Overexpression level of stromelysin 3 is related to lymph node involvement in non-small cell lung cancer. *Clin. Cancer Res.* **6**, 1086–1092.
12. Nawrocki, B., Polette, M., Marchand, V., Monteau, M., Gillery, P., Tournier, J.-M., and Birembaut, P. (1997) Expression of matrix metalloproteinases and their inhibitors in human bronchopulmonary carcinomas: quantificative and morphological analyses. *Int. J. Cancer* **72**, 556–564.
13. Trump, B. F., Dowell, E. M., Glaxin, F., Barret, L. A., Becci, P. J., Schurch, W., et al. (1978) The respiratory epithelium. III. Histogenesis of epidermoid metaplasia and carcinoma in situ in the human. *J. Natl. Cancer Inst.* **61**, 563–575.
14. Bolon, I., Brambilla, E., Vandenbunder, B., Robert, C., Lantuejoul, S., and Brambilla, C. (1996) Changes in the expression of matrix proteases and of

transcription factor c-ets-1 during progression of precancerous bronchial lesions. *Lab. Investig.* **75(1)**, 1–13.

15. Ellis, S. M., Nabeshima, K., and Biswas, C. (1989) Monoclonal antibody preparation and purification of a tumor cell collagenase-stimulatory factor. *Cancer Res.* **49**, 3385–3391.

16. Prescott, J., Troccoli, N., and Biswas, C. (1989). Coordinate increase in collagenase mRNA and enzyme levels in human fibroblasts treated with tumor cell factor, TCSF. *Biochem. Intl.* **19**, 257–266.

17. Kataoka, H., DeCastro, R., Zucker, S., and Biswas, C. (1993) Tumor cell-derived collagenase stimulating factor increases expression of interstitial collagenase, stromelysin, and 72-kDa gelatinase. *Cancer Res.* **53**, 3154–3158.

18. Lim, M., Martinez, T., Jablons, D., Cameron, R., Guo, H., Toole, B., et al. (1998) Tumor-derived EMMPRIN (extracellular matrix metalloproteinase inducer) stimulates collagenase transcription through MAPK p38. *FEBS Lett.* **441**, 88–92.

19. Bolon, I., Devouassoux, M., Robert, C., Moro, D., Brambilla, C., and Brambilla, E. (1997) Expression of urokinase-type plasminogen activator, stromelysin 1, stromelysin 3, and matrilysin genes in lung carcinomas. *Am. J. Pathol.* **150**, 1619–1629.

20. Anderson, I. C., Shipp, M. A., Docherty, A. J. P., and Teicher, B. A. (1996) Combination therapy including a gelatinase inhibitor and cytotoxic agent reduces local invasion and metastasis of murine Lewis lung carcinoma. *Cancer Res.* **56**, 715–718.

21. Prontera, C., Mariani, B., Rossi, C., Poggi, A., and Rotilio, D. (1999) Inhibition of gelatinase A (MMP-2) by batimastat and captopril reduces tumor growth and lung metastasis in mice bearing Lewis lung carcinoma. *Int. J. Cancer* **81**, 761–766.

22. Itoh, T., Tanioka, T., Matsuda, H., Nishimoto, H., Yoshioka, T., Suzuki, R., and Uehira, M. (1999) Experimental metastasis is suppressed in MMP-9-deficient mice. *Clin. Exp. Mets.* **17**, 177–181.

23. Brown, P. D. and Giavazzi, R. (1995) Matrix metalloproteinase inhibition: a review of antitumor activity. *Ann. Oncol.* **6**, 967–974.

24. Yip, D., Ahmad, A., Karapetis, C. S., Hawkins, C. A., and Harper, P. G. (1999) Matrix metalloproteinase inhibitors: applications in oncology. *Invest. New Drugs* **17**, 387–399.

25. Parsons, S. L., Watson, S. A., and Steele, R. J. (1997) Phase I/II trial of batimastat, a matrix metalloproteinase inhibitor, in patients with malignant ascites. *Eur. J. Surg. Oncol.* **23**, 526–531.

26. Macaulay, V. M., O'Byrne, K. J., Saunders, M. P., Braybrooke, J. P., Long, L., Gleeson, F., et al. (1999) Phase I study of intrapleural batimastat (BB-94), a matrix metalloproteinase inhibitor, in the treatment of malignant pleural effusions. *Clin. Cancer Res.* **5(3)**, 513–520.

27. Steward, W. P. (1999) Marimastat (BB2516): current status and development. *Cancer Chemother. Pharmacol.* **43(Suppl.)**, S56–S60.

28. Wojtowicz-Praga, S., Torri, J., Johnson, M., Steen, V., Marshall, J., Ness, E., et al. (1998) Phase I trial of marimastat, a novel matrix metalloproteinase inhibitor,

administered orally to patients with advanced lung cancer. *J. Clin. Oncol.* **16,** 2150–2156.

29. British Biotech PLC. (1999) Results of marimastat trial 128-pancreatic cancer monotherapy trial. Press release, February.
30. British Biotech PLC. (2000) Results of marimastat study 193 in advanced pancreatic cancer. Press release, January.
31. British Biotech PLC. (1999) Results of marimastat study 145 in gastric cancer. Press release, August.
32. Shalinsky, D. R., Shetty, B., Pithavala, Y., Bender, S., Neri, A., Webber, S., et al. (2000) Prinomastat: a selective matrix metalloprotease inhibitor-preclinical and clinical development for oncology, in *Cancer Drug Discovery and Development: Matrix Metalloproteinase Inhibitors in Cancer Therapy* (Clendennin, N. J. and Appelt, K., eds.), Humana Press, Inc., Totowa, NJ, pp. 143–173.
33. Shalinsky, D. R., Brekken, J., Zou, H., McDermott, C.D., Forsyth, P., Edwards, D., et al. (1999) Broad antitumor and antiangiogenic activities of AG3340, a potent and selective MMP inhibitor undergoing advanced oncology clinical trials. *Ann. NY Acad. Sci.* **878,** 236–270.
34. Shalinsky, D. R., Brekken, J., Zou, H., Bloom, L.A., McDermott, C. D., Zook, S., et al. (1999) Marked antiangiogenic and antitumor efficacy of AG3340 in chemoresistant non-small cell lung cancer tumors: single agent and combination chemotherapy studies. *Clin. Cancer Res.* **5,** 1905–1917.
35. Agouron Pharmaceuticals, Inc. (2000) Pfizer discontinues phase III trials of prinomastat in advanced cancers but continues multiple phase II trials. Press release, August 4. New York and La Jolla, CA www.agouron.com/pages/press_releases/pr080400.html

26

Vascular Endothelial Growth Factor Expression in Non-Small Cell Lung Cancer

Kenneth J. O'Byrne, Jonathan Goddard, Alexandra Giatromanolaki, and Michael I. Koukourakis

1. Introduction

Lung cancer is the most common cause of cancer-related death in the western world. Of patients with lung cancer, in the region of 90% are either current or ex-cigarette smokers. Non-small cell lung cancer (NSCLC) accounts for approx 80% of these cases. Despite improvements in the diagnostic evaluation and treatment of the disease, the prognosis for lung cancer patients remains appalling, with a 5-yr survival of 4–14% in developed countries *(1–3)*. An increased understanding of the biology of lung cancer is essential to develop novel approaches for the management of the disease.

Angiogenesis plays a central role in the growth and metastasis of malignant disease, being essential for tumor to grow beyond 1–2 mm in diameter. The intensity of angiogenesis, as assessed by microvessel counting methods, is an important prognostic factor in patients who have undergone surgical resection with curative intent for NSCLC. In both retrospective and prospective studies, high microvessel counts or microvessel density (MVD) have been found to be associated with disease spread and a poor survival *(4–8)*.

Angiogenesis is regulated by pro- and inhibitory angiogenic growth factors. The pro-angiogenic growth factors include vascular endothelial growth factor (VEGF). The VEGF family includes VEGF-A, -B, -C, -D, and -E and placental growth factor. All are dimeric glycoproteins with homologous amino acid sequences shared with platelet-derived growth factor (PDGF)-A and -B. These factors bind to similar tyrosine kinase receptors. VEGF-A is a potent and specific endothelial cell mitogenic, migratory, and vascular permeability factor.

From: *Methods in Molecular Medicine, vol. 74: Lung Cancer, Vol. 1: Molecular Pathology Methods and Reviews*
Edited by: B. Driscoll © Humana Press Inc., Totowa, NJ

Although produced from the same gene, a number of different isoforms of VEGF-A are created by differential splicing of RNA. These include variants of 121, 145, 148, 165, 189, and 206 amino acids. The most studied isoforms are $VEGF_{121}$, $VEGF_{165}$, $VEGF_{189}$, and $VEGF_{206}$. All have different characteristics. $VEGF_{121}$ is acidic and the most soluble. $VEGF_{165}$, is the most abundant isoform and, like $VEGF_{121}$, is soluble. $VEGF_{189}$ and $VEGF_{206}$ are more basic and remain close to the membrane, strongly bound to heparin sulphate (9–14).

VEGF binds with high affinity to two tyrosine kinase receptors, VEGFR-1 (Flt-1) and VEGFR-2 (Flk-1/KDR). VEGF receptors are present both on vascular endothelium and nonvascular epithelium. Ligand binding causes receptor dimerization, phosphorylation, and signal transduction (15–18).

VEGF expression is regulated by other angiogenic growth factors, such as basic fibroblast growth factor (bFGF), epidermal growth factor (EGF) and PDGF, inflammatory cytokines, including interleukin-1β (IL-1β) and hypoxia, all of which stimulate VEGF secretion (19–22). VEGF is also regulated by tumor-suppressor genes such as p53. Wild-type p53 downregulates VEGF promoter activity, whereas mutant p53 has the opposite effect (23,24).

VEGF plays a major role in remodeling of the extracellular matrix (ECM) by increasing vascular permeability. This results in the leakage of plasma proteins and fibrin deposition into the ECM. Fibrin acts as a scaffold for vascular structures. VEGF induces tissue-factor production, which promotes the conversion of thrombin from prothrombin. This in turn leads to matrix metalloproteinase-2 (MMP-2) activation and endothelial cell proliferation. VEGF also facilitates the activation of the plasmin cascade through the upregulation of urokinase and tissue plasminogen activator (tPA), plasminogen activator inhibitor-1 (PAI-1), and interstitial collagenase expression, allowing ECM degradation around the capillary bud. The coagulation and fibrinolysis pathways may also be involved in VEGF-associated angiogenesis. Platelets transport VEGF in the circulation and release it when activated. In tumors, blood-flow, particularly in tumor microvessels, may be impaired and platelet-binding proteins increased through microvessel hyperpermeability, stromal remodelling and/or the release of von Willebrand factor. This may result in increased platelet adherence and/or extravasation, activation, release of VEGF and increased local concentrations of the angiogenic growth factor, leading to further angiogenesis (reviewed in **ref.** 13).

Finally, recent work indicates a clear inverse correlation between angiogenesis and cell-mediated immunity in malignant diseases, including lung cancer (25). This contention is supported by the observation that VEGF causes a defect in the functional maturation of dendritic cells, which is associated with impaired activation of the nuclear transcription factor NF-κB (26,27).

1.2. Analysis of VEGF Expression in Normal and Malignant Tissues

There is accumulating evidence that high VEGF expression plays an important role in the pathogenesis of solid tumors. VEGF expression is associated with angiogenesis and/or a poor prognosis in breast *(28)*, colorectal *(29)*, esophegeal *(30)*, gastic *(31)*, and epithelial ovarian cancer *(32)* among others. Recent studies have confirmed that VEGF is associated with high microvessel counts and a poor prognosis in NSCLC *(7,33–39)*. Furthermore, different patterns of tumor angiogenesis have been identified by counting vessels both in the invading edge and inner areas of the tumor separately. Those with high vessel counts in both areas appear to have a worse prognosis. There is a significant correlation between high microvessel counts in the inner tumor areas and high tumor cell VEGF expression, indicating that VEGF plays an important role in endothelial cell survival in these areas *(40)*.

1.2.1. Importance of Different VEGF Isoforms

The VG1 monoclonal antibody (MAb) used in our studies detects the $VEGF_{121}$, $VEGF_{165}$, and $VEGF_{189}$ isoforms (*see* later) *(41)*. Current evidence would suggest that these are the most important isoforms of VEGF in malignant disease. For example, employing reverse transcription-polymerase chain reaction (RT-PCR), $VEGF_{121}$, $VEGF_{165}$, and $VEGF_{189}$, but not $VEGF_{206}$ have been found to be the predominant isoforms of VEGF expressed by lung and colonic tumors *(42)*. A number of studies have indicated that $VEGF_{121}$, $VEGF_{165}$ and/or $VEGF_{189}$ are associated with angiogenesis and/or a poor prognosis in NSCLC *(35,37,43–45)*. Of the 4 isoforms examined, including $VEGF_{206}$, Oshika and colleagues identified $VEGF_{189}$ mRNA in 90.5% of NSCLC tumours. Immunohistochemistry confirmed the presence of VEGF protein in 33 of the 76 cases studied. Cases with $VEGF_{189}$ mRNA and protein had a significantly poorer outcome than those without. Introducing a hammerhead-type ribosome into the NSCLC cell line OZ-6/VR to downregulate $VEGF_{189}$, tumor cell proliferation was not affected in vitro. In contrast, OZ-A/VR cells xenografted into nude mice were unable to form tumors, thus supporting an important role for this isoform in the growth of some NSCLC tumors *(46)*.

1.3. The Role of Apoptosis Regulators in Angiogenesis

Regulators of apoptosis, such as bcl-2 and p53, appear to have a role in the angiogenic process. We have reported that bcl-2 expression, associated with a favorable outcome in NSCLC, is inversely correlated with angiogenesis *(47)* and this contention has recently been supported by others *(48)*. Although not a uniform finding in all studies *(49)* a positive correlation has been reported between nuclear p53 and VEGF expression in solid tumors including colorectal cancer and NSCLC *(7,29,48,50)*. In keeping with these results we have shown an inverse correlation between VEGF and cytoplasmic/perinuclear p53 expression, a feature suggestive of the wild-type protein, in NSCLC *(51)*.

1.4. The Role of Platelet-Derived Growth Factors in Angiogenesis

Platelet-derived endothelial cell growth factor (PD-ECGF) is a 90 kDa homodimer, nonheparin binding angiogenic factor initially isolated from platelets. Transfection of PD-ECGF cDNA into transformed fibroblasts results in neo-angiogenesis. PD-ECGF stimulates endothelial cell migration in vitro and tumor growth in vivo. Subsequent studies showed that PD-ECGF is thymidine phosphorylase *(52–54)*. The mechanism by which PD-ECGF induces angiogenesis is unclear. PD-ECGF hydrolyzes thymidine to thymine 2′-deoxy-D-ribose-1-phosphate, which is subsequently dephosphorylated to 2′ deoxy-D-ribose. The sugar moiety is angiogenic in the chicken-chorioallantoic membrane assay *(54,55)*. In normal lung, PD-ECGF expression is invariably seen in alveolar macrophages and occasionally in bronchiolar epithelium. Weak immunoreactivity is seen in bronchial basal and differentiated columnar cells and also in stromal fibroblasts *(56)*. PD-ECGF overexpression is seen in breast *(57)*, colorectal *(58–60)*, esophageal *(61)*, ovarian *(62)*, and renal cell *(63)* cancers associated with angiogenesis, and/or advanced disease and, less commonly, with a poor outcome. We have demonstrated high PD-ECGF tumor cell immunoreactivity in 72/223 (32.3%) cases that correlated with angiogenesis and a poor prognosis on univariable analysis *(39)*. We have previously shown that PD-ECGF expression by stromal fibroblasts is independent of tumor cell PD-ECGF immunoreactivity and is itself associated with angiogenesis. However, high fibroblast PD-ECGF has no prognostic significance apart from a subgroup of patients with low vascular grade tumors where high expression was associated with a favorable outcome. Fibroblast PD-ECGF expression was associated with abundant stroma, suggesting that the growth factor may be a marker of an active ECM remodeling. Intense macrophage infiltration was associated with PD-ECGF expression in fibroblasts suggesting a role for these inflammatory cells in the activation of stromal fibroblasts *(64)*.

1.4.1. Significance of VEGF and PD-ECGF Co-Expression

Recent work has indicated that the co-expression of VEGF and PD-ECGF may enhance neovascularization in tumors such as breast and gastric cancer *(65,66)*. A significant association of co-expression of both VEGF and PD-ECGF has been shown to correlate with the presence of hepatic metastases *(67)*. A correlation between tumor cell VEGF and PD-ECGF positive CD68 infiltrating inflammatory cells has been observed in gastric cancer, the vessel count being significantly higher in tumors expressing both growth factors as compared to those expressing each growth factor alone *(31)*. A positive correlation between VEGF and PD-ECGF has also been reported in colorectal cancer *(59)*. In our study in NSCLC, a weak positive correlation between tumor VEGF and PD-ECGF expression was seen ($r = 0.21$; $p = 0.002$). However co-expression of the angiogenic growth factors by tumor cells was not associated with an increase in microvessel density or a worse outcome when compared to those tumors that expressed either VEGF or PD-ECGF alone analysis *(39)*. VEGF expression has also been found to correlate with that of other angiogenic growth factors such as bFGF *(68)* and tissue factor (TF) *(69)* in NSCLC where, in the latter case, co-expression was found to correlate with enhanced angiogenesis. In a further study, the expression of VEGF, PD-ECGF, and bFGF in 168 NSCLC tumors indicated that a combination of these angiogenic factors improved prognostic information. Only 43% of negative cases had lymph node metastases compared to 77% of those expressing all three growth factors *(70)*.

1.5. Analysis of VEGF Expression in Tumor Samples by Immunohistochemistry

Collectively, these results indicate that VEGF plays a central role in the pathogenesis of a significant proportion of NSCLC tumours. At present the most important isoforms of VEGF-A appear to be $VEGF_{121}$, $VEGF_{165}$, and $VEGF_{189}$ which are detectable by the VG1 MAb *(41)*. In our series high VG1 immunoreactivity correlates with the intensity of angiogenesis, as assessed by microvessel counts, and a poor prognosis (*see* later) *(39)*. Inhibition of VEGF activity with MAbs *(71)*, soluble VEGF receptors *(72)*, VEGF-receptor 2 (Flk-1/KDR) MAbs *(73)*, and selective VEGF tyrosine kinase inhibitors has shown promise in experimental in vivo models (reviewed in **ref.** *74*) and in patients *(75)* with inhibition of angiogenesis, tumor growth, and/or tumor cell invasion being recorded. These agents used alone, in combination with or following cytotoxic chemotherapy may have a role to play in the treatment of NSCLC.

We also observed that neither high VEGF or PD-ECGF expression were seen in a proportion of tumors with high MVD, emphasizing the importance of other angiogenic factors such as bFGF *(68)*, TF *(69)*, heparin-binding growth-associated molecule (HB-GAM) *(76)*, and CXC chemokines *(77)* in the induction of angiogenesis and the growth and spread of NSCLC. As such, other novel anti-angiogenic agents, including angiostatin, endostatin, TNP-470, and thalidomide, may have a role to play in the treatment of NSCLC *(74,78)*.

In all, using method 1 described herein, tissue sections were examined from 223 patients who had undergone surgery with curative intent. There were

156 squamous cell carcinomas and 67 adenocarcinomas. Forty-three tumors were stage 1a; 77, stage 1b; 22, stage IIa; 52, stage IIb; and 29, stage IIIa. Of these 183 were included in the survival analysis, patients dying within 60 d of surgery being excluded to avoid peri-operative mortality bias. The median follow-up at the time of analysis for patients alive was 3.5 yr (range 1.5–7 yr).

1.5.1. Observed VG1 Immunoreactivity Using Method 1

Using method 1, VEGF was found to be expressed by bronchiolar and differentiated columnar epithelium and alveolar macrophages in the normal lung. In contrast, stromal fibroblasts and macrophages are rarely positive. In NSCLC tumours, VEGF immunoreactive blood vessels are identified in >50% of cases. In contrast VEGF expression is seen in <10% of infiltrating lymphocytes *(41,52)*.

Using as cut-off points the 33rd and 66th percentile of the obtained scores, cases are divided into three categories, low vs medium vs high VEGF reactivity. According to the scores obtained, the low reactivity cases had 0–29% positive cells; the intermediate reactivity cases, 30–69% positive cells; and high reactivity cases, 70–100% positive cells. Using this method, the interobserver variability for VEGF immunointensity has been shown to be remarkably low ($r > 0.93, p < 0.0001$) *(39,52)*.

High VEGF immunoreactivity was seen in 104 of the 223 (46.6%) cases examined. Eighty-nine of the 223 (39.9%) were of high MVD tumors. High microvessel counts were associated with advanced T-stage ($p = 0.007$) and node-positive ($p = 0.0005$) disease. As mentioned earlier, a correlation was found between VEGF expression and high MVD ($p = 0.009$). No association was found with any of the other parameters evaluated including histology and tumor grade *(39)*.

1.6. Impact of VEGF on Overall Survival

Survival data was available on 189 patients (*see* **Fig. 1**). Univariable analysis of survival showed that T-stage (T2 vs T1; $p = 0.01$: T3 vs T2 and T1; $p = 0.0001$), N-stage (N2 vs N1; $p = 0.02$: N2 vs N0; $p = 0.0001$: N1 vs N0; $p = 0.002$); vascular grade (high vs low; $p = 0.0001$); and high tumor cell VEGF ($p = 0.02$) were of prognostic significance. T-stage ($p < 0.02$) and MVD ($p < 0.04$) remained significant on multivariable analysis.

2. Materials

2.1. Horseradish Peroxidase (HRP) Technique

1. Routinely processed, paraffin-embedded tissues, cut in 5-μm sections and mounted onto Superfrost slides.

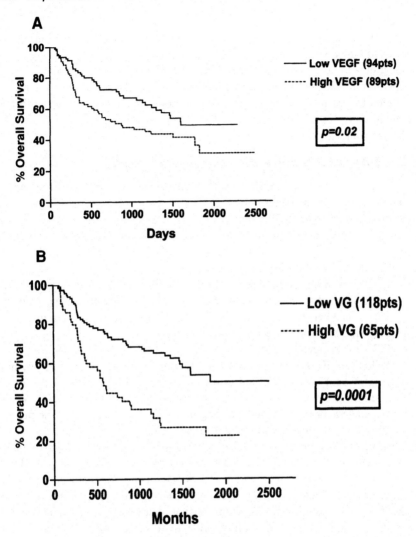

Fig. 1. Kalpan Meier's survival curves of high tumor cell VEGF vs low VEGF expressing tumors using method 1.

2. Microwave-safe plastic slide staining rack.
3. Citroclear®.
4. Dewaxing solutions: Xylene, xylene, xylene, 99% ethanol, 99% ethanol, 95% ethanol.
5. Quenching solution: 0.5% H_2O_2 in methanol (100 mL methanol containing 500 μL H_2O_2).
6. Phosphate-buffered saline (PBS).
7. Citrate buffer: 2.1 g citric acid monohydrate/L adjusted to pH 6.0 with NaOH.

8. DakoPen.
9. Primary antibody: VG1 undiluted supernatant (Clinical Sciences Laboratories, Oxford University).
10. Goat-anti-mouse immunoglobulin (Dako, Denmark). Use at 1:200.
11. HRP-conjugated rabbit anti-goat immunoglobulins (Dako). Use at 1:100.
12. Diamiobenzidine: Fast tablets (Sigma, St. Louis, MO). Use according to manufacturer's instructions.
13. Mayer's haematoxylin.

2.2. The DAKO EnVision+ Developing Technique

1. Routinely processed, paraffin-embedded tissues, cut in 5-μm sections and mounted onto Silane slides.
2. Warming oven(s) set at 37°C and 60°C.
3. Dewaxing solutions: Xylene, xylene, xylene, 99% ethanol, 99% ethanol, 95% ethanol.
4. EnVision Reagents (Dako).
   a. DAB+ substrate-chromogen solution: To each 1 mL of EnVision buffered substrate, 1 drop of EnVision DAB+ chromogen is added. The solution is mixed on a bench agitator and left at room temperature until required.
   b. EnVision blocking solution.
   c. EnVision secondary complex.
5. TRIS/EDTA, pH 9.0, buffer: Dissolve 12.12g of Trisma base (hydroxymethyl aminomethane) in 2 L distilled water on a magnetic stirrer. Once the Tris has fully dissolved, add 1.48 g EDTA (ethylenediaminetetra-acetic acid). Wearing gloves and eye protection, and working in a fume cupboard, adjust the pH of the solution to 9.0 with concentrated hydrochloric acid.
6. Tris-buffered saline (TBS): Dissolve 71.0 g of Trisma base (hydroxymethyl aminomethane) in 500 mL distilled water on a magnetic stirrer. Once the Tris has fully dissolved, add 85.0 g sodium chloride and continue to stir until dissolved. Wearing gloves and eye protection and working in a fume cupboard, adjust the pH of the solution to 7.6 with concentrated hydrochloric acid. Return to stirrer and add 4.0 g magnesium chloride and dissolve. Add 10 g bovine serum albumin (BSA) and dissolve. Half fill a 10 L container with distilled water, add concentrate and make the volume up to 10 L with distilled water.
7. Primary antibody solution: VG-1 (Oxford). Make up in TBS to a dilution of 1 in 2, mix on a bench agitator, and store at 5°C in a refrigerator until required.
8. Humidity tray.
9. Baytec® automated cover-slipper.

3. Methods

3.1. Horseradish Peroxidase (HRP) Technique

1. Cut 5-μm tissue sections from routinely processed paraffin-embedded tissues and mount onto Superfrost slides (*see* **Note 1**).

2. Perform deparaffinization using Citroclear® for 10 min and rehydrate sections in graded alcohols.
3. Incubate section in quenching solution at room temperature for 30 min, to block endogenous peroxidase activity.
4. Wash sections in PBS × 1 for 5 min.
5. Antigen retrieval is performed by immersing the tissue section slides in citrate buffer in a microwave oven for 4 min × 3 at a setting of 650W. After microwaving, slides are left for 20–30 min to cool at room temperature.
6. Apply the primary antibody to cover the whole tissue section (100–200 μL) after drawing a circle around the tissue area with a DakoPen to avoid leakage of the antibody. Incubation time is 1 h (*see* **Notes 2** and **3**).
7. Wash the section 3 times in PBS for 5 min/wash.
8. Incubate with goat-anti-mouse immunoglobulin for 30 min at room temperature.
9. Wash the section again 3 times in PBS for 5 min. The section is then incubated with HRP-conjugated rabbit anti-goat immunoglobulins for 30 min at room temperature and then washed 3 times in PBS for 5 min.
10. Develop the peroxidase reaction using diamiobenzidine as chromogen. Sections can be lightly counterstained, for 1–10 s, in haematoxylin.

3.2. The DAKO EnVision+ Developing Technique (see Note 4)

1. Cut 5-μm sections from routinely processed paraffin-embedded blocks and mounted on Silane slides.
2. Dry the slides in a warming oven at 37°C for 24 h.
3. Place the slides in a plastic staining rack suitable for use in a microwave, and dewax in an oven at 60°C for 10 min.
4. Rehydrate the slides by immersing the rack in 300 mL of graded alcohols for 3 min in each dish in the following order: xylene, xylene, xylene, 99% ethanol, 99% ethanol, 95% ethanol (*see* **Note 5**).
5. Wash the slides in running tap water for 5 min.
6. Place the rack in a plastic microwavable tray in 400 mL of Tris/EDTA, pH 9.0, buffer. Antigen retrieval is performed by microwaving the slides at full power (750W) for 15 min.
7. Place the microwavable tray in running tap water and leave the slides in the buffer until completely cool. This takes approx 20 min.
8. Prepare the EnVision DAB+ substrate-chromogen solution and the primary antibody solution.
9. When cool, the rack of slides can be washed in TBS with agitation on a magnetic stirring bench for 5 min.
10. Carefully wipe off excess buffer surrounding the tissue for each slide and place the slides in a humidity tray. The slides must not be allowed to dry out.
11. Apply two drops (or sufficient liquid to cover the whole tissue area) of EnVision blocking solution to each slide.
12. Incubate the slides at room temperature for 10 min.

13. Re-rack the slides and wash in TBS with agitation for 5 min.
14. Carefully wipe off excess buffer off each slide and place back in the humidity tray. Apply primary antibody to each slide (*see* **Note 6**). Incubate the slides at room temperature for 30 min.
15. Re-rack the slides and wash in TBS with agitation for 5 min.
16. Carefully wipe off excess buffer off each slide and place back in the humidity tray. Two drops (or sufficient liquid to cover the whole tissue area) of EnVision secondary complex are applied to each slide. Incubate the slides at room temperature for 30 min.
17. Re-rack the slides and wash in TBS with agitation for 5 min. Excess buffer is drained from the slides by pressing one edge into tissue paper and the slides are placed on glass staining racks over a sink. The slides must not be allowed to dry out.
18. Sufficient EnVision DAB Solution should be applied to each slide to flood the whole tissue. Incubate the slides at room temperature for 10 min.
19. Wash the slides thoroughly with distilled water (*see* **Note 7**).
20. Wash the racked slides in running tap water for a few seconds to remove the excess DAB.
21. Counterstain slides in 300 mL of Mayer's haematoxylin for 5 s and then immediately wash in running tap water for 3 min.
22. Dehydrate the slides by washing the rack in 300 mL of graded alcohols for 3 min in each dish in the following order: 95% ethanol, 99% ethanol, 99% ethanol, xylene, and xylene. The rack should be thoroughly drained of excess solvent between dishes.
23. Apply coverslips to each slide and allow to dry (*see* **Note 8**).

3.3. Quantitation of VEGF Immunohistochemical Analysis

The percentage of cancer cells with VEGF reactivity is assessed in all optical ×200 fields and the mean percentage is calculated, which was the final VEGF score per case (*see* **Fig. 2**).

4. Notes

1. VEGF expression has been evaluated in 5-µm tissue sections of normal lung and NSCLC tumor specimens. These were cut from routinely processed, paraffin-embedded tissue blocks retrieved from the archives of the histopathology departments from the centers involved in the study.
2. The development of anti-VEGF antibodies and the optimization of effective immunohistochemical techniques has allowed the localization of VEGF protein in normal and malignant tissues. The VG1 MAb, which recognizes the 121, 165, and 189 isoforms of VEGF, was developed in the Clinical Sciences Laboratories at Oxford University being raised using recombinant VEGF189 protein. The specificity of the antibody was confirmed using COS cells transfected with cDNA

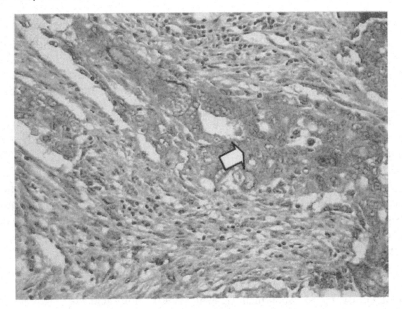

Fig. 2. High VEGF expression in a non-small cell lung cancer tumor using method 2. White arrows indicate positively stained cells.

coding for the $VEGF_{121}$, $VEGF_{165}$, and $VEGF_{189}$ isoforms of VEGF protein and by Western-blot studies *(41,51)*.

3. In our experience the antibody should be kept at 4–5°C until use and, if transported, should be placed in a cool box.
4. Method 2 is routinely employed in Leicester to utilize the quicker DAKO EnVision+ developing technique.
5. For the most efficient rehydration, the rack should be thoroughly drained of excess solvent between dishes.
6. Sufficient antibody should be used to cover the whole tissue area. In our experience, 120 µL can be used.
7. For best results, direct a slow jet of water to the end of each slide, taking care to avoid damaging the tissue.
8. In our laboratory we use the Baytec automated cover-slipper. This allows a more even application of adhesive, giving less variation in a series of slides.

References

1. van Zandwijk, N. and Giaccone, G. (1996) Treatment of metastatic non-small cell lung cancer. *Curr. Opin. Oncol.* **8,** 120–125.
2. Boyle, P. (1997) Cancer, cigarette smoking and premature death in Europe: a review including the recommendations of European Cancer Experts Consensus Meeting, Helsinki, October 1996. *Lung Cancer* **17,** 1–60.

3. Wingo, P. A., Ries, L. A. G., Giovino, G.A., et al. (1999) Annual report to the nation on the status of cancer, 1973–1996, with a special section on lung cancer and tobacco smoking. *J. Natl. Cancer Inst.* **8,** 675–690.

4. Macchiarini, P., Fontanini, G., Hardin, J. M., Squartini, F., and Angeletti, C. A. (1992) Relation of neovascularisation to metastasis of non-small cell lung cancer. *Lancet* **340,** 45–46.

5. Fontanini, G., Lucchi, M., Vignati, S., et al. (1997) Angiogenesis as a prognostic indicator of survival in non-small cell lung carcinoma: a prospective study. *J. Natl. Cancer Inst.* **89,** 881–886.

6. Giatromanolaki, A., Koukourakis, M., O'Byrne, K., et al. (1996) Prognostic value of angiogenesis in operable non-small cell lung cancer. *J. Pathol.* **179,** 80–88.

7. Fontanini, G., Vignati, S., Lucchi, M., et al. (1997) Neoangiogenesis and p53 protein in lung cancer: their prognostic role and their relation with vascular endothelial growth factor (VEGF) expression. *Br. J. Cancer* **75,** 1295–1301.

8. Cox, G., Walker, R. A., Andi, A., Steward, W. P., and O'Byrne, K. J. (2000) Prognostic significance of platelet and microvessel counts in non-small cell lung cancer. *Lung Cancer* **29,** 169–178.

9. Conn, G., Bayne, M., Soderman, L., et al. (1990) Amino acid and cDNA sequence of a vascular endothelial cell mitogen homologous to platelet-derived growth factor. *Proc. Natl. Acad. Sci. USA* **87,** 2628–2632.

10. Houck, K. A., Ferrara, N., Winer, J., et al. (1991) The vascular endothelial cell growth factor family: identification of a fourth molecular species and characterization of alternative splicing of RNA. *Mol. Endocrinol.* **5,** 1806–1814.

11. Ferrara, N. and Davis-Smyth, T. (1997) The biology of vascular endothelial growth factor. *Endocr. Rev.* **18,** 4–25.

12. Whittle, C., Gillespie, K., Harrison, R., Mathieson, P. W., and Harper, S. J. (1999) Heterogeneous vascular endothelial growth factor (VEGF) isoform mRNA and receptor mRNA expression in human glomeruli, and the identification of VEGF148 mRNA, a novel truncated splice variant. *Clin. Sci. (Colch)* **97,** 303–312.

13. Cox, G., Jones, J. L., Walker, R. A., Steward, W. P., and O'Byrne, K. J. (2000b) Angiogenesis and non-small cell lung cancer. *Lung Cancer* **27,** 81–100.

14. Clauss, M. (2001) Molecular biology of the VEGF and VEGF receptor family. *Semin. Thromb. Hemost.* **26,** 561–569.

15. deVries, C., Escobedo, J. A., Ueno, H., et al. (1992) The fms-like tyrosine kinase, a receptor for vascular endothelial growth factor. *Science* **255,** 989–991.

16. Terman, B. I., Dougher, V. M., Carrion, M. E., et al. (1992) Identification of the KDR tyrosine kinase as a receptor for vascular endothelial cell growth factor. *Biochem. Biophys. Res. Commun.* **187,** 1579–1586.

17. Gitay-Goren, H., Soker, S., Vlodavsky, I., et al. (1992) The binding of vascular endothelial growth factor to its receptors is dependent on cell surface-associated heparin-like molecules. *J. Biol. Chem.* **267,** 6093–6098.

18. Boocock, C. A., Carnock-Jones, D. S., Sharkey, A. M., et al. (1995) Expression of vascular endothelial growth factor and its receptors flt and KDR in ovarian carcinoma. *J. Natl. Cancer Inst.* **87,** 506–516.

19. Semenza, G. L. (1996) Transcriptional regulation by hypoxia-inducible factor 1-molecular mechanisms in oxygen homeostasis. *Trends Cardiovasc. Med.* **6,** 151–157.

20. Tsai, J.-C., Goldman, C. K., and Gillespie, G. Y. (1995) Vascular endothelial growth factor in human glioma cell lines: induced secretion by EGF, PDGF-BB, and bFGF. *J. Neurosurg.* **82,** 864–873.

21. Li, J., Perella, M. A., Tsai, J.-C., et al. (1990) Induction of vascular endothelial growth factor gene expression by interleukin-1β in rat aortic smooth muscle cells. *J. Biol. Chem.* **270,** 308–312.

22. Waltenberger, J., Mayr, U., Pentz, S., et al. (1996) Functional upregulation of vascular endothelial growth factor receptor KDR by hypoxia. *Circulation* **94,** 1647–1654.

23. Mukhopadhyay, D., Tsiokas, L., and Sukhatme, V. P. (1995) Wild-type p53 and v-Src exert opposing influences on human vacular endothelial growth factor gene expression. *Cancer Res.* **55,** 6161–6165.

24. Keiser, A., Weich, H. A., Brandner, G., et al. (1994) Mutant p53 potentiates protein kinase C induction of vascular endothelial growth factor expression. *Oncogene* **9,** 964–969.

25. O'Byrne, K. J. and Dalgleish, A. G. (2001) Chronic immune activation and inflammation as the cause of malignancy. *Br. J. Cancer* **17,** 473–483.

26. Gabrilovich, D. I., Ishida, T., Nadaf, S., Ohm, J. E., and Carbone, D. P. (1999) Antibodies to vascular endothelial growth factor enhance the efficacy of cancer immunotherapy by improving endogenous dendritic cell function. *Clin. Cancer Res.* **5,** 2963–2970.

27. Ohm, J. E. and Carbone, D. P. (2001) VEGF as a mediator of tumor-associated immunodeficiency. *Immunol. Res.* **23,** 263–272.

28. Gasparini, G., Toi, M., Gion, M., et al. (1997) Prognostic significance of vascular endothelial growth factor protein in node-negative breast carcinoma. *J. Natl. Cancer Inst.* **89,** 139–147.

29. Takahashi, Y., Bucana, C. D., Cleary, K. R., and Ellis, L. M. (1998a) p53, vessel count, and vascular endothelial growth factor expression in human colon cancer. *Int. J. Cancer* **79,** 34–38.

30. Inoue, K., Ozeki, Y., Suganuma, T., Sugiura, Y., and Tanaka, S. (1997) Vascular endothelial growth factor expression in primary esophegeal squamous cell carcinoma. Association with angiogenesis and tumor progression. *Cancer* **77,** 858–863.

31. Takahashi, Y., Bucana, C. D., Akagi, Y., et al. (1998) Significance of platelet-derived endothelial cell growth factor in the angiogenesis of human gastric cancer. *Clin. Cancer Res.* **4,** 429–434.

32. Hartenbach, E. M., Olson, T. A., Goswitz, J. J., Mohanraj, D., Twiggs, L. B., Carson, L. F., and Ramakrishnan, S. (1997) Vascular endothelial growth factor (VEGF) expression and survival in human epithelial ovarian carcinomas. *Cancer Lett.* **121,** 169–175.

33. Volm, M., Koomagi, R., and Mattern, J. (1996) Interrelationships between microvessel density, expression of VEGF and resistance to doxoresistance of non-small cell lung carcinoma. *Anticancer Res.* **16,** 213–218.

34. Mattern, J., Koomagi, R., and Volm, M. (1996) Association of vascular endothelial growth factor expression with intratumoral microvessel density and tumour cell proliferation in human epidermoid lung carcinoma. *Br. J. Cancer* **73,** 931–934.
35. Oshika, Y., Nakamura, M., Tokunaga, T., et al. (1998) Expression of cell-associated isoform of vascular endothelial growth factor 189 and its prognostic relevance in non-small cell lung cancer. *Int. J. Oncol.* **12,** 541–544.
36. Volm, M., Rittgen, W., and Drings, P. (1998) Prognostic value of ERBB-1, VEGF, cyclin A, FOS, JUN and MYC in patients with squamous cell lung carcinomas. *Br. J. Cancer* **77,** 663–669.
37. Fontanini, G., Boldrini, L., Chine, S., Pisaturo, F., Basolo, F., Calcinai, A., et al. (1999) Expression of vascular endothelial growth factor mRNA in non-small cell lung carcinomas. *Br. J. Cancer* **79,** 363–369.
38. Han, H., Silverman, J. F., Santucci, T. S., et al. (2001) Vascular endothelial growth factor expression in stage I non-small cell lung cancer correlates with neoangiogenesis and a poor prognosis. *Ann. Surg. Oncol.* **8,** 72–79.
39. O'Byrne, K. J., Koukourakis, M. I., Giatromanolaki, A., et al. (2000) Vascular endothelial growth factor, platelet-derived endothelial cell growth factor and angiogenesis in non-small cell lung cancer. *Br. J. Cancer* **82,** 1427–1432.
40. Giatromanolaki, A., Koukourakis, M. I., Sivridis, E., O'Byrne, K., Gatter, K. C., and Harris, A. L. (2000) 'Invading edge vs inner' (edvin) patterns of vascularisation: an interplay between angiogenic and vascular survival factors defines the clinical behaviour of non-small cell lung cancer. *J. Pathol.* **192,** 140–149.
41. Turley, H., Scott, P. A. E., Watts, V. M., Bicknall, R., Harris, A. L., and Gatter, K. C. (1998) Expression of VEGF in routinely fixed material using a new monoclonal antibody VG1. *J. Pathol.* **186,** 313–318.
42. Cheung, N., Wong, M. P., Yeun, S. T., Leung, S. Y., and Chung, L. P. (1998) Tissue-specific expression pattern of vascular endothelial growth factor isoforms in the malignant transformation of lung and colon. *Hum. Pathol.* **29,** 910–914.
43. Ohta, Y., Endo, Y., Tanaka, M., et al. (1996) Significance of vascular endothelial growth factor messanger RNA expression in primary lung cancer. *Clin. Cancer Res.* **2,** 1411–1416.
44. Yuan, A., Yu, C. J., Chen, W. J., et al. (2000) Correlation of total VEGF mRNA and protein expression with histologic type, tumor angiogenesis, patient survival and timimg of relapse in non-small cell lung cancer. *Int. J. Cancer* **89,** 475–483.
45. Baillie, R., Carlile, J., Pendleton, N., and Schor, A. M. (2001) Prognostic value of vascularity and vascular endothelial growth factor expression in non-small cell lung cancer. *J. Clin. Pathol.* **54,** 116–120.
46. Oshika, Y., Nakamura, M., Tokunaga, T., et al. (2000) Ribozyme approach to downregulate vascular endothelial growth factor (VEGF) 189 expression in non-small cell lung cancer (NSCLC). *Eur. J. Cancer* **36,** 2390–2396.
47. Koukourakis, M. I., Giaromanolaki, A., O'Byrne, K. J., Whitehouse, R. M., Talbot, D. C., Gatter, K. C., and Harris, A. L. (1997b) Potential role of bcl-2 as a suppressor of tumour angiogenesis in non-small cell lung cancer. *Int. J. Cancer* **74,** 565–570.

48. Fontanini, G., Boldrini, L., Vignati, S., et al. (1998) Bcl-2 and p53 regulate vascular endothelial growth factor (VEGF)-mediated angiogenesis in non-small cell lung carcinoma. *Eur. J. Cancer* **34,** 718–723.

49. Ambs, S., Bennett, W. P., Merriam, W. G., et al. (2000) Vascular endothelial growth factor and nitric oxide synthase expression in human lung cancer and the relation to p53. *Br. J. Cancer* **78,** 233–239.

50. Kang, S. M., Maeda, K., Onoda, N., et al. (1997) Combined analysis of p53 and vascular endothelial growth factor expression in colorectal carcinoma for determination of tumor vascularity and liver metastasis. *Int. J. Cancer* **74,** 502–507.

51. Giatromanolaki, A., Koukourakis, M. I., Kakolyris, S., et al (1998) Vascular endothelial growth factor, wild-type p53 and angiogenesis in early operable non-small cell lung cancer. *Clin. Cancer Res.* **4,** 3017–3024.

52. Ishikawa, F., Miyazono, K., Hellman, U., et al. (1989) Identification of angiogenic activity and the cloning and expression of platelet-derived endothelial cell growth factor. *Nature* **338,** 557–562.

53. Moghaddam, A. and Bicknell, R. (1992) Expression of platelet-derived endothelial cell growth factor in *Escherichia coli* and confirmation of its thymidine phosphorylase activity. *Biochemistry* **31,** 12141–12146.

54. Moghaddam, A., Zhang, H. T., Fan, T. P. D., et al. (1995) Thymidine phosphorylase is angiogenic and promotes tumour growth. *Proc. Natl. Acad. Sci. USA* **92,** 998–1002.

55. Haraguchi, M., Miyadera, K., Uemura, K., et al. (1994) Angiogenic activity of enzymes. *Nature* **368,** 198.

56. Giatromanolaki, A., Koukourakis, M., Comley, M., et al. (1997a) Platelet derived endothelial cell growth factor (thymidine phosphorylase) expression in lung cancer. *J. Pathol.* **181,** 196–199.

57. Toi, M., Hosina, S., Taniguchi, T., Yamamoto, Y., Ishitsuka, H., and Tominaga, T. (1995a) Expression of platelet-derived endothelial cell growth factor/thymidine phosphorylase in human breast cancer. *Int. J. Cancer* **64,** 79–82.

58. Saeki, T., Tanada, M., Takashima, S., et al. (1997) Correlation between expression of platelet-derived endothelial cell growth factor (thymidine phosphorylase) and microvessel density in early-stage human colon carcinomas. *Jpn. J. Clin. Oncol.* **27,** 227–230.

59. Amaya, H., Tanigawa, N., Lu, C., et al. (1997) Association of vascular endothelial growth factor expression with tumor angiogenesis, survival and thymidine phosphorylase/platelet derived endothelial cell growth factor expression in human colorectal cancer. *Cancer Lett.* **119,** 227–235.

60. Takebayashi, Y., Akiyama, S., Akiba, S., et al. (1996) Clinicopathologic and prognostic significance of an angiogenic factor, thymidine phosphorylase, in human colorectal carcinoma. *J. Natl. Cancer Inst.* **88,** 1110–1117.

61. Igarashi, M., Dhar, D. K., Kubota, H., Yamamoto, A., El-Assal, O., and Nagasue, N. (1998) The prognostic significance of microvessel density and thymidine phosphorylase expression in squamous cell carcinoma of the esophagus. *Cancer* **82,** 1225–1232.

62. Fujimoto, J., Ichigo, S., Sakaguchi, H., Hirose, R., and Tamaya, T. (1998) Expression of platelet-derived endothelial cell growth factor (PD-ECGF) and its mRNA in ovarian cancers. *Cancer Lett.* **126,** 83–88.

63. Imazano, Y., Takebayashi, Y., Nishiyama, K., et al. (1997) Correlation between thymidine phosphorylase expression and prognosis in human renal cell carcinoma. *J. Clin. Oncol.* **15,** 2570–2578.

64. Koukourakis, M. I., Giatromanolaki, A., Kakolyris, S., et al. (1998) Different pattern of stromal and cancer cell thymidine phosphorylase reactivity in non small cell lung cancer. Impact on tumour neoangiogenesis and survival. *Br. J. Cancer* **77,** 1696–1703.

65. Toi, M., Hosina, S., Taniguchi, T., Yamamoto, Y., Ishitsuka, H., and Tominaga, T. (1995) Vascular endothelial growth factor and platelet derived endothelial cell growth factor are frequently coexpressed in highly vascularized human breast cancer. *Clin. Cancer Res.* **1,** 961–964.

66. Giatromanolaki, A., Koukourakis, M. I., Stathopoulos, G. P., et al. (2000) Angiogenic interactions of vascular endothelial growth factor, of thymidine phosphorylase, and of p53 protein expression in locally advanced gastric cancer. *Oncol. Res.* **12,** 33–41.

67. Maeda, K., Kang, S. M., Ogawa, M., et al. (1997) Combined analysis of vascular endothelial growth factor and platelet-derived endothelial cell growth factor expression in gastric carcinoma. *Int. J. Cancer* **74,** 545–550.

68. Mattern, J., Koomagi, R., and Volm, M. (1997) Coexpression of VEGF and bFGF in human epidermoid lung carcinoma is associated with increased vascular density. *Anticancer Res.* **17,** 2249–2252.

69. Koomagi, R. and Volm, M. (1998) Tissue-factor expression in human non-small-cell lung carcinoma measured by immunohistochemistry: correlation between tissue factor and angiogenesis. *Int. J. Cancer* **79,** 19–22.

70. Volm, M., Koomagi, R., and Mattern, J. (1999) PD-ECGF, bFGF, and VEGF expression in non-small cell lung carcinomas and their association with lymph node metastsis. *Anticancer Res.* **19,** 651–655.

71. Kim, K. J., Li, B., Winer, J., et al. (1993) Inhibition of vascular endothelial growth factor-induced angiogenesis suppresses tumour growth in vivo. *Nature* **362,** 841–844.

72. Lin, P., Sanka, S., Shan, S., et al. (1998) Inhibition of tumor growth by targeting tumor endothelium using a soluble vascular endothelial growth factor receptor. *Cell Growth Diff.* **9,** 49–58.

73. Skobe, M., Rockwell, P., Goldstein, N., Vosseler, S., and Fusenig, N. E. (1997) Halting angiogenesis suppresses carcinoma cell invasion. *Nature Med.* **3,** 1222–1227.

74. O'Byrne, K. J. and Steward, W. P. (2001) Tumour angiogenesis: a novel therapeutic target in patients with malignant disease. *Emerg. Drugs* **6,** 155–174.

75. Thomas, A. L., Morgan, B., Drevs, J., et al. (2001) Pharmacodynamic results using dynamic contrast enhanced magnetic resonance imaging, of 2 phase I studies of

the VEGF inhibitorPTK787/ZK 222584 in patients with liver metastases from colorectal cancer. *Proc. Am. Soc. Clin. Oncol.* **20,** abstract 279.

76. Jager, R., Noll, K., Havemann, K., et al. (1997) Differential expression and biological activity of the heparin-binding growth-associated molecule (HB-GAM) in lung cancer cell lines. *Int. J. Cancer* **73,** 537–543.

77. Arenberg, D. A., Polverini, P. J., Kunkel, S. L., et al. (1997) The role of CXC chemokines in the regulation of angiogenesis in non-small cell lung cancer. *J. Leukoc. Biol.* **62,** 554–562.

78. Harris, A. L. (1998) Are angiostatin and endostatin cures for cancer? Commentary. *Lancet* **351,** 1598–1599.

27

Regulation of Angiostatin Mobilization by Tumor-Derived Matrix Metalloproteinase-2

Marsha A. Moses and Michael S. O'Reilly

1. Introduction

In recent years, the observation that many endogenous angiogenesis inhibitors are fragments of larger molecules has driven significant research efforts to understand the mechanisms by which these cryptic angiogenesis inhibitors are liberated. Our interest in this area stemmed from our discovery of angiostatin *(1)*, a 38 kDa internal fragment of plasminogen that is a specific inhibitor of capillary endothelial cell proliferation in vitro and angiogenesis in vivo. By inhibiting angiogenesis, angiostatin can induce the regression of a wide variety of malignant tumors *(2)* and can induce tumor dormancy defined by a dynamic equilibrium of tumor cell apoptosis and proliferation *(3)*. Angiostatin and other angiogenesis inhibitors are currently being evaluated in cancer patients in early clinical trials in the United States and around the world *(4)*. In this chapter, we will outline the reasoning and describe the experimental strategies that we employed in the course of identifying the enzymatic processing system that results in biologically active angiostatin. We will also discuss the clinical implications of our work with regards to the ongoing clinical trials of metalloproteinase inhibitors.

In our original studies of the suppression of tumor growth by tumor mass *(1)*, we developed a variant of Lewis lung carcinoma (LLC-LM) in which a primary tumor could completely suppress the growth of its metastases by generating the angiogenesis inhibitor angiostatin from plasminogen. Angiostatin is a 38 kDa internal fragment of plasminogen and was purified from the serum and urine of mice bearing LLC-LM xenografts *(1)*. Subsequently, we have found that

From: *Methods in Molecular Medicine, vol. 74: Lung Cancer, Vol. 1: Molecular Pathology Methods and Reviews*
Edited by: B. Driscoll © Humana Press Inc., Totowa, NJ

the systemic administration of angiostatin can potently inhibit angiogenesis and can regress a wide variety of malignant tumors in vivo without resistance or toxicity *(2,3)*. However, at the time of our initial discovery of angiostatin, the source of the protein was unclear. We hypothesized that the tumor or stromal cells might produce an enzyme that could cleave plasminogen sequestered by the primary tumor into angiostatin. Alternatively, we speculated that the tumor cells might express angiostatin. By Northern analysis of the LLC-LM cells, we could find no evidence that the tumor cells expressed angiostatin or other fragments of plasminogen suggesting that angiostatin was derived from the cleavage of plasminogen by an undetermined proteinase *(1,5)*.

A review of the literature revealed support for the former hypothesis, i.e., that the LLC-LM tumor itself was producing an angiostatin-processing enzyme. Through the mid-1990s, an increasing number of studies demonstrated that a number of angiogenesis inhibitors were fragments of larger parental molecules, which themselves had little or no inhibitory effects on neovascularization *(6)*. For example, an internal 16 kDa fragment of prolactin was shown to inhibit angiogenesis, whereas the parent molecule, intact prolactin, does not *(7–10)*. Other inhibitors of EC proliferation that are fragments of larger molecules which were being reported at the time included fragments of platelet factor 4 *(11)* with enhanced antiangiogenic activity as compared to the intact molecule *(12)*, thrombospondin *(13)*, epidermal growth factor (EGF) *(14)*, laminin *(15)*, fibronectin *(16)*, and endostatin *(17,18)*.

Simultaneously, a second literature was emerging that documented that members of a family of metal-dependent endopeptidases, the metalloprotein-ases, could process precursor or parent proteins into their bioactive form. Metalloproteinases (MMPs) were implicated in the processing of the tumor necrosis factor-α (TNF-α) precursor protein *(19,20)*, transforming growth factor-α (TGF-α) *(21)*, the Aβ precursor protein (APP) *(22)*, the lymphocyte L-selectin adhesion molecule *(23–25)*, the interleukin-6 (IL-6) receptor ectodomain *(26)*, the human thyrotropin receptor ectodomain *(27)*, the fibroblast growth factor receptor 1 (FGFR1) ectodomain *(28)*, and EGF-like growth factor *(29)*. Taken together, these studies show that MMPs can process a wide range of substrates, many of which play an indirect role in angiogenesis. We therefore chose to study the role that MMPs might play in the processing of plasminogen into the angiogenesis inhibitor angiostatin.

It was essential that we first determine whether or not LLC-LM cells were secreting metalloproteinase activity. We identified active gelatinase A (matrix metalloproteinase-2; MMP-2) in the conditioned media from the tumor's cells and then determined that it could process plasminogen into angiostatin that was nearly identical to that which we originally described *(1,5)*. In order to do this, it was necessary for us to actually purify to homogeneity that angiostatin and demonstrate that, on the basis of its amino acid sequence and its biological activity in vitro, it was similar to the angiostatin we had previously isolated. Finally, and perhaps most importantly, we confirmed that by specifically neutralizing the enzymatic activity, we could block the mobilization of angiostatin from plasminogen by the tumor cells in our in vitro systems.

The production of angiostatin by gelatinase A from the tumor cells helps to resolve the question as to why a primary tumor might be producing angiostatin. By increased production of gelatinase A, the tumor may become more locally invasive. However, our findings clearly demonstrate that gelatinase A can also mobilize angiostatin (5). It may therefore be prudent to consider gelatinase A and other metalloproteinase inhibitors and metalloproteinases themselves as angiogenesis modulators instead of merely inhibitors or stimulators. We propose that angiogenesis may depend not only on the balance of endothelial stimulators and inhibitors but also on the balance of matrix-degrading proteases and their endogenous inhibitors. In addition, the increased permeability of the tumor vessels may lead to the sequestration of circulating plasminogen into the tumor's neostroma (30,31) that could then be cleaved into active angiostatin.

Subsequent work has demonstrated that a variety of metalloproteinases and other enzymes that are important in tumor progression can cleave angiostatin from plasminogen (32–37). Thus, metalloproteinases and other enzymes can play a central role in the regulation of tumor angiogenesis and potentially act in an inhibitory (38,39) or a stimulatory capacity. By studying and defining the coordinate regulation of angiogenesis and metalloproteinase activity in biological systems, a better understanding of the control of angiogenesis will be possible. Further, the finding that angiogenesis inhibitors can be mobilized and/or activated by metalloproteinases suggests that therapeutic strategies for using inhibitors of metalloproteinase and other enzymatic activities must be carefully designed to consider both the clinical context and the cumulative effect on angiogenesis. It will also be necessary to develop a variety of directly relevant diagnostic and clinical strategies (40,41) in order that these inhibitors can be successfully incorporated into clinical practice.

It has been widely suggested that the limited clinical success of broad-spectrum MMP inhibitors is due, at least in part, to their lack of specificity and associated side effects. However, we have suggested that an alternate explanation is that the regulation of MMP activity may, in some cases, decrease the release of angiogenesis inhibitors. This possibility suggests that it will be important to define, for each different tumor type, the precise roles of MMPs and their inhibitors in the modulation of angiogenesis and malignancy.

2. Materials

All chemicals used should be of highest quality and purity. Double-distilled and autoclaved water should be used in all cases except as noted. Buffers are made fresh from stock solutions, sterile-filtered, and then stored at 4°C, with the exception of the 0.3 M phosphate buffer, which is stored at room temperature. Buffers are typically used within 1–2 d of preparation. Calcium- and magnesium-free phosphate-buffered saline (PBS) is used in all studies.

2.1. Isolation and Maintenance of LLC-LM Cell Lines

1. 6–8-wk-old C57Bl/6 mice (Jackson Laboratories) bearing 2,000 mm³ LLC-LM tumors of the subcutaneous dorsa. All mice were obtained from Jackson Laboratories and were maintained in the animal facility of Children's Hospital, Boston. Institutional and governmental guidelines and policies were strictly followed. Mice were maintained in groups of 4 or less and were given water and food ad libitum. During all studies, mice were monitored on a daily basis.
2. Ethanol.
3. Betadiene.
4. Dissection instruments (scalpel, dissecting scissors, iris scissors, fine forceps).
5. Cellector fine sieve (VWR Scientific).
6. Phosphate-buffered saline (PBS, calcium- and magnesium-free): 1X powder (Sigma).
7. 20-, 22-, 23-, 25-, 26-, and 30-gauge needles.
8. Antibiotic supplemented medium: Dulbecco's modified Eagle's medium (DMEM) with 3% glutamine penicillin and streptomycin (GPS), 25-fold dilution.
9. Culture medium: DMEM supplemented with 10% heat-inactivated fetal calf serum (FCS, 56°C for 20 min) and 1% GPS.
10. FCS should be used for the Lewis lung carcinoma cells. Serum should be heat-inactivated in a water bath at 56°C for 20 min with frequent mixing. Once cooled, serum can be stored at –20°C.

2.2. Collection of Conditioned Media

1. Trypsin-EDTA: 0.05% trypsin, 0.53 mM EDTA in PBS.

2.3. Substrate Gel Electrophoresis (Zymography)

1. Type I gelatin or commercially available pre-cast gels for zymography.
2. Standard Laemmli acrylamide polymerization mixture.
3. Substrate sample buffer: 10% sodium dodecyl sulfate (SDS), 4% sucrose, 0.25 M Tris-HCl, pH 6.8, and 0.1% bromophenol blue.
4. 2.5% Triton X-100.
5. Substrate buffer: 50 mM Tris-HCl buffer, pH 8, 5 mM CaCl$_2$ and 0.02% NaN$_3$.
6. Zymogram stain: 0.5% Coomassie Blue R-250 in acetic acid:isopropyl alcohol:water (1:3:6, v:v:v).

7. Destain in acetic acid: isopropyl alcohol: water (1:3:6).
8. 10 m*M* aminophenylmercuric acetate (APMA).

2.4. Endothelial Cell Proliferation Assay

Only double-distilled autoclaved water should be used to prepare reagents (PBS, 1.5% gelatin, and media) for endothelial cell culture.

1. Gelatinized coated 6-well tissue culture plastic dishes and 24-well culture plates: Incubate dishes with 1.5% gelatin (Gibco) in PBS for 12–24 h at 37°C and 10% CO_2 and then wash with 0.5 mL of PBS. PBS and 1.5% gelatin in PBS should be autoclaved immediately after they are made and can then be stored at room temperature under sterile conditions.
2. Endothelial growth medium: DMEM supplemented with 10% heat-inactivated bovine calf serum (BCS; serum should be heat-inactivated in a water bath at 56°C for 20 min with frequent mixing. Once cooled, serum can be stored at –20°C.), 1% GPS, and 3 ng/mL human recombinant basic fibroblast growth factor (bFGF, obtained commercially and stored at –80°C after aliquoting). Medium should be fresh when needed but can be stored at 4°C for periods of up to 72 h if serum is in the media.
3. Hematall (Coulter Corporation or Fisher).

2.5. Isolation and Purification of Human Plasminogen

All reagents should be of high-performance liquid chromatography (HPLC)-grade only used for the purposes of purification. Reagents should be stored at room temperature and kept tightly sealed when not in use.

1. Recovered outdated human plasma.
2. 0.45-µm filter.
3. Lysine Sepharose HPLC column (2 mL lysine Sepharose, Pharmacia, Uppsala, Sweden).
4. 0.3 *M* phosphate buffer, 0.003 *M* EDTA, pH 7.4.
5. 0.2 *M* aminocaproic acid, pH 7.4.
6. Chloroform.
7. Dialysis tubing: MWCO = 6–8,000.
8. 20 m*M* Tris-HCl, pH 7.6.
9. Reducing SDS-polyacrilamide gel electrophoresis (PAGE) gel, 12% acrylamide (Bio-Rad).
10. Nonreducing SDS-PAGE gel, 12% acrylamide (Bio-Rad).
11. Silver stain (any standard reagent and technique will suffice).

2.6. Processing and Purification of Angiostatin

1. MMP-2 (Provided by Dr. William G. Stetler-Stevenson).
2. 50 m*M* phosphate buffer, pH 7.4.
3. Spin concentrator, 4,000 MW cut off (Gelman Scientific).

4. SynChropak RP-4 (100 mm × 4.6 mm) reverse-phase HPLC column.
5. 0.1% trifluoroacetic acid (TFA) in H_2O.
6. TFA in acetonitrile (CH_3CN).

2.7. MMP-2 Neutralization Experiments

1. Rabbit anti-gelatinase A (anti-IVase) (Provided by Dr. William G. Stetler-Stevenson).

3. Methods

The focus of these chapters is to provide detailed procedures that will assist scientists to conduct similar studies in a particular subject area. We have therefore expanded the descriptions of the methods utilized in our original report identifying gelatinase A (Matrix Metalloproteinase-2; MMP-2), produced directly by the LLC-LM cells, as being responsible for the production of angiostatin in our in vivo model *(5)* described below.

3.1. Isolation and Maintenance of LLC-LM Cell Lines

1. LLC-LM lines are isolated from tumors growing in 6–8-wk-old C57Bl/6 mice (Jackson Laboratories) using aseptic technique as has been previously described *(1,42)*. Mice bearing 2,000 mm³ LLC-LM tumors of the subcutaneous dorsa are screened for evidence of visible lung metastases.
2. Mice without evidence of gross metastatic disease on autopsy are selected and the skin overlying the tumors is cleaned with three washes each of ethanol alternating with betadiene.
3. Tumor-bearing mice are then transferred to a laminar flow hood and the tumors draped with sterile gauze. The skin overlying the tumors is dissected sharply using a scalpel to expose the underlying tumor tissue.
4. The tumors are then visually inspected and removed in toto with dissecting scissors and transferred to a sterile field.
5. Viable tumor tissue (*see* **Note 1**), from the periphery of the tumors, is removed using iris scissors and fine forceps and then strained through a fine sieve.
6. Add approx 1 mL PBS for each 100 mg of tumor tissue and the pass the tumor cell suspension sequentially through a series of 20-, 22-, 23-, 25-, 26-, and 30-gauge needles (*see* **Note 2**).
7. Add the tumor cell suspension to antibiotic supplemented DMEM and centrifuge at 200g for 10 min.
8. Resuspend the cell pellet in culture medium and place in a 37°C in a 10% CO_2 incubator. Replace the media 12 h later and then at intervals of 3 d thereafter. Subculture cells when confluent.

3.2. Collection of Conditioned Media

1. Wash cells with PBS. Add trypsin-EDTA (0.05% trypsin, 0.53 m*M* EDTA) until the cells start to disperse.

2. Add growth medium and re-plate cells in T25 or T75 flasks and return to the incubator.
3. Prepare serum-free CM by washing nearly confluent cells with sterile PBS (3 washes) and then adding DMEM (2–3 mL of media for a T25 flask or 6–8 mL of media for a T75 flask) and 1% GPS for 24 h (*see* **Note 3**).
4. Collect the conditioned media and centrifuge at 2500*g* for 20 min.
5. Filter supernatant through a 0.45-µm filter and store at 4°C if it is to be used within 72 h or frozen at –20°C.

3.3. Substrate Gel Electrophoresis (Zymography)

Substrate gel electrophoresis is conducted according to the method of Herron and coworkers as modified by us *(43,44)*. If necessary, activate latent MMPs by incubating samples with APMA at a final concentration of 2 m*M* for 1 h at 37°C (*see* **Note 4**).

1. Add Type I gelatin to the standard Laemmli acrylamide polymerization mixture (10% acrylamide) to a final concentration of 1 mg/mL, or use commercially available zymography gel.
2. Mix samples with substrate sample buffer and load without boiling into wells of the zymography gel. Run gel at approx 15 mA/gel while stacking and at 20 mA/gel during the resolving phase at 4°C.
3. After electrophoresis, soak the gels in 2.5% Triton X-100 with gentle shaking for 30 min at ambient temperature with one change of detergent solution.
4. Rinse the gel and incubate overnight at 37°C in substrate buffer.
5. Stain the gel for 15–30 min then destain and photograph.

3.4. Endothelial Cell Proliferation Assay

Primary cultures of bovine capillary endothelial cells (BCE) were derived from the adrenal gland *(37,45)*. Please consult references, as a description of the methods for isolation of endothelial cells is beyond the scope of this chapter. The inhibition assay was performed as previously described *(1,37,44)*.

1. Maintain cells on gelatin coated 6-well tissue culture plastic dishes in endothelial growth medium (*see* **Note 5**). Media should be replaced every 3 d and cells split with a dilution of 1:6 or less when confluent.
2. Near confluent or confluent endothelial cells growing in 6-well dishes are washed with PBS (2 mL/well) and then 0.5 mL/well of trypsin-EDTA is added until the cells just start to disperse.
3. Add DMEM supplemented with 10% BCS and 1% GPS to cells and plate onto gelatinized 24-well culture plates (12,500 cells/well confirmed by hemocytometer count) and incubate at 37°C in 10% CO_2 for 24 h.
4. Replace media with 0.25 mL of DMEM supplemented with 5% BCS and 1% GPS and add test samples. After 20 min incubation, add 0.25 mL of DMEM supple-

mented with 5% BCS and 1% GPS and 2 ng/mL bFGF to each well to obtain
a final volume of 0.5 mL of DMEM with 5% BCS and 1% GPS and 1 ng/mL
bFGF.

5. After incubation for 72 h, aspirate media and disperse cells by adding 0.5 mL
   trypsin-EDTA.
6. Resuspend dispersed capillary endothelial cells in Hematall to achieve a final
   volume of 10 mL, and count electronically with a Coulter cell counter. Each
   sample should be tested at least in triplicate and all procedures reproduced at
   least once.

3.5. Isolation and Purification of Human Plasminogen

Human plasminogen is purified from outdated human plasma (obtained
from the blood bank of Children's Hospital Boston) *(46,47)* using a method
modified from those previously described *(48–50)*.

1. Centrifuge recovered outdated human plasma (*see* **Note 6**) at 9000g for 30 min.
   Filtered supernatant through a 0.45-μm filter and dilute twofold with cold PBS.
2. Apply diluted plasma a lysine Sepharose column at 4°C that has been equilibrated
   with PBS at a flow rate of 150–200 mL/h.
3. After applying the diluted plasma, re-equilibrate column with PBS at 4°C,
   followed by 0.3 M phosphate buffer in 0.003 M EDTA, pH 7.4, at room
   temperature.
4. Elute bound plasminogen using 0.2 M aminocaproic acid, pH 7.4, at 4°C. It
   should elute as a single peak.
5. Dilute the eluant with an equal volume of chloroform and centrifuge the mixture
   at 200g to separate the aqueous phase.
6. Remove the aqueous phase and dialyze extensively against 20 mM Tris-HCl,
   pH 7.6.
7. Confirm the purity of the plasminogen by SDS-PAGE with silver stain as greater
   than 99% under both reducing and non-reducing conditions.

3.6. Processing and Purification of Angiostatin

Having demonstrated that LLC-LM cells produce gelatinase A, they can
next be tested for the ability of the conditioned media to process human
plasminogen to angiostatin.

1. Incubate purified plasminogen with 125 ml of serum-free LLC-LM conditioned
   media (*see* **Note 7**) obtained as described (*see* **Subheading 3.4.**), or serum-free
   control media not conditioned by cells but identically treated otherwise as a
   control. Controls may also include MMP-2 *(44)*. It is imperative that the MMP-2
   to be utilized be tested by zymography to determine its activity status, i.e., the
   enzyme must be in its active form during the incubation. To the extent that
   the preparation is in its latent form, it should then be activated as described

(*see* **Subheading 3.3.**), before incubation with the plasminogen. Employ sterile technique throughout. Incubate samples at 37°C for 72 h with gentle rocking.

2. Following incubation, place test samples or control samples on ice and then apply to a lysine-Sepharose column equilibrated with 50 mM phosphate buffer, pH 7.4, at 4°C. Following application of the sample, re-equilibrate column with 50 mM phosphate buffer, pH 7.4, followed by PBS until the baseline (A_{280}) is stable.

3. Samples are fractionated by elution with 0.2 M aminocaproic acid and bound plasminogen should elute as a single broad peak from the column.

4. All fractions eluted from the lysine affinity column which contain protein as measured spectrophotometrically at A_{280} are pooled, and concentrated to a volume of less than 1 mL in a spin concentrator.

5. Apply concentrated sample to a SynChropak RP-4 reverse-phase HPLC column that was first equilibrated with 0.1% TFA.

6. Elute protein using a continuous gradient of 0.1% TFA in H_2O to TFA in acetonitrile (CH_3CN) (*see* **Notes 8 and 9**).

7. Immediately concentrate aliquots of each fraction by vacuum centrifugation and then resuspend in H_2O or PBS. Test aliquots for the ability to inhibit BCE cell proliferation stimulated by bFGF in an in vitro endothelial cell-proliferation bioassay as described in **Subheading 3.4.** (*see* **Note 10**).

8. Fractions should also be analyzed on SDS-PAGE gels under reducing and nonreducing conditions followed by silver staining according to standard protocols (*see* **Note 8**).

9. Purified angiostatin can also be subjected to protein microsequencing (*see* **Note 11**).

3.7. MMP-2 Neutralization Experiments

It is absolutely essential that the possibility that other enzymes in the conditioned media might be responsible for the production of angiostatin be addressed. Among the most rigorous approaches to accomplishing this is via the use of monospecific, immunoneutralizing antibodies to the enzyme of interest, in this case, gelatinase A. A series of neutralization experiments using a blocking polyclonal antibody (PAb) raised against gelatinase A (anti-IVase), which has been shown to specifically block the proteolytic activity of MMP-2 *(44)*, is described.

1. LLC-LM conditioned media is preincubated with anti-IVase) *(44)*, at a ratio of 1:50 (antibody:CM) at 37°C, for 10 min.

2. Incubate this mixture with intact human plasminogen as described (*see* **Subheading 3.5.**) Controls should include a sample of LLC-LM conditioned media preincubated and incubated with human plasminogen under the same conditions but in the absence of the neutralizing antisera.

3. Following the incubation with human plasminogen, samples from each of the treatment groups are fractionated over a lysine Sepharose affinity column,

followed by reverse-phase HPLC chromatography using a SynChropak RP-4 (100 mm × 4.6 mm) column (*see* **Note 8**) as described (*see* **Subheading 3.5.**).

4. Immediately concentrate aliquots of each fraction by vacuum centrifugation and then resuspend in H_2O or PBS. Test aliquots for the ability to inhibit BCE cell proliferation stimulated by bFGF in an in vitro endothelial cell proliferation bioassay as described in **Subheading 3.4.** (*see* **Note 10**).

5. Fractions should also be analyzed on SDS-PAGE gels under reducing and nonreducing conditions followed by silver staining according to standard protocols (*see* **Notes 8** and **12**).

4. Notes

1. It is critical to select viable tumor tissue and to avoid tumor that may have had small ulcerations or compromise. Tumors should be visually inspected and then dissected sharply. Viable tumor tissue is generally found at the periphery and appears as a gray solid tissue. Necrotic and fibrotic tissue should be carefully dissected away and tumor tissue then rinsed with sterile PBS. Tumor isolation should be performed under laminar flow using meticulous sterile technique

2. The tumor cell suspension should be passed through a series of sequentially smaller diameter needles as described. The final needle, 30-gauge, acts as a filter and should be changed when it becomes clogged. Difficulties with passing the suspension through the larger diameter needles can occur if necrotic of fibrotic tissue is not removed as described in **Note 1**.

3. For the production of serum-free conditioned media, the use of fully confluent cells or leaving the media on the cells for periods greater than 24 h or with lower volumes of media than described was associated with diminished cell viability.

4. Zymographic analysis (method described in **Subheading 3.3.**) of conditioned media of these LLC-LM cells revealed a prominent zone of clearance, which migrated at an apparent molecular weight of approx 64 kDa, consistent with it being gelatinase A or MMP-2. Treatment with APMA did not result in a decrease in molecular weight of this proteolytic activity, suggesting that the Lewis lung carcinoma cells secrete an active MMP-2 species. It is essential to verify the identity of MMP activities using monospecific antibodies. In this case, immunoblot analysis using MMP-2-specific antibodies (Oncogene Sciences, Cambridge, MA) verified the identification of this proteolytic species as being gelatinase A. A second immunoblot using the MMP-2 specific antibody, anti-IVase *(44)* verified this identification. Treatment with 1,10 phenanthroline resulted in a total abrogation of proteolytic activity demonstrating that the 64 kDa enzyme was a metal-dependent protease *(51)*.

5. The BCE cell proliferation assay can be difficult to work with because it relies upon primary endothelial cells. Only early passage cells should be used for this assay. This is the same assay that has been used previously to characterize native and recombinant angiostatins. In our studies of angiostatin, an IC_{50} of 200 ng/mL

has been observed for native angiostatin but recombinant human angiostatin may require a significantly higher concentration.

6. For the purification of human plasminogen, recovered human plasma that had been stored for periods of less than 2 mo resulted in the optimal yield and purity of plasminogen. Citrated plasma was obtained in plastic bags containing 200–250 ml from the blood bank and kept at 4°C at all times. Plasma was pooled immediately before commencing purifications for a total volume of 1.5–2.5 L. A 2.6 × 35 cm lysine Sepharose column was optimal for this range of plasma volumes.

7. Optimal processing of plasminogen into angiostatin was obtained by combining 1 mg of human plasminogen with 125 mL of conditioned media. The mixture was incubated on a shaker at 37°C for 72 h as described in **Subheading 3.6.**

8. Angiostatin elutes from the SynChropak RP-4 reverse-phase HPLC column at a concentration of approx 25% CH_3CN, consistent with the pattern of elution that would be expected for native angiostatin. Residual plasminogen elutes at a concentration of approx 35% CH_3CN. SDS-polyacrylamide gel electrophoresis and silver staining of purified angiostatin should result in a single band migrating at 38 kDa under reducing conditions, consistent with its identification as human angiostatin. As with angiostatin derived from the urine of tumor-bearing mice, the band should migrate at approx 28 kDa when run under nonreducing conditions.

9. Gelatinase A digestion of plasminogen will generate angiostatin as a single 38 kDa peptide identical to that seen after incubation of plasminogen with the conditioned media of Lewis lung carcinoma. This is in contrast to the multiple bands with angiostatin activity seen with the digestion of plasminogen using other approaches *(32–36)*.

10. Upon assay of the fractions containing protein from the final step of each of the purifications described, we found that only the fractions containing angiostatin inhibited EC proliferation. We did not detect any significant antiproliferative activity in any of the other fractions tested. Intact plasminogen or plasmin did not have any significant effect in the endothelial cell proliferation assay.

11. The 38 kDa protein obtained from LLC-LM CM processing is purified to homogeneity as described earlier, resolved by SDS-PAGE, and electroblotted onto PVDF. Purified protein is detected by Ponceau S staining, and excised from the membrane. N-terminal sequence was determined by William S. Lane, Harvard Microchemistry Facility (Cambridge, MA) using automated Edman degradation on a PE/ABD Model 470A protein sequencer (Foster City, CA) operated with gas-phase delivery of TFA.

    Interestingly, protein microsequencing of the angiostatin mobilized from plasminogen by LLC-LM conditioned media or gelatinase A revealed an N-terminus of residues 98–99, in comparison to that reported in the original angiostatin study (amino acid residues 97–98) *(1)*. One explanation for this difference may be that the angiostatin reported in the original study was derived from murine plasminogen, whereas human plasminogen was used as a substrate in these studies. A similar shift in the N-terminal residue has been consistently observed in our studies of mouse and human angiostatin and does not affect the in vitro activity of angiostatin in the capillary endothelial cell proliferation assay.

12. SDS-PAGE analysis of the samples obtained using the method described in **Subheading 3.6.** followed by silver staining can be used to verify the presence of angiostatin or plasminogen in the samples. Angiostatin can be identified as a single 38 kDa band (reducing conditions) or 28 kDa (nonreducing conditions) and should only be detected in the conditioned media samples where plasminogen was incubated in the absence of neutralizing antibody. In contrast, angiostatin should be absent and a band corresponding to intact plasminogen at 92 kDa (reducing or nonreducing conditions) should be observed in the conditioned media of samples that were incubated in the presence of the neutralizing gelatinase A antibody.

Acknowledgments

The authors gratefully acknowledge the support of the American Cancer Society (RPG 83821) and the National Cancer Institute, National Institutes of Health (R01 CA83106).

References

1. O'Reilly, M. S., Holmgren, L., Shing, Y., Chen, C., Rosenthal, R. A., Moses, M., et al. (1994) Angiostatin: a novel angiogenesis inhibitor that mediates the suppression of metastases by a Lewis lung carcinoma. *Cell* **79**, 315–328.

2. O'Reilly, M. S., Holmgren, L., Chen, C., and Folkman, J. (1996) Angiostatin induces and sustains dormancy of human primary tumors in mice. *Nature Med.* **2**, 689–692.

3. Holmgren, L., O'Reilly, M. S., and Folkman, J. (1995) Dormancy of micrometastases: balanced proliferation and apoptosis in the presence of angiogenesis suppression. *Nature Med.* **1**, 149–153.

4. Libutti, S. K. and Pluda, J. M. (2000) Antiangiogenesis: clinical applications, in *Principles and Practice of the Biologic Therapy of Cancer*, 3rd ed. (Rosenberg, S. A., ed.), Lippincott Williams & Wilkins, Philadelphia, pp. 844–864.

5. O'Reilly, M. S., Wiederschain, D., Stetler-Stevenson, W. G., Folkman, J., and Moses, M. A. (1999) Regulation of angiostatin production by matrix metalloproteinase-2 in a model of concomitant resistance. *J. Biol. Chem.* **274**, 29568–29571.

6. O'Reilly, M. S. (2000) Antiangiogenesis: basic principles, in *Principles and Practice of the Biologic Therapy of Cancer*, 3rd ed. (Rosenberg, S. A., ed.), Lippincott Williams & Wilkins, Philadelphia, pp. 827-843.

7. Clapp, C., Martial, J. A., Guzman, R. C., Rentier-Delrue, F., and Weiner, R. I. (1993) The 16-kilodalton N-terminal fragment of human prolactin is a potent inhibitor of angiogenesis. *Endocrinology* **133**, 1292–1299.

8. D'Angelo, G., Struman, I., Martial, J., and Weiner, R. I. (1995) Activation of mitogen-activated protein kinases by vascular endothelial growth factor and basic fibroblast growth factor in capillary endothelial cells is inhibited by the antiangiogenic factor 16-kDa N-terminal fragment of prolactin. *Proc. Natl. Acad. Sci. USA* **92**, 6374–6378.

9. Ferrara, N., Clapp, C., and Weiner, R. I. (1991) The 16K fragment of prolactin specifically inhibits basal or FGF stimulated growth of capillary endothelial cells. *Endocrinology* **129**, 896–900.

10. Struman, I., Bentzien, F., Lee, H., Mainfroid, V., D'Angelo, G., Goffin, V., et al. (1999) Opposing actions of intact and N-terminal fragments of human prolactin/growth hormone family members on agniogenesis: an efficient mechanism for the regulation of angiogenesis. *Proc. Natl. Acad. Sci. USA* **96**, 1246–1251.

11. Maione, T. E., Gray, G. S., Petro, J., Hunt, A. J., Donner, A. L., Bauer, S. I., et al. (1990) Inhibition of angiogenesis by recombinant human platelet factor-4 and related peptides. *Science* **247**, 77–79.

12. Gupta, S. K., Hassel, T., and Singh, J. P. (1995) A potent inhibitor of endothelial cell proliferation is generated by proteolytic cleavage of the chemokine platelet factor 4. *Proc. Natl. Acad. Sci. USA* **92**, 7799–7803.

13. Tolsma, S. S., Volpert, O. V., Good, D. J., Frazier, W. A., Polverini, P. J., and Bouck, N. (1993) Peptides derived from two separate domains of the matrix protein thrombospondin-1 have anti-angiogenic activity. *J. Cell Biol.* **122**, 497–511.

14. Nelson, J., Allen, W. E., Scott, W. N., Bailie, J. R., Walker, B., and McFerran, N. V. (1995) Murine epidermal growth factor (EGF) fragment (33-42) inhibits both EGF- and laminin-dependent endothelial cell motility and angiogenesis. *Cancer Res.* **55**, 3772–3776.

15. Grant, D. S., Tashiro, K.-I., Sequi-Real, B., Yamada, Y., Martin, G. R., and Kleinman, H. K. (1989) Two different laminin domains mediate the differentiation of human endothelial cells into capillary-like structures in vitro. *Cell* **58**, 933–943.

16. Homandberg, G. A., Williams, J. E., Grant, D., Schumacher, B., and Eisenstein, R. (1985) Heparin-binding fragments of fibronectin are potent inhibitors of endothelial cell growth. *Am. J. Path.* **120**, 327–332.

17. O'Reilly, M. S., Boehm, T., Shing, Y., Fukai, N., Vasios, G., Lane, W. S., et al. (1997) Endostatin: an endogenous inhibitor of angiogenesis and tumor growth. *Cell* **88**, 277–285.

18. Boehm, T., Folkman, J., Browder, T., and O'Reilly, M. S. (1997) Antiangiogenic therapy of experimental cancer does not induce acquired drug resistance. *Nature* **390**, 404–407.

19. McGeehan, G. M., Becherer, J. D., Bast, R. C., Jr., Boyer, C. M., Champion, B., Connolly, K. M., et al. (1994) Regulation of tumour necrosis factor-alpha processing by a metalloproteinase inhibitor. *Nature* **370**, 558–561.

20. Gearing, A. J., Beckett, P., Christodoulou, M., Churchill, M., Clements, J., Davidson, A. H., et al. (1994) Processing of tumour necrosis factor-alpha precursor by metalloproteinases. *Nature* **370**, 555–557.

21. Arribas, J., Coodly, L., Vollmer, P., Kishimoto, T. K., Rose-John, S., and Massague, J. (1996) Diverse cell surface protein ectodomains are shed by a system sensitive to metalloprotease inhibitors. *J. Biol. Chem.* **271,** 11376–11382.

22. Arribas, J. and Massague, J. (1995) Transforming growth factor-alpha and beta-amyloid precursor protein share a secretory mechanism. *J. Cell Biol.* **128,** 433–441.

23. Walcheck, B., Kahn, J., Fisher, J. M., Wang, B. B., Fisk, R. S., Payan, D. G., et al. (1996) Neutrophil rolling altered by inhibition of L-selectin shedding in vitro. *Nature* **380,** 720–723.

24. Feehan, C., Darlak, K., Kahn, J., Walcheck, B., Spatola, A. F., and Kishimoto, T. K. (1996) Shedding of the lymphocyte L-selectin adhesion molecule is inhibited by a hydroxamic acid-based protease inhibitor. Identification with an L-selectin-alkaline phosphatase reporter. *J. Biol. Chem.* **271,** 7019–7024.

25. Bennett, T. A., Lynam, E. B., Sklar, L. A., and Rogelj, S. (1996) Hydroxamate-based metalloprotease inhibitor blocks shedding of L-selectin adhesion molecule from leukocytes: functional consequences for neutrophil aggregation. *J. Immunol.* **156,** 3093–3097.

26. Mullberg, J., Durie, F. H., Otten-Evans, C., Alderson, M. R., Rose-John, S., Cosman, D., et al. (1995) A metalloprotease inhibitor blocks shedding of the IL-6 receptor and the p60 TNF receptor. *J. Immunol.* **155,** 5198–5205.

27. Couet, J., Sar, S., Jolivet, A., Hai, M. T., Milgrom, E., and Misrahi, M. (1996) Shedding of human thyrotropin receptor ectodomain. Involvement of a matrix metalloprotease. *J. Biol. Chem.* **271,** 4545–4552.

28. Levi, E., Fridman, R., Miao, H. Q., Ma, Y. S., Yayon, A., and Vlodavsky, I. (1996) Matrix metalloproteinase 2 releases active soluble ectodomain of fibroblast growth factor receptor 1. *Proc. Natl. Acad. Sci. USA* **93,** 7069–7074.

29. Suzuki, M., Raab, G., Moses, M. A., Fernandez, C. A., and Klagsbrun, M. (1997) Matrix metalloproteinase-3 releases active heparin-binding EGF-like growth factor by cleavage at a specific juxtamembrane site. *J. Biol. Chem.* **272,** 31730–31737.

30. Dvorak, H. F. (1986) Tumors: wounds that do not heal. *N. Engl. J. Med.* **315,** 1650–1659.

31. Dvorak, H. F., Nagy, J. A., Dvorak, J. T., and Dvorak, A. M. (1988) Identification and characterization of the blood vessels of solid tumors that are leaky to circulating macromolecules. *Am. J. Pathol.* **133,** 95–109.

32. Gately, S., Twardowski, P., Stack, M. S., Patrick, M., Boggio, L., Cundiff, D. L., et al. (1996) Human prostate carcinoma cells express enzymatic activity that converts human plasminogen to the angiogenesis inhibitor, angiostatin. *Cancer Res.* **56,** 4887–4890.

33. Stathakis, P., Fitzgerald, M., Matthias, L. J., Chesterman, C. N., and Hogg, P. J. (1997) Generation of angiostatin by reduction and proteolysis of plasmin. *J. Biol. Chem.* **272,** 20641–20645.

34. Patterson, B. C. and Sang, Q. X. A. (1997) Angiostatin-converting enzyme activities of MMP-7 and MMP-9. *J. Biol. Chem.* **272,** 28823–28825.

35. Falcone, D., Khan, K. M. F., Layne, T., and Fernandes, L. (1998) Macrophage formation of angiostatin during inflammation. *J. Biol. Chem.* **273,** 31480–31485.
36. Dong, Z., Kumar, R., Yang, X., and Fidler, I. J. (1997) Macrophage-derived metalloelastase is responsible for the generation of angiostatin in Lewis lung carcinoma. *Cell* **88,** 801–810.
37. Lay, A. J., Jiang, X. M., Kisker, O., Flynn, E., Underwood, A., Condron, R., and Hogg, P. J. (2000) Phosphoglycerate kinase acts in tumour angiogenesis as a disulphide reductase. *Nature* **408,** 869–873.
38. Moses, M. A., Sudhalter, J., and Langer, R. (1990) Identification of an inhibitor of neovascularization from cartilage. *Science* **248,** 1408–1410.
39. Moses, M. A. (1997) The regulation of neovascularization by matrix metalloproteinases and their inhibitors. *Stem Cells* **15,** 180–189.
40. Moses, M. A., Wiederschain, D., Loughlin, K. R., Zurakowski, D., Lamb, C. L., and Freeman, M. R. (1998) Increased incidence of matrix metalloproteinases in urine of cancer patients. *Cancer Res.* **58,** 1395–1399.
41. Camphausen, K., Moses, M. A., Beecken, W., Khan, M. K., Folkman, J., and O'Reilly, M. S. (2001) Radiation therapy to a primary tumor accelerates metastatic growth in mice. *Cancer Res.* **61,** 2207–2211.
42. O'Reilly, M., Rosenthal, R., Sage, E. H., Smith, S., Holmgren, L., Moses, M., et al. (1993) The suppression of tumor metastases by a primary tumor. *Surg. Forum* **44,** 474–476.
43. Braunhut, S. J. and Moses, M. A. (1994) Retinoids modulate endothelial cell production of matrix-degrading proteases and tissue inhibitors of metalloproteinases (TIMP). *J. Biol. Chem.* **269,** 13472–13479.
44. Fridman, R., Fuerst, T. R., Bird, R. E., Hoyhtya, M., Oelkuct, M., Kraus, S., et al. Domain structure of human 72-kDa gelatinase/type IV collagenase. Characterization of proteolytic activity and identification of the tissue inhibitor of metalloproteinase-2 (TIMP-2) binding regions. *J. Biol. Chem.* **267,** 15398–15405.
45. Folkman, J., Haundenschild, C. C., and Zetter, B. R. (1979) Long-term culture of capillary endothelial cells. *Proc. Natl. Acad. Sci. USA* **76,** 5217–5221.
46. O'Reilly, M. S., Holmgren, L., Shing, Y., Chen, C., Rosenthal, R. A., Cao, Y., et al. (1994) Angiostatin: a circulating endothelial cell inhibitor that suppresses angiogenesis and tumor growth. *Cold Spring Harbor Symp. Quant. Biol.* **59,** 471–482.
47. O'Reilly, M. S., Shing, Y., Cao, Y., and Folkman, J. (1996) Endogenous inhibitors of angiogenesis (Meeting abstract). Proceedings of the Annual Meeting of the American Association for Cancer Research. Cadmus Journal Services, Linthicum, MD, p. 669.
48. Bok, R. A. and Mangel, W. F. (1985) Quantitative characterization of the lysine binding of plasminogen to intact fibrin clots, lysine-sepharose, and fibrin cleaved by plasmin. *Biochemistry* **24,** 3279–3286.
49. Machovich, R. and Owen, W. G. (1989) An elastase-dependent pathway of plasminogen activation. *Biochemistry* **28,** 4517–4522.

50. Sottrup-Jensen, L., Claeys, H., Zajdel, M., Petersen, T. E., and Magnusson, S. (1978) The primary structure of human plasminogen: isolation of two lysine-binding fragments and one mini-plasminogen (MW, 38,000) by elastase-catalyzed-specific limited proteolysis, in *Progress in Chemical Fibrinolysis and Thrombolysis*, vol. 3 (Davidson, J. F., Rowan, R. M., Samama, M. M., and Desnoyers, P. C., eds.), Raven Press, New York, pp. 191–209.

51. Herron, G. S., Banda, M. J., Clark, E. J., Gavrilovic, J., and Werb, Z. (1986) Secretion of metalloproteinases by stimulated capillary endothelial cells. II. Expression of collagenase and stromelysin activities is regulated by endogenous inhibitors. *J. Biol. Chem.* **261,** 2814–2818.

28

In Vitro and In Vivo Assays for the Proliferative and Vascular Permeabilization Activities of Vascular Endothelial Growth Factor (VEGF) and Its Receptor

Seiji Yano, Roy S. Herbst, and Saburo Sone

1. Introduction

Angiogenesis, the formation of new blood vessels from the endothelium, develops in response to metabolic demands of tissues and tumors, and is thought to play an essential role in progression of solid tumors, including lung cancer *(1)*. It is observed in early stages of lung carcinogenesis, such as bronchial dysplasia and carcinoma *in situ*, which display increased vascularity when compared with normal bronchial epithelium and hyperplasia *(2)*. In addition, several reports have shown that microvascular density in primary tumors confers a poor prognosis in early-stage non-small cell lung cancer (NSCLC) *(3,4)*.

Large numbers of growth factors and cytokines are known to be involved in angiogenesis *(5)*. Among them, vascular endothelial growth factor (VEGF) is an important multifunctional cytokine that promotes developmental, physiological, and pathogenical neovascularization *(6–8)*. VEGF consists of at least four isoforms (VEGF$_{121}$, VEGF$_{165}$, VEGF$_{189}$, and VEGF$_{206}$) arising through alternate splicing of RNA from a single gene. VEGF$_{165}$ is the most potent and abundant isoform. VEGF can be produced by various cell types, including many tumor cells and activated macrophages *(6)*. VEGF binds with high affinity to two tyrosine kinase receptors, VEGF-R1 (Flt-1) and VEGF-R2 (Flk-1/KDR). Ligand binding causes receptor dimerization, autophosphorylation, and signal transduction. VEGF has been shown to stimulate the proliferation and migration of endothelial cells, and induce the expression of metalloproteinases and plasminogen activity by these cells *(6)*. There is direct correlation between angiogenesis and VEGF expression in NSCLC. High levels of expression of

From: *Methods in Molecular Medicine, vol. 74: Lung Cancer, Vol. 1: Molecular Pathology Methods and Reviews*
Edited by: B. Driscoll © Humana Press Inc., Totowa, NJ

VEGF and its receptors are found in lung adenocarcinoma and are associated with a poor prognosis *(9)*.

VEGF was initially identified as vascular permeablity factor (VPF), and is the most potent inducer of vascular hyperpermeability *(10)*. Malignant pleural effusions are frequently associated with advanced lung cancer. Recently, we reported that malignant pleural effusions of lung cancer patients contained a high level of VEGF *(11)*. We developed an animal model for pleural effusions, which we produced by iv injection of human lung adenocarcinoma PC-14 and its highly metastatic variant PC14PE6 *(12,13)*. In this model of pleural effusion, we demonstrated that VEGF is responsible for the formation of malignant pleural effusions of lung cancer via induction of localized vascular hyperpermeablity *(12)*. Therefore, VEGF is a key molecule not only in angiogenesis but also in the formation of malignant pleural effusions, suggesting that VEGF is an ideal target for treatment of lung cancer. In fact, various compounds that inhibit the function of VEGF and/or VEGF receptors, including humanized neutralization antibody for VEGF and VEGF-R2, dominant-negative VEGF, soluble VEGF/VPF receptors, and VEGF/VPF receptor tyrosine kinase inhibitors, have been developed and have shown their anti-angiogenic activities *(13–15)*.

In this chapter, methods for evaluating VEGF activity and the effect of anti-VEGF molecules on, such as endothelial proliferation and vascular permeability, are described.

2. Materials

2.1. Cell-Proliferation Assay

1. Cell line: Human dermal microvascular endothelial cells (HDMEC; Cascade Biologics, Portland, OR). For proliferation assays, cells at passage 2–5 should be used (*see* **Note 1**). Other endothelial cell lines can be used. Cells are maintained under standard culture conditions at 37°C in 5% CO_2-95% air.
2. Phosphate-buffered saline (PBS) (Life Technologies, Rockville, MD).
3. Medium 131 with Microvascular Growth Supplement (MVGS) (Cascade Biologics, Portland, OR): MVGS contains fetal calf serum (FCS) (5% v/v) (*see* **Note 2**), hydrocortisone, human fibroblast growth factor (FGF), heparin, human epidermal growth factor (EGF), and dibutyryl cyclic AMP. Store at 4°C. Protect from light.
4. MEM: Minimum Essential Medium (Life Technologies, Rockville, MD) with 5% FCS (*see* **Note 2**).
5. Trypsin/EDTA solution: PBS containing 0.025% trypsin and 0.01% EDTA.
6. 96-well flat-bottom plate (MICROEST 96, Becton Dickinson, Franklin Lakes, NJ).
7. 1.5% Gelatin solution: Place 0.6 g gelatin in 40 mL H_2O and dissolve the gelatin by microwaving for 1 min. Sterililize the resultant solution by filtration

(45-μm pore size). After use, it can be stored at 4°C (gel form). Before use, microwave for 1 min.

8. Test samples: Conditioned media or cytokines. Conditioned media is prepared by incubating tumor cells ($1–5 \times 10^5$/mL) in MEM with 0.5% BSA for 24–48 h. Cytokines should be diluted in MEM with 0.5% BSA.

9. MTT solution (2 mg/mL): Place 400 mg MTT (3-(4,5-dimethylthiazol-2-yl)-2.5-diphenyl-tetrazolium bromide, Sigma) in 200 mL PBS and dissolve with stirring while protecting from light. Sterilize the resultant solution by filtration (45-μm pore size). Store at 4°C in the dark.

10. Dimethyl sulfoxide (DMSO).

11. MR-5000 96-well microtiter plate reader.

2.1.1. Determination of the Effect of anti-VEGF Neutralizing Antibodies and VEGF Receptor Inhibitors

1. Goat anti-human VEGF polyclonal antibody (PAb) (R&D Systems, Minneapolis, MN): Reconstituted antibody is stable for at least 1 mo at at 2–4°C or at –20–70°C for more than 3 mo. Avoid repeated freeze-thaw cycles.

2. Control goat IgG (R&D Systems, Minneapolis, MN).

2.2. Vascular Permeability Assay

1. Nude mice: Male athymic BALB/c nude mice (Animal Production Area of the National Cancer Institute, Frederick Cancer Research Facility, Frederick, MD).

2. 0.5% Evans blue dye solution: Dissolve 250 mg Evans blue dye (Sigma Chemical Co., St. Louis, MO) in 50 mL PBS.

3. Recombinant human (rh)VEGF165 (R&D Systems, Minneapolis, MN): Reconstitute with sterile PBS. $VEGF_{165}$ can be stored under sterile conditions at 2–4°C for 1 mo or at –20–70°C for more than 3 mo.

4. PBS supplemented with 0.5% bovine serum albumin (BSA).

5. Fine needle (27–30-gauge) for intradermal injections.

6. Instruments for dissection.

7. Formamide: (CH_3NO, Sigma).

3. Methods

3.1. Cell-Proliferation Assay

Cell proliferation can be evaluated by cell number counting, the ^{3}H-thymidine-incorporation assay *(16)*, and the MTT assay *(17)*. As a nonradioisotope procedure, protocol for MTT assay is described here (*see* **Fig. 1**).

1. Add 50 μL gelatin solution into individual wells of 96-well plates and incubate for 30 min at room temperature.

2. Wash wells twice with PBS.

3. Add human dermal microvascular endothelial cells (HDMEC) (5×10^3/100 μL/ well in supplemented M131 medium) to wells in triplicate (*see* **Note 3**).

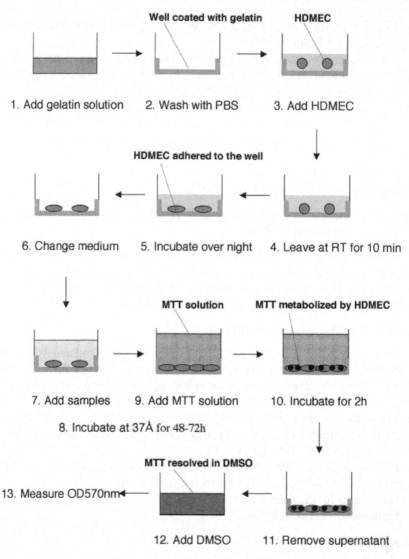

Fig. 1. Cell proliferation assay.

4. Leave the plate for 10 min at room temperature to allow homogenous cell distribution (*see* **Note 4**).
5. Place plates in an incubator overnight. After the overnight incubation, viable HDMEC will be tightly adherent to the plate.
6. Wash the culture twice with PBS to remove dead cells, and add MEM (100 μL) supplemented with 5% FCS immediately (*see* **Note 5**). Do not allow the cultures to dry out.

7. Add test samples (50–100 μL) (e.g., cytokines, culture supernatants).
8. Incubate at 37°C for 48–72 h, depending on the experimental protocol for the test sample being examined.
9. Add MTT solution (50 μL) and incubate for 2 h at 37°C. After the 2-h incubation in MTT, black particles in HDMEC will be observed under the microscope.
10. Remove the supernatant completely.
11. Add DMSO (100 μL) and shake the plate gently for 5 min to lyse the cells completely.
12. Measure the OD at 570 nm using with an MR-5000 96-well microtiter plate reader.

3.1.1. Determination of the Effect of Anti-VEGF Neutralizing Antibodies and VEGF Receptor Inhibitors

1. Pre-treat the sample (e.g., cytokines, culture supernatants) with anti-VEGF neutralizing antibody or control antibody, or any of the myriad possible VEGF receptor inhibitors, such as inhibitors of receptor tyrosine kinases, for 1 h at 37°C. If the samples contain high concentration of VEGF, dilute samples with MEM with 5% FCS.
2. Add the pre-treated sample to HDMEC cultures as in **Subheading 2.1., step 7** and continue assay as described.

3.2. Vascular Permeability Assay

This assay uses intradermal injection of test substances and intravascular injection of Evans blue dye (which binds to endogenous serum albumin) as a tracer to assay permeability in peripheral vessels. The assay is performed essentially as described *(10,18)* with minor modification (*see* **Fig. 2**).

1. Inject 200 μL 0.5% Evans blue dye solution iv into nude mice (*see* **Note 6**).
2. Ten minutes later, choose mice that do not exhibit nonspecific staining of the skin with Evans blue dye. (Approximately 20–40% of mice will exhibit nonspecific staining.)
3. Inject 50-μL boluses of samples with a fine needle, intradermally, on the dorsal skin in rows. Inject PBS (50 μL) with 0.5% BSA (negative control) and 20–100 ng/mL (rh)VEGF165 with 0.5% BSA (50 μL) (positive control) in the same mice (*see* **Note 7**).
4. Sacrifice mice 30 min after the injection of samples by cervical dislocation.
5. Photograph injection sites on the skin.
6. For quantitation of vascular permeability, remove the skin and resect wheals, which should be approx 5 mm in diameter.
7. Place the wheals in 500 μL formamide and incubate at 37°C for 48 h to extract the Evans blue dye.
8. Measure OD of the extracts at 630 nm in a spectrophotometer.

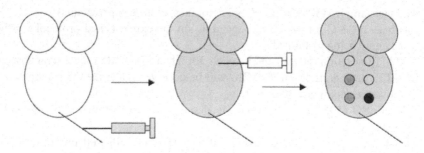

1. Inject Evans blue dye i.v.   3. Inject samples s.c.   5. Take the picture

2. Ten min later, choose the mouse   4. Thirty min later,
   without nonspecific staining   kill the mouse

Quantitative procedure

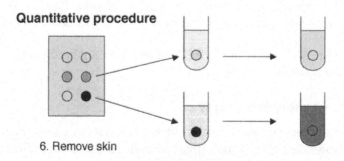

6. Remove skin

7. Resect wheals   8. Incubate wheals in   9. Measure OD630nm
                        formamide for 48h

Fig. 2. Vascular permeability assay.

4. Notes

1. Cells at passage less than 10 should be used. VEGF receptor, especially KDR, is highly expressed in fetal endothelial cells and its expression decreases during in vitro culture.
2. In the medium, 5% FCS is necessary for survival of HDMEC. FCS should be heat-inactivated.
3. Triplicate cultures are recommended to obtain reproducible results.
4. For the cell proliferation assay, the even distribution of cells during plating (**Subheading 3.1., steps 3** and **4**) is critical for reproducible results.
5. To explore endothelial growth activity, supplemented M131 medium should not be used because it contains a high concentration of growth factors, such as basic FGF (bFGF) and EGF. MEM supplemented with 5% FCS is therefore substituted for the duration of the assay.

6. To reduce individual variation, nude mice without hair should be carefully chosen and each mouse should be housed separately during the assay. Prepare some spare mice, in case of adverse reaction to assay.

7. When the effect of VEGF receptor inhibitors (VEGF receptor antibody, inhibitors of receptor tyrosine kinases) is to be assessed, pretreat the mice with VEGF receptor inhibitors for several days. Consider using pharmacokinetics, to get the maximal effect of the drug, the assay should start several hours after the last treatment with VEGF receptor inhibitors.

References

1. Fidler, I. J. and Ellis, L. M. (1994) The implications of angiogenesis for the biology and therapy of cancer metastasis. *Cell* **79**, 185–188.
2. Fontanini, G., Vignati, S., Bigini, D., Lucchi, M., Mussi, A., Basolo, F., et al. (1996) Neoangiogenesis: a putative marker of malignancy in non-small-cell lung cancer (NSCLC) development. *Int. J. Cancer* **67**, 615–619.
3. Macchiarini, P., Fontanini, G., Hardin, M. J., Squartini, F., and Angeletti, C. A. (1992) Relation of neovascularisation to metastasis of non-small-cell lung cancer. *Lancet* **340**, 145–146.
4. Yuan, A., Yang, P. C., Yu, C. J., Lee, Y. C., Yao, Y. T., Chen, C. L., et al. (1995) Tumor angiogenesis correlates with histologic type and metastasis in non-small-cell lung cancer. *Am. J. Respir. Crit. Care Med.* **152**, 2157–2162.
5. Herbst, R. S. and Fidler, I. J. (2000) Angiogenesis and lung cancer: potential for therapy. *Clin. Cancer Res.* **6**, 4604–4606.
6. Ferrara, N. (1997) The role of vascular endothelial growth factor in the regulation of blood vessel growth, in *Tumor Angiogenesis* (Bicknell, R., Lewis, C. E., and Ferrara, N., eds.), New York, Oxford University Press, pp. 185–199.
7. Carmeliet, P., Ferreira, V., Breier, G., Pollefeyt, S., Kieckens, L., Gertsenstein, M., et al. (1996) Abnormal blood vessel development and lethality in embryos lacking a single VEGF allele. *Nature* **380**, 435–439.
8. Yano, S., Shinohara, H., Herbst, R. S., Kuniyasu, H., Bucana, C. D., Bucana, C. D., et al. (2000) Expression of vascular endothelial growth factor is essential but not sufficient for production and growth of brain metastasis. *Cancer Res.* **60**, 4959–4967.
9. Takanami, I., Tanaka, F., Hashizume, T., and Kodaisra, S. (1997) Vascular endothelial growth facotr and its receptor correlate with angiogenesis and survival in pulmonary adenocarcinoma. *Anticancer Res.* **17**, 2811–2814.
10. Senger, D. R., Galli, S. J., Dvorak, A. M., Perruzzi, C. A., Harvey, V. S., and Dvorak, H. F. (1983) Tumor cells secrete a vascular permeability factor that promotes accumulation of ascites fluid. *Science* **219**, 983–985.
11. Yanagawa, H., Takeuchi, E., Suzuki, Y., Ohmoto, Y., Bando, H., and Sone, S. (1999) Vascular endothelial growth factor in malignant pleural effusion associated with lung cancer. *Cancer Immunol. Immunother.* **48**, 396–400.
12. Yano, S., Shinohara, H., Herbst, R. S., Kuniyasu, H., Bucana, C. D., Ellis, L. M., and Fidler, I. J. (2000) Production of experimental pleural effusions is

dependent on invasion of the pleura and expression of vascular endothelial growth factor/vascular permeability factor by human lung cancer cells. *Am. J. Pathol.* **157,** 1893–1903.

13. Yano, S., Herbst, R. S., Shinohara, S., Knighton, B., Bucana, C. D., Killion, J. J, et al. (2000) Treatment for malignant pleural effusion of human lung adenocarcinoma by inhibition of vascular endothelial growth factor receptor tyrosine kinase phosphorylation. *Clin. Cancer Res.* **6,** 957–965.

14. Gordon, M. S., Margolin, K., Talpaz, M., Sledge, G. W., Holmgren, Jr., E., Benjamin, R., et al. (2001) Phase I safety and pharmakokinetics study of recombinant human anti-vascular endothelial growth facotr in patients with advanced cancer. *J. Clin. Oncol.* **19,** 843–850.

15. Fong, T. A., Shawver, L. K., Sun, L., Tang, C., App, H., Powell, T. J., et al. (1999) SU5416 is a potent and selective inhibitor of the vascular endothelial growth factor receptor (Flk-1/KDR) that inhibits tyrosine kinase catalysis, tumor vascularization, and growth of multiple tumor types. *Cancer Res.* **59,** 99–106.

16. Sone, S., Inamura, N., Nii, A., and Ogura, T. (1988) Heterogeneity of human lymphokine (IL-2)-activated killer (LAK) precursors and regulation of their LAK induction by blood monocytes. *Int. J. Cancer* **42,** 428–434.

17. Green L. M., Reade, J. L., and Ware, C. F. (1984) Rapid colorimetric assay for cell viability: application to the quantitation of cytotoxic and growth-inhibitory lymphokines. *J. Immunol. Methods* **70,** 257–268.

18. Heiss, J. D., Papavassiliou, E., Merrill, M. J., Nieman, L., Knightly, J. J., Walbridge, S., et al. (1996) Mechanism of dexamethasone suppression of brain tumor-associated vascular permeability in rats: involvement of the glucocorticoid receptor and vascular permeability factor. *J. Clin. Invest.* **98,** 1400–1408.

III

MOLECULAR ABNORMALITIES IN LUNG CANCER

F. DETECTION OF ALTERATIONS IN DNA REPLICATION AND REPAIR

29

Detection of Telomerase Activity in Lung Cancer Tissues

Keiko Hiyama and Eiso Hiyama

1. Introduction

Cancer cells continue cell division and proliferation until they kill the host. Human germline cells have the capacity to undergo repeated cell divisions for millions of years, living on in descendants. However, most normal somatic cells can divide no more than several dozens of times. Recent research has shown that telomerase, a highly conserved reverse-transcriptase that adds G-rich nucleotide repeats onto the ends of chromosomal DNAs (i.e., telomeres), is the key that makes this difference *(1,2)*. Several thousands of clinical samples derived from human malignant neoplasms have been investigated for telomerase activity, and about 85% of them have been found to be positive for telomerase expression and activity *(3)*. In addition, almost all cancer cell lines established from human malignancies, all proliferating germline cells, most proliferating stem/progenitor cells (e.g., hematopoietic progenitor cells, intestinal crypt cells, skin epithelia, hair follicles, and endometrial cells), and activated lymphocytes exhibit telomerase activity. These findings would indicate that activation of telomerase is a prerequisite for human cells to prolong their life span of cell division. Therefore, detection of telomerase activity in clinical samples, which may be a marker of the presence of immortal cells, may be helpful for cancer diagnosis and inference of the malignant potential of tumors.

Telomerase activity was first detected in Tetrahymena in 1985 *(4)*. The activity of human telomerase was first detected by Morin in HeLa cells *(5)*. However, because the sensitivity of the conventional assay used in these studies was low, it was difficult to apply to clinical materials, whose telomerase activity

From: *Methods in Molecular Medicine, vol. 74: Lung Cancer, Vol. 1: Molecular Pathology Methods and Reviews*
Edited by: B. Driscoll © Humana Press Inc., Totowa, NJ

is lower than that in immortal cancer cell lines. In 1994, a highly sensitive, polymerase chain reaction (PCR)-based method for detecting telomerase activity, called TRAP (telomeric repeat amplification protocol) assay was developed *(6)*. Using this method, telomerase activity can be detected even with 10 cells, and we found that 80% of non-small cell lung cancer (NSCLC) and all small cell lung cancer tissues examined showed positive telomerase activity *(7)*. In addition, high telomerase activity was associated with small cell lung cancer and allelic deletions of *RB1* and *TP53*. We present here our original protocol for detecting telomerase activity in cancer tissues *(7–9)*, a modified protocol to avoid false-negatives owing to TRAP assay inhibitors, and a protocol using a commercial kit (TRAPeze™ telomerase detection kit, Intergen, NY).

2. Materials

2.1. Original TRAP Assay

1. Lysis buffer stock: 10 mM Tris-HCl, pH 7.5, 1 mM MgCl$_2$, 1 mM EGTA (ethylene glycol-bis(β-aminoethyl ether)-N,N,N′,N′-tetraacetic acid, pH 8.0), 0.5% CHAPS (3-[(3-cholamidopropyl)-dimethyl-ammonio]-1-propanesulfonate, Pierce, Rockford, IL), and 10% glycerol in diethyl pyrocarbonate (DEPC)-treated water. Store at room temperature.
2. β-mercaptoethanol (14.4 M): Stored at 4°C and 3.5 μL is added to 10-mL lysis buffer (final 5 mM) just prior to extraction.
3. 0.1 mM AEBSF (4-(2-aminoethyl)-benzenesulfonyl fluoride hydrochlorine, ICN, Costa Mesa, CA): Store at –20°C in small aliquots (~300 μL) and 10 μL is added to 10 mL lysis buffer (final 0.1 mM) just prior to extraction.
4. Determination of protein concentration: BCA Protein Assay Reagent™ (Pierce), store at room temperature. Spectrophotometer capable of measuring absorbance at 562 nm. 3.5 mL disposable cuvets (BioRad, Hercules, CA).
5. HotStart 50™ PCR tube (Gibco-BRL, Gaithersburg, MD): Store at room temperature.
6. CX primer (50 ng/μL, 5′-CCCTTACCCTTACCCTTACCCTAA-3′). Synthesized, purified by high-performance liquid chromatography (HPLC), and dissolved in TE (10 mM Tris-HCl, 1 mM EDTA). Store at –20°C in small aliquots.
7. 10X PCR buffer: 200 mM Tris-HCl, pH 8.3, 15 mM MgCl$_2$, 680 mM KCl, 0.5% Tween 20, 10 mM EGTA, pH 8.0, in DEPC-treated water. Store at –20°C in small aliquots.
8. A mixture of 2.5 mM each dNTP (dATP, dTTP, dGTP, dCTP). Store at –20°C in small aliquots.
9. TS primer (50 ng/μL, 5′-AATCCGTCGAGCAGAGTT-3′): Synthesized, purified by HPLC, and dissolved in TE (10 mM Tris-HCl, 1 mM EDTA). Store at –20°C in small aliquots.
10. T4gene32protein (5 μg/μL, Boehringer Mannheim, Indianapolis, IN). Store at –80°C.

11. Taq DNA polymerase (5 U/μL, Takara, Tokyo, Japan). Store at –20°C.
12. Redivue™ [α-^{32}P]dCTP (110 TBq/mmol, Amersham Pharmacia Biotech, Buckinghamshire, UK). Store at 4°C (*see* **Note 1**).

2.2. Polyacrylamide Gel Electrophoresis (PAGE)

Because acrylamide is a potent neurotoxin and is absorbed through the skin, it should be handled with gloves.

1. 40% acrylamide (C = 5%): Dissolve 190 g acrylamide and 10 g bisacrylamide with deionized water to a final volume of 500 mL at room temperature, and store shaded from light.
2. 5X TBE buffer stock: To make 1 L, mix 54 g Tris base (final 450 mM), 27.5 g boric acid, and 20 mL of 0.5 M EDTA, pH 8.0, and adjust the pH to ~8.3. Store at room temperature.
3. 10% Ammonium persulfate (APS): Dissolve 1 g of APS in 10 mL of deionized water. Prepare fresh or store at 4°C within a week. Wear gloves in handling.
4. TEMED (N,N,N′,N′-tetramethylethylenediamine). Store at room temperature. Wear gloves when handling.
5. Loading buffer stock: 2 mL of 1% xylene cyanol (XC)/DDW (final 0.05%), 2 mL of 1% bromophenol blue (BPB)/100 mM Tris-HCl, pH 8.0, final 0.05%, 20 mL glycerol (final 50%), and 16 mL DDW. Store at 4°C.
6. Electrophoresis apparatus: 20 × 20 cm glass plates and vertical electrophoresis apparatus. Spacers of 1 mm in thickness.

2.3. Modified TRAP Assay

In addition to the reagents listed above:

1. ITAS (internal telomerase assay standard) *(10)*: 150-bp internal control template to be amplified by CX and TS primers. Dilute to 10 attg (10^{-17} g)/μL and store at –20°C.
2. Phenol saturated with buffer (Nacalai Tesque, Kyoto, Japan). Store at 4°C, shaded from light.
3. CIAA: chloroform containing 4% isoamyl alcohol. To a 500-mL bottle of chloroform, add 20.8 mL of isoamyl alcohol. Store at room temperature.
4. 5 M NaCl. Store at room temperature.
5. 99.9% ethanol. Store at room temperature.

2.4. TRAPeze™ Telomerase Detection Kit

1. TRAPeze™ Telomerase Detection Kit (Intergene, NY): PCR-grade water, 1X lysis buffer, 10X TRAP reaction buffer, primer mix (RP primer, K1 primer) with a template for amplification of a 36-bp short internal control (TSK1), 50X dNTP mix, TS primer, and TSR8 (control template) are stored at –20°C. Positive control (immortalized cell pellet) is stored at –80°C. (TRAPeze™ Modified Reagent Set contains K2 primer instead of K1 primer and L-IC template instead of TSK1

so that the 173-bp long internal control band appears instead of the 36-bp short internal control band. *See* **Note 2**).
2. BCA Protein Assay Reagent™ (Pierce). Store at room temperature.
3. [γ-^{32}P]ATP (110 TBq/mmol, DuPont NEN, Boston, MA). Store at 4°C.
4. T4 polynucleotide kinase with 5X kinase buffer (Takara, Tokyo, Japan). Store at –20°C.
5. Taq DNA polymerase (5 U/µL, Takara). Store at –20°C.

3. Methods

3.1. Original TRAP Assay (Fig. 1A, 2A) (7–9)

Because telomerase contains an RNA component (hTR), all reagents should be free of RNase. DEPC-treated water, gloves and sterilized tips and tubes should be used for all methods and materials. Aerosol-resistant tips are recommended to avoid contamination.

3.1.1. DEPC-treated Water

1. Add 0.5 mL DEPC solution to 500 mL distilled, deionized water (0.1%).
2. Incubate overnight at 37°C (or at room temperature), and then autoclave so that the DEPC is destroyed completely.

3.1.2. Lysis Buffer

1. Add β-mercaptoethanol and AEBSF into ice-cold lysis buffer stock at final concentrations of 5 mM and 0.1 mM, respectively, just prior to extraction.

3.1.3. Protein Extracts

1. Place a 50–100 mg fresh or frozen (–80°C) tissue sample in a sterile 1.5-mL microcentrifuge tube containing 200 µL ice-cold lysis buffer.
2. Homogenize the tissue sample using a matching disposable pestle rotated at 450–500 rpm by an electric drill until the tissue is dispersed (~10 s).
3. Place the tube on ice for 25 min, and then centrifuge at 13,000g for 20 min at 4°C in a microcentrifuge.
4. Collect the supernatant in a new tube and freeze it immediately using liquid nitrogen or dry-ice, and then store it at –80°C. A 5 µL aliquot of the supernatant may be stored separately at –20°C for BCA protein assay. (We also store the remaining pellet separately at –80°C for future DNA extraction.)

Fig. 1. *(opposite page)* Procedures for the original TRAP assay **(A)**, TRAPeze™ assay, and modified TRAP assay **(B)**. In general, the TRAPeze™ assay is more sensitive than the original TRAP assay (*see* **Note 2**). The modified TRAP assay should be used for samples containing PCR inhibitors.

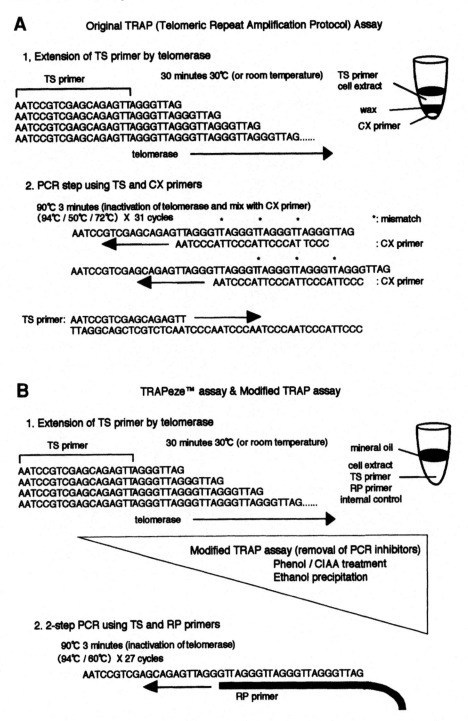

A Original TRAP (Telomeric Repeat Amplification Protocol) Assay

1, Extension of TS primer by telomerase

TS primer 30 minutes 30℃ (or room temperature) TS primer / cell extract

AATCCGTCGAGCAGAGTTAGGGTTAG
AATCCGTCGAGCAGAGTTAGGGTTAGGGTTAG wax
AATCCGTCGAGCAGAGTTAGGGTTAGGGTTAGGGTTAG CX primer
AATCCGTCGAGCAGAGTTAGGGTTAGGGTTAGGGTTAGGGTTAG......

telomerase ⟶

2. PCR step using TS and CX primers

90℃ 3 minutes (inactivation of telomerase and mix with CX primer)
(94℃ / 50℃ / 72℃) X 31 cycles   *   *   *   *: mismatch

AATCCGTCGAGCAGAGTTAGGGTTAGGGTTAGGGTTAGGGTTAG
⟵ AATCCCATTCCCATTCCCAT TCCC : CX primer

*   *   *
AATCCGTCGAGCAGAGTTAGGGTTAGGGTTAGGGTTAGGGTTAGGGTTAG
⟵ AATCCCATTCCCATTCCCATTCCC : CX primer

TS primer: AATCCGTCGAGCAGAGTT ⟶
TTAGGCAGCTCGTCTCAATCCCAATCCCAATCCCATTCCC

B TRAPeze™ assay & Modified TRAP assay

1. Extension of TS primer by telomerase

TS primer 30 minutes 30℃ (or room temperature) mineral oil

AATCCGTCGAGCAGAGTTAGGGTTAG cell extract
AATCCGTCGAGCAGAGTTAGGGTTAGGGTTAG TS primer
AATCCGTCGAGCAGAGTTAGGGTTAGGGTTAGGGTTAG RP primer
AATCCGTCGAGCAGAGTTAGGGTTAGGGTTAGGGTTAGGGTTAG...... internal control

telomerase ⟶

Modified TRAP assay (removal of PCR inhibitors)
Phenol / CIAA treatment
Ethanol precipitation

2. 2-step PCR using TS and RP primers

90℃ 3 minutes (inactivation of telomerase)
(94℃ / 60℃) X 27 cycles

AATCCGTCGAGCAGAGTTAGGGTTAGGGTTAGGGTTAGGGTTAG
⟵ RP primer

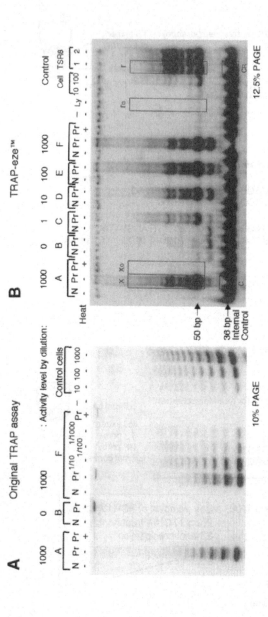

Fig. 2. Telomerase activity in lung cancer tissues (cases A-F) using original TRAP assay (**A**) and TRAPeze™ kit (**B**). Relative telomerase activity level using TRAPeze™ kit is expressed as the "Total Product Generated (TPG)," calculated by the following formula: TPG (units) = $\{(x-x_o)/c\}/\{(r-r_o)/c_R\} \times 100$

x: signal intensity of 6-bp ladders in a sample

x_o: that in heat-treated sample

r: that in TSR8 control

r_o: that in lysis buffer

c: signal intensity of 36-bp internal control in the sample

c_R: that in TSR8 control

Activity level determined by serial dilution using the original TRAP assay correlates well with that determined using the TRAPeze™ kit.

N: Noncancerous tissue

Pr: Primary lesion

Ly: Lysis buffer

3.1.4. Bicinchonic Acid (BCA) Protein Assay

1. Freshly prepare reagents within a few days of use. Make BCA working reagent by mixing reagents A and B at 50:1 (e.g., 50 mL of reagent A and 1 mL of reagent B for 18 samples).
2. Prepare albumin standard samples of 20, 40, 60, 80, 100 µg/100 µL by diluting bovine serum albumin (BSA) with DDW.
3. To 5 µL aliquots of sample protein extract, lysis buffer (negative control), or DDW (blank sample), add 95 µL DDW.
4. To each 100-µL sample and the albumin standard, add 2.0 mL BCA working reagent (1:20 vol).
5. Incubated at 37°C for 30 min, cool, transfer to a 3.5 mL disposable cuvet, and measure for the absorption at A_{562} by spectrophotometer. By comparing with the standard curve drawn for the albumin standards, protein concentration of each sample extract can be determined.

3.1.5. CX Tube

1. Place 2 µL of 50 ng/µL CX primer in the bottom of a HotStart 50™ PCR tube and heat to 80°C for 3 min using thermalcycler.
2. The CX tube can be used for TRAP assay after 10 min cooling at room temperature, which allows the CX primer to be sealed below the wax barrier. These tubes can be stored at 4°C for several days.

3.1.6. Negative Control

1. Negative controls must be included in each experiment.
2. Negative control one: Use lysis buffer instead of protein extract.
3. Negative control two: RNase to destroy hTR. Add 0.5 µL of RNase to a 5 µL aliquot of protein extract and incubate at 37°C for 20 min.
4. Negative control three: Heat protein extract at 85°C for 10 min.

3.1.7. PCR

1. For 10 assays, combine 50 µL 10X PCR buffer (final 1X), 10 µL of 2.5 mM 4 dNTP (final 50 µM), 20 µL of 50 ng/µL TS primer (final 344 nM), 2 µL of 5 µg/µL T4gene32protein (final 0.5 µM), 4 µL of 5 U/µL Taq polymerase (Takara, final 2 U/assay), 4 µL of Redivue™ [α-^{32}P]dCTP (final 4 µCi/assay), and 390 µL of DEPC-water (*see* **Note 1**).
2. Place 48 µL each of the PCR mix and up to 2 µL of CHAPS extract containing 6 µg of protein into the HotStart tubes with the sealed CX primer.
3. Incubate samples at 30°C for 30 min for extension of TS primer.
4. Subject each sample to PCR: after 90°C for 3 min, 31 cycles of 94°C for 40 s, 50°C for 40 s, and 72°C for 45 s, followed by 72°C for 3 min.
5. Store at 4°C until electrophoresis.

3.2. Polyacrylamide Gel Electrophoresis (PAGE)

3.2.1. Polyacrylamide Gel

1. For one 20×20 cm PAGE gel (10%, 1 mm thickness), combine 26 mL deionized water, 10 mL 40% acrylamide stock, and 4 mL 5X TBE buffer.
2. Mix well and de-aerated by applying vacuum. Add 100 μL of 10% APS and 36 μL of TEMED just before pouring between glass plates.
3. Immediately insert the comb into the gel and allow the acrylamide to polymerize for 1 h or more (*see* **Note 3**).

3.2.2. Polyacrylamide Gel Electrophoresis

1. Prepare 600 mL of 0.5X TBE buffer for one gel.
2. Add 4 μL loading buffer to 16 μL of each PCR product, and subject to electrophoresis for 4 h at 200 V or overnight at 80 V, until BPB comes to the bottom of the gel.
3. Remove the gel from between the glass plates, seal in Saran Wrap, and subject to autoradiography at –80°C overnight or expose to an imaging plate at room temperature for 1 h.

3.3. Modified TRAP Assay (Fig. 1B) (11)

Tissue extracts sometimes contain inhibitors for the TRAP assay. These inhibitors mainly affect the PCR step rather than the telomerase-mediated extension of the TS primer. When existence of inhibitors is suspected, they should be removed before the PCR step.

3.3.1. Detection of TRAP Assay Inhibitors

1. To the TRAP reaction mixture, add 5 μL of 10^{-17} g (10 attg)/μL ITAS for 10 assays.
2. Run TRAP assay and analyze result. If both 150-bp ITAS band and 6-bp telomerase ladder are absent in any sample, they should be considered to contain TRAP assay inhibitors.

3.3.2. Removal of TRAP Assay Inhibitors

1. Carry out the primer extension step in a 1.5-mL microcentrifuge tube instead of the HotStart tube.
2. For 1 assay, combine 40 μL DEPC-water, 5 μL 10X PCR buffer (final 1X), 1 μL 2.5 m*M* 4 dNTP (final 50 μ*M*), 2 μL 50 ng/μL TS primer (final 344 n*M*), and 2 μL protein extract and incubate at 30°C for 30 min.
3. After incubation, add 5 μL (1/10 volume) 5 *M* NaCl and 25 μL (1/2 volume) each of phenol and CIAA, mix well, and centrifuge at 10,000 rpm for 10 min at room temperature.
4. Transfer the supernatant to a new microcentrifuge tube and add 125 μL (2.5-fold volume) ethanol, mix well, and store at –20°C overnight or at –80°C for 20 min.

5. Centrifuge at 12,000 rpm for 20 min at 4°C. After the supernatant is removed, rinse pellet with 70% ethanol, centrifuge at 12,000 rpm for 10 min, and again remove supernatant.
6. Briefly dry pellet and dissolve in 5 μL DDW.

3.3.3. PCR

1. In a 0.5-mL PCR tube, combine 5 μL 10X PCR buffer (final 1X), 1 μL 2.5 m*M* 4 dNTP (final 50 μ*M*), 2 μL each of 50 ng/μL TS and CX primers (final 344 n*M* each), 0.2 μL of 5 μg/μL T4gene32protein (final 0.5 μ*M*), 0.4 μL of 5 U/μL Taq polymerase (final 2 U/assay), 0.4 μL of Redivue™ [α-^{32}P]dCTP (final 4 μCi/assay), and 34 μL of DDW.
2. Add 5 μL of resolved TS primer extension products to the reaction mixture and subject to PCR using conditions described for the original TRAP assay.

3.4. Protocol for Using the TRAPeze™ Telomerase Detection Kit (see Fig. 1B,2B) (12)

In this kit, β-mercaptoethanol or AEBSF need not be added to the lysis buffer. In the PCR step, using the modified CX primer (RP) allows elimination of T4gene32protein or HotStart tubes. For quantitation of the telomerase activity level and detection of TRAP assay inhibitors, a short internal control is already included. (TRAPeze™ Modified Reagent Set contains the long internal control.)

3.4.1. End-labeling of TS Primer (see **Note 2**)

1. For 10 assays, combine 2.5 μL [γ-^{32}P]ATP, 10 μL of TS primer, 2 μL 10X kinase buffer, 0.5 μL T4 polynucleotide kinase, and 5 μL of DEPC-water (total 20 μL).
2. Incubate at 37°C for 20 min for phosphorylation, then heat-inactivate at 85°C for 5 min.

3.4.2. TRAP Assay

1. For 10 assays, combine 50 μL 10X PCR buffer, 10 μL 50X dNTPs, 20 μL [γ-^{32}P]-labeled TS primer, 10 μL TRAP primer mix, 4 μL 5 U/μL Taq polymerase, and 386 μL of DEPC-water for master mix.
2. Place 48 μL aliquots of master mix into PCR tubes. To each tube, add 1–2 μL of protein extract (containing up to 2 μg of protein) and incubate at 30°C for 30 min for telomerase-mediated extension of TS primer.
3. Subject each sample to two-step PCR: after 90°C for 3 min, 27 cycles of 94°C for 40 s and 60°C for 40 s, followed by 72°C for 3 min.
4. Store samples at 4°C until electrophoresis.
5. TRAPeze™ samples are electrophoresed on a 12.5% PAGE gel (23.5 mL of deionized water, 12.5 mL of 40% acrylamide stock, and 4 mL of 5X TBE buffer) at 500V for about 1 h, until BPB dye reaches bottom of gel.

6. Gel is subjected to autoradiography as for original assay (*see* **Subheading 3.2.2.**).

3.5. Analysis of Result

1. Confirm that negative controls (lysis buffer and RNase- or heat-treated sample) show no ladder, and that positive samples (immortal cancer cell lines or TSR8 of TRAPeze™ kit) show 6-bp ladders.
2. False-positive has occurred if negative controls show 6-bp ladders. Possible causes are:
   a. primer-dimers (degraded T4gene32protein in original TRAP assay), or low annealing temperature in the PCR step, or
   b. contamination of telomerase positive extracts or PCR products.
3. False-negative has occurred if both the internal control and the 6-bp ladder signals are negative. Possible causes are:
   a. existence of TRAP assay inhibitors (usually PCR inhibitors),
   b. inappropriate PCR conditions, or
   c. degraded Taq polymerase.
      If the ladder signals in positive controls are also negative, suspect b. or c. If they are positive, it means probable presence of TRAP assay inhibitors in the sample extract, and use of the modified TRAP assay is strongly recommended. When a sample has excessively high telomerase activity (strong signal of the 6-bp ladder) the internal control bands (ITAS, the short internal control of TRAPeze™ kit, or the long internal control of Modified Reagent Set) may not be visible due to competitive PCR.
4. Relative telomerase activity level can be estimated by serial dilution of the protein extract. When 6-bp ladder signal is positive using 6 µg of protein but not 0.6 µg (10X dilution), the sample is considered to have a low level of telomerase activity. When positive using 0.6 µg of protein but not using 0.06 µg of protein (100X dilution), the sample is considered to have a moderate level of telomerase activity. The sample with positive 6-bp ladder signal using 0.06 µg protein is considered to have high telomerase activity.
5. Quantitation of telomerase activity level using the TRAPeze™ kit: By using a PhosphorImager™ (Molecular Dynamics, Sunnyvale, CA) or BAS2000™ (Fuji, Tokyo, Japan), signal intensities of 6-bp ladders in a sample (x), in the inactivated (RNase- or heat-treated) sample (x_0), in a TSR8 control (r), and in a negative control (lysis buffer, r_0), as well as those of 36-bp internal controls in the sample (c) and in the TSR8 control (c_R) can be measured. Relative telomerase activity level (TPG: total product generated) is expressed as the following formula:

$$\text{TPG (units)} = \{(x-x_0)/c\}/\{(r-r_0)/c_R\} \times 100 \qquad (\textit{see } \textbf{Fig. 2B})$$

4. Notes

1. The telomerase ladder signal can also be detected by a nonisotopic method, The PAGE gel can be stained with SYBR™ Green I (Molecular Probes) and

signal intensities can be estimated using a CCD Imaging System. However, the sensitivity is higher using the isotopic protocol. Quantitation of hTERT (catalytic component of telomerase) mRNA by reverse transcriptase (RT)-PCR can also be considered to represent the telomerase activity level. However, mRNA expression level does not always correlate with telomerase activity level, due to alternative splicing *(13)* or epigenetic mechanisms *(14)*. hTERT protein can be detected *in situ* by immunohistochemistry *(15)*, and the percentage of positive cells in the tissue correlates well with telomerase activity level.

2. In general, the sensitivity of the TRAPeze™ kit is higher than that of the original TRAP assay. However, since the TRAPeze™ kit includes a short internal control template (36-bp) in primer mix, and shorter fragments have higher PCR efficiency, samples with weak telomerase activity sometimes fail to show the 6-bp ladder signal (50 bp and more) due to competition with the internal control. In that case, original TRAP assay with ITAS (150 bp), TRAPeze™ Modified Reagent Set using a long internal control (173 bp), or TRAPeze™ kit protocol modified by incorporation of [α-^{32}P]dCTP instead of end-labeling with [γ-^{32}P]ATP is recommended (more ^{32}P molecules are incorporated in longer fragments by incorporation method, while only one ^{32}P molecule is labeled on every fragments by the end-labeling method) *(12)*.

3. Though gel may polymerize within 5–15 min, allow it to polymerize for 1 h or more, so that the background is reduced. It can be stored for a few days at 4°C or room temperature, sealed in Saran Wrap, until use.

Acknowledgments

We would like to acknowledge Drs Jerry W. Shay and Mieczyslaw A. Piatyszek for their generous help in setting up the protocols. A part of this work was carried out at the Research Center for Molecular Medicine, Hiroshima University School of Medicine.

References

1. Prescott, J. C. and Blackburn, E. H. (1999) Telomerase: Dr Jekyll or Mr Hyde? *Curr. Opin. Genet. Dev.* **9,** 368–373.
2. Shay, J. W., Zou, Y., Hiyama, E., and Wright, W. E. (2001) Telomerase and cancer. *Hum. Mol. Genet.* **10,** 677–685.
3. Shay, J. W. and Bacchetti, S. (1997) A survey of telomerase activity in human cancer. *Eur. J. Cancer* **33,** 787–791.
4. Greider, C. W. and Blackburn, E. H. (1985) Identification of a specific telomere terminal transferase activity in Tetrahymena extracts. *Cell* **43,** 405–413.
5. Morin, G. B. (1989) The human telomere terminal transferase enzyme is a ribonucleoprotein that synthesizes TTAGGG repeats. *Cell* **59,** 521–529.
6. Kim, N. W., Piatyszek, M. A., Prowse, K. R., Harley, C. B., West, M. D., Ho, P. L. C., et al. (1994) Specific association of human telomerase activity with immortal cells and cancer. *Science* **266,** 2011–2015.

7. Hiyama, K., Hiyama, E., Ishioka, S., Yamakido, M., Inai, K., et al. (1995) Telomerase activity in small-cell and non-small-cell lung cancers. *J. Natl. Cancer Inst.* **87,** 895–902.

8. Hiyama, E., Hiyama, K., Yokoyama, T., Matsuura, Y., Piatyszek, M. A., and Shay, J. W. (1995) Correlating telomerase activity levels with human neuroblastoma outcomes. *Nature Med.* **1,** 249–255.

9. Piatyszek, M. A., Kim, N. W., Weinrich, S. L., Hiyama, K., Hiyama, E., Wright, W. E., and Shay, J. W. (1995) Detection of telomerase activity in human cells and tumors by a telomeric repeat amplification protocol (TRAP). *Methods Cell Sci.* **17,** 1–15.

10. Wright, W. E., Shay, J. W., and Piatyszek, M. A. (1995) Modifications of a telomeric repeat amplification protocol (TRAP) result in increased reliability, linearity and sensitivity. *Nucleic Acids Res.* **23,** 3794–3795.

11. Hiyama, E., Hiyama, K., Tatsumoto, N., Kodama, T., Shay, J. W., and Yokoyama, T. (1996) Telomerase activity in human intestine. *Int. J. Oncol.* **9,** 453–458.

12. Holt, S. E., Norton, J. C., Wright, W. E., and Shay, J. W. (1996) Comparison of the telomeric repeat amplification protocol (TRAP) to the new TRAP-eze telomerase detection kit. *Methods Cell Sci.* **18,** 237–248.

13. Ulaner, G. A., Hu, J. F., Vu, T. H., Giudice, L. C., and Hoffman, A. R. (1998) Telomerase activity in human development is regulated by human telomerase reverse transcriptase (hTERT) transcription and by alternate splicing of hTERT transcripts. *Cancer Res.* **58,** 4168–4172.

14. Liu, K., Schoonmaker, M. M., Levine, B. L., June, C. H., Hodes, R. J., and Weng, N. P. (1999) Constitutive and regulated expression of telomerase reverse transcriptase (hTERT) in human lymphocytes. *Proc. Natl. Acad. Sci. USA* **96,** 5147–5152.

15. Hiyama, E., Hiyama, K., Yokoyama, T., and Shay, J. W. (2001) Immunohistochemical detection of telomerase (hTERT) protein in human cancer tissues and a subset of cells in normal tissues. *Neoplasia* **3,** 17–26.

30

Analysis of Alterations in a Base-Excision Repair Gene in Lung Cancer

Nandan Bhattacharyya and Sipra Banerjee

1. Introduction

Cellular DNA is continuously exposed to a variety of insults induced by different endogenous or exogenous agents, including ionizing radiation, ultraviolet (UV) light, chemicals, and by-products of oxidative stress *(1)*. Damaged DNA, if not repaired, can cause cell death, aging and cancer. Therefore, a highly efficient network of DNA repair systems is necessary to remove DNA lesions and to restore and maintain the correct genetic information. DNA lesions can be repaired by three major pathways *(see* **Fig. 1**): a) a direct reversal pathway, which undoes a harmful reaction and restores the original DNA by transferring a methyl group from O^6-methylguanine by O^6-Methylguanine-DNA methyltransferase *(2)*; b) an excision-repair pathway, which involves the removal of the endogenous damaged DNA; and c) a postreplication pathway, which allows cells to complete the replication process without removing the lesion. There are three major categories of excision repair *(see* **Fig. 1**): the nucleotide-excision repair (NER) pathway, the base-excision repair (BER) pathway, and the mismatch-repair (MMR) pathway *(3–9)*. Which of these is used depends on their mechanism of repair and the nature of the damaged substrate. The NER pathway can repair a 25–32 bp lesion *(5,9)*, whereas the BER pathway repairs a short patch (1–14 bp) of altered bases *(10)*. Mismatch repair is responsible for removing mis-paired DNA sequences and involves excision of a long, single-stranded fragment spanning the mismatch, with resynthesis of the segment *(9)*.

From: *Methods in Molecular Medicine, vol. 74: Lung Cancer, Vol. 1: Molecular Pathology Methods and Reviews*
Edited by: B. Driscoll © Humana Press Inc., Totowa, NJ

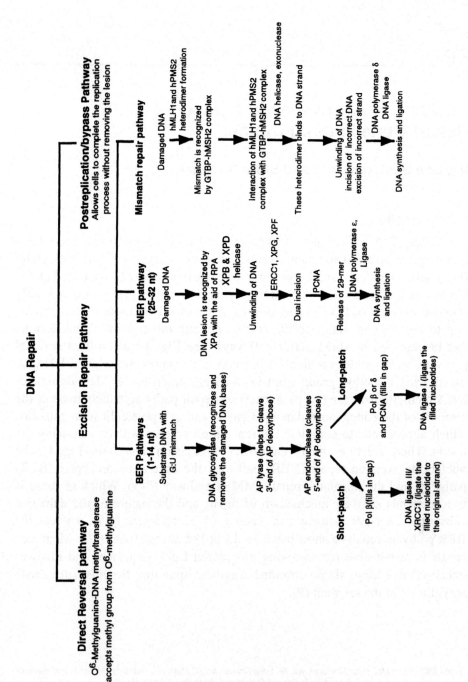

1.1. DNA Repair and Disease

A number of genetic diseases have been associated with defects in one or more DNA repair genes. Xeroderma pigmentosum (XP), a hereditary skin disease, is associated with a deficiency in replication of UV-damaged DNA. Patients with XP may also have severe neurological abnormalities. Cockayne syndrome (CS), an autosomal recessive inheritance syndrome characterized by severe neuronal degeneration, is associated with defects in the NER pathway. Patients with CS have an average life span of 12 years. Ataxia telangiectasia (AT), a rare autosomal recessive inheritance disease, is also associated with the deficiency of repair in a double-strand break. BRCA1 and BRCA2, breast and ovarian cancer susceptible genes, are also associated with a defect in double-strand repair. Defective DNA replication and repair are also associated with a rare autosomal recessive condition, Bloom's syndrome. Werner's syndrome, involving premature aging of the young, has also been associated with defects in the DNA repair machinery. It has been shown that most cases of hereditary nonpolyposis colon cancer are caused by defective MMR genes (11–15). Deficiencies of mismatch binding protein in a small group of lung cancer patients have been implicated in carcinogenesis (16). Previously, no known diseases were found to be associated with defects in BER. Several reports have suggested a possible role of repair genes in lung cancer. One report suggested that individuals having lower DNA repair capacity may have an increased risk of cancer (17). Very recently, in a case-control study, another group has found low expression levels of certain NER genes in lung cancer patients (18), which may have increased their risk of disease. Recently, it has been suggested that persons with polymorphisms of X-ray cross complementing group 1 (XRCC1), a DNA repair gene involved in the BER pathway, may be more susceptible to lung cancer (19,20). All this evidence suggests a possible involvement of these repair genes in lung cancer.

1.2. Base-Excision Repair

In BER, 1-14 nucleotide-damaged bases are removed, leaving a gap in the DNA strand. This gap is filled in by DNA synthesis and finally ligated by DNA ligase. Previously it was thought that BER repaired only a single-nucleotide gap (21). Frosina et al. (10) first postulated two distinct BER pathways in

---

Fig. 1. (*see facing page*) Schematic representation of the different pathways of DNA repair. Human Mut S homolog 2, hMSH2; Human Mut L homolog 1, hMLH1; human postmeoitic segregation 2, hPMS2; G/T binding protein, GTBP; Proliferating Cell Nuclear Antigen, PCNA; X-Ray Cross Complementing 1, XRCC1, Xeroderma Pigmentosum, XP; Base-excision repair, BER; Nucleotide excision repair, NER.

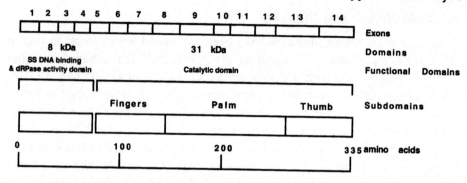

Fig. 2. Diagrammatic representation of the structure and function of mammalian DNA polβ.

the mammalian system (*see* **Fig. 2**). Supporting this hypothesis, Klungland and Lindahl *(22)* have shown that the BER pathway consists of two branches, "short-patch" and "long-patch" (*see* **Fig. 1**).

1.2.1. Steps in Base-Excision Repair

Human AP endonuclease (Ape), polymerase β (polβ), XRCC1, and DNA ligase III are sufficient for activation of the short-patch (also known as single nucleotide insertion) repair pathway (*see* **Fig. 1**) at the apurinic/apyrimidinic (AP) site. The long-patch repair pathway is also known as the proliferating cell nuclear antigen (PCNA) dependent pathway (*see* **Fig. 1**). Polβ and the PCNA-dependent polymerases δ and ε are involved in this pathway. In both, the first enzyme in the BER pathway is DNA glycosylase, which cleaves off the deoxyribose from mismatched or damaged DNA. AP deoxyribose is released by sequential action of an AP lyase, which cleaves 3′, and an Ape that cleaves 5′ to the AP site leaving a 5′ deoxyribose phosphate, dRP *(8)*. The AP sites inhibit replication and are mutagenic *(8)*. Ape is expressed abundantly in the nuclei of human cells. The next step of the BER pathway is removal of the dRP, followed by DNA gap-filling synthesis. DNA polβ has the ability to remove this dRP by its dRP lyase activity, and it also fills in the gap *(8)*. The final step is the ligation by DNA ligase to complete the repair process (*see* **Fig. 1**).

1.3. What is polβ?

DNA polβ is a single-copy 33-kb gene consisting of 14 exons *(23,24)*. The polβ gene encodes a 39-kDa protein consisting of 335 amino acids with two distinct functional domains, of 8-kDa and 31-kDa (*see* **Fig. 2**) *(8)*. The catalytic property of polβ resides in the carboxyl terminal region of the 31-kDa domain (~260 residues), whereas the amino terminal 8-kDa domain (75 residues)

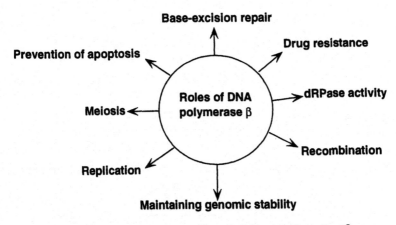

Fig. 3. Schematic representation of different roles of polβ.

shows a strong affinity for the DNA template (*see* **Fig. 2**). The catalytic domain consists of fingers, palm, and thumb subdomains *(8)*.

1.3.1. Roles of Polβ

A recent report from Sanderson and Mosbaugh *(25)* supports the concept that most uracil-mediated DNA repair synthesis occurs by the BER pathway. Polβ can remove dRP by its dRPase activity during the repair process *(26,27)*. In eukaryotic cells, polβ provides most of the gap-filling repair synthesis *(28)*. The polβ gene is presumably involved in both short-patch and long-patch BER pathways *(10,22)*. Recent reports have shown that polβ is essential for the embryonic viability of mice *(29)*. An embryonic fibroblast cell line, homozygous for a polβ deletion mutation, is reported to be defective in uracil-mediated BER *(28,30)*. Additional reports provide evidence that polβ has a contributing role in mammalian DNA replication, recombination, and meiosis and in conferring a drug-resistant phenotype *(31–33)*. It is interesting to note that during apoptosis, cell lines replace polα with polβ for DNA synthesis *(34)*. Also it has been shown recently that polβ has a role in the prevention of apoptosis *(35)*. Reichenberger and Pfeiffer *(36)* have reported that polβ has a role in nonhomologous DNA-end joining in *Xenopus laevis*. Hence, the accumulated evidence (summarized in **Fig. 3**) strongly supports the role of polβ in overcoming threatened DNA damage by repair and replication and thus in maintaining normal cellular survival in eukaryotic cells.

1.3.2. Alterations in DNA Polβ in Human Cancer

It has been demonstrated by this laboratory that the coding sequence of polβ is altered in sporadic primary colorectal, breast, and prostate carcinomas

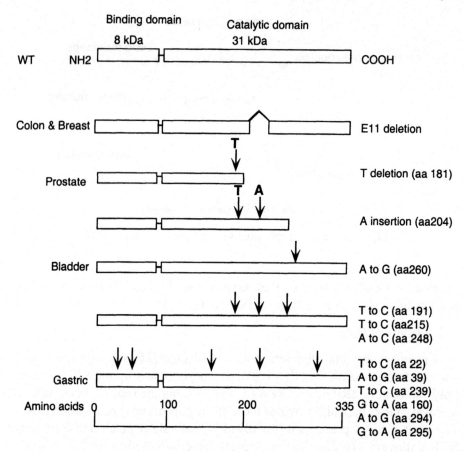

Fig. 4. Alterations of polβ in human tumor.

(37,38). An 87-bp deletion (polβΔ), which may arise either through a mutation or alternate splicing in the mRNA of polβ, occurs frequently (50–60%) in breast and colorectal tumors (*see* **Fig. 4**). Both wild-type (WT) and polβΔ proteins are expressed in colorectal and breast tumors and in a primary culture of renal cell carcinoma *(39–41)*.

An alteration in polβ is also detected at a low frequency (14–17%) in prostate adenocarcinoma; a single-base T deletion occurs, causing termination of polβ protein synthesis at codon 181 *(38)*. In contrast, sequences of polβ cDNA in normal corresponding prostate tissues matched the published sequence perfectly. Similarly, Dobashi et al. *(42)* reported a deletion of T in the polβ gene of prostate cancer. A report from Matsuzaki et al. *(43)* showed missense point mutations and a single base insertion in the cDNA of polβ in bladder cancer. Interestingly, the variant form of polβ has also been reported to be expressed in normal cells *(44)*. A presumptive role of polβ in gene therapy against colorectal cancer was suggested by Shadan and Villarreal *(45)*. This accumulating evidence suggests that polβ contributes to human carcinogenesis.

We provided evidence for the possible involvement of polβ in human carcinogenesis. An 87-bp deletion in the coding sequence of polβ occurs in colorectal and breast cancers *(37,38,40)*. This deletion encodes amino acid residues 208–236 in the catalytic domain of the polβ enzyme. Sadakane et al. *(46)* reported an identical deletion encoding amino acids 208–236 of polβ in blood samples of patients with Werner's syndrome. The Werner's syndrome gene (WRN) has been identified and localized on chromosome 8p12 *(47)* to which the polβ gene has also been mapped. The link between WRN and polβ, however, remains to be established.

1.3.3. Lung Cancer and DNA Polβ

Lung cancer is a major cause of cancer deaths in United States. It has been estimated that 156,900 people may have died from lung cancer in 2000 in the United States alone, accounting for 28% of all cancer deaths in this country.

To our knowledge, alterations in polβ have not been reported in the setting of lung cancer. Of all cancers, lung cancer has become the deadliest in both men and women. An important source for the development of lung cancer is environmental factors, including chemicals and radiation. Epithelial cells of the lung are continuously exposed to exogenous mutagenic and carcinogenic agents. Because polβ is involved in the sensitivity of cells to chemicals and in the repair of chemical-induced DNA damage *(28,39)*, we proposed to investigate a potential alteration in pol? of lung cancer cells. RNA from 11 primary lung cancers and corresponding normal lung tissues from the same patients was reverse transcribed, and the first strand of cDNA was amplified by polymerase chain reaction (PCR) and sequenced. In addition, normal lung tissues from healthy nonsmoking and smoking individuals were examined for polβ variants. An insertion of 105 bp in the mRNA sequence corresponding to sequences between exons 6 and 7 of polβ was first reported in human cells and named exon α *(24)*. However, expression of exon α in lung-cell RNA has not been reported. Thus, we also have examined a potential expression of exon α in lung tumors and normal lung tissues.

1.4. Examination of Alterations of Polβ in Lung Cancer

1.4.1. Patient Population

The clinical data of lung cancer patients used in this study are summarized in **Table 1**. The lung specimens were from both men and women, ages 59–74. The patients were either current or recent smokers with an average >40 pack-

Table 1
Variant Forms of Polβ in Lung Tumors and Lung Tissues

	Alterations in cDNA Sequence	
Cancer patient #	N[a]	T[b]
23	87 bp deletion	87 bp deletion
	140 bp deletion	140 bp deletion
	105 insertion	105 insertion
29	Unaltered	87 bp deletion
35	Unaltered	Unaltered
42	Unaltered	Unaltered
51	Unaltered	87 bp deletion
65	87 bp deletion	87 bp deletion
	140 bp deletion	140 bp deletion
	105 insertion	105 insertion
75	Unaltered	Unaltered
84	87 bp deletion	87 bp deletion
	140 bp deletion	140 bp deletion
	105 insertion	105 insertion
302	Unaltered	Unaltered
333	Unaltered	546 bp deletion
344	Unaltered	Unaltered
Healthy volunteer #		Normal lung tissue
NS326[c]		Unaltered
NS451		Unaltered
NS454		Unaltered
S212[d]		Unaltered
S298		87 bp deletion
S301		Unaltered
S330		87 bp deletion

[a]N: RNA from matched normal lung tissue from lung cancer patient.
[b]T: RNA from lung tumor tissue.
[c]NS: Non-smoker.
[d]S: Smoker.

year smoking history. Tumors were diagnosed as squamous, non-small, or large-cell carcinomas, and were well to poorly differentiated with stages I to III. All cancer patients were smokers except patient #75. Patient #75 had multiple malignancies identified 2 yr prior to the development of his lung cancer. He had a small cell carcinoma in the left lung, treated by chemotherapy, and prior to that, an adrenal adenoma, suggesting mutation other than polβ

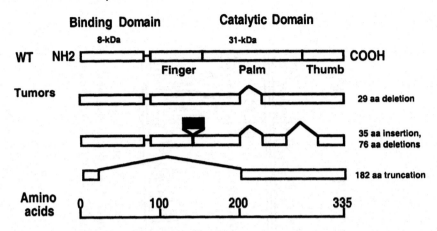

Fig. 5. Schematic illustrations of the wild-type and variant polβ in lung carcinomas. The locations of deletion of 87-bp (29 amino acid truncation) and deletions of 140-bp (76 amino acid truncation) and insertion of 105-bp (35 amino acid insertion) found in lung tumors are shown. Symbol ∧ represents deletion and symbol ■ represents insertion. Deletions of 182 amino acids in patient #333 are also shown. The predicted truncated proteins are localized in the catalytic domain of polβ.

leading to predisposition to multiple neoplasia. Patient #75 revealed an unaltered polβ sequence.

1.4.2. Characteristic Alterations in Polβ Exons

The 34-kb polβ gene is composed of 14 exons *(23)*. Exon 11 consists of 87-bp encoding amino acid residues 208–236. The length of exon 13 is 140-bp which encodes amino acid residues 259–304. The primary structure of wild-type polβ protein consists of 335 amino acid residues (*see* **Figs. 2,5**). The predominant variant form found in lung tumor is a deletion of 87-bp in the 3′ region of the coding sequence that would correspond to exon 11 (found in tumor #23,#29,#51,#65, and #84, *see* **Fig. 6**). The wild-type 1-kb transcript in tumor (T, **Fig. 7**) is 85% of 1-kb transcript of the normal matched tissue (N) (Adobe Photoshop and Image Quant programs were used to quantitate the transcript intensity level). It is interesting to observe that all tumors tested expressed the wild-type polβ transcript. The 913-bp transcript expressed in tumor is 493% of normal tissue transcript, indicating this is upregulated by 393%. This is the trend we have seen in tumors #23, 29, 51, 65, and 84. The smallest transcript (639-bp) is expressed in tumor at a level of 80% of the normal. The 639-bp transcript would correspond to exons 11 and 13 and insertion of 105-bp or exon α. It is possible that due to mutations at the exon-intron junctions of exons 11 (87-bp) and 13 (140-bp), these two exons will

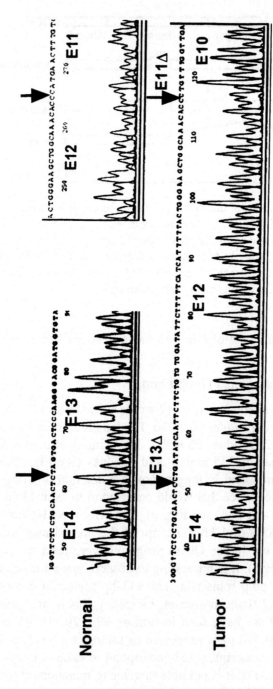

Fig. 6. Partial nucleotide sequence of polβ cDNA in lung carcinoma. The lower panel, designated Tumor, shows the sequence indicating deletions of 87 bp (E11Δ) and 140 bp (E13Δ) of the PCR product obtained from patient #23. The position is shown by an arrow (↓). The upper panel (Normal) shows wild-type cDNA sequences corresponding to exons 11 and 13 of a normal matched lung tissue obtained from patient #29.

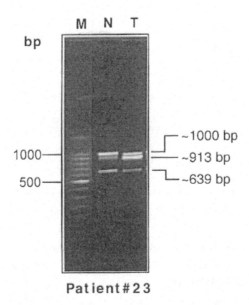

Fig. 7. PCR amplification of coding sequence of human polβ gene in lung tumor. Lanes N and T represent normal and lung tumor tissues (patient #23). Sizes of transcripts in base pairs (bp) are shown on the right side of the panel. Lane M shows molecular-weight markers in base pairs (bp).

be deleted from the polβ gene. A report from this laboratory showed a unique 0.8-kb allele in the polβ gene along with a wild-type 1.3-kb allele in colorectal tumors using genomic probe encompassing intron 10-exon 11-intron 11 (partial) of polβ gene (**Fig. 8**). The normal corresponding mucosa exhibited only the wild-type 1.3-kb allele *(49)*. This Southern-blot analysis suggests that an allelic alteration has occurred at this region of polβ of tumor DNA. Alternatively, it is highly possible that an error in splicing of polβ message has occurred in tumors.

1.5. Summary

Six of the 11 lung cancer patients exhibited variant forms of polβ at a frequency of 54.5%. A polβ variant with 87-bp or exon 11 deletion may express 306 amino acid residues. Identical deletions in polβ cDNA have been described in colorectal and breast cancers *(37,38,40)* and in blood specimens of Werner's syndrome patient *(46)*. Furthermore, a truncated polβ protein of 294 amino acids is expected to be expressed in tumor exhibiting deletions of 87-bp and 140-bp with an insertion of 105-bp. All the alterations in polβ identified in lung tumors are in the catalytic domain of the polβ protein and are in-frame alterations (**Fig. 9**), except tumor #333, in which the deletion extends from the

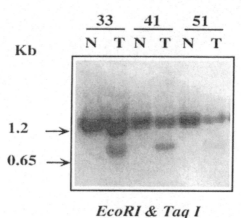

Fig. 8. Allelic alterations in the polβ gene. Lane T shows restriction fragments for tumors. Lane N shows fragments from corresponding normal tissues. The genomic probe consists of a 315-bp product.

binding domain to the catalytic domain. The truncated protein would consist of 182 amino acids (**Fig. 9**). Previously, others and we have demonstrated that all polβ variants are located in the catalytic domain of the protein in colorectal, breast, prostate, bladder carcinomas, and Werner's disease *(37,38,42,43,46)*. The polβ variant with deletions of 87- and 140-bp with an insertion of 105-bp between exons 6 and 7 is expected to express a truncated protein of 214 amino acid residues (tumor #23, #65, and #84). Interestingly, the normal tissue from same patients shows the same variant type as revealed by their counterpart. Although earlier reports have documented the occurrence of altered polβ cDNA in normal tissue *(24,44)*, the origin of these alterations in polβ in normal lung tissues of lung cancer patients is unclear. It may be owing to a predisposing mutation in noncancerous lung related to malignant transformation. These last two variants, detected in lung tumors, have not been observed in other tumors such as colorectal, prostate, breast, or bladder *(37,38,40,42,43)*. An expected 155-bp product was noticed in tumors #23, #65, and #84 (*see* **Fig. 9**). We reported exon α insertion in breast tumors and matched normal breast tissues as well as in human colon tumor cell lines (LoVo, HCT116, and DLDI), MCF7 (mammary tumor cell line) and in a primary culture of renal cell carcinoma *(50)*. The variants identified in this study have also been identified in other tumors, including those of the colon and breast, and in blood samples from WRN patients except one variant (exon 11 and 13 deletion along with exon α insertion). Because none of these other diseases has a profoundly smoking-related etiology, it cannot be strongly argued that these variants are directly related to smoking in lung cancer. Moreover, most lung cancer cases have

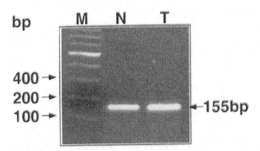

Fig. 9. RT-PCR products of 105-bp insertion (exon α) obtained from lung tumor (T) and normal matched lung tissue in patient #23. Lane M represents molecular-weight markers in base pairs. The sizes of the products are 155-bp.

a history of cigarette smoking, so it is not surprising that most of the lung cancer cases, where variants were observed, were smokers. The expression of a 29-amino-acid truncated polβ protein (87-bp deleted cDNA) has been reported in colorectal tumors *(39)*. Additionally, this truncated polβ markedly inhibits the gap-filling synthesis and DNA binding activities of the wild-type enzyme, indicating that the variant form of polβ acts as a dominant-negative mutant *(39)*. Furthermore, cells overexpressing truncated polβ are hypersensitive to N-methyl-N′-nitro-N-nitrosoguanidine, a potent DNA-damaging carcinogenic agent. A potential role of polβ in gene therapy against cancer has been suggested *(45)*. An altered polβ gene may be implicated in increasing susceptibility of individuals to develop cancer *(51)*.

2. Materials

2.1. Preparation of Tumor and Normal Lung Specimens

Lung tumor and matched normal lung tissues from the same patient, both snap-frozen in liquid nitrogen and formalin fixed immediately after surgery. Tissue analysis performed by The Cleveland Clinic's Department of Anatomic Pathology.

2.2. RNA Preparation

2.2.1. Total RNA Isolation

1. Bio-pulverizer (Biospec products, Inc.).
2. Liquid N_2 (**Be careful when using liquid N2 because it can cause severe skin burn**).
3. Aluminum foil (Bake at 250°C for 2 h).
4. Stainless steel spoon (Bake at 250°C for 2 h).
5. Spatula (teflon-coated; bake at 250°C for 2 h).
6. Eppendorf tubes (1.5-mL, RNase, DNase free).

7. Pipet tips (RNase, DNase free).
8. Chloroform.
9. RNA-Bee (TEL-TEST, TX).
10. Centrifuge, ice, gloves, and so on.

2.2.2. Reverse Transcription

1. SuperScript Preamplification System (Invitrogen, Rockville, MD). Includes random hexamers (50 ng/μL), 10X RT buffer containing 200 m*M* Tris-HCl, pH 8.4, and 500 m*M* KCl, 25 m*M* MgCl$_2$, 0.1 *M* DTT, 10 m*M* each of dATP, dCTP, dGTP, dTTP, Superscript II RT (50 U/μL), RNASEOUT (40 U/μL), RNase H (2 U/μL), DEPC treated water, control RNA, and control primers A & B.
2. Thin walled PCR tubes.
3. Two primers specific for DNA polymerase beta total cDNA:
   [Asym A, 5′-GGAATCACCGACATGCTC-3′
   Asym B, 5′-GTCCTTGGGTTCCCGGTA-3′],
4. Thermal cycler (MJ Research, Inc., Watertown, MA).
5. 37°C, 42°C, 65°C, and 70°C water baths.
6. Gloves, tips, pipets, and so on.

2.3. PCR Amplification

1. GeneAmp PCR Reagent Kit (Roche, Branchburg, NJ).

2.3.1. Separation and Purification of PCR Products

1. Agarose: High-strength analytical grade (Bio-Rad Laboratories, Hercules, CA).
2. 10X TBE buffer: 108 gm of Trizma base, 55 gm of Boric acid, and 7.4 gm EDTA/L.
3. 6X Loading dye: 0.25% bromophenol blue, 0.25% xylene cyanol FF, and 15% Ficoll in water.
4. Geneclean II kit (BIO 101 Inc., Vista, CA).
5. Sharp blade (Take proper precaution).
6. UV transilluminator (Take proper precaution).
7. Protective glasses for UV.
8. Water bath (55°C).

2.4. Subcloning and Sequencing

1. Reagents for re-amplification PCR as described in **Subheading 2.3.**
2. TA cloning system (Invitrogen, Carlbad, CA). Includes 10X Ligation buffer, PCR Vector, T4 DNA ligase, SOC medium, and competent cells.
3. Water bath (42°C).
4. LB agar plates with 100 μg/mL of ampicillin.
5. X-gal solution: 40 mg/mL in dimethylformamide.
6. 12°C cooler.
7. Pasteur pipet.
8. Flame.

2.5. Specific Exon Analysis

2.5.1. Amplification of Exon α

1. Primers used are those described by Chyan et al. *(24)*. Two primers that were used for the amplification of exon alpha are:
   5'-primer, GCTCACAGCTGGATTCATGCCCAG
   3'-primer CAGCCCAATTCGCTGATGATGGTTC.

2.5.2. Amplification of Exons of polβ

1. Reagents for PCR of entire coding sequence of polβ including primer set as described in **Subheading 2.2.2.**
2. Agarose: Nusieve GTG low melting agarose (FMC Bioproducts, Rockland, NE): 1.5% Nusieve GTG low melting temperature agarose gel in 1X TBE buffer.

3. Methods

3.1. Preparation of Tumor and Normal Lung Specimens

Lung tumor and matched normal lung tissues from the same patient are snap-frozen in liquid nitrogen after surgery at The Cleveland Clinic hospital. Ten-μm sections fixed in formalin from both tumors and matched normal lung tissues from the same patient are examined and evaluated by histopathology of hematoxylin-eosin stained sections by the Clinic's Department of Anatomic Pathology. Tumor specimens showing at least 95% tumor cells and normal tissues devoid of tumor cells are chosen for study. The specimens are transferred to the laboratory and RNA isolated *(37)*. Normal lung tissues from healthy volunteers are also obtained at fiberoptic bronchoscopy by bronchial brushing of the airway of healthy smoking and nonsmoking individuals. The Cleveland Clinic Foundation's Institutional Review Board approved this study and informed written consent was obtained from healthy volunteers.

3.2. RNA Preparation

Reverse Transcriptase-Polymerase Chain Reaction (RT-PCR) is a method in which the starting material is mRNA. The mRNA is then reverse transcribed into complementary DNA (cDNA) by reverse transcriptase. This strand is also known as first-strand. **Figure 10** shows the schematic diagram of different steps of reverse transcription. This first-strand is used as the substrate for subsequent amplification by polymerase chain reaction.

3.2.1. Total RNA Isolation

1. Total RNA can be prepared using RNA-Bee following the manufacturer's protocol (*see* **Note 1**). The first step is to break the tissue into fine powder. Measure tissue weight, then wrap in aluminum foil and chill in liquid N_2 for

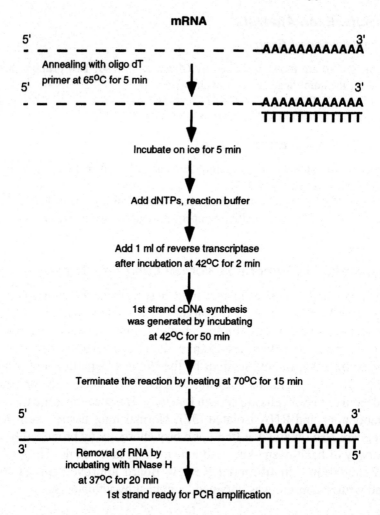

Fig. 10. Diagrammatic representation of different steps for reverse transcription.

at least 15 min. In addition, chill the bio-pulverizer with mortar and piston and
spatulas in liquid N_2 for at least 20 min before use.

2. Place the tissue in the mortar. Pulverize by pressing for 5 blows at a time. Repeat
this step two times until tissue becomes fine powder (*see* **Note 2**).

3. Place powdered tissue in a 1.5-mL eppendorf tube with the help of spatula
(*see* **Note 3**).

4. Add RNA-Bee according to the manufacturer's instruction (2 mL/100 mg of
tissue). Mix lysate thoroughly.

5. Add chloroform (0.2 mL/2 mL of homogenate). Shake the homogenate vigorously for 1 min.

6. Incubate the homogenate on ice for 15 min, then centrifuge for 15 min at 12,000g. Collect the supernatant in a fresh tube.
7. Add isopropanol (0.6 volume) to the supernatant and incubate on ice for 15 min.
8. Precipitate RNA by centrifugation at 12,000g for 15 min at 4°C. Wash the RNA pellet twice with 70% ethanol to remove salts. Dry the pellet. At this stage, RNA can be dissolved either in DEPC treated water or in 0.5% SDS solution (*see* **Note 5**).

3.2.2. Reverse Transcription

RT-PCR is a method in which the starting material is mRNA. For DNA polβ analysis from lung tissue, five microgram of total RNA was reverse transcribed *(37–39)* into complementary DNA (cDNA) by reverse transcriptase using the SuperScript Preamplification System (Invitrogen). **Figure 10** shows the schematic diagram of different steps of reverse transcription. This strand is also known as first-strand (**Note 6**). This first strand is used as the substrate for subsequent amplification by PCR. For DNA polβ analysis as described, first-strand c DNA was amplified (*see* **Fig. 11**) using a Gene Amp PCR Reagent Kit (Roche).

1. Reverse transcribe 5 µg total RNA *(37–39)* using the SuperScript Preamplification System according to manufacturer's instructions (Invitrogen). For DNA polβ analysis, use primers Asym A (5′-GGAATCACCGACATGCTC-3′) and Asym B (5′-GTCCTTGGGTTCCCGGTA-3′). These primers amplify the entire coding sequence of human polβ cDNA *(37,38)*.

3.3. PCR Amplification

1. Amplify first-strand cDNA using a GeneAmp PCR Reagent Kit (Roche) (*see* **Fig. 11**). For DNA polβ amplification, one cycle of denaturation at 96°C for 2 min is followed by 30 cycles of denaturation at 96°C for 1 min, annealing at 55°C for 1 min, and 72°C for 1 min. Finally, perform one extension cycle for 10 min.

3.3.1. Separation and Purification of PCR Products

PCR products are separated and purified PCR products as previously described *(37,38)*.

1. Make a 1% agarose gel with 1X TBE buffer.
2. Separate the samples by running through the gel along with a DNA molecular-weight marker.
3. Place the gel on a piece of Saran wrap on UV transilluminator. Wear protective glass and turn UV light on. Cut the band out of the gel and place in an Eppendorf tube.

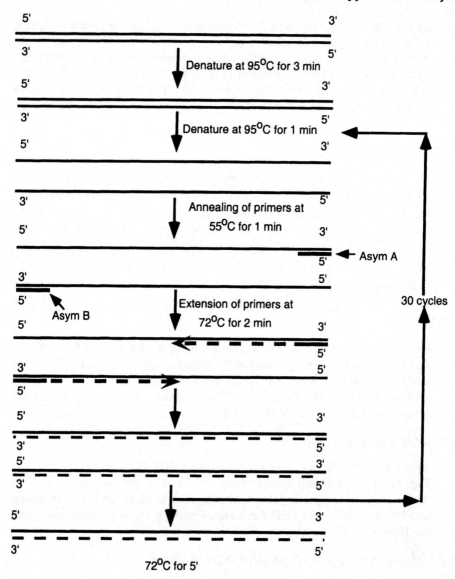

Fig. 11. Schematic representation of the different steps of PCR.

4. Purification uses reagents from the Geneclean II kit. Add 3 volumes of NaI to the gel. Place the tube in a 55°C waterbath. Incubate for at least 5 min (*see* **Note 7**).

5. Once gel pieces are completely dissolved, add 1–2 µL glassmilk. Before addition of any glassmilk, dissolve the glassmilk well by gentle shaking. Shake the suspension in a shaker for at least 15 min.

6. Centrifuge the suspension gently for a couple seconds (do not spin hard, as the silica granules can break). Wash the pellet twice with the wash buffer supplied. Take the same precautions for every spin.

7. Elute the DNA with 20 μL water.

3.4. Subcloning and Sequencing

1. Use the first PCR product for re-amplification. Briefly, 1 μL of the second PCR product is used as the template for second PCR in a 100 μL reaction volume.

2. Clone the re-amplified product into the TA cloning system (Invitrogen). Set up the ligation reaction according to the protocol provided by Invitrogen. Briefly, one μL of 10X ligation buffer, 2 μL PCR vector, one μL of T4 DNA ligase, 2 μL of PCR product, and 5 μL of distilled water are combined in a total volume of 10 μL. Incubate the reaction mixture at 12°C overnight.

3. Perform transformation according to the instructions provided by the supplier. Briefly, thaw 50 μL of one shot *Escherichia coli* competent cells on ice. Add 2 μL ligation mixture and incubate on ice 30 min. Heat-shock cells for 30 s at 42°C. Place back on ice immediately for another 30 min.

4. Add 250 μL of SOC medium to the transformed cells and then place in a 37°C shaker incubator for at least 1 h at a speed of 250 rpm. While the cells are shaking, spread 50 μL of X-gal on each LB plates with ampicillin with the help of a spreader. Place the plates in a 37°C incubator upside down for an hour.

5. After one hour, plate 10 μL of the transformed *E. coli* per plate. Place the plates in a 37°C incubator overnight.

6. Pick up white colonies from the plate next day and let them grow overnight in LB medium with ampicillin (100 μg/mL).

7. Isolate plasmid DNAs from these colonies and verify inserts by digesting with restriction endonuclease *Eco*RI and then separating on a 1% agarose gel.

8. Sequence re-amplified product. For DNA polβ analysis, direct nucleotide sequencing of the rest of the PCR product was analyzed by our sequence core facility (*see* **Note 8**).

3.5. Specific Exon Analysis

3.5.1. Exon α

To determine whether exon α is expressed in lung cells, use PCR to amplify this region in RNA obtained from normal and lung tumor tissues and sequenced (*see* **Subheadings 3.1.–3.4.**). The primers used are those described by Chyan et al. *(24)*.

1. Set up PCR conditions as follows: denaturation at 96°C for 2 min for one cycle followed by a 30 cycles of the following program: denaturation at 96°C for 30 s, annealing at 70°C for 30 s, and extension at 72°C for 1 min. Follow these 30 cycles by another extension cycle for 10 min at 72°C.

3.5.2. Other Exons of Polβ

1. To determine potential alterations in the polβ of lung tumors, the entire coding sequence of polβ mRNA from 11 cancer patients and their corresponding normal lung tissues is amplified by PCR as described in **Subheading 3.3.**
2. Analyze the PCR products, represented by data from patient #23, by low melting agarose gel electrophoresis (**Fig. 7**). Separate PCR products on a 1.5% Nusieve GTG low melting temperature agarose gel in 1X TBE buffer. A product of approx 1 kb each should be obtained from normal lung tissue (N) and lung tumor (T). In this particular patient, #23, two other PCR products (~913- and ~639-bp) were found in both normal and tumor tissues.
3. Excise the band of interest with a blade under UV light. Remove the excess agarose with the blade and purify the DNA from the gel as described in **Subheading 3.3.1.** using a GeneClean II kit.
4. Sequence the ~1 kb product (*see* **Subheading 2.4.**) from both normal and tumor tissues. In our hands, these sequences match the published human wild-type polβ sequence, represented in **Fig. 6 (48)** (*see* **Notes 9, 10**).
5. To compare with lung tumors, we also examined normal lung tissues from seven healthy young adult volunteers, 20–40 yr old. Total RNA is obtained and analyzed as described (*see* **Subheadings 3.2.–3.4.**).

4. Notes

1. Isolation of RNA from tissue is very tricky process, so extreme caution should be taken in order to avoid RNase contamination. All utensils, including the bio-pulverizer, Eppendorf tubes, aluminum foil, and so on, should be baked. Water should be treated with diethylpyrocarbonate (DEPC) overnight and then autoclaved. There are several good commercial kits available for the isolation of RNA from tissue.
2. Be careful of liquid N_2, as the splash can burn skin and eyes. Wear protective clothing, eye glasses, and use appropriate gloves for handling liquid N_2. Because of blow, aluminum foil might be punctured and the tissue might touch the well of the mortar. Therefore, it is advisable to bake the whole bio-pulverizer every single time it is being used to destroy RNase.
3. This step is important in terms of time factor. This process must be quick in order to avoid melting of the powder, thus avoiding the chance of degradation of RNA.
4. At this stage, it is important to make sure that all powders are solubilized. If not, an additional 0.5 mL of RNA-Bee should be added.
5. Note that at times the pellet might be loose, so care must be taken not to lose the pellet during the washing steps. Do not dry the pellet completely. This will make RNA difficult to dissolve. If the RNA does not dissolve completely incubate the solution at 60°C in a water bath for 15 min. It is advisable to test the purity of RNA by running on a formaldehyde agarose gel and then staining the gel with

ethidium bromide before using this RNA in RT-PCR analysis. You should see two distinct intact bands of 28S and 18S ribosomal RNA in a stained gel. If you notice fuzzy bands, the RNA must be degraded. The purity of the RNA can also be tested by taking the OD at 260 and 280 nm by UV spectrophotometry. If the ratio of OD at 260 and 280 nm is above 2.0, the RNA is pure.

6. Before starting any addition of chemicals, make sure all the frozen chemicals are completely thawed). Note that different commercial kits are available in the market and most work fine. Make sure to read the specifications before starting the experiment. It is a good idea to amplify the control primers provided by the supplier with RNA provided. This is the control experiment.

7. The time of incubation depends on the volume of gel. You should check whether the gel is completely dissolved before proceeding with purification. This is critical, because any undissolved particles will be precipitated in the next step.

8. One of the most important factors for direct sequencing is to provide homogeneous product. PCR products that show a single band on a gel were sent out for sequencing. Care must be taken to purify the PCR reaction products by using a Centricon-100 column or other purification system to remove free dNTPs and primers before sequencing. BigDye terminator chemistry is used for routine sequencing in the core.

9. The 913-bp and 639-bp products, nucleotide sequences showed: a) deletions of 87-bp and b) deletions of 87 bp and 140-bp with insertion of 105-bp, respectively (*see* **Fig. 6**). Analyzing the polβ cDNA sequence in 11 primary lung tumors and corresponding normal lung tissues revealed variant forms of polβ in six tumors. Five tumors (#23, #29, #51, #65, and #84) revealed an 87-bp deletion in the cDNA sequence of polβ. Three of these tumors (#23, #65, and #84) also showed deletions in cDNA corresponding to exons 11 and 13 and an insertion of 105-bp. The results are summarized in **Table 2**. Interestingly, matched normal lung tissues of patients #23, #65 and #84 revealed the same alterations in polβ as did their tumors. Tumor #333 exhibited a deletion of 546-bp at nucleotide positions 59 to 604 in polβ cDNA. Thus, these results demonstrate three variant forms in lung tumors (schematically shown in **Fig. 5**).

Besides deletions, an insertion of 105-bp (corresponding to exon α) was identified in three tumors, (#23, #65, and #84). An expected 155-bp PCR product in matched normal lung and tumor tissues is shown in **Fig. 9**. Nucleotide sequencing of this 155-bp PCR product confirmed that it is similar to the 105-bp sequence between exons 6 and 7 (**24**).

10. The mRNA sequence of the polβ gene was unaltered in individuals #NS326, NS451, and NS454, nonsmokers (*see* **Table 1**). A definition for "nonsmoker" means they have never smoked cigarettes in their lifetime. In contrast, lung tissues from individuals #S298 and S330 showed a deletion of 87-bp in the polβ cDNA; two others (#S212 and S301) exhibited an unaltered sequence. These individuals are smokers.

Table 2
Clinical Characteristics of Lung Cancer Patients

Patient #	Age	Sex	Smoker/ nonsmoker	Side	Type	Stage
23	74	F	Smoker	Left	Sq. cell carcinoma[a]	$T_1N_0M_0$ (I)
29	57	M	Smoker	Right	Non-small cell carcinoma	$T_2N_1M_0$ (II)
35	71	M	Smoker	Right	Sq. cell carcinoma	$T_3N_0M_0$ (IIa)
42	65	M	Smoker	Right	Sq. cell carcinoma (mod. diff.)[b]	$T_2N_0M_0$ (II)
51	74	M	Smoker	Left	Sq.cell carcinoma (well diff.)	$T_1N_0M_0$ (I)
				Right	Sq. cell carcinoma (poorly diff.)	
65	59	F	Smoker	Right	Sq. cell carcinoma (mod. to poorly diff.)	$T_1N_0M_0$ (I)
75[c]	66	M	Non-Smoker	Right	Sq. cell carcinoma (poorly diff.)	$T_1N_0M_0$ (I)
84	69	M	Smoker	Left	Sq. cell carcinoma	$T_2N_0M_0$ (I)
302	62	M	Smoker	Left	Large cell carcinoma (poorly diff.)	$T_2N_0M_0$ (I)
333	60	M	Smoker	Right	Large cell carcinoma	$T_2N_0M_0$ (II)
344	62	M	Smoker	Right	Sq. cell carcinoma	$T_4N_0M_0$ (III)

[a]Squamous cell carcinoma.
[b]Moderately differentiated.
[c]Non-small cell carcinoma 3 yr earlier in left lung.

434

Acknowledgment

This work was supported by a NIH grant RO1 CA83768 to S.B and a ACS grant to NB. We thank H.-C. Chen for Southern analysis of colorectal tumors. We extend our appreciation to Christine Kassuba for editing this manuscript.

References

1. Friedberg, E. C., Walker, G. C., and Siede, W. (1995) DNA Repair and Mutagenesis. American Society for Microbiology Press, Washington, DC.
2. Mitra, S. and Kaina, B. (1993) Regulation of repair of alkylation damage in mammalian genomes. *Prog. Nucl. Acids Res. Mol. Biol.* **44,** 109–142.
3. Jiricny, J. (1996) Mismatch repair and cancer. *Cancer Surv.* **28,** 47–68.
4. Kolodner, R. D. (1995) Mismatch repair: mechanisms and relationship to cancer susceptibility. *Trends Biochem. Sci.* **20,** 397–401.
5. Sancar, A. (1995) DNA repair in humans. *Annu. Rev. Genet.* **29,** 69–105.
6. Seeberg, E., Eide, L., and Bjoras, M. (1995) The base excision repair pathway. *Trends Biochem. Sci.* **20,** 391–397.
7. Wilson, D. M. III and Thompson, L. H. (1997) Life without DNA repair. *Proc. Natl. Acad. Sci. USA* **94,** 12754–12757.
8. Wilson, S. H. (1998) Mammalian base excision repair and DNA polymerase β. *Mut. Res.* **407,** 203–215.
9. Wood, R. D., Mitchell, M., Sgouros, J., and Lindahl, T. (2001) Human DNA repair genes. *Science* **291,** 1284–1289.
10. Frosina, G., Fortini, P., Rossi, O., Carrozzino, F., Raspaglio, G., Cox, L. S., et al. (1996) Two pathways for base excision repair in mammalian cells. *J. Biol. Chem.* **271,** 9573–9578.
11. Bronner, C. E., Baker, S. M., Morrison, P. T., Warren, G., Smith, L. G., Lescoe, M. K., et al. (1994) Mutation in the DNA mismatch repair gene homologue hMLH1 is associated with hereditary non-polyposis colon cancer. *Nature* **368,** 258–261.
12. Eshleman, J. R. and Markowitz, S. D. (1996) Mismatch repair defects in human carcinogenesis. *Hum. Mol. Genet.* **5,** 1489–1494.
13. Fishel, R., Lescoe, M. K., Rao, M. R., Copeland, N. G., Jenkins, N. A., Garber, J., et al. (1993) The human mutator gene homolog MSH2 and its association with hereditary nonpolyposis colon cancer. *Cell* **75,** 1027–1038.
14. Fishel, R. and Kolodner, R. D. (1995) Identification of mismatch repair genes and their role in the development of cancer. *Curr. Opin. Genet. Dev.* **5,** 382–395.
15. Lynch, H. T. and de la Chapelle, A. (1999) Genetic susceptibility to non-polyposis colorectal cancer. *J. Med. Genet.* **36,** 801–818.
16. Zienolddiny, S., Ryberg, D., Gazdar, A., and Haugen, A. (1999) DNA mismatch binding in human lung tumor cell lines. *Lung Cancer* **26,** 15–25.
17. Wei, Q., Cheng, L., Hong, W. K., and Spitz, M. R. (1996) Reduced DNA repair capacity in lung cancer patients. *Cancer Res.* **56,** 4103–4107.
18. Cheng, L., Spitz, M. R., Hong, W. K., and Wei, Q. (2000) Reduced expression levels of nucleotide excision repair genes in lung cancer: a case-control analysis. *Carcinogenesis* **21,** 1527–1530.

19. Abdel-Rahman, S. Z. and El-Zein, R. A. (2000) The 399Gln polymorphism in the DNA repair gene XRCC1 modulates the genotoxic response induced in human lymphocytes by the tobacco-specific nitrosamine NNK. *Cancer Lett.* **159**, 63–71.

20. Divine, K. K., Gilliland, F. D., Crowell, R. E., Stidley, C. A., Bocklage, T. J., Cook, D. L., and Belinsky, S. A. (2001) The XRCC1 399 glutamine allele is a risk factor for adenocarcinoma of the lung. *Mutat. Res.* **461**, 273–278.

21. Dianov, G., Price, A., and Lindahl, T. (1992) Generation of single-nucleotide repair patches following excision of uracil residues from DNA. *Mol. Cell. Biol.* **12**, 1605–1612.

22. Klungland, A. and Lindahl, T. (1997) Second pathway for completion of human DNA base excision-repair: reconstitution with purified proteins and requirement for DNase IV (FEN1). *EMBO J.* **16**, 3341–3348.

23. Chyan, Y. J., Ackerman, S., Shepherd, N. S., McBride, O. W., Widen, S. G., Wilson, S. H., and Wood, T. G. (1994) The human DNA polymerase β gene structure. Evidence of alternative splicing in gene expression. *Nucleic Acids Res.* **22**, 2719–2725.

24. Chyan, Y. J., Strauss, P. R., Wood, T. G., and Wilson, S. H. (1996) Identification of novel mRNA isoforms for human DNA polymerase β. *DNA Cell Biol.* **15**, 653–659.

25. Sanderson, R. J. and Mosbaugh, D. W. (1998) Fidelity and mutational specificity of uracil-initiated base excision DNA repair synthesis in human glioblastoma cell extracts. *J. Biol. Chem.* **273**, 24822–24831.

26. Matsumoto, Y. and Kim, K. (1995) Excision of deoxyribose phosphate residues by DNA polymerase β during DNA repair. *Science* **269**, 699–702.

27. Prasad, R., Beard, W. A., Strauss, P. R., and Wilson, S. H. (1998) Human DNA polymerase β deoxyribose phosphate lyase, Substrate specificity and catalytic mechanism. *J. Biol. Chem.* **273**, 15263–15270.

28. Sobol, R. W., Horton, J. K., Kuhn, R., Gu, H., Singhal, R. K., Prasad, R., Rajewsky, K., and Wilson, S. H. (1996) Requirement of mammalian DNA polymerase-β in base-excision repair. *Nature* **379**, 183–186.

29. Sugo, N., Aratani, Y., Nagashima, Y., Kubota, Y., and Koyama, H. (2000) Neonatal lethality with abnormal neurogenesis in mice deficient in DNA polymerase beta. *EMBO J.* **19**, 1397–1404.

30. Gu, H., Marth, J. D., Orban, P. C., Mossmann, H., and Rajewsky, K. (1994) Deletion of a DNA polymerase β gene segment in T cells using cell type-specific gene targeting. *Science* **265**, 103–106.

31. Ali-Osman, F., Berger, M. S., Rairkar, A., and Stein, D. E. (1994) Enhanced repair of a cisplatin-damaged reporter chloramphenicol-O-acetyltransferase gene and altered activities of DNA polymerases α and β, and DNA ligase in cells of a human malignant glioma following *in vivo* cisplatin therapy. *J. Cell. Biochem.* **54**, 11–19.

32. Sweasy, J. B. and Loeb, L. (1993) Detection and characterization of mammalian DNA polymerase β mutants by functional complementation in *Escherichia coli. Proc. Natl. Acad. Sci. USA* **90,** 4626–4630.

33. Plug, A. W., Clairmont, C. A., Sapi, E., Ashley, T., and Sweasy, J. B. (1997) Evidence for a role for DNA polymerase β in mammalian meiosis. *Proc. Natl. Acad. Sci. USA* **94,** 1327–1331.

34. Miscia, S., Di Baldassarre, A., Alba Rana, R., Di Pietro, R., and Cataldi, A. (1997) Engagement of DNA polymerases during apoptosis. *Cell Prolif.* **30,** 325–340.

35. Ochs, K., Sobol, R. W., Wilson, S. H., and Kaina, B. (1999) Cells deficient in DNA polymerase β are hypersensitive to alkylating agent-induced apoptosis and chromosomal breakage. *Cancer Res.* **59,** 1544–1551.

36. Reichenberger, S. and Pfeiffer, P. (1998) Cloning, purification and characterization of DNA polymerase β from *Xenopus laevis*: studies on its potential role in DNA-end joining. *Eur. J. Biochem.* **251,** 81–90.

37. Wang, L., Patel, U., Ghosh, L., and Banerjee, S. (1992) DNA polymerase β mutations in human colorectal cancer. *Cancer Res.* **52,** 4824–4827.

38. Wang, L. and Banerjee, S. (1995) Mutations in DNA polymerase β occur in breast, prostate, and colorectal cancer. *Int. J. Oncol.* **6,** 459–463.

39. Bhattacharyya, N. and Banerjee, S. (1997) A variant of DNA polymerase β acts as a dominant negative mutant. *Proc. Natl. Acad. Sci. USA* **94,** 10324–10329.

40. Bhattacharyya, N., Chen, H.-C., Grundfest-Broniatowski, S., and Banerjee, S. (1999) Alteration of hMSH2 and DNA polymerase β genes in breast carcinomas and fibroadenomas. *Biochem. Biophys. Res. Comm.* **259,** 429–435.

41. Chen, H.-C., Bhattacharyya, N., Wang, L., Recupero, A. J., Klein, E. A., Harter, M. L., and Banerjee, S. (2000) Defective DNA repair genes in a primary culture of human renal cell carcinoma. *J. Cancer Res. Clin. Oncol.* **126,** 185–190.

42. Dobashi, Y., Shuin, T., Tsuruga, H., Uemura, H., Torigoe, S., and Kubota, Y. (1994) DNA polymerase β gene mutation in human prostate cancer. *Cancer Res.* **54,** 2827–2829.

43. Matsuzaki, J., Dobashi, Y., Miyamoto, H., Ikeda, I., Fujinami, K., Shuin, T., and Kubota, Y. (1996) DNA polymerase β gene mutations in human bladder cancer. *Mol. Carcin.* **15,** 38–43.

44. Nowak, R., Bieganowski, P., Konopinskir, R., and Siedlecki, J. A. (1996) Alternative splicing of DNA polymerase β mRNA is not tumor-specific. *Int. J. Cancer* **68,** 199–202.

45. Shadan, F. F. and Villarreal, L. P. (1996) Potential role of DNA polymerase beta in gene therapy against cancer: a case for colorectal cancer. *Med. Hypoth.* **47,** 1–9.

46. Sadakane, Y., Maeda, K., Kuroda, Y., and Hori, K. (1994) Identification of mutations in DNA polymerase β mRNAs from patients with Werner syndrome. *Biochem. Biophys. Res. Commun.* **200,** 219–225.

47. Yu, C.-E., Oshima, J., Fu, Y.-H., Wijsman, E. M., Hisama, F., Alisch, R., et al. (1996) Positional cloning of the Werner's syndrome gene. *Science* **272,** 258–262.

48. Sengupta, D. N., Zmudzka, B. Z., Kumar, P., Cobianchi, F., Skowronski, J., and Wilson, S. H. (1986) Sequence of human DNA polymerase β mRNA obtained through cDNA cloning. *Biochem. Biophys. Res. Comun.* **136,** 341–347.

49. Banerjee, S., Chen, H. C., and Bhattacharyya, N. (1996) Role of DNA β polymerase in human cancer. Cold Spring Harbor Laboratory Meeting on Cancer Genetics and Tumor Suppressor Genes, p. 257.

50. Chen, H.-C. and Banerjee, S. (1997) Mutational heterogeneity of DNA polymerase β in human tumor cell lines. *Proc. Am. Assoc. Cancer Res.* **38,** 511.

51. Loeb, L. A. (1998) Cancer cells exhibit a mutator phenotype. *Adv. Cancer Res.* **72,** 25–56.

IV

LUNG CANCER MODEL SYSTEMS

A. ANIMAL MODELS FOR LUNG CANCER

31

Induction of Lung Cancer by Passive Smoking in an Animal Model System

Hanspeter Witschi

1. Introduction

In 1930, a German physician wrote a paper in which he most strongly suggested that smoking of cigarettes is a cause of lung cancer (1). In the same year, Mertens (2) published the results of a study in which he had exposed individual mice to cigarette smoke. He used a compressible rubber bulb to force cigarette smoke into a glass desiccator. Exposures were from 1–4 h daily, for up to 15 mo. Upon histological examination, he observed inflammatory changes in the lungs, although he was quick to point out that large areas of the lungs showed no pathological alterations. Neoplastic lung lesions were found in two animals. In one mouse, multiple small nodules, classified as adenocarcinomas, were considered to have been pre-existing. The second animal showed several small nodules and, in addition, one large adenocarcinoma, 4 mm in diameter, originating in a bronchus and invading the adjacent parenchyma. The author summarized his findings by stating that he had found one bronchial cancer, but that it was doubtful whether it had been caused by tobacco smoke.

1.1. Equivocal Results from Early Animal Models for Tobacco Smoke Inhalation-Induced Tumorigenesis

This early study proved to be predictive of later developments. During the next five decades, numerous attempts were made to produce lung cancer in experimental animals by inhalation of tobacco smoke. However, such a carcinogenic response proved to be a rare event, difficult to observe. Although multiple histopathological changes, such as inflammation, were seen in the

From: Methods in Molecular Medicine, vol. 74: Lung Cancer, Vol. 1: Molecular Pathology Methods and Reviews
Edited by: B. Driscoll © Humana Press Inc., Totowa, NJ

respiratory tracts of mice, rats, hamsters, and dogs, evidence for deposition of particulate material and subsequent engulfment by macrophages was rare. In addition, metaplastic changes in the airway epithelia and tumor response to these early inhalation treatments were practically nil. In a most comprehensive review of all the available evidence in 1978, the conclusion was reached: "No researcher has succeeded as yet in producing a significant incidence of pulmonary tumors" *(3)*. In 1986, the International Agency for Research on Cancer (IARC) *(4)* summarized the evidence. Out of four rat studies that were judged to be adequate for critical analysis, only one yielded unequivocal evidence for the carcinogenicity of tobacco smoke; however, tumor incidence in the exposed group was below 10%. In similar studies, hamsters developed laryngeal tumors, but no tumors in the lower respiratory tract. The IARC document also discussed six mouse studies. Disregarding differences in strain, number of animals, or duration of exposure between the different experiments, the aggregated data show that out of a total of 1703 mice exposed to tobacco smoke in various laboratories, only 108 animals (6.3%) developed lung tumors. In control animals, the overall incidence was 3.9% (39 out of 998). Though the overall incidence was low, the difference was still statistically significant because of the large number of animals involved. It was concluded, from this combined data, that tobacco smoke increased lung tumor incidence by more than 50%. In another large study, involving several hundred animals and conducted in a single laboratory, lung tumor incidence in the exposed animals was again low (5% as opposed to 4.3% in controls), although smoke inhalation seemed to shorten the time for tumor development *(5,6)*. In addition to studies with full tobacco smoke, experiments were conducted in which mice were exposed to the gas phase only of tobacco smoke *(7–9)*. These studies were of much interest, as one of them conclusively showed that the gas phase of tobacco smoke is as carcinogenic as is unfiltered smoke *(8)*.

However, two newer studies, one in mice and one in rats, again failed to demonstrate significant increases in lung tumor development attributable to the inhalation of tobacco smoke *(10,11)*. As recently as 1998, a review of the results of 14 chronic inhalation studies with mainstream cigarette smoke emphasized that "significant increases in the numbers of malignant tumors were not produced in the respiratory tract of rats or mice exposed chronically by inhalation of cigarette smoke" *(12)*. Thus, most animal inhalation studies failed to provide unequivocal evidence that exposure to tobacco smoke produces lung cancer in experimental animals. To date, the Syrian golden hamster is considered the most reliable animal model for the production of tobacco smoke-induced lung cancers *(13)*. It should be noted, however, that tobacco smoke only produced carcinomatous lesions in the larynx of hamsters but never in the deep lung. There are several possibilities to explain why rodents fail to develop cancers in the bronchial tree at all or only with very low incidence, usually below 10%. It has been noted that rodents are obligatory nose breathers and their nasal passages constitute an effective filtering system, preventing penetration of carcinogens into the deep lung. Although some early studies have convincingly shown the penetration of particulate matter into the lung periphery of rats, accumulation in the peripheral lung was dependent on concentration of particulate matter in the smoke *(14,15)*. If exposed to puffs of tobacco smoke in nose-only inhalation chambers, as were used in many of the older studies, animals also tend to hold their breath, a factor that conceivably might inhibit delivery of carcinogenic agents to the respiratory tract.

1.2. Improved Models for Tobacco Smoke Carcinogen-Induced Tumorigenesis

1.2.1. Whole Body Exposure Models

Some newer studies on the carcinogenicity of tobacco smoke used whole body exposure of animals *(10,11,16,17)*. Whole body exposure is open to some criticism. It has usually been assumed that the preferred method is to expose animals by a nose-only inhalation system, because this prevents particulate material, loaded with carcinogens, from being deposited on the fur of the animals which then, by grooming, can be ingested. However, in view of the observation that the gas phase of cigarette smoke is as carcinogenic as is the full smoke including particulate matter *(8,18)*, deposition of material on the fur of animals seems not to be an important confounding factor in whole body inhalation studies. One systematic study that examined the acute effects of inhaled cigarette smoke when delivered to the animals in nose-only exposure systems compared to whole body exposure systems showed few significant differences between the two exposure systems *(19)*.

1.2.2. Establishment of Strain A/J Mice as a Model for Tobacco Smoke-Induced Carcinogenesis

The realization that environmental tobacco smoke is a human carcinogen *(20)* triggered a renewed interest in animal inhalation studies, including carcinogenicity experiments. In 1997, we published the results of the first of several studies that showed that it is possible to produce lung tumors in strain A mice by inhalation of tobacco smoke *(17)*. This strain is particularly sensitive to developing lung tumors following carcinogen exposure, most notably following intraperitoneal injection or administration of the carcinogen in the diet *(21)*. This strain had already been used before in several inhalation studies with tobacco smoke. An early experiment *(22)* was negative. In 1952, Essenberg observed significantly increased lung tumor incidence in A/J mice exposed for 1 yr to cigarette smoke (incidence: 91%), compared to an incidence of 59% in controls *(23)*. In one subsequent study this finding was reproduced, whereas in another it was not *(24,25)*. Two later studies using strain A mice also gave negative results *(11,16)*. However, increased tumor multiplicities and incidences were successfully produced by exposing strain A mice to a variety of toxic industrial airborne agents and common air pollutants *(26–28)*. A 9-mo exposure of strain A mice to ozone *(29)* essentially confirmed the results of a larger, lifetime study in mice and rats *(30)*, thus indicating that lung tumors in strain A mice represent an adequate model for inhalation toxicology.

1.2.3. Nonconventional Inhalation Models

It now appears that a key element in the development of lung tumors following exposure to tobacco smoke, as reported in 1997 *(17)*, was the design of a nonconventional protocol. Instead of being exposed for the total lifespan to tobacco smoke, animals were exposed for 5 mo only. After cessation of smoke exposure, they were allowed to recover in air for another 4 mo, before being evaluated for tumor development. This modification of the more conventional protocol, in which animals are usually exposed for life, proved to be crucial for the production of lung tumors in an experimental animal model of tobacco smoke carcinogenesis. Results of a series of experiments in which we exposed animals to a mixture of cigarette sidestream and mainstream smoke are given in **Tables 1** and **2**. **Table 1** gives the results for lung tumor multiplicity in environmental tobacco smoke (ETS) exposed animals and the corresponding controls and **Table 2** shows lung tumor incidences. The data can be summarized as follows:

1. In every experiment the average number of tumors per lung was significantly higher in the ETS-exposed animals than it was in the animals that breathed filtered air.
2. In no experiment did we find more than 1.2 tumors per lung in the filtered air-exposed animals, whereas, in the ETS-exposed animals, the average number of tumors per lung was always greater than 1. The rigorous criteria for a positive lung tumor assay are thus met: A positive carcinogenic response in the strain A/J mouse lung tumor assay is obtained when lung tumor multiplicity in the treated animals is significantly increased, preferably to 1 or more lung tumors per mouse. The mean number of lung tumors in the appropriate controls should approximate the anticipated number for untreated mice of the same age. Additionally, for marginally positive compounds, positive results in an initial test must be repeatable in a second test *(21,31)* (*see* **Note 1**).
3. In animals exposed to a concentration of 80–90 mg/m^3 of total suspended particulate (TSP), the average number of tumors per lung was approximately

Table 1
Summary of Control Data: Tumor Multiplicities

Exposure (mg/m³ of TSP)	Lung tumor multiplicity[a]		Reference[b]
	Filtered air	Smoke	
87	0.5 ± 0.2 (24)	1.4 ± 0.2 (24)[c]	*(17)*
79	0.5 ± 0.1 (24)	1.3 ± 0.3 (26)[c]	*(18)*
83	0.9 ± 0.2 (29)	1.3 ± 0.2 (33)[c]	*(55)*
132	0.6 ± 0.1 (30)	2.1 ± 0.3 (38)[c]	*(35)*
137	0.9 ± 0.2 (30)	2.8 ± 0.2 (38)[c]	*(36)*
137	1.0 ± 0.1 (54)	2.4 ± 0.3 (28)[c]	*(36)*
134	1.2 ± 0.2 (25)	2.3 ± 0.3 (26)[c]	Unpublished data

[a]Mean ± SE, number of animals in parenthesis.
[b]Data reproduced with permission from Oxford University Press.
[c]Significantly different ($p < 0.05$) compared to air controls by Welch's alternate test.

half the number counted in animals exposed to the higher concentration of 130–140 mg/m³. This indicates a dose response.

Table 2 lists the lung tumor incidence for the same experiments. It shows that in 5 of the 7 experiments, the lung tumor incidence (percentage of tumor bearing animals) was significantly higher in the ETS exposed animals when compared to filtered air controls.

1.2.3.1. ANALYSIS OF RESULTS OF NONCONVENTIONAL INHALATION PROTOCOLS

Selected tumors were examined under the light microscope in order to confirm the diagnosis. Proliferative pulmonary lesions were morphologically similar between control mice and those exposed to ETS and were typical of pulmonary lesions commonly observed in strain A mice.

Lesions were categorized as focal alveolar epithelial hyperplasia, alveolar/bronchiolar adenomas, and alveolar/bronchiolar adenocarcinomas. The majority of adenomas had a solid growth pattern with contiguous neoplastic cells filling alveolar spaces. There was no difference in the relative distribution of adenocarcinomas and of adenomas between the two groups. In the ETS exposed animals, 17% of all tumors had a pattern consistent with the diagnosis of adenocarcinoma and in the controls 20% did so. Of 4 carcinomas observed, 2 had a solid growth pattern, 1 had a mixed solid and papillary growth pattern, and 1 was a papillary neoplasm arising within a solid adenoma. Diagnosis of malignancy was based primarily on presence of nuclear atypia (hyperchromatic and pleomorphic nuclei) and cellular crowding. Tumor progression appeared to occur along a continuum from hyperplasia to adenoma to carcinoma *(17,18)*.

Table 2
Summary of Control Data: Tumor Incidence

Exposure	Lung tumor multiplicity[a]		
(mg/m³ of TSP)	Filtered air	Smoke	Reference[b]
87	38%	83%[c]	*(17)*
79	42%	58%	*(18)*
83	69%	73%	*(55)*
132	50%	86%[c]	*(35)*
137	60%	100%[c]	*(36)*
137	65%	89%[c]	*(36)*
134	60%	88%[c]	Unpublished

[a]No. of tumor bearing animals as percentage of all animals at risk.
[b]Data reproduced with permission from Oxford University Press.
[c]Significantly different ($p < 0.05$) from filtered air animals by Fisher's exact test.

1.2.4. Conclusions from Nonconventional Inhalation Studies

We conclude from these data that exposure to ETS during 5 mo, followed by a 4-mo recovery period, produces benign and malignant tumors in the lungs of strain A mice. A key factor in the model development was to allow the animals to recover for 4 mo in air following explore to tobacco smoke. The importance of the recovery period is illustrated by the following experiment: One group of animals was exposed for 4 mo to approx 140 mg/m³ of TSP, followed by the usual recovery period in air. A second group of animals was exposed for the full 9 mo to ETS. **Table 3** shows that in animals exposed for the full 9 mo, substantially fewer lung tumors developed, although the percentage of animals with lung tumors was similar to the incidence found in animals exposed for 5 mo only. This suggests that smoke may inhibit or delay the development of tumors. The practical implication of the finding is that a recovery phase in air is necessary to allow for full tumor development. The observation is reminiscent of the well-established phenomenon that in smokers who recently quit, there is, for a certain length of time, an increased risk to develop lung cancer *(32–34)*. From an experimental standpoint, this observation allows us to study the effects of chemopreventive agents separately in smokers (e.g., during the exposure phase) and in "quitters" (e.g., during the recovery phase). It has recently been found that a mixture of myoinositol and dexamethasone prevents the development of tobacco smoke-induced lung cancers when given during smoke exposure *(35)* and also when given after smoke exposure *(36)*.

In summary, a workable and reproducible animal model is available that allows to study the carcinogenic effects of tobacco smoke in mouse lung.

Table 3
Lung Tumors in Animals Exposed for 5 or 9 Mo to Tobacco Smoke[a]

Treatment (Group)[b]	Lung tumor multiplicity[c]	Lung tumor incidence[d]
Filtered air[d] (1)	1.0 ± 0.1 (84)	53/84 (63%)
Tobacco smoke 5 mo (2)	2.6 ± 0.3 (66)[e]	63/66 (95%)[e]
Tobacco smoke 9 mo (3)	1.5 ± 0.2 (27)[f]	23/27 (85%)[e]

[a]Table reproduced by permission from **ref. 56**.
[b]Animals exposed to 137 mg/m³ of TSP.
[c]Average number of tumors per lung, including nontumor-bearing animals. Data are given as means ± SE with the number of animals in parenthesis.
[d]Number of tumors bearing animals per total number of animals at risk.
[e]Significantly higher ($p < 0.05$) than animals kept in filtered air (1).
[f]Significantly lower ($p < 0.05$) compared to animals exposed to smoke for 5 mo only (2).

This opens the possibility to examine mechanisms and the effects of putative chemopreventive or therapeutic agents.

2. Materials

2.1. Exposure System

1. Male strain A/J mice, 6–8 wk old (Jackson Laboratory, Bar Harbor, ME) (*see* **Note 1**). Upon arrival, sentinel animals are checked for of their health status. After a 2-wk acclimatization period, the animals can be assigned by a random procedure to the different experimental groups.
2. Conditioned Kentucky 1R4F reference cigarettes (Tobacco and Health Research Institute, Lexington, KY). Store until needed at 4°C.
3. Smoking machine (*see* **Note 2**).
4. Glycerin/water: 76/24.
5. Glass and stainless-steel Hinners-type exposure chamber (volume: 0.44 m³).
6. Monitor for TSP: Piezobalance (TSI Instruments, St. Paul, MN), plus a PDM-3 MiniRam forward light scattering device (MIE, Inc., Billerica MA), calibrated by gravimetric method (weight of particles collected on Teflon filters). Particle size distribution is determined using a Royco 236 Laser particle counter (HIAC/Royco Instruments, Menlo Park, CA).
7. Carbon monoxide monitor: Model 880 non-dispersive-infrared (NDIR) analyzer (Beckmann Industries, La Habra, CA).

2.2. Tumor Analysis

1. Sodium pentobarbital.
2. Tellyesniczky's fluid: 640 mL ethanol, 55 mL phosphate-buffered saline (PBS) at pH 7.4, 87 mL formaldehyde, 44 mL glacial acetic acid, and 174 mL of water for a total of 1 L.
3. Set up for paraffin embedding, sectioning, and hematoxylin/eosin staining.

2.3. Materials for Measuring Nicotine Concentrations

1. Sorbent tubes (SKC, Eighty Four, PA).
2. HPLC-grade ethyl acetate containing 0.1% triethylamine.
3. Gas chromatograph (Varian 3740).
4. DB-5 30 m × 0.53 mm column (film thickness 1.5 μm) (Varian Analytical Instruments).
5. Nitrogen-selective thermionic specific detector. (Varian Analytical Instruments).
6. Temperature and relative humidity probes (Rustrack, St. Paul, MN).

3. Methods

3.1. Exposure System

The technical details for construction and operation of the tobacco smoke exposure system used in our own experiments have been described in detail elsewhere and only a summary of principles can be given here *(37)*. Originally, the system was designed to expose animals to a surrogate of environmental tobacco smoke (*see* **Note 2**). With suitable modifications, it also would lend itself to the study of mainstream cigarette smoke. Essentially, it is a whole body exposure system.

3.1.1. Tobacco Smoke Exposure System

1. At least 48 h prior to use, place cigarettes in a closed chamber at 23°C, along with a mixture of glycerin/water to establish a relative humidity of 60%.
2. The cigarettes are smoked with standardized 35 mL puffs of 2-s duration, once every minute, for a total of eight puffs per cigarette.
3. Keep the animals, within their cages, for the entire experimental period in the smoke inhalation chamber. Control animals are kept in a similar chamber that is ventilated with filtered air. Animals should have access to food and water ad libitum. Check general health daily and weigh weekly (*see* **Notes 3** and **4**).
4. For exposure, the sidestream smoke (SS) given off the tip of the smoldering cigarette between puffs is drawn, after dilution and aging (2 min), into a glass and stainless-steel Hinners-type exposure chamber (volume: 0.44 m³). The sidestream smoke can, if so desired, be reinforced every 58 s with a 2-s puff of mainstream smoke (*see* **Notes 5** and **6**).
5. Monitor the chamber atmosphere continuously monitored for CO, nicotine, and TSP. CO and TSP can be monitored using the instruments listed in the Materials section (**Subheading 2.1.**).
6. Monitor temperature and relative humidity within the chambers with an appropriate probe.

3.1.1.1. METHOD FOR MEASURING NICOTINE CONCENTRATIONS

1. Draw exposure air samples through sorbent tubes.
2. Extract tubes with high-performance liquid chromatography (HPLC)-grade ethyl acetate containing 0.1% triethylamine.

3. Analyze the extract in a gas chromatograph equipped with a DB-5 30 m × 0.53 mm column (film thickness 1.5 μm) and a nitrogen-selective thermionic specific detector.

3.1.2. Recovery

1. Remove animals, in their cages, from the exposure chamber to a facility where they can breathe room air for up to 4 mo. Animals should be monitored for general health and weight as described (*see* **Subheading 3.1.1.**).

3.2. Tumor Analysis

1. At the end of the experiment, sacrifice animals by sodium pentobarbital overdose.
2. Instill the lungs intratracheally with Tellyesniczky's fluid, the preferred fixative for tumor counting (*see* **Note 7**).
3. After 24–48 h in fixative at room temperature, the tumors can be counted. A surface count will accurately reflect the over-all tumor count *(52,57)* (*see* **Note 8**).
4. Histological analysis of lung tumors can be performed by embedding lungs or individual tumors into paraffin, cutting conventional 5-μm sections and staining by hematoxylin/eosin.
5. Tumor data are calculated as recommended by Shimkin and Stoner *(21)*. Tumor incidence is defined as the percentage of animals in any given experimental group showing one or several lung tumors. Tumor incidences are compared using Fisher's exact test. A *p*-value of 0.05 or less is usually considered to be significant.
6. Tumor multiplicity is calculated as the average number of tumors per lung in each experimental group, including nontumor-bearing animals. This number is obtained by listing individually the number of tumors for each animal (and assigning a value of 0 to no-tumor bearing animals) and by calculating from these individual numbers the mean and SD or SEM of the group. Comparisons of tumor multiplicity between different treatment groups are made by either by Welch's alternate test or, in case of multiple comparisons by analysis of variance (ANOVA), followed by the Tukey-Kramer multiple comparison test post-test.

4. Notes

1. Strain A mice have now been used for more than seven decades in studies on lung tumor development. The strain is highly sensitive to multiple classes of carcinogens, particularly polycyclic aromatic hydrocarbons and nitrosamines, major constituents of cigarette smoke. However, there is usually a much poorer response to aromatic amines or metals injected intraperitoneally *(53,54)*. Nevertheless, over years of study by multiple laboratories, the susceptibility of the strain A mouse to carcinogens has been found to be remarkably constant. In each assay it should therefore be monitored as to whether the particular batch of

mice being used develop a spontaneous lung tumor incidence (dependent on their age) as historical controls show *(31)*. In addition, the sensitivity to carcinogens is best monitored by including a group of positive controls injected with urethane, usually at a dose of 1000 mg/kg. In a 25 g mouse, this should produce, within 4 mo, an average of 25 tumors per lung (1 tumor per mg of urethane). It should be noted that this number will only been found approx 4–5 mo after urethane injection *(21)*. Over a longer incubation period, some tumors become confluent and are no longer recognizable as individual enmities.

2. Information on the inhalation system used in our studies and originally developed by Teague et al. *(37)* is available at http://www.teague-ent.com.

3. In our experiments we never have found any deaths that might have been caused by tobacco smoke exposure, even at nicotine and CO concentrations as high as 20–25 mg/m^3 and 200–300 ppm, respectively. While in the smoke atmosphere, the animals may not gain weight at the same rate as do air exposed controls; however, upon removal from the smoke, they rapidly will gain weight and, at the end of the experiment, usually have reached the same weight as have controls kept in filtered air throughout.

4. The animals, while in smoke, may develop a yellowing of their fur. While this may be in part due to deposition of some particulate material, it is more likely that the discoloration is caused by the presence of formaldehyde in the smoke atmosphere.

5. There are many other detailed descriptions of similar inhalation systems available in the literature. For a general overview and highly useful general characterization of inhalation technology, *see* the chapters by Wong, Hext or Kennedy, and Valentine *(38–40)*. References that specifically describe exposure of small laboratory animals to cigarette mainstream smoke tobacco smoke include the following: Dontenwill depicts a comparatively early system with useful photographs *(41)*. The design of a machine that continuously smokes cigarettes under controlled conditions was reported by Baumgartner and Coggins in 1980 *(42)*. The machine has since been further refined and developed and integrated into a complete and versatile exposure inhalation system. Information about this versatile system is available at http://www.inhalation.net or http://www.toxics.com.

6. More recently there has been interest in exposing laboratory animals to surrogates for environmental tobacco smoke. ETS is a mixture of cigarette sidestream smoke, the smoke curling off the end of a lit cigarette between puffs, and mainstream exhaled by smokers. ETS contains about 80–90% of sidestream smoke, which is generated at lower burning temperatures than is mainstream smoke; as a result, the concentration of certain carcinogens is higher in sidestream smoke than it is in mainstream smoke *(43)*. The mainstream smoke exhaled by smokers has been scrubbed of many of its ingredients, mostly nicotine and CO. Since in practice it is not possible to use, in animal experiments, mainstream smoke that has passed through human lungs, a surrogate for ETS is usually sidestream smoke alone aor a mixture of sidestream smoke and cigarette mainstream

smoke as generated by a smoking machine. Detailed information on design and construction of a system that allows to exposed animals to ETS is provided by Ayres et al. *(44)*. Results of 14- and 90-d inhalation studies in rats with ETS are available *(12,45,46)*.

A particular feature of ETS is that its chemical composition changes with aging of the smoke. It also may be influenced by the surroundings; for example, certain surfaces will adsorb nicotine and other constituents of the smoke. A system has been developed that takes these events into account and allows to compare, in experimental animals, the effects of fresh as compared to the effects of room aged sidestream smoke *(47,48)*. Finally it should be mentioned that a system is available that allows to expose cell cultures or small laboratory animals simultaneously to mainstream and sidestream cigarette smoke *(49–51)*.

7. This fixative is useful because the acetic acid produces some shrinkage of the lung tissue, making small nodules stand out in better contrast *(21)*. However, Tellyesniczky's fluid may not be the best fixative for studies involving special staining procedures (e.g., immunohistochemistry).

8. It is not advisable to attempt a tumor count on unfixed lung tissue. Small tumors (diameter 0.5 mm and less) can only be seen if tissues are fixed long enough (24–48 h) so that tumors begin to stand out as whitish nodules against a darker background. After 5 mo in tobacco smoke and 4 mo recovery, the average tumor diameters are between 1 and 3 mm. Larger tumors are usually observed only after longer exposure and/or recovery periods. If large tumors are required (e.g., for biochemical/molecular analysis), animals should be maintained in recovery for a longer time before sacrifice.

Acknowledgments

I wish to thank Imelda Espiritu, Dale Uyeminami, and Robert R. Maronpot for their help in performing these experiments. This publication was made possible by grants number ES07908, ES07499 and ES05707 from the National Institute of Environmental Health Sciences (NIEHS). Its contents are solely the responsibility of the authors and do not necessarily represent the official views of the NIEHS, NIH.

References

1. Lickint, F. (1930) Tabak und Tabakrauch als aetiologischer Faktor des Carcinoms. *Zeitschrift fuer Krebsforschung* 30, 349–365.
2. Mertens, V. E. (1930) Zigarettenrauch eine Ursache des Lungenkrebses? (Eine Anregung). *Zeitschrift fuer Krebsforschung* 32, 82–91.
3. Mohr, U. and Reznik, G. (1978) Tobacco Carcinogenesis, in Pathogenesis and Therapy of Lung Cancer (Harris, C. C., ed.), Marcel Dekker, Inc., New York, pp. 263–368.
4. International Agency for Research on Cancer (IARC) (1986) Biological Data Relevant to the Evaluation of Carcinogenic Risk to Humans. 1. Carcinogenicity

Studies in Animals, in *IARC Monographs on the Evaluation of the Carcinogenic Risk of Chemicals to Humans. Tobacco Smoking* Vol. 38 (WHO IARC, ed.), IARC, Lyon, pp. 127–139.

5. Henry, C. J. and Kouri, R. E. (1984) *Chronic Exposure of Mice to Cigartte Smoke. Final Report, The Council for Tobacco Research—USA, Inc. Contract CTR-030, "Smoke Inhalation in Mice."* Field, Rich & Associates, New York.

6. Henry, C. J. and Kouri, R. E. (1986) Chronic inhalation studies in mice. II. Effects of long-term exposure to 2R1 cigarette smoke on (C57BL/Cum x C3H/AnfCum)F1 mice. *J. Natl. Cancer Inst.* **77**, 203–212.

7. Leuchtenberger, C. and Leuchtenberger, R. (1970) Effects of chronic inhalation of whole fresh cigarette smoke and of its gas phase on pulmonary tumorigenesis in Snell's mice, in *Morphology of Experimental Respiratory Carcinogenesis.* (Nettesheim, P., Hanna, M. G., Jr., and Deatherage, J. W., Jr., eds.) Proceedings of a Biology Division, Oak Ridge National Laboratory, Conference held in Gatlinburg, Tennessee, May 13–16, 1970. US Atomic Energy Commission, Division of Technical Information, Washington, DC, pp. 329–346.

8. Leuchtenberger, C. and Leuchtenberger, R. (1974) Differential response of Snell's and C57 black mice to chronic inhalation of cigarette smoke. Pulmonary carcinogenesis and vascular alterations in lung and heart. *Oncology* **29**, 122–138.

9. Harris, R. J., Negroni, G., Ludgate, S., Pick, C. R., Chesterman, F. C., and Maidment, B. J. (1974) The incidence of lung tumours in c57bl mice exposed to cigarette smoke: air mixtures for prolonged periods. *Int. J. Cancer* **14**, 130–136.

10. Finch, G. L., Nikula, K. J., Barr, E. B., Bechtold, W. E., Chen, B. T., Griffith, W. C., et al. (1995) Lung tumor synergism between 239PuO2 and cigarette smoke inhaled by Fisher 344 rats. *Toxicologist* **15**, 47 (Abstract).

11. Finch, G. L., Nikula, K. J., Belinsky, S. A., Barr, E. B., Stoner, G. D., and Lechner, J. F. (1996) Failure of cigarette smoke to induce or promote lung cancer in the A/J mouse. *Cancer Lett.* **99**, 161–167.

12. Coggins, C. R. E. (1998) A review of the chronic inhalation studies with mainstream cigarette smoke in rats and mice. *Toxicol. Pathol.* **26**, 307–314.

13. Hecht, S. S. (1999) Tobacco smoke carcinogens and lung cancer. *J. Natl. Cancer Inst.* **91**, 1194–1210.

14. Binns, R., Lugton, W. G., and Dyas, B. J. (1978) The effect of exposure conditions on cigarette smoke deposition in the respiratory system of male rats, in *Clinical Toxicology* (Duncan, W. A. and Leonard, B. J., eds.), Excerpta Medica, Amsterdam, pp. 267–269.

15. Binns, R., Lugton, W. G., Wilton, L. V., and Dyas, B. J. (1978) Inhalation toxicity studies on cigarette smoke. V. Deposition of smoke particles in the respiratory system of rats under various exposure conditions. *Toxicology* **9**, 87–102.

16. Witschi, H. P., Oreffo, V. I. C., and Pinkerton, K. E. (1995) Six month exposure of strain A/J mice to cigarette sidestream smoke: cell kinetics and lung tumor data. *Fundam. Appl. Toxicol.* **26**, 32–40.

17. Witschi, H. P., Espiritu, I., Peake, J. L., Wu, K., Maronpot, R. R., and Pinkerton, K. E. (1997) The carcinogenicity of environmental tobacco smoke. *Carcinogenesis* **18**, 575–586.

18. Witschi, H. P., Espiritu, I., Maronpot, R. R., Pinkerton, K. E., and Jones, A. D. (1997) The carcinogenic potential of the gas phase of environmental tobacco smoke. *Carcinogenesis* **18**, 2035–2042.

19. Mauderly, J. L., Bechtold, W. E., Bond, J. A., Brooks, A. L., Chen, B. T., Cuddihy, R. G., Harkema, J. R., Henderson, R. F., Johnson, N. F., and Rithidech, K. (1989) Comparison of 3 methods of exposing rats to cigarette smoke. *Exp. Pathol.* **37**, 194–197.

20. National Cancer Institute (1999) *Health Effects of Exposure to Environmental Tobacco Smoke: The Report of the California Environmental Protection Agency.* Smoking and Tobacco Control Monograph No. 10. U.S. Department of Health and Human Services, National Institutes of Health, National Cancer Institute, NIH Pub. No. 99-4645, Bethesda MD.

21. Shimkin, M. B. and Stoner, G. D. (1975) Lung tumors in mice: application to carcinogenesis bioassay. *Adv. Cancer Res.* **21**, 1–58.

22. Lorenz, E., Stewart, H. L., Daniel, J. H., and Warren, S. (1943) The effects of breathing tobacco smoke on strain A mice. *Cancer Res.* **3**, 123. (Abstract.)

23. Essenberg, J. M. (1952) Cigarette smoke and the incidence of primary neoplasm of the lung in the albino mouse. *Science* **116**, 561–562.

24. Essenberg, J. M., Horowitz, M., and Gaffney, E. (1955). The incidence of lung tumors in albino mice exposed to the smoke from cigarettes low in nicotine content. *West. J. Surg. Obstet. Gynecol.* **63**, 265–267.

25. Essenberg, J. M. (1957) Further study of tumor formation in the lungs of the albino mice. *West. J. Surg. Obstet. Gynecol.* **65**, 161–163.

26. Adkins, B. J., Van Stee, E. W., Simmons, J. E., and Eustis, S. L. (1986) Oncogenic response of strain A/J mice to inhaled chemicals. *J. Toxicol. Environ. Health* **17**, 311–322.

27. Pepelko, W. E. and Peirano, W. B. (1983) Health effects of exposure to Diesel exhaust emissions. *J. Am. Coll. Toxicol.* **2**, 253–306.

28. Leong, B. K., MacFarland, H. N., and Reese, W. H., Jr. (1971) Induction of lung adenomas by chronic inhalation of bis (chloromethyl) ether. *Arch. Environ. Health* **22**, 663–666.

29. Witschi, H., Espiritu, I., Pinkerton, K. E., Murphy, K., and Maronpot, R. (1999) Ozone Carcinogenesis Revisited. *Toxicol. Sci.* **52**, 162–167.

30. Boorman, G. A., Sills, R. C., Grumbein, S., Hailey, R., Miller, R. A., and Herbert, R. A. (1995) Long-term toxicity studies of ozone in F344/N rats and B6C3F1 mice. *Toxicol. Lett.* **82–83**, 301–306.

31. Stoner, G. D. and Shimkin, M. B. (1985) Lung tumors in strain A mice as a bioassay for carcinogenicity, in *Handbook of Carcinogen Testing* (Milman, H. and Weisburger, E. K., eds.), Noyes Publications, Park Ridge, NJ, pp. 179–214.

32. Hammond, E. C. (1966) Smoking in relation to the death rates of one million men and women. *Natl. Cancer Inst. Monogr.* **19**, 127–204.

33. Wynder, E. L. and Stellman, S. D. (1977) Comparative epidemiology of tobacco-related cancers. *Cancer Res.* **37,** 4608–4622.
34. Postmus, P. E. (1998) Epidemiology of lung cancer, in *Fishman's Pulmonary Diseases and Disorders* (Fishman, A. P., Elias, J. A., Fishman, J. A., Grippi, M. A., Kaiser, L. R., and Senior, R. M., eds.), McGraw-Hill, New York, pp. 1707–1717.
35. Witschi, H., Espiritu, I., and Uyeminami, D. (1999) Chemoprevention of tobacco smoke-induced lung tumors in A/J strain mice with dietary myo-inositol and dexamethasone. *Carcinogenesis* **20,** 1375–1378.
36. Witschi, H., Uyeminami, D., Moran, D., and Espiritu, I. (2000) Chemoprevention of tobacco-smoke lung carcinogenesis in mice after cessation of smoke exposure. *Carcinogenesis* **21,** 977–982.
37. Teague, S. V., Pinkerton, K. E., Goldsmith, M., Gebremichael, A., Chang, S., Jenkins, R. A., and Moneyhun, J. H. (1994) Sidestream cigarette smoke generation and exposure system for environmental tobacco smoke studies. *Inhal. Toxicol.* **6,** 79–93.
38. Wong, B. A. (1999) Inhalation systems design, methods and operation, in *Toxicology of the Lung* (Gardner, D. E., Crapo, J. D., and McClellan, R. O., eds.), Taylor & Francis, Philadelphia, PA, pp. 1–53.
39. Hext, P. M. (1999) Inhalation Toxicology, in *General and Applied Toxicology* (Ballantyne, B., Marrs, T. C., and Syversen, T., eds.), Grove's Dictionaries, Inc., New York, pp. 587–602.
40. Kennnedy, G. L. and Valentine, R. (1994) Inhalation Toxicology, in *Principles and Methods of Toxicology* (Hayes, A. W., ed.), Raven Press, New York, pp. 805–838.
41. Dontenwill, W. (1970) Experimental investigations on the effect of cigarette smoke inhalation on small laboratory animals, in *Morphology of Experimental Respiratory Carcinogenesis* (Nettesheim, P., Hanna, M. G., Jr., and Deatherage, J. W., Jr., eds.), Proceedings of a Biology Division, Oak Ridge National Laboratory, conference held in Gatlinburg, Tennessee, May 13–16, 1970. U.S. Atomic Energy Commission, Division of Technical Journals, Washington, DC, pp. 389–412.
42. Baumgartner, H. and Coggins, C. R. (1980) Description of a continuous-smoking inhalation machine for exposing small animals to tobacco smoke. *Beitr. Tabakforsch. Int.* **10,** 169–174.
43. Guerin, M. R., Jenkins, R. A., and Tomkins, B. A. (1992) *The Chemistry of Environmental Tobacco Smoke: Composition and Measurement. Indoor Air Research Series.* Lewis Publishers, Boca Raton, FL.
44. Ayres, P. H., Mosberg, A. T., and Coggins, C. R. (1994) Design, construction, and evaluation of an inhalation system for exposing experimental animals to environmental tobacco smoke. *Am. Ind. Hyg. Assoc. J.* **55,** 806–810.
45. Coggins, C. R., Ayres, P. H., Mosberg, A. T., Ogden, M. W., Sagartz, J. W., and Hayes, A. W. (1992) Fourteen-day inhalation study in rats, using aged and diluted sidestream smoke from a reference cigarette. I. Inhalation toxicology and histopathology. *Fundam. Appl. Toxicol.* **19,** 133–140.

46. Lee, C. K., Brown, B. G., Reed, E. A., Coggins, C. R., Doolittle, D. J., and Hayes, A. W. (1993) Ninety-day inhalation study in rats, using aged and diluted sidestream smoke from a reference cigarette: DNA adducts and alveolar macrophage cytogenetics. *Fundam. Appl. Toxicol.* **20**, 393–401.
47. Haussmann, H. J., Anskeit, E., Becker, D., Kuhl, P., Stinn, W., Teredesai, A., et al. (1998) Comparison of fresh and room-aged cigarette sidestream smoke in a subchronic inhalation study on rats. *Toxicol. Sci.* **41**, 100–116.
48. Haussmann, H. J., Gerstenberg, B., Goecke, W., Kuhl, P., Schepers, G., Stabbert, R., et al. (1998) 12-Month inhalation study on room-aged cigarette sidestream smoke in rats. *Inhal. Toxicol.* **10**, 663–697.
49. Griffith, R. B. (1984) A simple machine for smoke analytical studies and total particulate matter collection for biological studies. *Toxicology* **33**, 33–41.
50. Griffith, R. B. and Hancock, R. (1985) Simultaneous mainstream-sidestream smoke exposure systems I. Equipment and procedures. *Toxicology* **34**, 123–138.
51. Griffith, R. B. and Standafer, S. (1985) Simultaneous mainstream-sidestream smoke exposure systems II. The rat exposure system. *Toxicology* **35**, 13–24.
52. Witschi, H. P. (1981) Enhancement of tumor formation in mouse lung by dietary butylated hydroxytoluene. *Toxicology* **21**, 95–104.
53. Maronpot, R. R., Shimkin, M. B., Witschi, H. P., Smith, L. H., and Cline, J. M. (1986) Strain A mouse pulmonary tumor test results for chemicals previously tested in the National Cancer Institute carcinogenicity tests. *J. Natl. Cancer Inst.* **76**, 1101–1112.
54. Maronpot, R. R. (1991) Correlation of data from the strain A mouse bioassay with long-term bioassays. *Exp. Lung Res.* **17**, 425–431.
55. Witschi, H., Espiritu, I., Yu, M., and Willits, N. H. (1998) The effects of phenethyl isothiocyanate, N-acetylcysteine and green tea on tobacco smoke-induced lung tumors in strain A/J mice. *Carcinogenesis* **19**, 1789–1794.
56. Witschi, H. (2000) Successful and not so successful chemoprevention of tobacco smoke-induced lung tumors. *Exp. Lung Res.* **26**, 743–756.
57. John, L. C. H. (2001) Assessment of murine lung tumour development: a comparison of two techniques. *Br. J. Biomed. Sciences* **58**, 159–163.

32

Metastatic Orthotopic Mouse Models of Lung Cancer

Robert M. Hoffman

1. Introduction

A number of xenograft models have been developed for human lung cancer. These include subcutaneous (sc)-implant models and implantation under the renal capsule, but these models have not been sufficiently representative of the clinical situation (1). The studies of McLemore et al. (2,3) have utilized the orthotopic concept to develop more relevant lung-tumor models in nude mice. The first model developed by McLemore et al. (2) utilized the growth of human lung cancer cell lines in the bronchioloalveolar region of the right lung of nude mice implanted via an intrabronchial injection. Suspensions of disaggregated fresh tumor specimens were also implanted intrabronchially (ib) by this group. These tumors grew intrabronchially much more extensively than the same tumors inoculated sc. However, most of the tumors propagated ib were localized to the right lung, with only 1% metastasizing to the left lung, 2% to the trachea, 6% to the peritracheal area, and only 3% spreading distantly to lymph nodes, liver, or spleen. McLemore et al. (3) subsequently developed a second model by injecting lung tumor cells via an intrathoracic route into the pleural space. This model seems similar to the intrabronchial model in that extensive local growth occurs with little metastatic spread.

Ten years ago, we described a method that utilizes histologically intact tumor tissue implanted into the left lung by a novel thoracotomy procedure. We have demonstrated that this method results not only in extensive local growth in nude and severe combined immunodeficient (SCID) mice but also in development of regional and distant metastases (4–6). This corroborates the

From: *Methods in Molecular Medicine, vol. 74: Lung Cancer, Vol. 1: Molecular Pathology Methods and Reviews*
Edited by: B. Driscoll © Humana Press Inc., Totowa, NJ

findings from numerous other tumor models developed by our group, in which the orthotopic transplantation of intact tissue leads to extensive local growth and metastasis, as in the clinical situation *(1)*.

We developed stable transfectants of lung tumor cells that express high-level green fluorescent protein (GFP) fluorescence in vivo. GFP expression in the surgical orthotopic implantation (SOI) models of lung cancer revealed the very extensive and widespread metastatic potential of lung cancer *(7,8)*. GFP fluorescence in SOI models will facilitate the understanding of metastatic processes including each step of the metastatic cascade including cancer. These models are reviewed in this chapter.

2. Materials

2.1. Green Fluorescent Protein Techniques

2.1.1. DNA Manipulations and Expression Vector Constructions

1. hGFP-S65T gene was purchased from CLONTECH Laboratories, Inc. (Palo Alto, CA).
2. RetroXpress vector pLEIN was purchased from CLONTECH Laboratories, Inc.
3. pLEIN vector expresses enhanced green fluorescent protein (EGFP) and the neomycin resistance gene on the same bicistronic message which contains an IRES site.

2.1.2. Packaging Cells and GFP Vector Production

1. PT67, an NIH3T3-derived packaging cell line, expressing the 10 Al viral envelope, was purchased from CLONTECH Laboratories, Inc.
2. DME (Irvine Scientific, Santa Ana, CA) supplemented with 10% heat-inactivated fetal calf serum (FCS) (Gemini Bio-products, Calabasas, CA).
3. DOTAP™ reagent (Boehringer Mannheim).
4. G418 (Life Technologies, Grand Island, NY).

2.1.3. Retroviral GFP Transduction of Cancer Cells

1. RPMI 1640 (GIBCO) containing 10% fetal calf serum (FCS) (Gemini Bio-products).
2. Trypsin/EDTA.
3. Cloning cylinders (Bel-Art Products, Pequannock, NJ).

2.1.4. Fluorescence Imaging of GFP Lung Carcinoma

1. Nikon microscope equipped with a xenon lamp power supply.
2. Leica stereo fluorescent microscope model LZ12 equipped with a mercury lamp power supply.
3. GFP filter set (Chroma Technology, Brattleboro, VT).

2.2. Surgical Orthotopic Implantation (SOI)

2.2.1. Tumor Models

1. Human patient lung tumors directly from surgery.
2. Human small-cell lung-carcinoma-xenograft Lu-24.
3. Human small-cell carcinoma xenograft Lu-130.
4. Human small-cell carcinoma xenograft H-69.
5. Human lung adenocarcinoma A549.
6. Human non-small cell carcinoma xenograft H460.

2.2.2. Implantation Surgery

1. 7× magnifying dissection microscope.
2. Male and female athymic nu/nu and SCID mice, approx 4–6 wk of age.
3. Glass chamber.
4. Isoflurane.
5. Glass tube.
6. Small animal surgical instruments.
7. 6-0, 7-0, 8-0 surgical sutures.
8. 3-mL syringe and 25 G1 1/2" needle.

3. Methods

3.1. Green Fluorescent Protein Techniques

3.1.1. DNA Manipulations and Expression Vector Constructions

1. Vectors required for retroviral production were prepared by standard DNA preparation methods. Plasmids included the expression vector containing the codon-optimized hGFP-S65T gene and the RetroXpress vector pLEIN. pLEIN vector expresses enhanced green fluorescent protein (EGFP) and the neomycin resistance gene on the same bicistronic message which contains an IRES site *(7)*.

3.1.2. Packaging Cells and GFP Vector Production

1. Culture PT67 cells in supplemented DME. For vector production, incubate cells, at 70% confluence, with a precipitated mixture of DOTAP™ and saturating amounts of pLEIN plasmid for 18 h.
2. Replenish cultures with fresh medium.
3. Examine cells by fluorescence microscopy after 48 h for GFP expression as an indication of successful transduction.
4. For selection of GFP transductants, culture cells in the presence of 500–2000 µg/mL G418 for 7 d *(7)*.

3.1.3. Retroviral GFP Transduction of Cancer Cells

1. For GFP gene transduction, incubate 20%-confluent cancer cells were with a 1 : 1 precipitated mixture of retroviral supernatants of PT67 cells and supplemented RPMI 1640 for 72 h.

2. Harvest cells using trypsin/EDTA 72 h postinfection, and subculture at a ratio of 1:15 into selective medium which contains 200 µg/mL G418.
3. Gradually increase the level of G418 to 800 µg/mL.
4. Isolate clones expressing GFP using trypsin/EDTA in cloning cylinders. Amplify and transfer clones by conventional culture methods (7).

3.1.4. Fluorescence Imaging of GFP Lung Carcinoma

1. Cells can be examined using a Nikon microscope equipped with a xenon lamp power supply and a GFP filter set.

3.2. Surgical Orthotopic Implantation

3.2.1. Implant Preparation

1. Before starting the operation, sew 1–6 tumor pieces (1 mm³ per piece) together with a 7-0 nylon surgical suture and fix by making one knot. Putting all pieces of the tumor on one suture in advance can ensure a quick operation, which is necessary for the survival of the animals.

3.2.2. Implantation Surgery

All the procedures described should be performed using a 7× magnifying microscope (4–6).

1. Place male and female athymic *nu/nu* and SCID mice in a glass chamber and anesthetize with an inhalation anesthetic, isoflurane.
2. When fully anesthetized, remove mice from the chamber and continue on inhalation anesthesia via a glass tube containing the anesthetic.
3. Transplant tumors into the left lung of experimental animals (*see* **Note 1**). Put animal in a position of right lateral decubitus, with the 4 limbs properly fixed.
4. Make a 0.8-cm transverse incision of skin in the left chest wall. Separate chest muscles by a sharp dissection, and expose costal and intercostal muscles.
5. Make an intercostal incision of 0.4–0.5 cm on the third or fourth costs on the chest wall and open.
6. Lift the left lung with a forceps and sew the tumor into the left upper lung with one suture. Make two knots and cut off the rest of the thread.
7. Return all the lung tissue into the chest cavity and close the chest-wall incision with a 6-0 surgical suture. Examine the closed condition of the chest wall immediately. If a leak exists, it must be closed by adding sutures until the incision is closed completely.
8. Following this procedure, make an intrathoracic puncture with a 3-mL syringe and 25 G11/2″ needle to withdraw the remaining air from the chest cavity. After the air has been withdrawn, a completely inflated lung should be seen through the thin chest wall.
9. Finally, close the skin and chest muscles with 6-0 surgical suture in one layer.

3.2.3. Nude Mouse Models of Metastatic Lung

Following implantation, examinaton of the experimental animals that reflected the clinical picture for this disease can be developed *(4–11)* (*see* **Note 2**).

1. Symptoms of tumor growth are determined from weight loss, respiratory distress, or debilitation.
2. Measure actual tumor growth and metastatic spread at autopsy (*see* **Notes 3–8**).

3.2.3.1. PATTERNS OF LUNG TUMOR METASTASES AFTER SOI VISUALIZED BY GFP EXPRESSION

1. Following SOI, the human ANIP-GFP non-small cell lung carcinoma grows in the operated left lung in all mice. GFP expression allows visualization of the advancing margin of the tumor spreading in the ipsilateral lung. Observe evidence of chest wall invasion and local and regional spread. Metastatic contralateral tumors involve the mediastinum, contralateral pleural cavity, and the contralateral visceral pleura.
2. While the ipsilateral tumor may have a continuous and advancing margin, the contralateral tumor seems to form by multiple seeding events. These observations are made possible by GFP fluorescence of the fresh tumors tissue.
3. Contralateral hilar lymph nodes are also involved, and cervical lymph nodes also show GFP expression.
4. When non-GFP-transfected ANIP is compared with GFP-transformed ANIP for metastatic capability, similar results were observed. The metastatic pattern of human lung adenocarcinoma visualized in exquisite detail by GFP expression in fresh tissue should eliminate all the artifacts of fixation or freezing *(11)*.

3.2.3.2. GFP-EXPRESSING LUNG AND BONE METASTASES IN NUDE MICE

1. Nude mice are implanted in the left lung by SOI with 1-mm^3 tissue cubes of the human non-small-cell lung carcinoma H460-GFP (**Subheading 3.2.2.**).
2. Sacrifice the implanted mice at 3–4 wk at the time of significant decline in performance status. All mice should have tumors in the left lung that metastasize to the contralateral lung, and chest wall.
3. A large majority of tumors should metastasize to the skeletal system. The vertebrae are the most involved skeletal site of metastasis. Skull metastases, as well as tibia and femur marrow metastases, can be visualized by GFP fluorescence. Examine the tumor lodged in the bone marrow for the beginnings of involvement of the bone as well (*see* **Note 9**).

3.2.3.3. METASTATIC PATTERN OF THE SOI LEWIS LUNG CARCINOMA IN NUDE MICE

The developments described here have enabled the widely-used Lewis lung carcinoma to become a far more powerful model to study the mechanism of tumor progression including regional and distant metastasis representative of lung cancer. These results contrast with orthotopic injection of cell suspension of the Lewis lung carcinoma, which show a very limited metastatic pattern (12,13).

1. Implant the Lewis lung-GFP carcinoma by SOI on the left lung of nude mice (see **Subheading 3.2.2.**).
2. Examine all animals by d 12, which is the median survival age for this model (far shorter than the median survival of 27 d in the subcutaneous transplant model).
3. Look for disseminated contralateral lung metastases, mediastinal lymph node metastases, and ipsilateral and contralateral diafragmatic surface metastases.
4. Other organ involvement should fall into the following pattern: heart metastases in 40% of the animals and brain metastases in 30%. Metastases in the contralateral lung, contralateral diafragmatic surface, heart, and brain will only be detectable by GFP expression and not detectable under bright-field microscopy in fresh tissue (8).

4. Notes

1. The left lung was used for two reasons: 1) the loss of lung function is relatively smaller than in right-lung operations, and the left-lung-operated animals survive better; and 2) the left lung in mice has only one lobe, and tumors can develop easily after implantation (4–6).
2. Tumor growth was initially assessed by symptomatology and survival: the median survival time was, respectively, 27.9 d and 31 d for visceral-pleural and parietal-pleural implanted groups. The comparison between the slopes of the mean weight curves of corresponding groups demonstrated that visceral-pleural implanted animals lost significantly more weight than the parietal-pleural implanted animals. Both in the visceral- and parietal-pleural implanted groups, post-mortem analysis revealed that tumor grew in all mice demonstrating local and regional spread mimicking clinical features. However, mediastinal lymph node metastases were observed only in mice with visceral pleural implantation. Tumor symptoms, growth, and spread as well as survival indicated that the parietal-pleural and visceral-pleural models represent, respectively, early- and advanced-stage disease (9,10).
3. When the poorly-differentiated, large-cell squamous-cell human patient lung tumor AC2268 was transplanted orthotopically to the left lung as histologically intact tissue directly from surgery, tumors grew locally in all mice and opposite-lung metastases occurred, as well as lymph node metastases. Histopathology of the primary tumor and metastases, demonstrated the tumor faithfully maintained its large cell squamous cell morphology. When grown sc, this tumor grew only locally in animals and no metastases were observed (4).
4. When the histologically-intact, human small-cell lung carcinoma cell line Lu-24 was transplanted into the left lung of nude mice via thoractomy after harvesting of sc-growing tissue from nude mice, all mice produced locally growing tumors. All

mice produced regional metastases, including tumor invasion of the mediastinum, chest wall and pericardium, and distant metastases involving the right lung, esophagus, diaphragm, parietal pleura, and lymph nodes *(4)*.

5. SCID mice were also implanted orthotopically with histologically-intact Lu-24 tissue via thoracotomy. All animals produced locally-growing tumors and developed regional metastases involving the mediastinum, left chest wall, and pericardium and distant metastases involving the opposite lung, lymph nodes, parietal pleura, and diaphragm. The time to morbidity in the nude mice after transplantation of Lu-24 via thoractomy was 24 d, but in the SCIDs it was only 17 d, with the tumor apparently growing and metastasizing more rapidly in the SCIDs. The tumor faithfully maintained its oat-cell morphology while growing locally, as well as metastasizing, in immunodeficient mice of both types *(4)*.

6. Human small-cell carcinoma xenograft Lu-130 was implanted into the left lung of nude mice as intact tissue via thoracotomy. Extensive local growth occurred with metastases to the contralateral lung and mediastinal lymph nodes. Average time to obvious symptoms in the mice was 62 d. Subcutaneous implantations of this tumor resulted in local growth with no metastases *(6)*.

7. Small cell carcinoma xenograft H-69 was implanted into the left lung of the nude mice via thoracotomy. Extensive local growth occurred with metastases to the mediastinum, chest wall, ipsilateral lung, contralateral lung, and mediastinal lymph nodes. The growth of this tumor was exceedingly rapid with time to symptoms only 18.5 d as compared to 62 d for Lu-130 *(6)*.

8. After orthotopic transplantation of histologically intact tissue of A549 human lung adenocarcinoma into the left lung of nude mice via thoractomy, the animals became symptomatic of apoxia with an elevated breathing rate and became cachectic. The primary tumor reached about 1 cm in diameter and also was found widely disseminated on the chest wall. The histopathology revealed an adenocarcinoma phenotype. Opposite lung metastases were also observed with the histopathology revealing an adenocarcinoma phenotype. The tumor also metastasized to lymph nodes. A mediastinal lymph node revealed an adenocarcinoma phenotype *(5)*.

9. The H460-GFP SOI model revealed the extensive skeletal metastasizing potential of lung cancer. Such a high incidence of skeletal metastasis could not have been previously visualized before the development of the GFP-SOI model, which provided the necessary tools.

References

1. Hoffman, R. M. (1999) Orthotopic metastatic mouse models for anticancer drug discovery and evaluation: a bridge to the clinic. *Investig. New Drugs* **17,** 343–359.
2. McLemore, T. L., Liu, M. C., Blacker, P. C., Gregg, M. G., Alley, M. C., Abbott, B. J., et al. (1987) Novel intrapulmonary model for orthotopic propagation of human lung cancers in athymic nude mice. *Cancer Res.* **47,** 5132–5140.

3. McLemore, T. L., Eggleston, J. C., Shoemaker, R. H., Abbott, B. J., Bohlman, M. E., Liu, M. C., et al. (1988) Comparison of intrapulmonary, percutaneous intrathoracic, and subcutaneous models for the propagation of human pulmonary and nonpulmonary cancer cell lines in athymic nude mice. *Cancer Res.* **48,** 2880–2886.

4. Wang, X., Fu, X., and Hoffman, R.M. (1992) A new patient-like metastatic model of human lung cancer constructed orthotopically with intact tissue via thoracotomy in immunodeficient mice. *Int. J. Cancer* **51,** 992–995.

5. Wang, X., Fu, X., and Hoffman, R. M. (1992) A patient-like metastasizing model of human lung adenocarcinoma constructed via thoracotomy in nude mice. *Anticancer Res.* **12,** 1399–1401.

6. Wang, X., Fu, X., Kubota, T., and Hoffman, R. M. (1992) A new patient-like metastatic model of human small-cell lung cancer constructed orthotopically with intact tissue via thoracotomy in nude mice. *Anticancer Res.* **12,** 1403–1406.

7. Yang, M., Hasegawa, S., Jiang, P., Wang, X., Tan, Y., Chishima, T., et al. (1998) Widespread skeletal metastatic potential of human lung cancer revealed by green fluorescent protein expression. *Cancer Res.* **58,** 4217–4221.

8. Rashidi, B., Yang, M., Jiang, P., Baranov, E., An, Z., Wang, X., et al. (2000) A highly metastatic Lewis lung carcinoma orthotopic green fluorescent protein model. *Clin. Exp. Metastasis.* **18,** 57–60.

9. Astoul, P., Colt, H. G., Wang, X., and Hoffman, R. M. (1994) A "patient-like" nude mouse model of parietal pleural human lung adenocarcinoma. *Anticancer Res.* **14,** 85–91.

10. Astoul, P., Colt, H. G., Wang, X., Boutin, C., and Hoffman, R. M. (1994) A "patient-like" nude mouse metastatic model of advanced human pleural cancer. *J. Cell. Biochem.* **56,** 9–15.

11. Chishima, T., Miyagi, Y., Wang, X., Baranov, E., Tan, Y., Shimada, H., et al. (1997) Metastatic patterns of lung cancer visualized live and in process by green fluorescent protein expression. *Clin. Exp. Metastasis.* **15,** 547–552.

12. Li, L., Shin, D. M., and Fidler, I. J. (1990) Intrabronchial implantation of the Lewis lung tumor cell does not favor tumorigenocity and metastasis. *Invasion Metastasis.* **10,** 129–141.

13. Doki, Y., Murakami, K., Yamaura, T., Sugiyama, S., Misaki, T., and Saiki, I. (1999) Mediastinal lymph node metastases model by orthotopic intrapolmonary implantation of Lewis lung carcinoma cells in mice. *Br. J. Cancer* **79,** 1121–1126.

33

Lung-Specific Expression of Mutant p53 as Mouse Model for Lung Cancer

Kam-Meng Tchou-Wong and William N. Rom

1. Introduction

The p53 tumor suppressor gene is the most commonly mutated gene in cancer *(1,2)* and is mutated in 50% non-small cell lung cancer (NSCLC) and 70% of small cell lung cancer (SCLC) *(3)*. Mutations in p53 commonly reflect exposures to environmental carcinogens, e.g., cigarette smoke and lung cancer or aflatoxin and liver cancer. In support for tobacco smoking as a major risk factor for lung cancer, as the content of tar and nicotine per cigarette has dropped by more than two-thirds, there has been a concomitant change in the histologic type of lung cancer *(4)*. While SCLC has persisted at about 20%, adenocarcinoma has increased to 45% with declines in squamous cell and large cell carcinoma. Thun and colleagues *(5)* have suggested that these changes are due to the design of the cigarette; e.g., filter-tip cigarettes are inhaled more deeply than earlier, unfiltered cigarettes (more toxic), and deeper inhalation transports tobacco-specific carcinogens more distally toward the bronchoalveolar junction where adenocarcinomas often arise. In human lung cancer, both the frequency and type of mutations in the p53 gene can act as fingerprints providing information about external etiological agents, carcinogen exposure, and host factors affecting the carcinogenesis process *(6)*.

p53 missense mutations are detected in about 60% of lung cancer *(7)* and occur in the DNA binding domain, resulting in the loss of the ability of p53 to act as a transcription factor *(8)*. Analysis of the distribution and nature of p53 mutations in 876 lung tumors confirms that G to T transversions are the predominant type of mutations (about one-third) in lung cancer from smokers, but not from nonsmokers *(3,7)*. G to T transversions are a molecular signature

From: *Methods in Molecular Medicine, vol. 74: Lung Cancer, Vol. 1: Molecular Pathology Methods and Reviews*
Edited by: B. Driscoll © Humana Press Inc., Totowa, NJ

of mutagenesis by benzo[a]pyrene (BaP), a potent DNA-damaging carcinogen found at significant concentrations in tobacco smoke. Several of the most frequently mutated codons (157, 248, 273) have been shown to correspond to sites of in vitro DNA adduct formation by metabolites of BaP *(9)*. Whereas <10% of smokers develop lung cancer, almost 50% of smokers with Li-Fraumeni Syndrome (LFS), an autosomal dominant disorder characterized by germline mutations in the p53 gene, develop lung cancer, suggesting that p53 plays a crucial role in the predisposition and development of human lung cancer *(10)*.

Genetic factors influence the susceptibility to lung tumors in both mice and humans. Mice develop lung tumors similar to peripheral adenocarcinomas in humans *(11)*. The reproducible natural history of these tumors in mice allows molecular characterization at each stage of progression, from premalignant to malignant lesions. Hence, inbred mice strains and their transgenic derivatives provide useful experimental tools for studying differences in susceptibility to lung tumorigenesis and sensitivity to carcinogens. Specific genetic alterations affecting tumor-suppressor genes and proto-oncogenes occur during mouse lung tumorigenesis *(12)*. Mutational activation of the K-ras gene occurs at a frequency of about 80% in both spontaneous and chemical-induced adenomas and adenocarcinomas of the lung, suggesting that it is an early event that persists into malignancy. Allelic loss of the p16 tumor-suppressor gene occurs at 50% in lung adenocarcinomas, but rarely in adenomas, suggesting that it may play a role during tumor progression or malignant conversion. The p16^{INK4a} locus contains an overlapping gene named ARF (p19^{ARF} and p14^{ARF} in mouse and human, respectively) and hence named INK4a/ARF locus. The INK4a/ARF locus is transcriptionally activated by oncogenic stresses such as Ras and Myc, resulting in cell-cycle arrest or apoptosis, and plays a role in murine tumorigenesis *(13)*.

The p14^{ARF}/p53 pathway is thought to be deregulated in the vast majority of human tumors. Deletion of the p14^{ARF} gene has been demonstrated in human breast, brain, and lung cancers, especially when the p53 gene is not mutated *(2)*. In response to oncogenic stresses, ARF is induced, which activates and stabilizes p53 both by neutralizing MDM2, which destabilizes p53, and by interacting directly with p53. This would lead to p53-dependent growth arrest or apoptosis, unless a second lesion occurred, such as a mutation in p14^{ARF} or p53 itself. The A/J mouse lung tumor model results in a high percent of lung adenomas that harbor K-ras mutations but interestingly, p53 mutations are uncommon *(14,15)*. Similarly, FVB/N mice have a relatively high incidence of spontaneous lung cancer and 75% of the carcinomas contained K-ras mutations *(16)*. In the murine model of lung tumorigenesis, the p53/ARF pathway may have been activated in response to the oncogenic stress induced by oncogenic

Table 1
Effects of p53^{val135} Transgene Expression on the Incidence and Spectrum of Tumor Development in 18-Mo-Old Mice

	p53$^{+/+}$		p53$^{+/-}$		p53$^{-/-}$	
	—	p53^{val135}	—	p53^{val135}	—	p53^{val135}
Lymphoma	0%	54%	27%	40%	83%	89%
Lung adenocarcinoma	0%	31%	2%	20%	2%	0%
Osteosarcoma	0%	0%	24%	9%	5%	0%
Hemangiosarcoma	0%	0%	12%	11%	0%	5%
Rhabdomyosarcoma	0%	7.5%	7%	3%	2%	5%

Data from **ref. *19***.

K-ras. This may put selective pressure on inhibiting the p53/ARF pathway to overcome p53-dependent growth arrest and apoptosis by dowregulating p19^{ARF} or mutating p53. Because in the majority of lung tumors in mice, mutations in p53 are rare events *(17)*, it remains to be determined whether p19^{ARF} is inactivated in these tumors, as in human cancers containing wild-type p53. Alternatively, other pathways upstream or downstream of p53 may be affected in murine lung tumorigenesis.

Because p53 is the guardian of the genome, mice with disrupted germline p53 alleles are more susceptible to the development of spontaneous tumors of various types, primarily lymphomas and sarcomas *(18)*. Because homozygous p53 knockout (p53$^{-/-}$) mice develop lymphomas and sarcomas by 6 mo of age *(18,19)* while heterozygous p53 knockout (p53$^{+/-}$) mice are more susceptible to carcinogens than normal mice *(20)*, heterozygous p53 knockout mouse offers a tool for studying both spontaneous and chemical-induced lung carcinogenesis. A second transgenic mouse containing a mutant p53^{val135} (alanine to valine change at codon 135) developed a high incidence of lung adenocarcinomas, osteosarcomas and lymphomas *(21)*. The p53^{val135} mutant is of particular interest because p53$^{+/+}$ mice expressing this mutant have a high incidence of spontaneous lung adenocarcinomas (31%), second to the incidence of lymphomas (54%) (*see* **Table 1**) *(22)*. In the absence of the transgene, the incidence of lymphoma and lung adenocarcinoma in the p53$^{+/-}$ heterozygous knockout mice was 27% and 2%, respectively. The p53val135 transgene increased the incidence of lymphoma to lung adenocarcinoma in p53$^{+/-}$ mice to 40% and 20%, respectively. Hence, in the presence of the mutant p53^{val135} transgene, animals homozygous (p53$^{+/+}$) and hemizygous (p53$^{+/-}$) for the endogenous wild-type p53 gene exhibited accelerated tumor development and an altered tumor spectrum compared to their nontransgenic counterparts.

Interestingly, in the absence of p53 function in p53$^{-/-}$ knockout mice, the p53^{val135} transgene has no effect on tumor development. This could be explained by the early deaths of p53$^{-/-}$ mice from lymphoma before the development of lung cancer. Alternatively, these results suggested that the p53^{val135} mutant may act in vivo in a dominant-negative manner in the presence of wild-type p53 (22). If the loss of wild-type p53 function alone enhances lung cancer development, one would expect to see increased incidence of the latter with the progressive loss of p53 function in p53$^{+/-}$ or p53$^{-/-}$ mice. However, only 2% of tumors in p53$^{+/-}$ or p53$^{-/-}$ mice were lung adenocarcinoma. Hence, it is conceivable that the mutant p53^{val135} protein produces a gain-of-function activity, altering tumor spectrum and promoting the development of lung adenocarcinomas.

Interestingly, the enhanced incidence of lung cancer conferred by the p53^{val135} transgene in mice is reminiscent of LFS patients who are at increased risk for smoking-related lung cancer. Whereas <10% of smokers develop lung cancer, almost 50% of males with LFS develop lung cancer. Support for the role of p53 mutations in enhancing the susceptibility of lung cancer in humans comes from the analysis of a database of germline p53 mutations in 448 cancer-prone individuals. Among these patients, two LFS patients harbor point mutations in the p53 gene at codon 138 (equivalent to codon 135 in mouse) (23) and one of the patients developed lung cancer. The preferential induction of lung adenocarcinomas, second to lymphoma, by the p53^{val135} mutant protein makes this an interesting mouse model for studying the role of p53 in the development of adenocarcinoma, the most common type of human lung cancer.

Expression of the p53^{val135} transgene under the control of the endogenous murine p53 promoter in FVB/N mice has also been shown to increase the incidence of lung cancer (53%) (16). Induction of the latter by expression of the p53^{val135} mutant was independent of the genetic background of the mouse (21,22). The p53^{val135} transgenic mouse also exhibited increased susceptibility to lung cancer induced by two major tobacco-related carcinogens, 4-(methylnitrosamino)-1-(3-pyridyl)-1-butanone (NNK) and BaP (23). The C57BL/6, A/J, or C3H/HeJ strains exposed intratracheally to BaP plus charcoal developed squamous cell carcinomas at early time points with a high dose (8 mg), followed by adenomas and adenocarcinomas at later time points with a lower dose (4 mg) (24). Charcoal was necessary for the development of squamous cell carcinomas by impeding clearance of BaP. Crossing the A/J mice with p53$^{+/-}$ heterozygous or p53^{135} mice resulted in increased adenomas after intraperitoneal injection of carcinogen, with the highest number of tumors in A/J × p53^{val135} mice (23). In contrast, lung-specific expression of a dominant-negative mutant form of p53^{his175} (arginine to histidine change at codon 175) did not lead to the development of lung tumors in mice (25). Mice expressing p53 transgenes with mutation at codon 248 (arginine to tryptophan) or codon 249 (arginine to serine) also failed to induce the lung tumor *(26)*. Hence, only specific mutations in p53, such as codon 135, may confer susceptibility to lung cancer while other changes (codons 175, 248, or 249) may not have an effect on lung tumorigenesis.

Strictly speaking, in order to examine the role of oncogene or tumor-suppressor gene in mouse model of lung tumorigenesis, one should utilize lung-specific promoters to control the expression of these transgenes. Transgenic mice with the viral oncogene SV40 large T antigen, which binds and inactivates both p53 and retinoblastoma (Rb) proteins, driven by the CC10 or SP-C promoter developed lung adenocarcinomas by 6 mo *(27–29)*. However, in the T-antigen transgenic mouse models, both the p53 and Rb pathways were inactivated. To examine specifically the p53 pathway in lung tumorigenesis, transgenic mouse models in which p53 function is compromised only in the lungs are needed. It has previously been demonstrated that both surfactant protein C (SP-C) and Clara cell 10 kD (CC10) promoters are lung-specific promoters. The SP-C promoter mainly functions in the type II pneumocytes and the CC10 promoter is active in Clara cells, the non-ciliated secretory bronchial epithelial cells. Since most NSCLCs are derived from bronchial epithelial cells and the murine respiratory epithelium contains 50–60% Clara cells *(30)*, the CC10 promoter was chosen to control the expression of a dominant-negative mutant form of p53 (dnp53). This mutant p53 lacks the transactivation and DNA binding domains (amino acids 15-301) but retains the C-terminal oligomerization domain which interacts with endogenous wild-type p53 to generate DNA binding-incompetent oligomers, thus acting in a dominant-negative fashion. It has been shown that this mutant p53 is able to form complex with wild-type p53 and enhances the transfoming activity of ras and myc in rat embryo fibroblasts *(31)*. We hypothesized that expression of dnp53 specifically in the Clara cells in the bronchial mucosa will antagonize the function of wild-type p53, thereby promoting the development of lung cancer.

1.1. Generation of Transgenic Mice and Lung-Specific Expression of Dominant-Negative Mutant p53

The murine CC10 promoter (mCC10) was cloned by PCR from a genomic DNA library (*see* **Notes 1** and **2**). Then the dnp53 construct was cloned downstream of the mCC10 promoter to generate pmCC10/dnp53 (*see* **Fig. 1A**) (*see* **Note 3**). To demonstrate the expression of dnp53 under the CC10 promoter, the pmCC10/dnp53 plasmid was transfected into H441 cells, which are human adenocarcinoma cells that display Clara cell-like phenotype *(32)* (*see* **Note 4**). Expression of dnp53 in three stably transfected clones was analyzed by

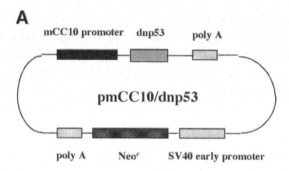

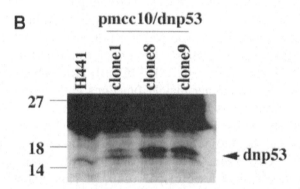

Fig. 1. Expression of dnp53 under the mCC10 promoter in H441 cells. (**A**) Schematic representation of the pmCC10/dnp53 plasmid. (**B**) H441 cells were transfected with the pmCC10/dnp53 plasmid and selected with G418. Expression of the 18-kD dnp53 protein in three G418-resistant clones was detected by immunoprecipitation with anti-p53 antibody followed by Western-blot analysis using the same antibody.

immunoprecipitation with anti-p53 antibody directed against the C-terminus (PAb421) followed by Western-blot analysis using the same antibody (*see* **Fig. 1B**).

To generate transgenic mouse, the dnp53 expression cassette containing the mCC10 promoter, dnp53 gene, and the poly A signal was isolated from the pmCC10/dnp53 plasmid and injected into fertilized zygotes from FVB/N mice (*see* **Notes 5** and **6**). Transmission of the transgene in founder mice was screened by polymerase chain reaction (PCR). Seven transgene-positive founder mice were identified and crossed with wild-type FVB/N mice to generate F1 mice. Expression of the transgene in the lungs of F1 mice from each of the seven founder lines (1506, 2005, 2008, 2501, 3503, 5004, 5503) was examined by Western-blot analysis using anti-p53 antibody. Expression

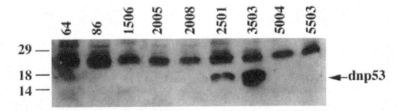

Fig. 2. Expression of the dnp53 transgene in the lungs of transgenic mice. Lung tissues from seven F1 lines (1506, 2005, 2008, 2501, 3503, 5004, and 5504) were homogenized and the expression of dnp53 was detected by Western blot analysis using anti-p53 antibody.

of dnp53 protein was detected in the lungs of two F1 lines 2501 and 3503 (*see* **Fig. 2**) but not in any other tissues including the brain, heart, intestine, kidney, liver, muscle, spleen, or uterus (data not shown). Hence, expression of the dnp53 transgene under the CC10 promoter was lung-specific.

1.2. Effects of dnp53 Expression on Lung Cancer Susceptibility

When expressed in the choroid plexus epithelium, the dnp53 transgene induced the development of brain tumor. On the other hand, expression of dnp53 in the liver had no adverse effect and the transgenic mice lived a normal life span *(33)*. To examine the effects of expression of dnp53 in lung tumorigenesis, FVB/N wild-type and CC10/dnp53 transgenic mice were kept for observation for approx 18 mo for the development of spontaneous lung cancer. Animals were sacrificed and lungs were fixed in formalin- and paraffin-embedded lung sections were stained with hematoxylin and eosin (H&E). The incidences of spontaneous lung tumors were 20% and 45% in wild-type and CC10/dnp53 mice, respectively. These lung tumors demonstrated histology of adenocarcinomas, as examined by H&E staining.

Because expression of dnp53 protein in the lungs increased the incidence of spontaneous lung cancer, the CC10/dnp53 transgenic mouse will also be a useful model for deciphering the role of p53 in smoking-related lung carcinogenesis. Wild-type and CC10/dnp53 mice can be exposed to the two major tobacco carcinogens, BaP or NNK, by intratracheal instillation or intraperitoneal (IP) injection. The incidence of lung cancer in solvent-treated and carcinogen-treated wild-type and CC10/dnp53 mice can be compared. The incidence of BaP-induced lung cancer after intratracheal injection was 39% and 73% in wild-type and CC10/dnp53 mice, respectively. All tumors were determined by histology to be adenocarcinomas. The absence of squamous cell carcinoma may be due to the low dose of BaP (5 mg) used. In addition, BaP was dissolved in tricarpylin in the absence of charcoal, which impedes

PCNA Ab   # p53 Ab

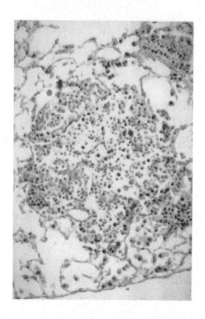 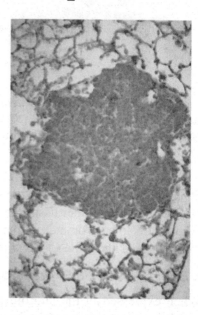

Fig. 3. Immunohistochemical staining of lung sections of CC10/dnp53 transgenic mice. PCNA nuclear staining was detected in lung adenocarcinomas, but no immuno-staining was detected with anti-p53 antibody.

lung clearance and may be necessary for the induction of squamous cell carcinomas *(24)*.

1.3. Characterization of Lung Tumors

For further characterization of lung tumors, immunohistochemistry was performed on paraffin-embedded lung sections. As shown in **Fig. 3**, spontaneous-derived lung adenocarcinomas were stained positive for proliferation cell nuclear antigen (PCNA), a marker for proliferating cells. In contrast, no immunostaining was detected in the tumors using anti-p53 antibody PAb122 (amino acids 370-378). In the lungs of CC10/dnp53 mice, there was intense immunostaining of dnp53 in the bronchial epithelial cells in the normal mucosa with anti-CC10 antibody and anti-p53 antibody. Interestingly, in tumors derived from both wild-type and CC10/dnp53 mice, there was no immunostaining with anti-p53 or anti-CC10 antibody (data not shown). Wild-type p53 has a short half-life and is not detected in normal tissues. Detection of p53 staining usually is indicative of expression of mutant p53, which generally has a longer half-life. Consistent with the absence of staining for p53, it has been demonstrated that mutations of p53 are not common in murine lung tumors. On the other hand, 75% of spontaneous lung carcinomas from FVB/N mice contained K-ras mutations *(16)*.

Since the endogenous CC10 protein was not expressed in tumors, it is not surprising that the dnp53 protein, which is under the control of the CC10 promoter, is also not expressed. This is consistent with the reduced and sporadic expression of the endogenous CC10 gene in tumors, in transformed Clara cells in vitro *(27)*, and in lung adenocarcinomas of CC10-T antigen transgenic mice. Pulmonary adenocarcinomas in humans have also been demonstrated to express predominantly surfactant protein rather than CC10 protein *(34)*. In fact, overexpression of CC10 in A549 cells has been shown to reduce anchorage-independent growth and cell transformation *(35)*. Exposure of hamsters and mice to NNK led to reduced CC10 expression and downregulation of CC10 has been suggested to contribute to carcinogenesis *(36)*. The absence of CC10 expression in lung adenocarcinomas suggests that its expression may be selected against in some tumors, perhaps by downregulation of the CC10 promoter activity. By the same token, the expression of dnp53 transgene under the CC10 promoter in adenocarcinomas may also be downregulated. Nevertheless, these data suggest that expression of the mutant p53 protein may be important for the initiation of lung carcinogenesis but is not required for the maintenance of the transformed phenotype in the tumor. Because the dnp53 transgene is expressed in normal Clara cells but lost in the tumor cells, it will be interesting to determine when the expression of the dnp53 transgene is turned off during the carcinogenesis process by examining early preneoplastic lesions.

In summary, transgenic mice in which the function of the p53 tumor-suppressor gene is specifically compromised in the lung provide useful animal models for lung cancer for multiple purposes including basic mechanistic studies, screening for potential carcinogens, and screening for chemopreventive or chemotherapeutic agents *(17)*.

2. Materials

All materials, excluding animals, are available through Sigma (St. Louis, MO).

2.1. Administration of Carcinogens

2.1.1. Intratracheal Instillation

1. Benzo(a)Pyrene (BaP): 1 mg in 50 μL tricaprylin.
2. Fiberoptic mouse mini-laryngoscope (prototype).
3. Two-month-old CC10/dnp53 mice.
4. Isofluorane.
5. Restraining board, rubber bands.
6. 1-mL Syringe fitted with a blunt 18-gauge needle.

2.1.2. Intraperitoneal Injection

1. BaP: 100 mg/kg body weight, dissolved in tricaprylin.
2. 4-(methylnitrosamino)-1-(3-pyridyl)-1-butanone (NNK): 100 mg/kg body weight, dissolved in phosphate-buffered saline (PBS).

2.2. Characterization of Lung Sections

1. 10% Buffered formalin.
2. H&E stain.
3. Anti-p53 antibodies: PAb 421, PAb 122 (Lab Vision Corp, Fremont, CA).
4. Anti-CC10 antibody (courtesy Franco DeMayo, PhD).
5. Anti-thyroid transcription factor-1 (TTF-1) antibody (Lab Vision Corp, Fremont, CA).
6. Avidin-biotin complex.
7. Ventana Medical Systems computer controlled NexES automated immunohistochemical staining instrument.

3. Methods

3.1. Administration of Carcinogens

To test the susceptibility of the CC10/dnp53 mice for carcinogen-induced lung cancer, BaP is administered via intratracheal instillation. The two most potent carcinogens found in cigarettes are BaP and NNK and therefore are chosen for the study of smoking-related lung carcinogenesis. These carcinogens can be administered by intratracheal instillation or intraperitoneal injection (*see* **Note 7**).

3.1.1. Intratracheal Instillation

1. Because BaP is a potent carcinogen, instillation should be performed in a chemical hood and all personnel should wear particulate masks, safety gowns, boots, and gloves. Dissolve BaP in tricaprylin. Check BaP/tricaprylin for contaminants by observing under a UV hand-held lamp.
2. A prototype fiberoptic mouse mini-laryngoscope has been developed for intratracheal instillation. Two-month-old mice are anesthetized in a plastic bag with gauze containing isofluorane until the animals do not respond to a tactile stimulus.
3. Place the animal on its dorsum on a restraining board with a rubber band to hold the mouth open. Pass a 1-mL syringe with a blunt 18-gauge needle via the mini-laryngoscope into the trachea and inject 50 μL of BaP dissolved in the tricaprylin solvent or tricaprylin alone.
4. Return the animal to the cage. It should wake in 1–2 min. Our first instillation attempt was at 2 mg BaP in 100 μL tricaprylin solvent. Because several mice died from the instillation, we suggest that the primary and three subsequent instillations be performed using 1 mg BaP in 50 μL tricaprylin.

5. Repeat instillations weekly for 4 wk (total of 5 mg BaP) and sacrifice animals 6 mo later, at the age of 9–10 mo old.

3.1.2. Intraperitoneal Injection

1. Give mice single or multiple intraperitoneal injections of BaP or NNK and sacrifice at various timepoints after injections.
2. Check mice at 4–5 mo after a single intraperitoneal injection of carcinogen for lung adenomas. At this time adenomas are to be expected, but longer time points may be needed for adenocarcinomas to develop *(23)*.

3.2. Characterization of Lung Sections

1. Sacrifice animals and fix whole lungs in 10% buffered formalin.
2. Cut paraffin-embedded lung sections at 1-mm intervals, immobilize on slides and stain with H&E for quantitation of lung tumors.
3. Perform immunohistochemical staining on unstained slides using a Ventana Medical Systems computer controlled NexES automated immunohistochemical staining instrument and avidin-biotin complex for development. The primary staining methods were preprogrammed for anti-p53, anti-CC10, and anti-thyroid transcription factor-1 antibodies.

4. Notes

1. For lung-specific expression of the transgene, the murine CC10 (mCC10) promoter was cloned. Previous studies have shown that the 3 kb full-length mCC10 promoter is active in the lung but also has weak activity in the uterus *(37)*. Further characterization of this promoter revealed that a basic core promoter containing 803 bp of the 3 kb mCC10 promoter is active only in the lung but not in any other organs *(38,39)*. Based on these results, primers were designed to clone the basic core mCC10 promoter from a murine liver genomic DNA library by PCR using the high fidelity enzyme *pfu*. The 898 bp PCR fragment containing the mCC10 promoter was subcloned into the mammalian expression vector pcDNA3 (Invitrogen), replacing the human CMV promoter and enhancer, to generate the pmCC10 vector. To test the activity of the mCC10 promoter, the β-galactosidase (βgal) reporter gene was inserted downstream of the mCC10 promoter to generate pmCC10-βgal. As control, the β-galactosidase gene was also cloned downstream of the constitutively active CMV promoter in the pcDNA3 vector, generating pCMV-βgal.
2. The use of lung-specific promoters is especially important for the expression of genes that may otherwise cause embryonic or perinatal lethality in mice when expressed ubiquitously. Ubiquitous expression of oncogenic ras frequently leads to lethality in mouse embryos, which is the major cause of failure for successful establishment of transgenic mice. Although we have success with expression of mutant p53 under the mC10 promoter in the lungs, we failed to overexpress oncogenic K-ras (codon 12 mutation) using the same mCC10 promoter, despite

transmission of the transgene. In the case of the CC10/dnp53 transgenic mouse model, since the dnp53 transgene was expressed in normal bronchial epithelium but turned off in adenocarcinomas, expression of the transgene may not be required for the maintenance of transformation. However, if expression of the transgene is continuously required for lung tumorigenesis, other lung-specific promoters such as SP-C should be used because the CC10 promoter may be selected against in some NSCLCs. Alternatively, an inducible system can be used in which expression of the transgene can be regulated in the lung *(41)*.

3. The dominant-negative mutant p53 gene (kindly provided by Dr. Moshe Oren), lacking the transactivation and sequence-specific DNA binding domain (amino acids 15-301) but retaining the C-terminal oligomerization domain (amino acids 302-393) *(31)*, was subcloned into the pmCC10 vector to generate pmCC10/dnp53 (*see* **Fig. 1A**). The pmCC10/dnp53 plasmid was transfected into H441 cells and uptake of the plasmid was selected for neomycin resistance with the drug G418. G418-resistant colonies were screened for expression of the 18-kD dnp53 protein by immunoprecipitation with anti-p53 antibody (PAb421) followed by Western-blot analysis. After immunoprecipitation, proteins were fractionated on 10% sodium dodecyl sulfate polyacrylamide gel electrophoresis (SDS-PAGE) gels and transferred onto Immobilon-P membrane (Millipore, Bedford, MA). The membrane was probed with anti-p53 antibody and anti-mouse IgG-HRP (PharMingen/Transduction Laboratories, San Diego, CA) and detected by enhanced chemiluminescence (Amersham, Piscataway, NJ).

4. To test for promoter activity, β-galactosidase activity was measured after transient transfection of pmCC10-βgal, pCMV-βgal or empty vector control into H441 lung adenocarcinoma cells. Transfection with pCMV-βgal and pmCC10-βgal yielded β-galactosidase activity fivefold and twofold, respectively, over that with empty vector. These results were consistent with previous reports that the mCC10 promoter is less active in in vitro cell culture systems but possibly acquires full activity in vivo *(38)*.

5. The FVB/N mouse strain created in the early 1970s has been used extensively in transgenic mouse research because of its well-defined inbred background, superior reproductive performance, and prominent pronuclei of fertilized zygotes, which facilitate microinjection of DNA. These are important properties for the successful generation of transgenic mice. Compared with other mouse strains, the incidences of tumors in FVB/N mice suggest a higher than usual rate of lung tumors and a lower incidence of liver tumors and lymphomas *(40)*. Hence, the FVB/N mice are more susceptible to lung tumorigenesis and are appropriate for the development of transgenic mouse models for lung cancer. Because the incidence of lung adenocarcinomas varies from strain to strain, the use of the same strain of mouse will eliminate the strain-dependent effect on lung tumorigenesis.

6. The dnp53 expression cassette fragment containing the mCC10 promoter, the dnp53 gene, and the poly A signal was isolated from the pmCC10/dnp53 plasmid and injected into the pronucleus of fertilized eggs of FVB/N mice. Transmission

of the transgene was verified using a PCR-based technique. DNA extracted from the tails of founder mice was screened by PCR using primers from the mCC10 promoter and p53 gene. Seven transgene-positive founder lines were identified. Each positive founder mouse was crossed with a wild-type FVB/N mouse to generate F1 mice. One mouse from each F1 line was sacrificed and the lungs homogenized for protein extraction. Expression of dnp53 protein was determined by Western-blot analysis using anti-p53 antibody. Since the level of dnp53 protein expression is higher in line 3503 than in line 2501, the 3503 line was maintained and used in all studies. Some mice were kept for observation for 18 mo for the development of spontaneous lung tumors.

7. To induce lung adenocarcinomas with carcinogens, single or multiple intraperitoneal injections of BaP or NNK is the preferred method because no specialized techniques or special equipments such as the laryngoscope, particulate masks, and safety gowns are needed as are required for intratracheal instillations. For the induction of squamous cell carcinomas, intratracheal instillation of higher doses of carcinogens in the presence of charcoal may be needed.

References

1. Levine, A. J., Momand, J., and Finlay, C. A. (1991) The p53 tumour suppressor gene. *Nature* **351**, 453–456.
2. Vogelstein, B., Lane, D., and Levine, A. J. (2000) Surfing the p53 network. *Nature* **408**, 307–310.
3. Greenblatt, M. S., Bennett, W. P., Hollstein, M., and Harris, C. C. (1994) Mutations in the p53 tumor suppressor gene: clues to cancer etiology and molecular pathogenesis. *Cancer Res.* **54**, 4855–4878.
4. Fielding, J. E. (1985) Smoking: health effects and control. *N. Engl. J. Med.* **313**, 491–498, 555–562.
5. Thun, M. J., Lally, C. A., Flannery, J. T., Calle, E. E., Flanders, W. D., and Heath, C. W. (1997) Cigarette smoking and changes in the histopathology of lung cancer. *J. Natl. Cancer Inst.* **89**, 1580–1586.
6. Bartsch, H. and Hietanen, E. (1996) The role of individual susceptibility in cancer burden related to environmental exposure. *Environ. Health Perspect.* **104S3**, 569–577.
7. Hernandez-Boussard, T. M. and Hainaut, P. (1998) A specific spectrum of *p53* mutations in lung cancer from smokers: review of mutations compiled in the IARC *p53* database. *Environ. Health Perspect.* **106**, 385–391.
8. Harris, C. C. (1996) Structure and function of the p53 tumor suppressor gene: clues for rational cancer therapeutic strategies. *J. Natl. Cancer Inst.* **88**, 1442–1455.
9. Denissenko, M. F., Pao, A., Tang, M. S., and Pfeifer, G. P. (1996) Preferential formation of benzo[a]pyrene adducts at lung cancer mutational hotspots in p53. *Science* **274**, 430–432.
10. Malkin, D., Li, F. P., Strong, L. C., Fraumeni, J. F., Jr., et al. (1990) Germ line p53 mutations in a familial syndrome of breast cancer, sarcomas, and other neoplasms. *Science* **250**, 1233–1238.

11. Malkinson, A. M. (1998) Molecular comparison of human and mouse pulmonary adenocarcinomas. *Exp. Lung Res.* **24,** 541–555.

12. Herzog, C. R., Lubet, R. A., and You, M. (1997) Genetic alterations in mouse lung tumors: implications for cancer chemoprevention. *J. Cell Biochem. Suppl.* **28–29,** 49–63.

13. Serrano, M. (2000) The *INK4α/ARF* locus in murine tumorigenesis. *Carcinogenesis* **21,** 865–869.

14. You, M., Candrian, U., Maronpot, R. R., Stoner, G. D., and Anderson, M. W. (1989) Activation of the Ki-*ras* protooncogene in spontaneously occurring and chemically induced lung tumors of the strain A mouse. *Proc. Natl. Acad. Sci. USA* **86,** 3070–3074.

15. Mass, M. J., Jeffers, A. J., Ross, J. A., Nelson, G., Galati, A. J., Stoner, G. D., and Nesnow, S. (1993) Ki-*ras* oncogene mutations in tumors and DNA adducts formed by benz[*j*]aceanthrylene and benzo[*a*]pyrene in the lungs of strain A/J mice. *Mol. Carcinogenesis* **8,** 186–192.

16. Shafarenko, M., Mahler, J., Cochran C., Kisielewski, A., Golding, E., Wiseman, R., and Goodrow, T. (1997) Similar incidence of K-*ras* mutations in lung carcinomas of FVB/N mice and FVB/N mice carrying a mutant p53 transgene. *Carcinogenesis* **18,** 1423–1426.

17. Lubet, R. A., Zhang, Z., Wiseman, R. W., and You, M. (2000) Use of p53 transgenic mice in the development of cancer models for multiple purposes. *Exp. Lung Res.* **26,** 581–593.

18. Donehower, L. A., Harvey, M., Slagle, B. L., McArthur, M. J., Montgomery, C. A., Jr., Butel, J. S., and Bradley, A. (1992) Mice deficient for p53 are developmentally normal but susceptible to spontaneous tumours. *Nature* **356,** 215–221.

19. Harvey, M., McArthur, M. J., Montgomery, C. A., Butel, J. S., Bradley, A., and Donehower, L. A. (1993) Spontaneous and carcinogen-induced tumorigenesis in p53-deficient mice. *Nature Genet.* **5,** 225–229.

20. Purdie, C. A. , Harrison, D. J., Peter, A., Dobbie, L., White, S., Howie, S. E. M., et al. (1994) Tumour incidence, spectrum and ploidy in mice with a large deletion in the p53 gene. *Oncogene* **9,** 603–609.

21. Lavigueur, A., Maltby, V., Mock, D., Rossant, J., Pawson, T., and Bernstein, A. (1989) High incidence of lung, bone, and lymphoid tumors in transgenic mice overexpressing mutant alleles of the p53 oncogene. *Mol. Cell. Biol.* **9,** 3982–3991.

22. Harvey, M., Vogel, H., Morris, D., Bradley, A., Bernstein, A., and Donehower, L. A. (1995) A mutant p53 transgene accelerates tumor development in heterozygous but not nullizygous p53-deficient mice. *Nature Genet.* **9,** 305–311.

23. Zhang, Z., Liu, Q., Lantry, L. E., Wang, Y., Kelloff, G. J., Anderson, M. W., et al. (2000) A germ-line *p53* mutation accelerates pulmonary tumorigenesis: p53-independent efficacy of chemopreventive agents green tea or dexamethasone/*myo*-inositol and chemotherapeutic agents taxol or adramycin. *Cancer Res.* **60,** 901–907.

24. Yoshimoto, T., Inoue, T., Iizuka, H., Nishikawa, H., Sakatani, M., Ogura, T., et al. (1980) Differential induction of squamous cell carcinomas and adenocarcinomas in mouse lung by intratracheal instillation of benzo(a)pyrene and charcoal powder. *Cancer Res.* **40,** 4301–4307.

25. Morris, G. F., Hoyle, G. W., Athas, G. B., Lei, W. H., Xu, J., Morris, C. B., and Friedman, M. (1998) Lung-specific expression in mice of a dominant negative mutant form of the p53 tumor suppressor protein. *J. LA. State Med. Soc.* **150,** 179–185.

26. Hosokawa, A. (1999) Generation and analyses of transgenic mice containing mutant p53 transgene. *Jukuoka Igaku Zasshi* **90,** 80–87.

27. Magdaleno, S. M., Wang, G., Mireles, V. L., Ray, M. K., Finegold, M. J., and DeMayo, F. J. (1997) Cyclin-dependent kinase inhibitor expression in pulmonary Clara cells transformed with SV40 Large T Antigen in transgenic mice. *Cell Growth Differ.* **8,** 145–155.

28. Wikenheiser, K. A., Clark, J. C., Linnoila, R. I., Stahlman, M. T., and Whitsett, J. A. (1992) Simian Virus 40 Large T Antigen directed by transcriptional elements of the human surfactant protein C gene produces pulmonary adenocarcinomas in transgenic mice. *Cancer Res.* **52,** 5342–5352.

29. Wikenheiser, K. A. and Whitsett, J. A. (1997) Tumor progression and cellular differentiation of pulmonary adenocarcinomas in SV40 Large T Antigen transgenic mice. *Am. J. Respir. Cell Mol. Biol.* **16,** 713–723.

30. Pack, R. J., Al-Ugaily, L. H., and Morris, G. (1981) The cells of the tracheobronchial epithelium of the mouse: a quantitative light and electron microscope study. *J. Anat.* **132 (Pt 1),** 71–84.

31. Shaulian, E., Zauberman, A., Ginsberg, D., and Oren, M. (1992) Identification of a minimal transformation domain of p53: negative dominance through abrogation of sequence-specific DNA binding. *Mol. Cell. Biol.* **12,** 5581–5592.

32. Sawaya, P. L., Stripp, B. R., Whitsett, J. A., and Luse, D. S. (1993) The lung-specific CC10 gene is regulated by transcription factors from the AP-1, octamer, and hepatocyte nuclear factor 3 families. *Mol. Cell. Biol.* **13,** 3860–3871.

33. Bowman, T., Symonds, H., Gu, L., Yin, C., Oren, M., and Van Dyke, T. (1996) Tissue-specific inactivation of p53 tumor suppression in the mouse. *Genes Dev.* **10,** 826–835.

34. Nomori, H., Morinaga, S., Kobayashi, R., and Torikata, C. (1994) Protein 1 and Clara cell 10-kDa protein distribution in normal and neoplastic tissues with emphasis on the respiratory system. *Virchows Arch.* **424,** 517–523.

35. Szabo, E., Goheer, A., Witschi, H., and Linnoila, R. I. (1998) Overexpression of CC10 modifies neoplastic potential in lung cancer cells. *Cell Growth Differ.* **9,** 475–485.

36. Linnoila, R. I., Szabo, E., DeMayo, F., Witschi, H., Sabourin, C., and Malkinson, A. (2000) the role of CC10 in pulmonary carcinogenesis: from a marker to tumor suppression. *Ann. NY Acad. Sci.* **923,** 249–267.

37. Margraf, L. R., Finegold, M. J., Stanley, L. A., Major, A., Hawkins, H. K., and DeMayo, F. J. (1993) Cloning and tissue-specific expression of the cDNA for

the mouse Clara cell 10 kD protein: comparison of endogenous expression to rabbit uteroglobin promoter-driven transgene expression. *Am. J. Respir. Cell Mol. Biol.* **9,** 231–238.

38. Ray, M. K., Magdaleno, S. W., Finegold, M. J., and DeMayo, F. J. (1995) cis-acting elements involved in the regulation of mouse Clara cell-specific 10-kDa protein gene. In vitro and in vivo analysis. *J. Biol. Chem.* **270,** 2689–2694.

39. Ray, M. K., Chen, C. Y., Schwartz, R. J., and DeMayo, F. J. (1996) Transcriptional regulation of a mouse Clara cell-specific protein (mCC10) gene by the NKx transcription factor family members thyroid transciption factor 1 and cardiac muscle-specific homeobox protein (CSX). *Mol. Cell. Biol.* **16,** 2056–2064.

40. Mahler, J. F., Stokes, W., Mann, P. C., Takaoka, M., and Maronpot, R. R. (1996) Spontaneous lesions in aging FVB/N mice. *Toxicol. Pathol.* **24,** 710–716.

41. Zhan, B., Magdaleno, S., Chua, S., Wang, Y. L., Burcin, M., Elberg, D., et al. (2000) Transgenic mouse models for lung cancer. *Exp. Lung Res.* **26,** 567–579.

34

Use of Nucleotide Excision Repair-Deficient Mice as a Model For Chemically Induced Lung Cancer

David L. Cheo and Errol C. Friedberg

1. Introduction

The combination of classical mouse genetics with mouse models derived from transgenic and gene-targeting technologies provides new opportunities to elucidate the functional roles of genes in normal and disease processes. Candidate disease genes can be systematically inactivated and tested individually or in combination with other mutations, alleles, or transgenes. Such new mouse models can also be examined in the context of different strain backgrounds that are relevant to the field of study. In our studies we have demonstrated how the combined effect of multiple gene knockout mutations involved in DNA repair and cell-cycle progression can be examined in classical tumor-induction protocols. The goal of this chapter is to serve as a guide for investigators who may be relatively new to the field of mouse genetics, but are interested in utilizing this vast and expanding resource in lung cancer research.

1.1. The Classical Mouse Model

The laboratory mouse has for many decades been one of the most important tools in which to study cancer in mammals and has long served as a bioassay for carcinogen testing. As a result, a plethora of specific tumor-induction protocols have been developed. Many of these protocols still serve as useful model systems with which to study specific types of cancer. In addition, a variety of inbred strains of mice that are highly predisposed to both spontaneous and chemical-induced carcinogenesis have emerged from conventional breeding studies. These strains have been extensively used to examine the

From: *Methods in Molecular Medicine, vol. 74: Lung Cancer, Vol. 1: Molecular Pathology Methods and Reviews*
Edited by: B. Driscoll © Humana Press Inc., Totowa, NJ

genetic components of cancer. The breeding of susceptible strains to resistant strains has revealed candidate disease genes from quantitative linkage analysis with microsatellite markers that are functionally linked to susceptibility and resistance *(1)*. The usefulness of this approach has been well-demonstrated in lung cancer *(2)*. For example, progenitors of strain A mice are highly susceptible to both spontaneous and chemical-induced pulmonary adenoma *(3)*. Crosses with resistant strains of mice have identified a complex set of genes involved in both susceptibility and resistance to lung cancer. Although the same loci are apparently involved in both spontaneous and chemical-induction of lung carcinogenesis, there appear to be separate pathways controlling lung tumor incidence and tumor multiplicity *(4)*. With the complete genetic maps and sequences of the human and mouse genomes in hand, unprecedented advances in our understanding of cancer genetics are sure to come.

1.2. A New Age of Mouse Modeling

Transgenic, knockout, knockin, and regulated or conditional mutant mouse models are being extensively used to investigate the roles of individual genes in carcinogenic processes. These approaches can be used to examine complex interactions among cancer genes and the functional roles they play in carcinogenesis. For example, mice carrying mutations in two or more genes known to play protective or causative roles in carcinogenesis can be generated by breeding, and the effect of multiple mutations examined in the context of specific tumor-induction models. This chapter will detail the use of a mouse model which is deficient in a DNA repair pathway known as nucleotide excision repair (NER), and its utility as a model system for investigating the process of chemically induced lung cancer.

1.3. DNA Repair Defective Mice

NER is an important DNA repair process that protects the genome from the persistence of DNA damage that may lead to mutations *(5)*. Humans with hereditary mutations in NER genes develop the skin cancer-prone disease xeroderma pigmentosum (XP). Such individuals are extremely sensitive to sunlight and typically develop skin cancer in sun-exposed areas at a very young age. Predisposition to cancers of internal organs has been documented in XP patients, but most succumb to skin cancer and other developmental and neurological abnormalities before internal tumors have developed. Like human XP patients, mice mutated in XP genes are highly predisposed to UV radiation-induced skin cancer *(6–8)*. To examine the influence of NER-deficiency on the predisposition to chemically-induced tumors of internal organs, *Xpc* mutant mice were treated with 2-acetylaminofluorene (AAF) or N-hydroxy-2-acetyl aminofluorene (N-OH-AAF), well-characterized lung and liver carcinogens *(9)*. From this study it was demonstrated that *Xpc* mutant mice are highly predisposed to chemically induced lung and liver tumors (*see* **Fig. 1** and **Table 1**).

1.4. Xpc Trp53 (p53) *Double Mutant Mice and Induction of Carcinogenesis*

The *p53* gene (*Trp53* in mice) plays a central role in modulating cellular responses to DNA damage. Mutations in the *p53* gene are among the most common mutations identified in human cancers. UVB radiation-induced skin cancer studies in mice have demonstrated that mutations in *Trp53* significantly shorten the latency time and alter the spectrum of skin tumors in *Xpc* mutant mice *(10,11)*. Introduction of a *Trp53* heterozygous mutation into the *Xpc* genetic background resulted in an acceleration of liver tumor progression following treatment with AAF or N-OH-AAF *(9)*. Interestingly, the *Trp53* heterozygous condition seemed to have much less influence on the phenotype of lung tumors induced in *Xpc* mutant mice (*see* **Table 1**). These studies demonstrate that *Xpc* mutant mice can serve as an important model system in which to study carcinogenesis in the lung. A growing list of DNA repair-defective mouse models has been compiled in a series of review articles *(12)* and the interested reader is referred to these. The remainder of this chapter is dedicated to defining the methods and procedures used to induce lung tumors in *Xpc* mutant and *Xpc Trp53* mutant mice. Important considerations in mouse breeding, genotyping, tumor induction, and techniques in collecting tissue samples with which to investigate the molecular pathology of lung cancer is presented (*see* **Note 1**).

2. Materials
2.1. Mouse Breeding and Genotyping

1. *Xpc* mutant mice were generated by us as described below *(8)* (*see* **Note 2**).
2. *Trp53* mutant mice were purchased from The Jackson Induced Mutant Resource, (Bar Harbor, ME).
3. 1.5-mL micro centrifuge tubes.
4. Ear tags, a pair of scissors (large) and a soldering iron.
5. Lysis buffer: 100 mM Tris-HCl pH 8.5, 5 mM EDTA, 0.2% sodium dodecyl sulfate (SDS), 200 mM NaCl, 100 µg/mL Proteinase K.
6. Isopropanol.
7. TE: 10 mM Tris-HCl, pH 8.0, 1 mM EDTA.
8. *Xpc* mutant mice were genotyped by PCR using the following set of PCR primers: mXpc ex10S (mouse *Xpc* exon 10 sense primer), ATTGCGTGCATACCTT GCAC, 10 pmoles/µL in TE. mXpc in 10AS (mouse *Xpc* intron 10 antisense

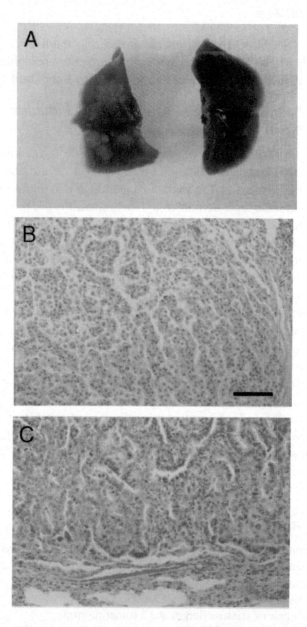

Fig. 1. Pathology of lung tumors in AAF-and N-OH-AAF-treated *XPC Trp53*
mutant mice. (**A**) Gross pathology of lungs from *Xpc$^{-/-}$ Trp53$^{+/+}$* (left) and *Xpc$^{+/-}$
Trp53$^{+/+}$* (right) mice treated with N-OH-AAF. Note the presence of multiple nodules
of varying size in the lung from the *Xpc$^{-/-}$* animal. (**B**) Histology of a low-grade
papillary neoplasm. (**C**) Histology of a papillary adenocarcinoma of the lung exhibiting
increased nuclear hyperchromasia, pleomorphism, nucleolar prominence, and mitotic
activity. Each photomicrograph was prepared at the same magnification and the scale
bar represents 50 micrometers.

Table 1
Incidence of Lung Tumors in *Xpc Trp53* Mutant Mice

Genotype Drug		*Trp53*⁺/⁺			*Trp53*⁺/⁻		
		PM[a]	M[b]	Total	PM	M	Total
Xpc⁺/⁺	AAF	0	1	1/3 33%	0	1	1/7 14%
	N-OH-AAF	1	0	1/9 11%	0	0	0/11 0%
	Total	1/12 8%	1/12 8%	2/12 17%	0/18 0%	1/18 6%	1/18 6%
Xpc⁺/⁻	AAF	0	0	0/14 0%	0	0	0/11 0%
	N-OH-AAF	0	2	2/18 11%	0	0	0/21 0%
	Total	0/32 0%	2/32 6%	2/32 6%	0/32 0%	0/32 0%	0/32 0%
Xpc⁻/⁻	AAF	1	2	3/7 43%	1	3	4/7 57%
	N-OH-AAF	3	3	6/8 75%	2	2	4/5 80%
	Total	4/15 27%	5/15 33%	9/15 60%	3/12 25%	5/12 42%	8/12 67%

[a]PM, pre-malignant (adenoma).
[b]M, malignant (adenocarcinoma).

primer), TATCTCCTCAAACCCTGCTC, 10 pmoles/μL in TE. Neo primer, CGCATCGCCTTCTATCGCCT, 10 pmole/μL in TE.

9. *Trp53* mutant mice are genotyped by polymerase chain reaction (PCR) using the following set of PCR primers as recommended by The Jackson Laboratory: oIMR0336 (*Trp53* exon 7 reverse primer), ATAGGTCGGCGGTTCAT, 10 pmole/μL in TE. oIMR0337 (*Trp53* exon 6 forward primer), CCCGAG TATCTGGAAGACAG, 10 pmoles/μL in TE. oIMR0013 (Neo1 primer) CTT GGGTGGAGAGGCTATTC, 10 pmole/μL in TE. oIMR140014 (Neo2 primer) AGGTGAGATGACAGGAGATC, 10 pmole/μL in TE.

10. PCR tubes and plates (Robbins Scientific, Sunnyvale, CA).

11. Reagents for PCR reactions: 25 mM MgCl$_2$, 2.5 mM dNTPs, PCR reaction buffer, H$_2$O and 5 U/μL Platinum Taq polymerase (Invitrogen, Carlsbad, CA), and a thermocycler.

12. Multichannel pipettor.

13. Sunrise 96 gel electrophoresis unit, power supply, agarose, electrophoresis buffer, 1 kb plus DNA size markers, and 6X gel loading buffer (Invitrogen).

2.2. Chemical Induction of Lung Tumors

1. Chemical carcinogens. 2-acetylaminofluorene (AAF) was purchased from Sigma Chemical Co., (St. Louis, MO). N-hydroxy-2-acetylaminofluorene (N-OH-AAF) was purchased from CCR, Inc., (Chanhassen, MN). Both chemicals (AAF and N-OH-AAF) are highly toxic, mutagenic, and carcinogenic and must be stored, and handled with a high standard of safety (*see* **Note 3**). AAF and N-OH-AAF are insoluble in water and thus are dissolved in dimethyl sulfoxide (DMSO) to a concentration of 100 mg/mL and 50 mg/mL, respectively, and stored in 100 μL aliquots at –70°C.

2. Tricaprylin (also known as trioctanoin) was purchased from Sigma and is a triglyceride used as a vehicle to further dilute the chemicals just prior to each ip injection.

3. Appropriate personal safety equipment: Tyvek suits, double gloves, face masks, and goggles should be worn when administering carcinogens to the mice and when handling treated animals or changing their bedding.

2.3. Preparation of Tumors for Histology and Molecular Studies

1. Surgical and dissection instruments: scissors (small and large), razor blades, and forceps.

2. 10% neutral-buffered formalin, pre-filled specimen jars and biopsy cassettes (Surgipath Medical Industries Inc., Richmond IL).

3. Liquid nitrogen.

4. Cryovials.

3. Methods

The breeding of *Xpc Trp53* double mutant mice is described below and serves as an example of how mice carrying multiple knockout mutations, can be generated and used in a chemical-induced lung tumor protocol. Homozygous mutant *Xpc* mice are first crossed with *Trp53* heterozygous mice (*see* **Note 4**). Progeny are weaned, genotyped, and mice heterozygous for both *Xpc* and *Trp53* are used in subsequent crosses to generate progeny used in chemically induced lung cancer studies. These mice will consist of all nine combinations of normal and mutant *Xpc* and *Trp53* alleles (*see* **Note 5**).

3.1. Mouse Breeding and Genotyping

Mice that are 3–4 wk old are weaned from their mothers, separated into male and female boxes, ear-tagged and processed for genotyping. Genomic DNA is isolated from tail biopsy samples using a simplified protocol *(13)* and used in PCR reactions that discriminate normal alleles from mutant alleles. Critical information such as, date of birth, sex, parents, strain background, and so forth are entered into record books and preferably into a computer database (*see* **Note 6**).

3.1.1. Tail Biopsy

1. Tail biopsies are obtained by cutting approx 1 cm off the tip of the tail with a pair of scissors. Mice are held firmly by the tail such that the mouse is inside a box and the end of its tail is accessible outside of a wire top while cutting the tip of the tail.
2. The end of the tail is cauterized by brief contact with a hot soldering iron just long enough to stop bleeding.
3. The biopsy is transferred to a labeled 1.5-mL microcentrifuge tube and either processed immediately or stored at –20°C for later processing.

3.1.2. Genomic DNA Preparation

1. Add 0.5 mL of lysis buffer to each tail biopsy tube.
2. Place the tubes in a 55°C water bath or incubator for several hours or overnight with agitation (*see* **Note 7**).
3. Following complete lysis, the samples are vortexed and spun in a microcentrifuge for 10 min at 12,000g to pellet the debris.
4. Supernatants are then poured into prelabeled tubes containing 0.5 mL of isopropanol.
5. The tubes are mixed and the DNA precipitate is recovered by lifting the aggregated precipitate from the solution using a disposable pipet tip and transferring it to a new tube containing 0.1 to 0.5 mL of TE depending on the size of the DNA precipitate (*see* **Note 8**).
6. The DNA may require incubation and agitation at 37°C or 55°C to ensure complete dissolution. It is important that the DNA becomes completely dissolved to ensure reproducible results in subsequent steps.

3.1.3. PCR Genotyping of Xpc Mutant Mice

1. Tail DNA is diluted to 200 ng/μL and boiled for 5 minutes. One μL is removed to a PCR tube containing a 5 μL mix of the following primers: 1 μL mXpc ex10S primer (10 pmole/μL), 2.5 μL mXpc in 10AS primer (10 pmole/μL) and 1.5 μL neo primer (10 pmole/μL).
2. A 19 μL aliquot of a PCR reaction mixture containing 11 μL of H_2O, 2 μL of $MgCl_2$ (25 mM stock), 3 μL of dNTPs (2.5 mM stock), 2.5 μL of a 10X PCR buffer and 0.5 μL of Platinum Taq Polymerase (5 U/μL stock). The PCR reaction tubes or plate is placed in the thermocycler and the following PCR profile is run (*see* **Note 9**): 94°C for 3 min, 5 cycles of 94°C for 30 s, 55°C for 30 s and 72°C for 45 s, 5 cycles of 94°C for 30 s, 53°C for 30 s and 72°C for 45 s, 20 cycles of 94°C for 30 s, 51°C for 30 s and 72°C for 45 s, 72°C for 10 min, 8°C hold. After the PCR cycling is complete, add 5 μL of a 6X loading dye and run 12 μL in a 1% agarose gel with 1 kb plus DNA size markers (*see* **Note 10**). The expected band sizes are 250 bp for the normal *Xpc* allele and 350 bp for the mutant *Xpc* allele.

3.1.4. PCR Genotyping of Trp53 Mutant Mice

1. Tail DNA is prepared as in **Subheading 3.1.3.** One µL is removed to a PCR tube containing a 5 µL mix of the following primers: 1 µL oIMR0013 primer (10 pmole/µL), 1 µL oIMR0014 primer (10 pmole/µL), 1.5 µL oIMR0336 primer (10 pmole/µL), and 1.5 µL oIMR337 primer (10 pmole/µL).

2. A 19 µL aliquot of a PCR reaction mixture containing 11 µL of H_2O, 2 µL of $MgCl_2$ (25 mM stock), 3 µL of dNTPs (2.5 mM stock), 2.5 µL of a 10X PCR buffer, and 0.5 µL of Platinum Taq Polymerase (5 units/µL stock). The PCR reaction tubes or plate is placed in the thermocycler and the following PCR profile is run: 94°C for 3 min, 13 cycles of 94°C for 35 s, 64°C (deceasing by 0.5°C per cycle) for 45 s and 72°C for 45 s, 26 cycles of 94°C for 35 s, 58°C for 30 s and 72°C for 45 s, 72°C for 2 min, 10°C hold. After the PCR cycling is complete, add 5 µL of a 6X loading dye and run 12 µL in a 1% agarose gel with 1 kb plus DNA size markers. The expected band sizes are 280 bp for the normal *Trp53* allele and 600 bp for the mutant *Trp53* allele.

3.2. Chemical Induction of Lung Tumors

Crosses are established among *Xpc Trp53* double heterozygous breeders. Pregnant females are noted, provided with nesting materials, observed and cared for daily. The date of birth of each litter is then noted and recorded. The progeny at 1–2 wk of age are given 0.1 cc injections ip of chemical carcinogen.

1. Chemicals are prepared for injection by diluting an appropriate number of 100 µL aliquots of AAF (mol. wt. 223.26 g/mole at 100 mg/mL) or N-OH-AAF (mol. wt. 239.26 g/mole at 50 mg/mL) with 900 µL of tricaprylin. The chemicals are then mixed well by vortexing.

2. Progeny between one and two weeks of age are injected ip with 0.1 cc of freshly prepared chemical (*see* **Note 11**). The average weight of a pup of this age is between 10 g and 20 g and thus, the dose of AAF and N-OH-AAF given to each pup is approx 400 nmole/g body weight and 200 nmole/g body weight, respectively.

3. Animals are weaned from mothers, separated into male and female boxes, ear-tagged and processed for genotyping as described earlier (*see* **Subheading 3.1.**). Critical data is recorded and entered into record books and databases.

4. Animals are observed at least 2 times per week, usually at times of feeding, watering, and bedding changes for signs of illness or disease. Animals can be sacrificed at regular intervals (every 2–3 mo) or longer up to 12–16 mo of observation for analysis of tumors.

3.3. Preparation of Tumors for Histology and Molecular Studies

1. Humanely euthanize animals by terminal CO_2 inhalation or by anesthetization followed by cervical dislocation.

2. The lungs along with other major internal organs are dissected from the animals and examined grossly by eye or with a dissecting microscope for signs of pathology. Lung tumors appear as pearly-white discrete round nodules dispersed throughout both sides of the lung (*see* **Fig. 1**).

3. Lung tissue and other representative tissues are sliced into approx 2–3 mm thick pieces using a razor. Selected tissue slices of lung tumors and other internal organs are placed into biopsy cassettes for histological examination. Several tissue pieces can be placed in each biopsy cassette so that the number of cassettes per mouse can be limited to one or two. Large tumors of approx 3 mm in diameter or greater can be trimmed free of nontumor tissue and frozen in liquid nitrogen. These frozen tumor samples can be stored in cryovials at –70°C for later preparations of DNA, RNA, or protein samples for molecular studies (*see* **ref.** *14*) (*see* **Note 12**).

4. Biopsy cassettes are labeled with pencil and placed into 10% neutral-buffered formalin for at least 24 h (*see* **Note 13**).

5. Routine histological staining of paraffin-embedded tissue should be performed by an established histology laboratory.

6. Microscopic examination of histology slides should be performed with an experienced pathologist. Lung tumors are classified as adenoma or adenocarcinoma based upon their presentation as benign or malignant lesions (*see* **Fig. 1**).

4. Notes

1. Since experiments with mice in general are very time-consuming and expensive to perform, careful planning is important in order to gather the most information possible from each experiment in the most efficient manner.

2. Mice deficient in the *Xpc* gene were generated by targeted gene replacement of a normal allele with a mutant allele using homologous recombination in mouse embryonic stem cells *(8)*. Embryonic stem cells heterozygous for the *Xpc* mutation were microinjected into blastocyst stage embryos to generate chimeric founder mice that passed the mutant *Xpc* allele to their offspring. A similar *Xpc* mutant mouse model is commercially available (Charles River Laboratories, Wilmington, MA). The genotyping method described here would not apply to this mouse. In addition, there are a wide variety of mice deficient in DNA repair pathways and cellular responses to DNA damage have been generated and are summarized in a recent review *(12)*.

3. AAF was being developed as an insecticide by the USDA in the 1940s and was soon shown to be highly carcinogenic. AAF is thus, one of the most extensively studied chemical mutagens and carcinogens. The genetic toxicity of AAF and its metabolites is the subject of a comprehensive review *(15)*.

4. *Xpc* homozygous mutant mice are fertile and can be used for breeding. On the other hand, *p53* homozygous mutant mice typically succumb to spontaneous tumors by 6 mo of age and thus, breeding of *p53* mutant mice should be restricted to heterozygotes.

5. The outcome of any carcinogenesis study in mice can be profoundly influenced by the choice of strain. Ideally, mice used in any study will be of pure genetic background or composed of the same mix of strain backgrounds. The influence of a targeted gene mutation can be examined in the context of any strain background by successive back crossing. Typically 5–10 back crosses (generating mice that are 97–99.9% pure genetic background, respectively) are performed before use in an experiment.

6. Entry of relevant mouse records into a computer database becomes an essential tool when breeding and managing large colonies of mice. Having critical mouse records linked to the experimental results of any given experiment in an extensive relational database is an extremely useful method to analyze the data.

7. Agitation of the tail biopsies is important to obtain complete lysis.

8. If the DNA does not aggregate you can pellet the DNA by spinning in a microcentrifuge for 10 min at 12,000g. Remove the isopropanol completely and dissolve the DNA in a smaller volume of TE.

9. Virtually every component of a PCR reaction including the tubes, reagents, and thermocycler can influence the quality of PCR results. The methods are ones that have been optimized for our lab. Slight modifications and/or optimizations may be required to adapt the protocol for use in another lab. Some critical factors are freshness of reagents such as dNTPs and primers. It is good practice to make single use aliquots of stocks to minimize the number of freeze-thaw cycles of these PCR reagents.

10. If running more than 24 samples it becomes useful to use PCR plates, a multichannel pipet and a Sunrise 96 gel electrophoresis unit. There are a large number of web sites containing useful information about working with mice. Two such recommended sites are: The Whole Mouse Catalog (www.rodentia.com/wmc) and The Jackson Laboratories (www.jax.org).

11. AAF and N-OH-AAF are highly insoluble and after dilution in tricaprylin they may come out of solution. A brief emersion in a 37°C water bath and vortex mixing will re-solubilize them.

12. Tumor tissue should be prepared and frozen as quickly as possible in order to preserve the molecular integrity of the samples. This is not so critical for DNA isolation but is especially true for RNA and protein isolation.

13. Be sure to label the biopsy cassettes with pencil since most lab markers will dissolve in the formalin fixative. Formalin fixation is suitable for most applications such as routine histological staining or immunohistochemistry, however, different fixation procedures may be required for more specialized applications.

References

1. Paterson, A. B. (ed.) (1998) *Molecular Dissection of Complex Traits*. CRC Press, Boca Raton, FL.
2. Pataer, A., Nishimura, M., Kamoto, T., Ichioka, K., Sato, M., and Hiai, H. (1998) Genetic resistance to urethane-induced pulmonary adenomas in SMXA recombinant inbred mouse strains. *Cancer Res.* **57**, 2904–2908.

3. Stoner, G. D., Adam-Rodwell, G., and Morse, M. A. (1993) Lung tumors in strain A mice: application for studies in cancer chemoprevention. *J. Cell Biochem. Suppl.* **17F**, 95–103.
4. Malkinson, A. (1999) Inheritance of pulmonary adenoma susceptibility in mice. *Prog. Exp. Tumor Res.* **35**, 78–94.
5. Friedberg, E. C., Walker, G. C., and Siede, W. (eds.) (1995) *DNA Repair and Mutagenesis.* American Society for Microbiology, Washington, DC.
6. Sands, A. T., Abuin, A., Sanchez, A., Conti, J. C., and Bradley, A. (1995) High susceptibility to ultraviolet-induced carcinogenesis in mice lacking XPC. *Nature* **377**, 162–165.
7. Nakane, H., Takeuchi, S., Yuba, S., Saijo, M., Nakatsu, Y., Murai, H., et al. (1995) High incidence of ultraviolet-B or chemical-carcinogen-induced skin tumours in mice lacking the xeroderma pigmentosum group A gene. *Nature* **377**, 169–173.
8. Cheo, D. L., Ruven, H. J. T., Meira, L. B., Hammer, R. E., Burns, D. K., Tappe, N. J., et al. (1997) Characterization of defective nucleotide excision repair in *Xpc* mutant mice. *Mutation Res.* **374**, 1–9.
9. Cheo, D. L., Burns, D. K., Meira, L. B., Houle, J. F., and Friedberg, E. C. (1999) Mutational inactivation of the xeroderma pigmentosum group C gene confers predisposition to 2-acetylaminofluorene-induced liver and lung cancer and to spontaneous testicular cancer in *Trp53*$^{-/-}$ mice. *Cancer Res.* **59**, 771–775.
10. Meira, L. B., Cheo, D. L., Hammer, R. E., Burns, D. K., Reis, A. M. and Friedberg, E. C. (1997) Genetic interaction between HAP1/REF-1 and p53. *Nature Genet.* **17**, 145.
11. Cheo, D. L., Meira, L. B., Burns, D. K., Reis, A. M., Issac, T., and Friedberg, E.C. (2000) Ultraviolet B radiation-induced skin cancer in mice defective in the *Xpc*, *Trp53*, and *Apex* (*Hap1*) genes: genotype-specific effects on cancer predisposition and pathology of tumors. *Cancer Res.* **60**, 1580–1584.
12. Meira, L. B. and Friedberg, E. C. (2000) Database of mouse strains carrying targeted mutations in genes affecting cellular responses to DNA damage. Version 4. *Mutation Res.* **459**, 243–274.
13. Laird, P. W., Zijderveld, A. Linders, K. Rudnicki, M. A., Jaenisch, R., and Berns, A. (1991) Simplified mammalian DNA isolation procedure. *Nucleic Acids Res.* **19**, 4293.
14. Reis, A. M., Cheo, D. L., Meira, L. B., Greenblatt, M. S., Bond, J. F., Nahari, D., and Friedberg, E. C. (2000) Genotype-specific *Trp53* mutational analysis in utraviolet B radiation-induced skin cancers in *Xpc* and *XpcTrp53* mutant mice. *Cancer Res.* **60**, 1571–1579.
15. Heflich, R. H. and Neft, R. E. (1994) Genetic toxicity of 2-acetlyaminofluorene, 2-aminofluorene and some of their metabolites and model metabolites. *Mutation Res.* **318**, 73–174.

IV

LUNG CANCER MODEL SYSTEMS

B. ANIMAL MODELS FOR TUMOR METASTASES TO THE LUNG

35

Nude Mouse Lung Metastases Models of Osteosarcoma and Ewing's Sarcoma for Evaluating New Therapeutic Strategies

Shu-Fang Jia, Rong-Rong Zhou, and Eugenie S. Kleinerman

1. Introduction

Osteosarcoma *(1,2)* and Ewing's sarcoma *(3,4)* are the two most common primary bone tumors in children. The 2-yr metastasis-free survival rate is 60–65% *(5–9)* and 41% *(10)* in patients having osteosarcoma and Ewing's sarcoma, respectively. These rates have not changed over the past 15 years despite numerous alterations in chemotherapy for these tumors *(7–9)*. The most common site of metastatic spread of both of these tumors is the lung. Additionally, salvage chemotherapy regimens have shown only limited efficacy against them *(11–13)*. Therefore, new treatment strategies are needed to control or prevent lung metastasis and improve the long-term survival rate.

The use of animal models that closely mimic clinical situations can be valuable in identifying potential new therapeutic agents. The ideal in vivo model for studying the biology of tumors and the metastatic process must allow for the interaction of tumor cells with the relevant organ environment. Transplantation of human tumors into immunodeficient athymic nude mice is one approach to studying both biology of and therapy for various human tumors *(14,15)*. Therefore, we developed both an osteosarcoma *(16)* and Ewing's sarcoma nude mouse lung metastasis model using intravenous injection or orthotopic implantation of tumor cells. Lung metastases developed several weeks after tumor inoculation in these models. These models allow for the evaluation of novel anti-tumor agents against established tumors in the relevant metastatic organ environment, i.e., the lung.

From: *Methods in Molecular Medicine, vol. 74: Lung Cancer, Vol. 1: Molecular Pathology Methods and Reviews*
Edited by: B. Driscoll © Humana Press Inc., Totowa, NJ

2. Materials

2.1. Osteosarcoma Lung Metastasis Model

1. Eagle's minimal essential medium (1X EMEM; and 2X EMEM) and Hanks' balanced salt solution (HBSS) without Ca^{2+} or Mg^{2+} purchased from Bio Whittaker Inc. (Walkersville, MD) and stored at room temperature (*see* **Note 1**).
2. Nonessential amino acids (NEAA; 100X) and sodium pyruvate (SP; 100 m*M*) purchased from Bio Whittaker Inc. and stored at 2–8°C.
3. MEM vitamins (100X) and L-glutamine (200 m*M*) purchased from Bio Whittaker Inc. and stored at –20°C.
4. Fetal bovine serum (FBS) purchased from Atlanta Biological (Norcross, GA) and stored at –20°C.
5. Trypsin (2.5%; 10X) purchased from GIBCO BRL (Grand Island, NY) and stored at –20°C.
6. Ethylenediamine tetraacetate (EDTA) purchased from Fisher scientific (Pittsburgh, PA) and stored at room temperature.
7. Agarose purchased from Sigma Chemical Co. (St. Louis, MO) and stored at room temperature.
8. Trypan blue solution (0.4%) purchased from Sigma Chemical Co. and stored at room temperature.
9. Hemacytometer (Fisher Scientific).
10. Dimethyl sulfoxide (DMSO) purchased from Sigma Chemical Co. and stored at room temperature.
11. Cell freezing medium: Mix 8.2 mL 10% FBS EMEM, 1 mL of FBS, and 0.8 mL of DMSO, then filter using a 0.2-μm syringe filter disc (Fisher Scientific).
12. Cryogenic vials (Corning Inc. Life Sciences).
13. 35-mm tissue culture dishes (Corning Glass Works, Corning, NY).
14. Type I collagenase purchased from Sigma Chemical Co. and stored at –20°C.
15. DNase purchased from Sigma Chemical Co. and stored at –20°C.
16. Gentamicin (50 mg/mL) purchased from Sigma Chemical Co. and stored at 2–8°C.
17. Cell line SAOS-2 human osteosarcoma cell line, purchased from the American Type Culture Collection (Rockville, MD). Cells were free of mycoplasma contamination and were also verified free of the following pathogenic murine viruses: reovirus type 3, pneumonia virus, K virus, Theiler's virus, Sendai virus, minute virus, mouse adenovirus, mouse hepatitis virus, lymphocytic choriomeningitis virus, ectromelia virus, and lactate dehydrogenase virus (assayed by Microbiological Associates, Inc., Rockville, MD) (*see* **Note 2**). Cell-maintenance medium is changed weekly, and when cells are 80 ± 5% confluent, they are split by trypsinization.
18. SAOS-2 cell maintenance medium: antibiotic-free 1X EMEM supplemented with 1X NEAA, 1 m*M* L-glutamine, 2X vitamins, and 10% heat-inactivated (56°C for 30 min) FBS.

19. Cells are maintained in 75-cm² tissue-culture flasks (Costar, Cambridge, MA) at 37°C in a humidified 5% CO_2 incubator.
20. Athymic nude mice, (T-cell-deficient) used at 4–5-wk-old and specified pathogen-free, purchased from Charles River Laboratories (Wilmington, MA) (*see* **Note 3**).
21. Belly Dancer shaker (Stovall Life Science Inc., Greensboro, NC).
22. Sterile gauze.

2.2. Ewing's Sarcoma Lung Metastasis Model

1. EMEM (stored at 15–30°C). Medium, HBSS, and supplements purchased from Bio Whittaker Inc.
2. HBSS without Ca^{2+} or Mg^{2+} (stored at 15–30°C).
3. Nonessential amino acids (NEAA) 100X, stored at 2–8°C.
4. Sodium pyruvate (SP) 100 m*M*, stored at 2–8°C.
5. 100X MEM vitamins stored at –5–20°C.
6. 200 m*M* L-glutamine (stored at –10–20°C).
7. Trypsin (2.5%, stored at –5–20°C) purchased from GIBCO-BRL.
8. FBS (stored at –20°C) purchased from Atlanta Biological.
9. DMSO purchased from Sigma Chemical Co.
10. Trypan blue solution (0.4%; stored at room temperature) purchased from Sigma Chemical.
13. Cell line TC71 human Ewing's sarcoma cells were kindly provided by Dr. P. Pepe (University of Southern California, Los Angeles, CA) (*see* **Notes 1** and **2**).
14. Cell maintenance medium: EMEM supplemented with 10% heat-inactivated (56°C for 30 min) FBS, 1 m*M* SP, 2X MEM vitamins, 1X NEAA, and 2 m*M* L-glutamine. Cells are subcultured twice weekly after detachment by 0.25% trypsin in 0.02% EDTA. The cell lines used in the in vivo experiments are from the third to tenth passages.
15. Cells maintained at 37°C in a humidified 5% CO_2 incubator.
16. Athymic male nude mice, purchased from Charles River Laboratories (*see* **Note 3**).
17. 70% EtOH.
18. 1-mL disposable syringes fitted with 30-gauge needles.
19. Pentobarbital, 5 mg/mL.
20. Iodine.
21. 1-mL disposable syringes fitted with 27-gauge needles (MPL, Chicago, IL).

3. Methods

3.1. Osteosarcoma Lung Metastasis Model

3.1.1. Reagent Preparation

1. Aliquot reagents. Thaw stock reagents in a 37°C water bath and then aliquot as follows: L-glutamine at 5 mL per tube, MEM vitamins at 10 mL per tube,

trypsin at 10 mL per tube (stored at –20°C), NEAA at 5 mL per tube, and SP at 5 mL per tube (stored at 2–8°C).

2. Heat-inactivate FBS in a 56°C water bath for 30 min and then aliquot at 25 or 50 mL per tube and stored at –20°C. All of these reagents are stable up to the expiration date.

3. Prepare a 0.02% (w/v) EDTA solution in phosphate-buffered saline, aliquot at 90 mL per bottle, autoclave at 121°C for 20 min, then store at 4°C for up to 1 yr.

4. Make a 2X solution of type I collagenase (400 U/mL) and DNase (540 U/mL) in unsupplemented, serum-free EMEM. This preparation is then aliquotted at 5–10 mL per tube and stored at –20°C for no longer than up to the expiration date.

5. Dilute trypan blue to 1:10 with HBSS or PBS and stored at room temperature for up to 2 yr.

6. Prepare 4.5% (w/v) and 3% (w/v) agarose. Dissolve agarose in distilled water, autoclave at 121°C for 20 min, and store at 2–8°C for up to 1 yr.

7. Prepare supplemented 10% FBS and 2X supplemented EMEM. Thaw aliquoted NEAA, SP, L-glutamine, MEM vitamins, heat-inactivated FBS, and 1X or 2X EMEM and warm in a 37°C water bath. Combine 50 milliliters of filtered heat-inactivated FBS, 5 mL of NEAA, 5 mL of SP, 5 mL of L-glutamine, and 10 mL of MEM vitamins, then filter using a 115-mL 0.22-μm filter system (Corning Inc., Life Sciences, Acton, MA). Add 500 mL 1X EMEM. Combine filtered 2X EMEM with filtered NEAA, SP, L-glutamine, and EMEM vitamins. These preparations can be stored at 2–8°C for up to 2 yr.

8. Prepare 0.25% trypsin in 0.02% EDTA. Thaw aliquoted 2.5% trypsin (w/v) and 0.02% EDTA (w/v) and warmed in a 37°C water bath. Combine 10 mL trypsin and 90 mL of EDTA, then filter using a 0.22-μm filter system. Stored at 2–8°C for up to 1 mo.

3.1.2. Thawing Frozen Cells

1. To obtain the maximum number of viable cells, they must be thawed quickly. A vial of cells should be removed from dry ice (packaging material) or liquid nitrogen and immediately placed in a 37°C water bath (*see* **Note 4**).

2. As soon as cells are thawed, the vial should be removed from the water bath and wiped with a WEBCOL towelette (alcohol prep; Kendall Co., Mansfield, MA).

3. Place thawed cells into a 14-mL tube containing 10 mL HBSS (37°C) and centrifuge at 259*g* for 10 min to wash out DMSO.

4. Resuspend cell pellet in 5 or 10 mL warmed EMEM containing 10% FBS and supplements. Maintain monolayer cell culture in T25 or T75 tissue-culture flasks (Costar) at 37°C in a humidified 5% CO_2 incubator. Change medium within 24 h of thawing.

3.1.3. Cell Maintenance

It is necessary to store aliquotted cells in liquid nitrogen for later use (*see* **Note 5**). All these procedures should be done in a laminar flow hood under sterile conditions.

1. Warm media in a 37°C water bath. The outside of the bottles should be sprayed with 70% alcohol and wiped dry.
2. When cells that are in the exponential growth phase and 80 ± 5% confluent they can be harvested by trypsinization. Briefly, remove medium from flasks, wash with 5 mL of HBSS. Next, add 2–3 mL 0.25% trypsin/0.02% EDTA and incubate 1.0–1.5 min at 37°C to allow the cells to loosen (cells appear round and bright under the microscope). Pour off as much trypsin/EDTA as possible, and shake flask (*see* **Note 6**). Resuspend cells in supplemented 10% FBS EMEM and pipet up and down to produce a single-cell suspension.
3. Because viable cells exclude trypan blue, it can be used to distinguish between viable and nonviable cells. Briefly, dilute the cell suspension at 1 : 10 in trypan blue (100-μL cell suspension; 900 μL of diluted trypan blue). Load 10 μL cell suspension into the chamber side of a hemacytometer, count cells, and calculate total cell number and % viability (*see* **Note 7**).

3.1.4. Cell Storage

1. Following trypsinization, pellet cell suspension at 259g for 10 min at 4°C.
2. Suspend pelleted cells in supplemented 20% FBS EMEM containing 0.8% DMSO (freezing medium, kept on ice) to a concentration of 1–2 × 10^6 cells/mL. Aliquot into cryogenic vials at 1 mL of cell suspension having greater than 80% cell viability per vial.
3. Place vials in a –20°C freezer for 24 h, –70°C freezer for 24 h, and then store in liquid nitrogen. To confirm product integrity, one vial of cells is thawed from the liquid nitrogen the next day to determine viability and growth properties and to confirm that cells are free of contamination.

3.1.5. Establishing Osteosarcoma Lung Metastases

All of the following procedures should be performed in a laminar flow hood under sterile conditions to prevent contamination. Note that SAOS-2 human osteosarcoma cells do not grow in nude mice when injected subcutaneously, intraosseously, or intravenously *(16,17)*. We developed SAOS-LM1 cells from a rare lung metastasis in nude mice that appeared 6 mo after intravenous injection with SAOS-2 cells collected from a 0.9% agarose gel. These SAOS-LM1 tumor cells were recycled in nude mice to establish the SAOS-LM2, -LM3, -LM4, -LM5, and -LM6 cell lines.

3.1.5.1. GROWTH OF SAOS-2 CELLS IN SEMISOLID AGAROSE *(17,18)*

1. Set base layer in 35-mm tissue-culture dishes with 1 mL 0.6% agarose (w/v) containing supplemented 10% FBS EMEM. Melt 3% agarose in a microwave for 90 s (high setting) and keep all reagents in a 39°C water bath. Mix 1 mL 3% agarose, 2.5 mL of 2X supplemented EMEM (no serum), 0.5 mL of FBS, and 1 mL of 1X EMEM. Keep this mixture in the 39°C water bath.

2. Set top layer with 1 mL 0.9% agarose containing supplemented 10% FBS EMEM and an SAOS-2 single-cell suspension (1000 cells).
3. After the top agarose layer containing the cells has solidified, add 1–2 mL of medium supplemented with 20% FBS.
4. Place the 35-mm dishes inside a 150-mm dish. One empty 35-mm dish inside the 150-mm dish should contain a sterile cotton ball moistened with autoclaved water. Cover the 150-mm dish, and incubate cultures at 37°C in a humidified 5% CO_2 incubator.
5. Check cultures during the growth phase, and add water if the cotton dries up. Add 0.1–0.2 mL of EMEM supplemented with 20% FBS to the cultures every 5 d or whenever needed.
6. After 30 d, collect colonies.

3.1.5.2. ESTABLISHING SAOS-LM–VARIANT CELL LINES

1. Collect SAOS-2 colonies from hard agarose, trypsinize with trypsin/EDTA, and resuspend in supplemented 10% FBS EMEM at a concentration of 1.0–1.5×10^6 cells/mL. Pipet up and down to produce a single-cell suspension (*see* **Note 8**).
2. Wash cells, pellet at $259g$ for 10 min at 4°C, then resuspend in Ca^{2+}- and Mg^{2+}-free HBSS (4°C) at 5×10^6 cells/mL. Verify viability by trypan blue exclusion staining.
3. Keep the SAOS-2 single-cell suspension, having greater than 90% viability, on the ice. In a laminar hood under sterile conditions, inject cells (10^6 cells/0.2 mL) intravenously into nude mice via the lateral tail vein.
4. Monitor mice daily for evidence of morbidity related to lung metastasis (*see* **Note 9**). Sacrifice moribund animals and examined for lung metastases.
5. Sacrifice surviving mice under sterile conditions 6 mo after inoculation. Remove lungs, isolate metastases, and placed in 10 mL of HBSS containing gentamicin (5 mg/100 mL) at 4°C.
6. Dissect each SAOS-LM1 lung metastasis nodule free of necrotic tissue, connective tissue, and blood clots. Rinse three times with HBSS containing gentamicin and chop into 1-mm cubes using sterile scalpel blades in a 100-mm dish.
7. Transfer chopped fragments to a 15-mL centrifuge tube and enzymatically digeste with type I collagenase (200 U/mL) and DNase (270 U/mL) in a Belly Dancer shaker at 37°C for 45 min.
8. Following enzymatic dissociation, filter cell suspension through four layers of sterile gauze and wash three times with supplemented 5% FBS EMEM containing gentamicin.
9. Resuspend cells in supplemented EMEM containing gentamicin and 10% FBS and maintain in T75 tissue-culture flasks at 37°C in a humidified 5% CO_2 incubator. Replace medium on the following day.
10. Grow SAOS-LM1 cells in culture for 4–6 wk.
11. Harvest cells and re-injected into nude mice as described above to develop an SAOS-LM2 cell line. Repeat this process four more times to establish SAOS-LM3, -LM4, -LM5, and -LM6 cell lines (*see* **Note 10**).

3.2. Ewing's Sarcoma Lung Metastasis Model

All procedures should be performed using sterile technique in a laminar flow hood.

3.2.1. Medium Preparation

All medium preparations should be performed in a sterile laminar flow hood.

1. Warm 500 mL EMEM, 5 mL of NEAA, 5 mL of SP, 5 mL of L-glutamine, 10 mL of vitamins, and 50 mL of FBS in a 37°C water bath. Filter supplements using a 0.2-μm filter system and add to 500 mL EMEM to obtain 10% FBS EMEM.
2. Thaw, warm, and filter 10 mL FBS. Filter 0.8 mL DMSO using a 0.2-μm syringe filter disc, add to 8.2 mL of 10% FBS EMEM to obtain 10 mL, and keep on ice.

3.2.2. Thawing Frozen TC71 Ewing's Sarcoma Cells and Standard Maintenance

1. Remove the microtube containing 3×10^6 cells/mL from liquid nitrogen and place in a 37°C water bath.
2. Remove thawed cells from tube and place into 75-cm cell culture flasks containing 10 mL warmed supplemented EMEM. Maintain cells at 37°C in a humidified 5% CO_2 incubator. Change medium after 24 h. When the cells grow to 80–90% confluency, trypsinize, and subculture.

3.2.3. Establishing Ewing's Sarcoma Lung Metastases

1. Harvest TC71 cells (third through tenth passages) in the mid-log growth phase by trypsinization using 0.25% trypsin/0.02% EDTA (wt/vol) (*see* **Note 11**).
2. Suspend cells in supplemented EMEM and pipetted so as to produce a single-cell suspension (*see* **Note 12**).
3. Centrifuge cells at 720*g* for 5 min at 4°C, resuspend in Ca^{2+}- and Mg^{2+}-free HBSS, and bring to a final concentration of 1.25×10^7 cells/mL (for intravenous implantation) or 10^7 cells/mL (for intratibial implantation). A single-cell suspension having greater than 90% viability (assessed using 0.04% trypan blue staining) is kept on ice (0–2 h) until ready for use.

3.2.4. Intravenous Implantation of TC71 Ewing's Sarcoma Cells

1. Clean mouse tails with 70% ethanol in water. Before the cell suspension is aspirated, vortex the microtube containing the cells. Aspirate the TC71 cells into a 1-mL disposable syringe fitted with a 30-gauge needle (*see* **Note 13**).
2. Insert the needle into the lateral tail vein of nude mice, and push plunger on syringe gently. No pressure should be felt when pushing the syringe, indicating that the needle is in the vein. Inject 200 μL per animal. Keep the needle in the

lateral vein for a few seconds to avoid cell escape, then remove from the vein. The syringe containing the remaining cell suspension is returned to the ice bath until the next animal is given an injection.

3. Following the injection, cover the needle hole with a 70% ethanol soaked cotton ball for a few seconds to prevent bleeding. Return the mouse to its cage and maintain under specific pathogen-free conditions.

4. Repeat the tail-vein injection weekly for 3 wk. Lung metastases should occur 7–8 wk after the first inoculation.

3.2.5. Intratibial (Orthotopic) Implantation of TC71 Cells

1. Anesthetize mice (see **Note 14**) using an intraperitoneal injection of pentobarbital (5 mg/mL; 10 µL/g body weight).

2. Clean the animal's left rear leg with iodine and 70% ethanol.

3. Aspirate the TC71 cell suspension into a 1-mL disposable syringe fitted with a 27-gauge needle.

4. Insert the tip of the needle through the cortex of the anterior tuberosity of the tibia using a gentle rotating "drill-like" movement in a direction parallel with the longitudinal axis of the tibia and at a 15–20° angle to the cortex. Once the bone cortex is traversed, insert the needle 1–3 mm down the diaphysis of the tibia. Inject 10 µL single-cell suspension (containing 10^5 cells).

5. Hold the needle in the tibia for a few seconds to prevent cells from escaping the needle hole. Remove the needle from the bone. The syringe containing the remaining cell suspension is returned to the ice bath until the next animal is given an injection.

6. After the injection, use a cotton swab saturated with 70% ethanol to sterilize the injection hole. Return the mouse to its cage and keep in a laminar flow cabinet.

7. X-ray the tibia 2–3 wk later to assess tumor growth.

8. When a tumor is detected in the tibia, sacrifice amputate the affected leg. Leg amputation is necessary; otherwise, the tumor will grow too large, ending the investigation. Lung metastasis should be evident 12–14 wk after the bone inoculation.

4. Notes

1. All reagents should be free of endotoxins as determined using the limulus amebocyte lysate assay (sensitivity limit, 0.025 mg/mL), which can be purchased from Sigma Chemical Co. All of these solutions should be prepared in a tissue-culture hood under sterile conditions to prevent contamination.

2. It is very important to prevent mice from becoming infected with pathogenic murine viruses or mycoplasma as it may interfere with the results of experiment. Cells are therefore established as free of mycoplasma contamination, and screened using the Gen-Probe mycoplasma screening assay (Gen-Probe, San Diego, CA).

3. Mice should be maintained in an animal facility approved by the American Association for Accreditation of Laboratory Animal Care and in accordance with the current regulations and standards of the U. S. Department of Agriculture, the Department of Health and Human Services, and the National Institutes of Health. Mice are housed five to a cage, and the cages are changed twice weekly. Cages, food, and water are sterilized in an autoclave. Mice should be kept in a laminar flow cabinet under specific pathogen-free conditions at 24 ± 1°C, and lit for 12 h each day. Animals should be housed for 1–2 wk before any experiments are initiated.

4. To decrease the chance of contamination, the cap of the vial of cells should not be immersed in the water bath. The vial should be gently agitated to allow uniform thawing.

5. Cells can be used for 12 and 8 wk from thawing for in vitro and in vivo experiments, respectively.

6. If trypsinization occurs for more than 2 min, the cells will completely detach. Do not remove trypsin/EDTA or cells will be lost. Instead, add medium to wash out the trypsin and spin the cells at 259g for 10 min. Resuspend the cell pellet with medium. Conversely, if cells are not loosened using this trypsinization procedure, put the flasks in an incubator at 37°C for an additional 1–2 min.

7. The volume of one large square of the hemacytometer chamber is 0.1 mm^3. The cell concentration is calculated using the following formula: number of cells/number of large squares × 10^5 cells/mL. For example, if the cell number in nine large squares is 90, then the cell concentration is 90/9 × 10^5 cells/mL. Also, cell viability is calculated using the following formula: $(A - B)/A \times 100\%$, in which A is the total cell number and B is the number of cells stained blue (dyed cells).

8. It is important to make a single-cell suspension. If a single-cell suspension cannot be made using a pipet, a syringe and 20-gauge needle shaken up and down three times may be used.

9. Moribundity evidenced by, weight loss, roughened fur, immobility, diarrhea, dyspnea, and cachexia.

10. In a previous study, the growth rate of SAOS-LM6 cells was fastest both in vitro and in vivo when compared with that of parental SAOS-2 cells and SAOS-LM2 cells *(16)*. The doubling time was 34.9 ± 1.4 vs 43.6 ± 4.2 h for SAOS-LM6 and parental SAOS-2 cells, respectively. Also, lung metastases developed 17 vs 12 wk following intravenous injection of the SAOS-LM1 and SAOS-LM5 cells, respectively. Microscopic lung metastases were present 6 wk after the injection of SAOS-LM6 cells, with visible metastases observed approx 8 wk after the injection. This recycling procedure allowed us to develop a mouse model of experimental osteosarcoma lung metastasis in which to evaluate therapeutic approaches. Specifically, the SAOS-LM6 cells are used to establish lung metastases. Therapeutic strategies are initiated 6–14 wk after intravenous injection of the cells to assess the activity against microscopic and macroscopic disease.

11. Because the TC71 Ewing's sarcoma cells are very easy to detach, trypsinization should take only 30–40 s.
12. A "single-cell" suspension must be used for injection. Otherwise, intravenous injection may result in death due to a pulmonary tumor embolis.
13. Take care that there is no air in the syringe to avoid injecting it into the vein.
14. Note that for this procedure, mice should be 4 wk old.

References

1. Mertens, W. C. and Bramwell, V. (1994) Osteosarcoma and other tumors of bone. *Curr. Opin. Oncol.* **6,** 384–390.
2. Zunino, J. H. and Johnston, J. (1998) Early results of lower limb surgery for osteogenic sarcoma of bone. *Orthopedics* **21,** 47–50.
3. Horocoitz, M. E., Malauzer, M. M., Woo, S. Y., and Hicks, M. J. (1997) Ewing's sarcoma family of tumors: Ewing's sarcoma of bone and soft tissue and the peripheral neuroectodermal tumors, in *Principles and Practice of Pediatric Oncology* (Pizzo, P. A. and Popladk, D. E., eds.), J.B. Lippincott, Co., Philadelphia, PA, pp. 831–863.
4. Landuzzi, L., De Giovanni, C., Nicoletti, G., Rossi, I., and Lollini, P-L. (2000) The metastatic ability of Ewing's sarcoma cells is modulated by stem cell factor and by its receptor C-kit. *Am. J. Pathol.* **157,** 2123–2131.
5. Ajiki, W., Hanai, A., Tsukuma, H., Hiyama, T., and Fujimoto, I. (1995) Survival rates of childhood cancer patients in Osaka, Japan, 1975–1984. *Jpn. J. Cancer Res.* **86,** 13–20.
6. Picci, P. (1992) Osteosarcoma and other cancers of bone. *Curr. Opin. Oncol.* **4,** 674–680.
7. Eiber, F., Giuliano, A. Eckardt, J., Patterson, K., Moseley, S., and Goodnight, J. (1987) Adjuvant chemotherapy for osteosarcoma: a randomized prospective trial. *J. Clin. Oncol.* **5,** 21–26.
8. Jaffe, N. (1986) Experimental and clinical progress in cancer chemotherapy, in *Advances and Controversies* (Muggia, F. M., ed.), Martinus Nijhoff Publishers, Boston, MA, pp. 223–233.
9. Link, M. P., Goorin, A. M., Miser, A. W., Green, A. A., Pratt, C. B., Belasco, J. B., et al. (1986) The effect of adjuvant chemotherapy on relapse-free survival in patients with osteosarcoma of the extremity. *N. Engl. J. Med.* **314,** 1600–1606.
10. Dorfman, H. D. and Czernick, B. (1994) Bone cancers. *Cancer* **75,** 203–210.
11. Skinner, K. S., Eilber, F. R., Holmes, C., Eckardt, J., and Rosen, G. (1992) Surgical treatment and chemotherapy for pulmonary metastases from osteosarcoma. *Arch. Surg.* **127,** 1065–1071.
12. Goorin, A. M., Shuster, J. J., Baker, A., Horowitz, M. E., Meyer, W. H., and Link, M. P. (1991) Changing pattern of pulmonary metastases with adjuvant chemotherapy in patients with osteosarcoma: results from a multi-institutional osteosarcoma study. *J. Clin. Oncol.* **9,** 600–605.
13. Putnam, J. B., Roth, J. A., and Wesly, M. N. (1986) Survival following aggressive resection of pulmonary metastases from osteogenic sarcoma. Analysis of prognostic factors. *Ann. Thorac. Surg.* **36,** 516–523.

14. Kjonmiksen, I., Winderens, M., Bruland, O., and Fodstas, O. (1994) Validity and usefulness of human tumor models established by intratibial cell inoculation in nude rats. *Cancer Res.* **54,** 1715–1719.

15. Manzotti, C., Audisio, R. A., and Pratesi, G. (1993) Importance of orthotopic implantation for human tumors as model system relevance to metastasis and invasion. *Clin. Exp. Metastasis* **11,** 5–14.

16. Jia, S.-F., Worth, L. L., and Kleinerman, E. S. (1999) A nude mouse model of human osteosarcoma lung metastases for evaluating new therapeutic strategies. *Clin. Exp. Metast.* **17,** 501–506.

17. Radinsky, R., Fidler, I. J., Price, J. E., Esumi, N., Tsan, R., Petty, C. M., et al. (1994) Terminal differentiation and apoptosis in experimental lung metastases of human osteogenic sarcoma cells by wild type p53. *Oncogene* **9,** 1877–1883.

18. Li, L., Price, J. E., Fan, D., Zhang, R.-D., Bucana, C. D., and Fidler, I. J. (1989) Correlation of growth capacity of human tumor cells in hard agarose with their *in vivo* proliferative capacity at specific metastatic sites. *J. Natl. Cancer Inst.* **81,** 1406–1412.

36

Tumor-Specific Metastasis to Lung Using Reporter Gene-Tagged Tumor Cells

Lloyd A. Culp, Wen-Chang Lin, Nanette Kleinman, Julianne L. Holleran, and Carson J. Miller

1. Introduction

1.1. Overview of Metastasis to Lung

The lung offers circulating tumor cells—after their initial development as primary tumors and their selection for metastasis to other organs of patients—several optimal conditions for survival and progression that may be unique to this organ. First, the lung is highly oxygenated and provides maximal oxygen tension required for the aggressive metabolism that occurs in most tumor cell populations. Second, the lung offers a vast array of small blood vessels that are required for oxygen: CO_2 exchange and for nutrient:catabolite exchange; this microvasculature serves the very active metabolic requirements of tumor cells very effectively. Third, the lung is the first or second organ encountered by tumor cells when they are "liberated" from primary tumors. Fourth, the endothelial/intimal linings of the small blood vessels of the lung may offer adhesion and/or migration sites for tumor cells that are more facile than blood vessels in many other organs. In these regards, a contrast is provided by micrometastases that develop in the lung vs those in bone where oxygen/nutrient/blood vessel availabilities are much more limited. For these and many other reasons, metastasis to the lung may be a more efficient process than metastasis to other organs.

However, these efficiencies have been difficult to quantitate in experimental model systems and in human patients for a variety of reasons. Experimental systems are usually based on ectopic injection of tumor cells into animals. Ectopic tumors do not necessarily reflect the efficiencies of metastasis to

From: *Methods in Molecular Medicine, vol. 74: Lung Cancer, Vol. 1: Molecular Pathology Methods and Reviews*
Edited by: B. Driscoll © Humana Press Inc., Totowa, NJ

multiple organs when compared with orthotopic injections (1–3). This is not surprising because most human carcinomas develop in their "native" epithelial beds and are quite foreign in the subcutis, the dermis, or intraperitoneal sites of animals. Efficiencies of metastasis based on tail vein injections (the experimental metastasis model [4,5]) provide some limited information but must be considered in light of obviating several demanding steps during selection of variants in the primary tumor and their subsequent intravasation.

1.2. Primary Tumors of the Lung vs Metastasis to the Lung

It is particularly surprising that investigators have yet to compare the cell division/outgrowth properties of carcinomas developing in the epithelium of the lung with metastases of other tumor classes, not originating in the lung, when they become established in this organ. Such a comparison has been made recently by Li et al. (6) comparing glioblastomas developing in the brain with metastases of other tumor classes that become established in the brain. They observed that glioblastomas, while highly invasive in brain architecture, do not metastasize outside the brain and only express the standard isoform of CD44 (CD44s); in contrast, tumors from other organs that metastasize to the brain express CD44variant isoforms when identified in brain tissue.

From such a comparison we might learn a great deal about the growth-enhancing and/or growth-retarding environmental cues that apply to both lung-based carcinomas and metastases of other carcinomas and other tumor classes once ensconced in the lung. (Some of these requirements for primary tumors developing in the lung are described in many other chapters of this volume and will not be reviewed here.) Do both tumor classes require similar growth factors or chemokines for cell division (3,7)? Do they grow in similar patterns close to or distant from small blood vessels indicating "chemoattraction" for higher oxygen tensions or growth retardation by oxygen leading to apoptosis or other cell-death mechanisms (8,9)? Do both tumor classes require effective angiogenesis inducers secreted by tumor cells (10–12)? Are the growth patterns of these two tumor classes very distinctive, such that cellular or molecular markers could be identified that are primary tumor-specific or metastasis-specific? Do "latent" primary tumors of the lung share gene-regulation patterns similar to "latent" micrometastases of other tumor classes in this organ? Or are the molecular/genetic bases of latency very different for these two tumor classes? These are the types of issues that require address during the next decade of experimentation into tumor development in the lung.

1.3. Rationale for Using Histochemical Marker Genes

In our own studies of mouse fibrosarcoma metastasis from subcutis-localized tumors to the lung (13), we had been frustrated with our inability to identify tumor cells as they developed the very earliest micrometastases. To overcome this obstacle, we adopted use of a histochemical marker gene (initially bacterial *lacZ*) which provides histochemical reactivity to an X-gal substrate making the cells stain intensively blue *(14,15)*. By this means, the earliest micrometastases developing in the lung could be identified at the level of single cells and the number of micrometastases quantitated readily *(15,16)*. This approach was then extended by use of two different histochemical marker genes to genetically tag two different tumor cell classes to track their metastatic behavior singly or together—*lacZ* vs human placental alkaline phosphatase gene *(17,18)*.

1.3.1. Fibrosarcoma Micrometastases in Lung

Experimental micrometastases in the lung were tracked after injecting *ras*-transformed and *lacZ*-tagged 3T3 cells into the tail veins of nude mice *(15)*. As early as 5 min after injection, a large number of foci could be identified in the lung and these persisted for at least 1 h. Then clearance of unstable micrometastases occurred over the next 24 h after which 1–1.5% of the original foci remained stably in lung tissue for 2 wk or more. Subcutaneous or footpad injections, in contrast, revealed a small number of micrometastases 2–3 wk after injection, indicating the slow selection that occurs for spontaneous metastasis. Some of these micrometastases persisted as such for many weeks while a few grew out into overt metastases that soon overwhelmed the organ. What makes these overt growers special remains to be investigated in the face of many micrometastases that fail to grow effectively but remain as viable foci over long periods of time.

These cells were then treated in tissue culture with different reagents (fixation, irradiation, or mitomycin C) prior to their injection into tail veins to test possible mechanisms of persistence *(16)*. Fixed-cell foci were large but were cleared completely from the lung within hours. In contrast, the DNA-targeted treatments led to heterogeneously sized foci, similar to those of live cells, which were cleared slowly and incompletely. These studies led us to hypothesize that altered deformability of the cell surface modulates the effectiveness of host-clearing mechanisms in the lung and can facilitate clearance of live tumor cells when the two cell classes are co-injected *(16)*.

In a similar vein, we tested the ability of *ras*-transformed cells tagged with *lacZ* to compete with or complement micrometastasis to the lung when co-injected with *sis*-transformed cells tagged with another marker gene, human placental alkaline phosphatase, which gives rise to reddish-brown or black stainability *(17,18)*. When the *sis* transformant is injected singly, it is incapable of forming any stable micrometastases; *ras* transformants readily establish stable micrometastases, many of which develop into overt metastases. When the two cells are co-injected, the *ras* transformant provides environmental cues that generate stable micrometastases for the *sis* transformant and eventually leads to overt metastases comprised of both cell types. This experiment demonstrates considerable synergy between two tumor cell classes in stabilizing and generating outgrowth of a tumor cell class that is normally not lung-metastatic by itself.

1.3.2. Neuroblastoma Micrometastases in Lung

The experiments described in **Subheading 1.3.1.** using mouse fibrosarcoma cells eventually led us to test a human tumor of different origin: neuroblastoma *(19)*. Human neuroblastoma cells were genetically tagged with *lacZ* and tested under similar conditions. When these cells were injected into the subcutis or the dermis, there was virtually no metastasis of these cells to the lungs of animals but foci were observed in other organs. Similarly, injection of these cells into tail veins to follow the experimental metastasis model led to very few foci at any time points; those that were observed were very transient and were ultimately cleared from lungs. This was the first indication to us that there was tumor cell-type specificity in establishment and persistence of lung micrometastases in two different systems, with the caveat that ectopic injections were being compared in all cases. Whether this is due to the particular cell type chosen or applies more generally to neuroblastoma will require tagging of many more types of neuroblastoma (from class I through class IV).

1.3.3. Prostate Carcinoma Micrometastases in Lung

Prostate carcinoma (PCA) studies in animal models have overwhelmingly used already-metastatic populations from human patients, specifically DU145, PC3, and LNCaP *(20–22)*. In order to evaluate the cellular and molecular mechanisms for generation of metastatic variants from the primary tumor population, it was critical that we study a population of human PCA cells from a primary tumor of a patient. Such a population became available with the description of the CWR22R xenograft developed at this University in athymic nude mice that was (a) derived from a human primary tumor in the prostate gland and (b) metastatic to the lungs of animals when carried as a subcutaneous xenograft *(23)*. This xenograft was adapted eventually to tissue culture *(24)*. Our laboratory subsequently transfected the *lacZ* gene into these cells and identified clone H as a highly stable expressor of the *lacZ* gene for >25 passages in culture *(25–27)*.

When LZ-CWR22R clone H cells were injected into the subcutis of nude mice in a PBS vehicle, approx one-half of the animals developed primary tumors as well as micrometastases in lung, liver, and bone *(25)*. These three organs are the primary sites of metastasis in human disease; therefore, this model offers significant parallels in targeting behavior between the actual disease progression in humans and animal model studies. Furthermore, injection of these cells in a matrigel vehicle led to 100% tumorigenicity at the subcutis and, again, micrometastasis development in all three organs, as well as some minor targeting of kidney and brain *(25)*. It was also notable that micrometastases persisted in the lung and bone for long periods of time but rarely developed into overt metastases. Examples of micrometastases are provided in **Fig. 1** for lung, liver, and kidney while **Fig. 2** displays several examples of micrometastases in bone at high magnification. Efficiency of overt metastasis outgrowth in the liver was quite high indicating differences in the enviromental conditions for stabilization and/or their outgrowth in these different organs. The molecular and cellular bases for these differences have yet to be resolved.

We then explored the fate of these LZ-CWR22R clone H cells when injected into the tail veins of animals *(28)*: the experimental metastasis model which obviates any selection in the primary tumor and which tests for competency to colonize various organs once the cultured cell population is introduced directly into the animal's circulation. In this case, a large number of micrometastases were observed in the lungs within 1 h but only persisted for a few hours before their complete clearance *(28)*. Serial sectioning of individual micrometastases revealed their size heterogeneity; most of them were comprised of 1–5 cells but some contained as many as 19 cells *(28)*. This was true even though extensive precautions were taken to inject a single-cell population. An example of serial sections across a 2-cell micrometastasis is shown in **Fig. 3**.

With this experimental metastasis model, micrometastases were also observed in liver and bone but these were consistently small when visualized with whole-organ X-gal staining *(28)*. Serial sections of 8 separate micrometastases in the liver indicated that they were all composed of only 1 or at most 2 cells. Therefore, these sites differ from those in the lung at the very same time point (again, within 1 h of injection). The size of the bone sites were also comparable to those of liver: homogeneously small.

The studies described in **Subheadings 1.3.1.**, **1.3.2.**, and **1.3.3.** reveal differences in micrometastases residing in the lungs of experimental animals from three different tumor classes. Whether these differences are truly tumor type-specific remains to be tested with other isolates of the same human tumor classes. In general, several differences were observed. First, fibrosarcoma micrometastases frequently grew out into overt metastases in lung. Neuroblastoma tumor cells were very labile in the lung as were many PCA cells; however, a small fraction of PCA cells persisted as micrometastases. What makes these latter cells special requires further analysis. Second, serial sectioning of both fibrosarcoma and PCA micrometastases at their earliest residence times, well before cell division could occur, indicated considerable heterogeneity in the

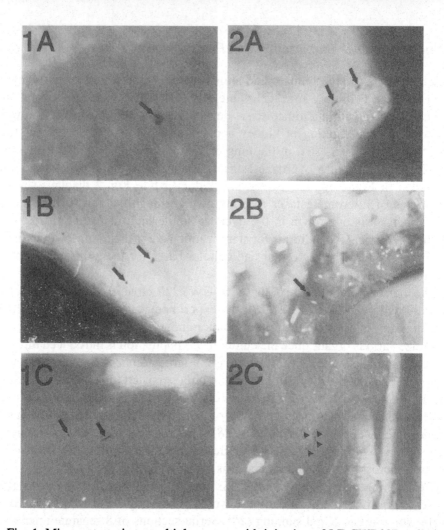

Fig. 1. Micrometastasis to multiple organs with injection of LZ-CWR22R cells in a matrigel vehicle. Matrigel-suspended clone H cells were injected sc into nude mice. When the primary tumors had become large, animals were sacrificed and many organs were excised, fixed, and X-gal-stained to evaluate development of micrometastases. (A) A lung micrometastasis (small arrow) at 44 d postinjection. Original magnification, ×102. (B) Liver micrometastases (small arrows) at 72 d postinjection. Original magnification, ×34. (C) Kidney micrometastases (small arrows) at 44 d postinjection. Original magnification, ×17. Adapted with permission from ref. 25.

Fig. 2. Micrometastasis to bone. Clone H cells were injected s.c. in either PBS or matrigel vehicles. When primary tumors had become large, the animals were sacrificed for excision of many bones, followed by bone fixation and X-gal staining. (A) Micrometastases (small arrows) in the long bone of the leg 17 days post-PBS-injection. Original magnification, ×42. (B) Micrometastases (small arrow) along the spinal column 113 d post-PBS-injection. Original magnification, ×13. (C) Micrometastases (small arrowheads) along the spinal column 44 days post-matrigel-injection. Original magnification, ×34. Adapted with permission from ref. 25.

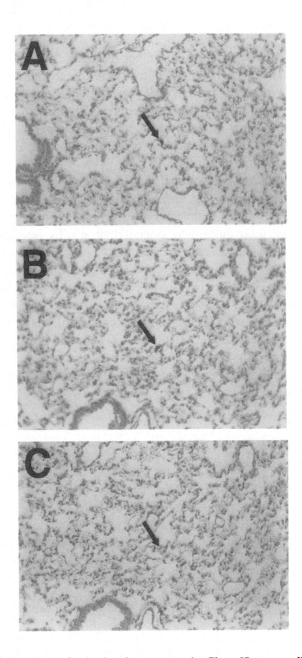

Fig. 3. Serial sections of a single micrometastasis. Clone H tumor cells were injected into the tail vein of an athymic nude mouse. At 30 min postinjection, the mouse was sacrificed; the lungs were excised, fixed, and X-gal-stained. Pieces of lung were cut out of the tissue, one of which was serially sectioned to give the sections (A–C) shown here harboring only one micrometastasis. Sections were 5 μm thick. Note that this micrometastasis is comprised of 2 cells (arrows). Several sections on either side of these three sections did not reveal any tumor cells. Magnification, ×65.

sizes of these sites in terms of cell number. Whether this is a result of cells accumulating at special sites of the lung microvasculature before extravasation into lung tissue or whether "pioneering" tumor cells generate tunnels into the tissue that other tumor cells can take advantage of remains to be determined *(28)*. Third, the efficiency of forming micrometastases per 1000 tumor cells varied considerably among these three tumor classes with fibrosarcoma>> prostate carcinoma>neuroblastoma.

In light of these findings, it would also be instructive to take different classes of human lung cancer cells (e.g., adenocarcinoma of the lung vs small-cell carcinoma of the lung), tag them with a histochemical marker gene such as *lacZ*, and then test their outgrowth when orthotopically injected into lungs or injected into tail veins as an experimental "metastasis" model. Do these cells behave similarly to any of the three heterologous tumor classes described earlier because this is their "native" tissue environment? Or do they differ from all of these foreign tumor classes? Alternatively, the lung cancer cells could be tagged with the placental alkaline phosphatase gene, these cells mixed with one of the *lacZ* transfectants described earlier, and then the two cell classes co-injected to determine any degree of synergy between the two *(17,18)*. Clearly, other scenarios using these various tumor classes can also be constructed and tested in animal models.

2. Materials

2.1. Transfection of Tumor Cells

2.1.1. Tissue Culture Medium

1. RPMI 1640 (Mediatech Inc., Herndon, VA). Store at 4°C.
2. Fetal calf serum (FCS) (Irvine Scientific, Santa Ana, CA). Store frozen at –20°C. Add 10% (v/v) to RPMI 1640.
3. Penicillin-streptomycin: Add 6.15 g/L penicillin G, sodium, 14.28 g/L streptomycin sulfate, and 8.5 g/L NaCl to distilled water. Sterile-filter, aliquot, and then freeze. Store at –20°C. Use at final concentration of 10,000 U penicillin/ mL and 10,000 µg streptomycin/ mL.
4. Phosphate-buffered saline (PBS), pH 7.4. Add penicillin and streptomycin (*see* 3 above). Store at 4°C.
5. Trypsin solution: 8 g/L NaCl, 0.4 g/L KCl, 1 g/L dextrose, 0.58 g/L NaHCO$_3$, 0.2 g/L EDTA, 0.5 g/L trypsin, 0.002 g/L phenol red to distilled water. Sterile-filter and store at 4°C.

2.1.2. Transfection Reagent

1. LipofectAMINE PLUS Reagent (Gibco, Grand Island, NY). Other transfection reagents available may be substituted as transfection efficiency may be cell

type-specific. Follow the Gibco protocol to determine transfection conditions for each cell line.

2. G-418 sulfate (Gibco). Store powder at room temperature. Add to RPMI 1640 with 10% FCS and store at 4°C. The optimal concentration should be re-evaluated for altered experimental conditions, different lot numbers, and different cell lines.

2.2. Stainability of Cultured Cells or Animal Tissues

1. PBS, pH 7.4.
2. Fix solution: 2% (v/v) formaldehyde in PBS. Store at 4°C.
3. Stain solution: 5 mM potassium ferricyanide, 5 mM potassium ferrocyanide, 2 mM magnesium chloride in PBS. Store at 4°C.
4. X-gal (Research Organics, Cleveland, OH): 40X stock solution: 40 mg/mL X-gal in dimethyl sulfoxide (DMSO). Store at –20°C. Light sensitive.
5. Nonidet P-40 (Sigma, St Louis, MO). Use at final concentration of 0.02% (v/v). Store at room temperature.
6. Sodium deoxycholate 1000x stock solution: 10% (w/v) sodium deoxycholate in distilled water. Store at –20°C.
7. Tissue rinse solution: 3% (v/v) DMSO in PBS.
8. Storage solution: 0.02% (w/v) sodium azide in PBS.

2.3. Animal Injection and Harvest

1. Matrigel (Collaborative Research, Bedford, MA). Store at –20°C. Thaw overnight on ice at 4°C. Gels rapidly and irreversibly at room temperature. Use precooled pipets and syringes.
2. PBS, pH 7.4.
3. Syringes (1 mL).
4. For subcutaneous injection: 22-gauge, 1 inch needles.
5. For tail vein injection: 25-gauge, 5/8 inch needles.
6. Sterile surgical ware for tumor harvest.
   a. scissors.
   b. forceps.
   c. hemostat.
   d. scapel.

2.4. Embedding and Sectioning of Tissues

All of the following products, as well as histological lab equipment, can be obtained from Fisher Scientific (Pittsburgh, PA).

1. 10% formalin neutral buffer.
2. Rapid decalcifier.
3. Processing/embedding cassettes.

4. EtOH: 70, 95, and 100%.
5. Xylene or xylene substitute.
6. Paraffin-embedding media.
7. Base molds.
8. Neutral red counterstain.
9. Mounting media.
10. Glass slides and slide covers.

3. Methods

3.1. Transfection of Tumor Cells

An important issue that had to be faced with transfection of a heterologous gene into animal or human tumor cells in culture is whether expression of the histochemical marker gene is sufficiently robust to provide excellent stainability of cells. Furthermore, the notable genetic instability of tumor cells raises a second issue as to whether expression would persist in a major fraction of cells over lengthy periods of cell culturing and subsequent outgrowth of tumors in various tissues of the animal (*see* **Subheading 4.1.** below). Both of these potential problems have been overcome in several tumor systems (*see* **Note 1**).

1. Because transfection can be based on several different methods, it is important for the investigator to test several different transfecting reagents in transient assays to maximize efficiency of introducing the foreign gene, whether it be bacterial *lacZ*, human placental alkaline phosphatase, or Drosophila alcohol dehydrogenase genes. Calcium phosphate turned out to be the method of choice for fibrosarcoma and neuroblastoma but was extremely poor with prostate carcinoma cells. In the latter case, lipofectamine was the optimal agent.
2. In addition, consideration must be given to the promoter driving expression of the marker gene. Some cells display higher levels of expression with an RSV-LTR promoter while others yield higher activities with a CMV promoter. This laboratory has routinely tested both these panels of genes on integrating plasmids regulated by both sets of promoters. In all stable transfectants that we have evaluated with integrating plasmids, only 1 or at most 2 copies were ever integrated into the genome of tumor cells.
3. When a population of cells has been transfected, it is critical that as many colonies be identified and isolated as possible to maximize the opportunity to pick a highly stable-expressing clone of transfectant cells. Many of these early colonies will be highly unstable and will lose expression within 2–5 passages. Some will have intermediate stability with 50% loss of stainability by passage 10–15. A fraction of colonies will be extremely stable with >85% of cells staining for as long as 25 passages (*see* **Note 2**).
4. Once a stable transfectant has been identified, a large bank of vials of this cell line should be frozen in liquid nitrogen to provide stocks for experiments over

many years of research effort. In our experience, freezing in liquid nitrogen has no adverse effect on the intensity or stability of staining of cells.

3.2. Stainability of Cultured Cells or Animal Tissues

3.2.1. Cultured Cell Staining

1. Cultured cells should be rinsed well with PBS and then fixed with either 2% formaldehyde in PBS or a mixture of formaldehyde/glutaraldehyde in which the glutaraldehyde concentration is kept relatively low. Cultured cells are fixed at 4°C or at room temperature for 5 min (10 min with the glutaraldehyde mixture). These conditions do not destroy histochemical marker enzyme activity but do destroy the cell's hydrolytic activities.
2. X-gal staining is performed at room temperature or at 37°C overnight. β-galactosidase activity can be evaluated qualitatively by eye under the microscope or quantitatively using luminometry *(29)*. Using fluorescein-digalactoside as the live-cell permeable substrate for *lacZ* activity, such cells can even be sorted into high-expressors vs low-expressors by flow cytometry.

3.2.2. Tissue Staining

1. Once euthanized, the investigator should dissect the animal as soon as possible for subsequent fixation and staining of tissues. However, we have found some success in immediately freezing tissues in liquid nitrogen and then fixing/staining them weeks or even months later. Optimally, tissues should be handled immediately to avoid necrotic activities, particularly in large tumors that are highly vascularized.
2. Tissues are then fixed for 1–2 h at 4°C.
3. X-gal staining is performed overnight at room temperature or, in cases where background staining can be a problem (e.g., bone; *see* **Subheading 4.2.**), staining is performed at 4°C (*see* **Notes 2** and **3**).

3.2.3. Storage

1. Cultured cells or animal tissues that have been stained with X-gal (or one of its analogs generating other colored products) or with substrates for placental alkaline phosphatase are stable in our hands at 4°C when stored in PBS:azide solution. We cannot detect any loss of color stain under these conditions. In fact, some of these specimens have been used for serial sectioning months later; an example for lung micrometastases is provided in **Fig. 3**.

3.3. Animal Injection and Harvest

3.3.1. Injection Into Animals: Formation of Primary Tumors

1. Tagged tumor cell populations are trypsinized off culture dishes by standard techniques, rinsed well with PBS, and then injected into ectopic or orthotopic sites of animals in either PBS or matrigel vehicles. The latter is essential for

prostate carcinoma to maximize efficiency of tumorigenicity but not necessary for fibrosarcoma or neuroblastoma.

2. In initial experiments, the investigator should remove primary tumors at various stages of growth to verify stability of expression of the marker gene after extensive growth in vivo. This is critical because some tagged clones, while stable expressors in culture, yield primary tumors with excellent stainability at their surface but have generated nonexpressing variants at their interiors and, therefore, no longer stain. If metastatic variants should arise from these nonstaining interior regions, then they will not be detected when assaying for micrometastases in target organs.

3. In our initial studies of any tumor system, we routinely take 1-cm diameter primary tumors after excision from the animal, slice them into halves or quarters, and then fix/stain to determine uniformity of stainability throughout the tumor. (In this regard, it is likely that substrates such as X-gal or X-phosphate can only penetrate 5–10 cell layers into dense tissues.) Therefore, it is essential that large fragments of tissue be fixed and stained only after fragmenting them.

3.3.2. Identification of Micrometastases

1. Organs being assayed for micrometastases should be excised immediately after euthanasia and assayed as soon as possible by fixation and histochemical staining.

2. When whole organs such as lung or brain are being evaluated, all areas at the surface of the organ should be carefully scanned by two different investigators under the dissecting microscope (in our case, a Nikon SMZU microscope operating at 5–25×). It should be noted that any micrometastases that are deeper into the tissue than a few hundred microns will not be detected by this approach because of limited permeability of the stain substrate.

3. Fragments of all tissues can be made prior to fixation and histochemical staining to investigate any asymmetric distribution of micrometastases in a particular organ (*see* **Note 4**). Bone poses a particularly "thorny" problem because soft connective tissue is bound to this hard tissue and must be carefully dissected away to evaluate whether micrometastases are truly bone-associated.

3.4. Embedding and Sectioning of Tissues

More detailed information on cellular composition and distributions can be acquired about primary tumors, micrometastases, and overt metastases after histochemical staining and serial sectioning. In particular, this approach can tell you whether tumors are homogeneous at specific locations, are interspersed with connective tissue cells of the particular organ, and are penetrated with blood vessels as a consequence of angiogenesis. Different classes of tumor can also be distinguished using a double-staining technique (*see* **Note 5**).

1. Both methacrylate and paraffin embedding have been used successfully in our hands; both methods fail to destroy the staining in tumor cells. However, embedding should always be executed after histochemical staining and not before

it (high temperatures destroy histochemical enzyme activity with the exception of human placental alkaline phosphatase activity, which is heat-resistant).

2. Serial sectioning can also be performed on organs that are already stained and have been stored for lengthy periods of time in PBS:azide at 4°C. However, we have found that soft tissues such as lung and liver are more effectively sectioned after lengthy storage with a second formalin treatment.

3. Individual stained cells can be readily identified in 4–5 μm-thick sections without any detectable leakage of histochemical product out of cells. Sectioning of bone micrometastases may be more effective with partial demineralization of bone architecture; however, we are currently undertaking a more exhaustive analysis of bone micrometastases.

4. Notes

1. Tumor cells exhibit notable genetic and epigenetic instability for a variety of reasons. This instability becomes a serious obstacle to generating transfectants of tumor cells with histochemical marker genes that are stable over lengthy periods of time in vitro and in vivo. It should also be remembered that there are no selective advantages for cells expressing marker genes. After their isolation, we do not routinely keep cultured cell populations in drug-selection medium because: a) we wish to evaluate the true genetic and epigenetic stability of the marker gene in vitro, and b) ultimately we cannot use drug selection in vivo (unless we move to a tet^R-responsive promoter system). We have sent these marker genes to over 120 laboratories worldwide and we can share some common experience at dealing with this instability issue.

   a. Our experiences in three different tumor systems and those of other laboratories have been that a sizable number of independent isolates of "stable" transfectants must be isolated initially to provide any measure of success in any tumor system. Many laboratories have contacted us with the frustration that they were unable to identify any long-term stable transfectants of their tumor system. When you ask them how many independent isolates they pursued in their initial experiments, they invariably say 1–3 isolates. This is exactly why they were unsuccessful.

   b. We routinely isolate 10–15 independent transfection events and then work each of these up independently *(26,27)*. As an example, out of 12 transfectants we routinely find that 5–6 of these are highly unstable and lose *lacZ* or alkaline phosphatase stainability over 3–5 passages in culture; 4 or 5 transfectants have intermediate stability with stainability lost over 10–15 passages; only 2 or at most 3 isolates have excellent stability with >85% of the cells staining for the marker gene beyond 20 passages in culture. Although we have not determined the molecular biological basis for loss of marker gene activity in these tumor cells, we can say that our *lacZ*-tagged prostate carcinoma cells do not lose this activity via hypermethylation of the *lacZ* gene promoter *(26,27)*.

2. Assessing the "faithfulness" of tumor progression by transfectants is an important issue raised in developing any new tumor-progression model. Does the

"stable" *lacZ* transfectant of a tumor cell population display the same tumor-forming/progressing properties of the population that was used as the starting material for the experiment? Because these stable transfectants are clones isolated under stringent selection conditions, investigators must provide evidence that ectopic or orthotopic injection of the cloned *lacZ*-tagged population leads to the same tumor formation as the original population.

   a. The issue of the "faithfulness" of progression and metastasis of these two different populations is even more difficult to address. Clearly, the *lacZ* transfectant provides ultrasensitive detection of micrometastases that cannot be duplicated by the original cultured cell population in which there is no marker gene for tracking. However, if the original population gives rise to overt metastases in the lung and/or the liver, then one would expect the *lacZ* transfectant to do the same. If it does not, then the model is analyzing a different class of cells with the transfectant. Gene-array analyses on the two populations should be highly beneficial in future studies for comparing and contrasting these two sets of cells.

3. It should also be noted that, even with the most stable stainers after cloning, a minority of cells in the population do not stain at any one time (usually 3–5% of the cells; this remains true with subsequent re-cloning indicating a cellular physiological property of expression of the marker gene). These nonstaining cells may be in a particular phase of the cell cycle where enzyme activity is unstable or lost or there are various other cellular physiological reasons for low-percentage nonexpressors. Our laboratory has not followed up on this property. In any case, it does not interfere with any tumor-progression studies.

4. When we undertook these genetic-marker experiments in the 1980s, we intentionally avoided the use of fluorescing genetic tags, such as luciferase and green fluorescent protein (GFP). While these latter tags provided excellent sensitivity for detecting tumor cells, they obviated our ability for examining the relationships between tumor cells in tissues and neighboring host-organ cells. Only histochemical marker genes could provide the very highest resolution and sensitivity for performing both functions in the light microscope.

   Perhaps the biggest surprise of our early studies in the 1980s using bacterial *lacZ* was the excellent contrast between blue-staining tumor cells using X-gal and the lack of stainability of most host tissues. This was based on the bacterial enzyme having a pH-optimum of 7.2 while the mammalian enzyme has a pH-optimum close to 4. Therefore, in most tissues background staining was minimal when PBS was used as the buffer for staining reactions.

   a. Two tissues were notable exceptions to this rule. First, the kidney does display some diffuse blue staining around the inner regions of the cortex. Second, the growth plate regions of the long bones of the animal also displayed some diffuse blue staining. Both of these backgrounds were eliminated by performing the staining reaction at 4°C where the bacterial enzyme remains quite active while the mammalian enzyme does not.

b. Background staining with substrates directed to another marker gene, human placental alkaline phosphatase, posed a more difficult problem. Alkaline phosphatase substrates frequently stain blood vessels because of the elevated levels of this gene product in endothelial cells. However, the enzyme product of the human placental gene is highly heat-resistant while the endogenous blood vessel enzyme is highly sensitive. Therefore, a heat treatment at 60°C for 10–15 min is usually sufficient to reduce background staining of blood vessels to an absolute minimum.

5. Care must be taken when staining the interior regions of dense organs. The lung is an unusual organ in that it is highly infiltrated with air sacs and blood vessels, which make it a highly penetrable organ for most histochemical substrates (e.g., X-gal, red-gal, X-phosphate, and other *lacZ* or alkaline phosphatase substrates). In contrast, the liver, kidney, brain, and bone are relatively dense and substrates can only penetrate a few hundred microns (probably even less for bone, although we have not evaluated this parameter specifically). To evaluate micrometastases at interior regions of these organs, it is essential that fresh organs be sliced into defined fragments or thick sections made with topological mapping for subsequent fixation and histochemical staining. Only this approach can define whether micrometastases appear throughout the organ or in localized regions, perhaps as a consequence of accessible blood vessels.

6. In **Subheading 1.3.1.**, we defined the use of different histochemical marker genes to track two different classes of tumor cells in vivo: in this case *lacZ* and human placental alkaline phosphatase genes. It took some effort on our part to sort out the sequence of staining reactions so that maximal efficiency of detection of both tumor cell classes could be effected. This was achieved as follows.

a. Because the heat step was required to eliminate background alkaline phosphatase staining, the staining reaction for *lacZ* was performed first after fixation of tissues. Then the heat step was executed, followed by alkaline phosphatase staining. When heating is performed prior to staining for *lacZ*, detection of this class of tumor cells becomes much poorer, so much so that small clusters of cells in micrometastases can be missed easily.

b. Another approach that could prove useful with two-marker systems is the use of the *lacZ* or alkaline phosphatase histochemical marker gene in one tumor class and luciferase or GFP in the second tumor class. Then cells could be examined under both light and epifluorescence illumination to determine the topological relationships among the two tumor cell classes and neighboring host-organ cells. We have not attempted this approach but would be interested in its possibilites, particularly in light of modern tumor-targeting strategies.

Acknowledgments

The authors acknowledge partial support for these studies from the Comprehensive Cancer Center of the Ireland Cancer Center at Case Western Reserve

University (NCI-supported via P30-CA43703) and the support of research grant DAMD 17-98-1-8587 from the U.S. Army. Athymic nude mouse experiments were conducted in the Athymic Animal Facility (AAALAC-I-approved) of the Case Western Reserve University/Ireland Cancer Center, assisted by Pamela Steele, and approved by the Animal Care and Use Committee of this University. The authors thank Drs. Thomas and Theresa Pretlow of the Department of Pathology for assistance with tumor and organ tissue sectioning and immunohistochemistry protocols, pathology consultation, consultation of PCA xenograft biology, and use of testosterone pellets implanted into nude mice. The assistance of Joseph Giaconia in the Pretlow lab is also acknowledged for implantation of testosterone pellets. The CWR22Rv1 cell line was kindly donated by Dr. James Jacobberger of the Cancer Center.

References

1. Fidler, I. J., Gersten, D. M., and Hart, I. R. (1978) The biology of cancer invasion and metastasis. *Adv. Cancer Res.* **28,** 149–250.
2. Singh, R. K., Tsan, R., and Radinsky, R. (1997) Influence of the host microenvironment on the clonal selection of human colon carcinoma cells during primary tumor growth and metastasis. *Clin. Exp. Metast.* **15,** 140–150.
3. Nicolson, G. L. (1993) Cancer progression and growth: relationship of paracrine and autocrine growth mechanisms to organ preference of metastasis. *Exp. Cell Res.* **204,** 171–180.
4. Fidler, I. J. and Hart, I. R. (1982) Biological diversity in metastatic neoplasms: origins and implications. *Science* **217,** 998–1003.
5. Fisher, B. and Fisher, E. R. (1967) The organ distribution of disseminated ^{51}Cr-labeled tumor cells. *Cancer Res.* **27,** 412–420.
6. Li, H., Hamou, M.-F., de Tribolet, N., Jaufeerally, R., Hofmann, M., Diserens, A.-C., and van Meir, E. G. (1993) Variant CD44 adhesion molecules are expressed in human brain metastases but not in glioblastomas. *Cancer Res.* **53,** 5345–5349.
7. Muller, A., Homey, B., Soto, H., Ge, N., Catron, D., Buchanan, M. E., et al. (2001) Involvement of chemokine receptors in breast cancer metastasis. *Nature* **410,** 50–56.
8. Tarin, D. and Price, J. E. (1981) Influence of microenvironment and vascular anatomy on "metastatic" colonization potential of mammary tumors. *Cancer Res.* **41,** 3604–3609.
9. Sperandio, S., de Belle, I., and Bredesen, D. E. (2000) An alternative, nonapoptotic form of programmed cell death. *Proc. Natl. Acad. Sci. USA* **97,** 14376–14381.
10. Fidler, I. J. and Ellis, L. M. (1994) The implications of angiogenesis for the biology and therapy of cancer metastasis. *Cell* **79,** 185–188.
11. Blood, C. H. and Zetter, B. (1990) Tumor interactions with the vasculature: angiogenesis and tumor metastasis. *Biochim. Biophs. Acta* **1032,** 89–118.
12. Folkman, J. (1995) Angiogenesis in cancer, vascular, rheumatoid and other disease. *Nature Med.* **1,** 27–31.

13. Radinsky, R., Kraemer, P. M., Raines, M. A., Kung, H.-J., and Culp, L. A. (1987) Amplification and rearrangement of the Kirsten *ras* oncogene in virus-transformed Balb/c 3T3 cells during malignant tumor progression. *Proc. Natl. Acad. Sci. USA* **84,** 5143–5147.

14. Lin, W.-C., Pretlow, T. P., Pretlow, T. G., and Culp, L. A. (1990) Bacterial *lacZ* gene as a highly sensitive marker to detect micrometastasis formation during tumor progression. *Cancer Res.* **50,** 2808–2817.

15. Lin, W.-C., Pretlow, T. P., Pretlow, T. G., and Culp, L. A. (1990) Development of micrometastases: earliest events detected with bacterial *lacZ* gene-tagged tumor cells. *J. Natl. Cancer Inst.* **82,** 1497–1503.

16. Lin, W.-C. and Culp, L. A. (1992) Altered establishment/clearance mechanisms during experimental micrometastasis with live and/or disabled bacterial *lacZ*-tagged tumor cells. *Invasion Metast.* **12,** 197–209.

17. Lin, W.-C., Pretlow, T. P., Pretlow, T. G., and Culp, L. A. (1992) High resolution analyses of two different classes of tumor cells *in situ* tagged with alternative histochemical marker genes. *Am. J. Pathol.* **141,** 1331–1342.

18. Lin, W.-C., O'Connor, K. L., and Culp, L. A. (1993) Complementation of two related tumour cell classes during experimental metastasis tagged with different histochemical marker genes. *Br. J. Cancer* **67,** 910–921.

19. Kleinman, N. R., Lewandowska, K., and Culp, L. A. (1994) Tumour progression of human neuroblastoma cells tagged with a *lacZ* marker gene: earliest events at ectopic injection sites. *Br. J. Cancer* **69,** 670–679.

20. Pretlow, T. G., Pelley, R. J., and Pretlow, T. P. (1994) Biochemistry of prostatic carcinoma, in *Biochemical and Molecular Aspects of Selected Cancers*, vol. 2 (Pretlow, T. G. II and Pretlow, T. P., eds.), Academic Press, Inc., San Diego, CA, pp. 169–237.

21. Lalani, E.-N., Lanaido, M. E., and Abel, P. D. (1997) Molecular and cellular biology of prostate cancer. *Cancer Met. Rev.* **16,** 29–66.

22. Lange, P. H. and Vessella, R. L. (1999) Mechanisms, hypotheses and questions regarding prostate cancer micrometastases to bone. *Cancer Met. Rev.* **17,** 331–336.

23. Nagabhushan, M., Miller, C. M., Pretlow, T. P., Giaconia, J. M., Edgehouse, N. L., Schwartz, S., et al. (1996) CWR22: the first human prostate cancer xenograft with strongly androgen-dependent and relapsed strains both *in vivo* and in soft agar. *Cancer Res.* **56,** 3042–3046.

24. Sramkoski, R. M., Pretlow, T. G., Giaconia, J. M., Pretlow, T. P., Schwartz, S., Sy, M.-S., et al. (1999) A new human prostate carcinoma cell line, 22Rv1. *In Vitro* **35,** 403–409.

25. Holleran, J. L., Miller, C. J., and Culp, L. A. (2000) Tracking micrometastasis to multiple organs with *lacZ*-tagged CWR22R prostate carcinoma cells. *J. Histochem. Cytochem.* **48,** 643–651.

26. Culp, L. A., Lin, W.-C., Kleinman, N. R., Campero, N. M., Miller, C. J., and Holleran, J. L. (1998) Tumor progression, micrometastasis, and genetic instabil-

ity tracked with histochemical marker genes. *Prog. Histochem. Cytochem.* **33,** 329–350.

27. Culp, L. A., Lin, W.-C., and Kleinman, N. R. (1999) Tagged tumor cells reveal regulatory steps during earliest stages of tumor progression and micrometastasis. *Histol. Histopathol.* **14,** 879–886.

28. Holleran, J. L., Miller, C. J., Edgehouse, N. L., Pretlow, T. P., and Culp, L. A. (2002) Differential experimental micrometastasis to lung, liver, and bone with *lacZ*-tagged CWR22R prostate carcinoma cells. *Clin. Exp. Metast.* **19,** 17–24.

29. O'Connor, K. L. and Culp, L. A. (1994) Quantitation of two histochemical markers in the same extract using chemiluminescent substrates. *BioTechniques* **17,** 502–509.

IV

LUNG CANCER MODEL SYSTEMS

C. MODELS FOR DEVELOPMENT OF TARGETED THERAPEUTICS

37

Cultures of Surgical Material from Lung Cancers

A Kinetic Approach

Bruce C. Baguley, Elaine S. Marshall, and Timothy I. Christmas

1. Introduction

Despite great advances in our understanding of the molecular basis of lung cancer, the efficacy of chemotherapy of lung cancer remains disappointingly low *(1)*. Most of the drugs with established activity against lung cancer were developed using mice with transplantable solid tumors of either murine or human origin. In the 1980s, methods were developed for semi-automated testing of drugs against multiple cell lines *(2,3)*. This allowed the feasibility of an alternative, in vitro approach to the discovery of new anticancer drugs to be explored. Thirty cell lines representing eight lung cancer pathologies, together with 76 other cell lines representing other carcinomas, gliomas, leukemias, melanomas, and sarcomas, were collected in a major initiative by the U.S. National Cancer Institute (NCI) *(4)*. Tens of thousands of new drugs have been screened against this panel and multiple relationships linking growth inhibition, resistance mechanisms, and other genetic characteristics have been elucidated *(5,6)*. However, recent studies have also highlighted the differences between cell lines and tumors growing in vivo. In particular, the patterns of gene expression of cell lines in the NCI cell line panel, when measured by microarray analysis, are more like each other than like those of tumors growing in vivo *(7)*.

One of the important differences between cell lines and in vivo tumors concerns their cytokinetics. The human lung cancer lines in the NCI panel have cell cycle times of 0.75–3.75 d with a median of 1.54 d *(8)*. In contrast, a study of 38 patients with lung cancer, where in vivo potential doubling times were

From: *Methods in Molecular Medicine, vol. 74: Lung Cancer, Vol. 1: Molecular Pathology Methods and Reviews*
Edited by: B. Driscoll © Humana Press Inc., Totowa, NJ

measured by following cells labeled with bromodeoxyuridine through the cell cycle, varied from 1.4 d to 19 wk with a median of 7.3 d *(9)*.

A second important difference between cell lines and tumors is in the rates of cell turnover. Early studies *(10)* drew attention to the fact that the doubling times for human solid tumors were generally much longer than the measured cycle times. Initially, it was thought that this discrepancy was a result of the growth of tumor cells away from the blood supply, thus depriving them of oxygen and nutrients and inducing growth arrest and necrosis. However, histological studies in lung cancer have demonstrated the presence of apoptotic cells at an incidence comparable to that of mitotic cells *(11)*. Because the duration of the process of apoptosis is quite short (a little longer than that for mitosis), the results suggest that although pockets of necrosis are prominent features of human tumors, apoptosis may play the major role in balancing cellular proliferation in cancer tissue. The incidence of spontaneous apoptosis in lung tumor cell lines is comparable to that observed in vivo *(12)* but because the proliferation rate is higher, the turnover rate is lower (*see* **Fig. 1**).

The aforementioned considerations emphasize the need for in vitro models of lung cancer with longer cell-cycle times. One potential solution is to grow cultures of cancer cells, taken from surgery.

We have developed methods in our laboratory to estimate cell-cycle times from such primary cancers *(13)*. In 15 samples of non-small cell lung cancer (NSCLC), estimated cycle times ranged from 2.8 to 12.2 d with a median of 5.1 d *(14,15)*. This result suggests that such primary cultures have an intrinsically lower proliferation rate than cells from established lines and may more closely resemble the original tumor.

In this chapter, we consider the practical aspects of growing lung cancer cells in primary culture from surgical specimens or pleural fluids. The information obtained may be used in the following directions:

- A method for the estimation of cycle times that may be related to in vivo cycle times.
- A potential method for estimating drug- or radiation-induced cell death (e.g., apoptosis).
- A better understanding of the basis for sensitivity or resistance of cultures from individual patients, potentially allowing tailoring of treatment to individual patients.
- Basic studies on the mechanisms involved in control of proliferation and responses of cells not adapted to rapid growth to radiation or chemotherapeutic drugs.
- A complementary testing system for the analysis of drugs with novel mechanisms of action, particularly those that might increase the rate of apoptosis rather than decrease the rate of proliferation.

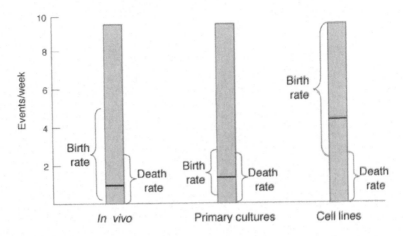

Fig. 1. Comparison of the ranges of proliferation rates (median values shown by the horizontal lines) of in vivo tumors, primary cultures and cell lines. Assumed "cell death" rates are also shown. A change in cell death rate will have a much greater effect in tumors in vivo and in primary cultures than in cell lines.

1.1. A Kinetic Model for the Analysis of Growth of Primary Cultures

The basic features of the model are shown in **Fig. 2**. Consider first the G_1-phase population before and after blocking cell division of a cycling population. In an exponentially growing population of cells, the rate of entry of cells into G_1-phase from cell division will be approximately twice the rate of departure of cells into S-phase, providing an exponential increase. If cell division is blocked, the rate of entry becomes zero and the rate of departure initially does not change, but then decreases as the pool of G_1-phase cells is reduced. Because of the way that G_1-phase transit times are distributed *(16,17)*, the G_1-phase population of the arrested population will decrease in approximately exponential fashion, rather like a radioactive decay. Conversely, the G_1-phase population of the control population will increase exponentially.

The effect of blocking cell division on the S-phase of the cell cycle, estimated by the incorporation of ^{3}H-thymidine into S-phase cells, can now be considered. Because the S-phase population is fed from G_1-phase cells, the arguments presented earlier will also apply to S-phase cells. We have tested this by measuring ^{3}H-thymidine incorporation with time in a series of early passage cell lines after addition of paclitaxel to block cell division. Incorporation decreases linearly with time on a semi-logarithmic plot, and the slope of the line should be a function of the cell cycle time, and the rate of decrease is inversely related to the measured doubling times *(13,15)*. In the example in

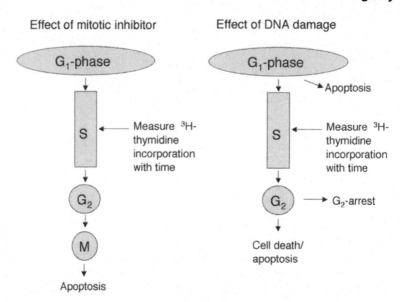

Fig. 2. Model used in this kinetic approach. Cell division is halted on the left-hand side by a mitotic poison and on the right by DNA damage. Both allow G_1-phase cells to feed the S-phase population, which decreases approximately exponentially with time. However, if the DNA damage leads to apoptosis in addition to G_2-phase arrest, there will be a greater rate of reduction of S-phase cells with time.

Fig. 3, the time courses of inhibition of cell division are compared for a primary culture and a cell line. The slopes of the two lines correspond to doubling times of 10 d and 1 d, respectively.

The next effect to consider is that of a cytotoxic agent (radiation or a cytotoxic drug). The main effects are the induction of cycle arrest in G_2-phase (thereby blocking cell division) and the induction of cell death *(18)*. If the application of the cytotoxic agent induces G_2-phase arrest alone, its effect will be similar to that of paclitaxel (*see* **Fig. 4**). If it induces loss of G_1- and/or S-phase cells in addition to causing G_2-phase arrest, the S-phase population will drop more rapidly than with a mitotic inhibitor (*see* **Fig. 4**). Cytotoxic agents can also induce G_1-phase arrest, which complicates the interpretation, but this is discussed later (**Subheading 4.2.**).

In summary, the application of this model permits one to estimate two quite different properties of cell populations: the rate of proliferation in the unperturbed state, and the degree of cell loss (e.g., apoptosis) induced by drugs or radiation. These are important parameters both at the level of the individual patient (for instance in the tailoring of therapy) and at the level of new drug development.

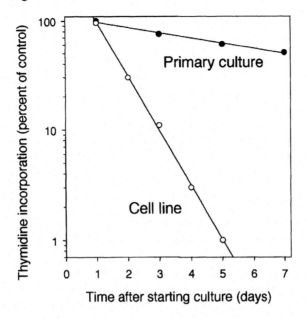

Fig. 3. Examples of the maximal reduction of incorporation of ^{3}H-thymidine by paclitaxel in a primary culture (●) and in a cell line (○) after different times of incubation. The steeper slope of the cell line reflects its higher proliferation rate.

2. Materials

2.1. Preparation of Tumor Samples

1. 50-mL sterile sample tubes.
2. Transport medium: α-modified minimal essential growth medium (Gibco BRL), supplemented with fetal bovine serum (FBS) (Life Technologies, New Zealand; 5%), insulin (10 µg/mL), transferrin (10 µg/mL), sodium selenite (10 ng/mL), penicillin (100 U/mL), and streptomycin (100 µg/mL). Insulin, transferrin, and sodium selenite were obtained from Boehringer Mannheim (Germany).
3. Sodium heparin (5 International U/mL).

2.2. Culture of Tumor Samples

1. Scalpels.
2. Stainless steel screen (0.65-mm mesh size).
3. Round-ended dental probe.
4. Centrifuge tubes.
5. ITS medium: α-modified minimal essential growth medium supplemented with FBS (5% v/v), insulin (10 µg/mL), transferrin (10 µg/mL), sodium selenite (10 ng/mL), penicillin (100 units/mL), streptomycin (100 µg/mL), hydrocortisone (50 nM), and epidermal growth factor (EGF; 5 ng/mL).
6. Hemacytometer.

7. Cytospin materials: microscope slides, slide holders, filter cards, 0.25% albumin, clinical centrifuge fitted with a cytospin rotor.
8. 100-mL clear centrifuge bottles.
9. Clinical centrifuge.

2.3. Culture Plate Setup

1. Cell-culture plates (96-well flat-bottom; Falcon).
2. Agarose (ultrapure grade; Gibco BRL).
3. Multichannel pipettor.
4. Low-oxygen incubator.

2.4. Drug Treatments

1. Paclitaxel, maximum concentration of 2 μM, clinical vial.
2. Vincristine, maximum concentration 30 nM, clinical vial.
3. Docetaxel, maximum concentration 2 μM, clinical vial.
4. Cisplatin, maximum concentration 15 μM, clinical vial.
5. Carboplatin maximum concentration 40 μM, clinical vial.
6. 4-Hydroperoxycyclophosphamide maximum concentration of 40 μM, kindly provided by Asta Medica (Germany).
7. Etoposide maximum concentration 10 μM, clinical vial.
8. Doxorubicin maximum concentration 0.2 μM, clinical vial.
9. Camptothecin maximum concentration 0.5 μM, Sigma Chemical Company.

2.5. Radiation Treatments

1. ^{60}Co source.

2.6. Endpoints

1. ^{3}H-thymidine (20 μCi/mmol).
2. Thymidine (0.1 μM).
3. 5-Fluorodeoxyuridine (0.1 μM).
4. Glass-fiber filter mats.
5. Multiple automated sample harvester.
6. Beta counter, vials, and liquid-scintillation fluid.

3. Methods

There is a great need for a better understanding of what controls the growth and response to treatment of lung cancer. Although a variety of molecular methods including genetic analysis and gene-expression analysis have been applied to this problem, they basically provide "snapshots" of the tumor at particular times. The methods described here allow the addition of a dynamic dimension, and have the capacity to be combined with molecular technologies to advance both prognosis and treatment.

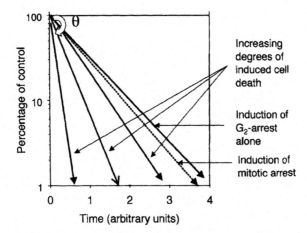

Fig. 4. Predicted changes in an S-phase population as a percentage of the control. The S-phase of a cell population treated with paclitaxel, expressed on a semi-logarithmic scale, will decrease linearly with time as shown in **Fig. 3**. If DNA damage induces G_2-phase arrest alone, its effect (i.e., the angle θ) will be similar to that of paclitaxel. If it induces loss of G_1- and/or S-phase cells in addition to causing G_2-phase arrest, the S-phase population will drop more rapidly than with a mitotic inhibitor. With increasing degrees of induced cell death, the slope of the line becomes progressively steeper (i.e., the angle θ will increase).

3.1. Preparation of Tumor Samples (see Note 1)

1. When samples of non-small cell lung cancers become available as a consequence of surgery, surgical material is sent fresh to the pathologist for diagnosis. Where possible, a sample of the tumor material is retained for research and placed in a sterile sample tube (*see* **Note 2**).
2. Samples of pleural fluid, obtained at paracentesis from patients with confirmed lung cancer, are treated with sodium heparin and stored upright, overnight (or for up to 3 d) in 2-L bottles at 4°C.

3.2. Culture of Tumor Samples (see Note 3)

3.2.1. Solid Tumor Cell Culture

1. Disaggregate solid tumor specimens either immediately or after overnight storage at 4°C. Remove normal, adipose, or grossly necrotic material and the mince tumor finely using crossed scalpels.
2. Pass tumor mince through a stainless steel screen (0.65 mm mesh size) using a round-ended dental probe (*see* **Note 4**).
3. The resulting small aggregates of tumor cells (5–100 cells) are pipetted into tubes, collected by low-speed centrifugation (30*g*, 2 min) to remove blood cells,

necrotic material and debris, washed twice in ITS medium ($30g$, 2 min) (*see* **Note 5**).

4. Estimate cell viability and density using a hemacytometer and phase contrast microscopy.

5. Prepare cytospins of isolated cells and have them checked by a pathologist to confirm the presence and proportion of malignant cells (*see* **Note 6**).

3.2.2. Pleural Fluid Cell Culture

1. Check the pleural fluids, which had been left to stand following collection to allow the sedimentation of cellular material, to ensure that they were clear of nucleated cells. Carefully decant the supernatants, thus eliminating the need to centrifuge large volumes of fluid.

2. Collect pleural fluid residue containing tumor and other cells, and centrifuge in 100-mL clear centrifuge bottles at $400g$ for 10 min.

3. Resuspend collected cells in ITS medium and centrifuge up to three times ($30g$ for 2 min) to minimize red blood cell contamination.

4. Estimate cell viability and density using a hemacytometer and phase-contrast microscopy. Prepare cytospins of isolated cells and have them checked by a pathologist to confirm the presence and proportion of malignant cells.

3.3. Culture Plate Setup

The general scheme for the culture technique is shown in **Fig. 5**.

1. Cells are grown in ITS medium in 96-well plates on a layer of agarose (*see* **Note 7**) *(19)*. Make sterile 0.15% agarose by boiling (microwave oven) in Milli-Q water.

2. After cooling agarose to 40°C, pipet an aliquot (40 µL) under sterile conditions into each well with a multichannel pipet.

3. Invert plate and flick once to remove excess agarose, leaving a thin film of agarose on the plate.

4. Allow plate to dry and store at room temperature for at least 24 h prior to use. The plates are stable for up to 1 mo.

5. A minimum of 10^6 cells is required to set up a full set of assays for each experiment. Set up cell suspensions in growth medium so that each well (125 µL) contains 940, 1875, 3750, and 7,500 cells. If the quantity of cells is limiting, only the top one or two cell densities can be used.

6. Maintain cultures under low oxygen conditions (*see* **Note 8**). Cultures were incubated for 7 d (unless otherwise required) in a low-oxygen incubator using an atmosphere of 5% O_2, 5% CO_2, and 90% N_2.

3.4. Drug Treatments

1. Prepare a dilution series of each of the test drugs in ITS medium in threefold dilution steps (each at 6 times the final concentration) in master 96-well plates (not agar-coated) using an 8-channel pipet. Cytotoxic drugs are generally used in the same clinical formulations used for treatment.

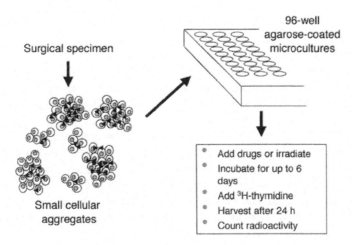

Fig. 5. General scheme for the culture method used in this study.

2. Add drug dilutions immediately (25 µL per well of the appropriate dilution) using an 8-channel pipet. Drugs tested by this assay include: Paclitaxel (*see* **Note 10**), vincristine, docetaxel, cisplatin, carboplatin, 4-hydroperoxycyclophosphamide, etoposide, doxorubicin, camptothecin (*see* **Note 9**).

3.5. Radiation Treatments

1. Set up cells in a final volume of 150 µL/well.
2. Irradiate plates at room temperature from a ^{60}Co source, using a lead wedge designed to produce a dose gradient across the plate with individual doses of between 1.7 and 9 Gy *(21,22)*.
3. Add control cells to the plates immediately after the radiation period.

3.6. Endpoints

1. The main endpoint used for the kinetic studies is thymidine incorporation (*see* **Note 11**). Add ^{3}H-thymidine (20 µCi/mmol; 0.04 µCi/well), together with unlabeled thymidine (0.1 µM) and 5-fluorodeoxyuridine (0.1 µM) to cultures (in growth medium; 20 µL/well) 24 h before harvesting.
2. Collect cells on glass fiber filter mats using a multiple automated sample harvester.
3. Quantitate radioactivity by liquid scintillation. A 7-d culture time for primary cell cultures is used (*see* **Notes 12–14**) and a dose-response curve to ensure linearity is routinely set up *(13,19)*. Samples are excluded if ^{3}H-thymidine incorporation is not linearly related to the number of cells added to the culture (*see* **Notes 15** and **16**).

4. Notes

1. Most hospitals require the written approval of the appropriate Human Ethics Committee prior to commencement of the research. In order to carry out this

work, it is important to provide an information sheet to patients, and to provide procedures so that staff can talk to patients prior to surgery and obtain formal consent for the use of their tumor material for research.

2. Sample tubes (50-mL capacity) are stored, ready for use, containing 25 mL transport medium. Sample tubes can be kept at 4°C for up to 2 mo at the histopathology laboratory. The tumor sample can be kept for up to 24 h at 4°C without loss of proliferative potential.

3. Many different techniques have been used to grow tumor tissue from surgical material *(26)*. While most early studies utilized clonogenic assays *(27,28)*, the time required for such assays (several months) limited their usefulness. A further key problem with clonogenic assays is that cell-cell and cell-matrix interactions are lost in the preparation of single-cell suspensions. A number of subsequent approaches have therefore utilized nonclonogenic assays, such as those presented here.

4. Cell survival requires not only a continuous supply of external growth factors but also survival signals from neighboring cells and the extracellular matrix, transmitted through integrins and other molecules *(34–36)*. Artificial extracellular matrices have been developed for selective tumor cell culture *(37–39)* and methods involving hanging collagen droplets have also been employed *(40)*. In our method, tumor tissue is disaggregated into clusters of cells that are small enough to be pipetted by standard multichannel pipets but large enough to include the natural extracellular matrix (ECM) and to allow cell-cell interactions. In earlier experiments we released cells as small clumps by digestion of tumor tissue with collagenase (1 mg/ml) and DNase (50 μg/mL) and continuous agitation at 37°C, with monitoring by phase-contrast microscopy. However, results from later experiments where tissue was disaggregated using a 0.65-mm mesh stainless steel sieve were found to be similar, and the nonenzymatic method is both simpler and quicker to perform.

5. Nonclonogenic assays must take into account the survival requirements of lung tumor specimens, and generally employ a rich growth medium containing FBS, supplemented by factors that might further improve cell survival. We have utilized ITS growth medium, which contains insulin to saturate the insulin-like growth factor (IGF-1) receptor *(29)*, transferrin to ensure adequate iron uptake *(30)* and selenite to ensure optimal glutathione peroxidase activity *(31)*, and EGF and hydrocortisone to improve survival *(32,33)*.

6. In order to ensure that the cells being cultured were tumor cells, cytospin preparations were prepared before cell culture and examined by a pathologist to confirm the presence of malignant cells. In some cases, control cultures were labeled with ^{3}H-thymidine (20 μCi/mmol; 0.04 μCi/well) over the last 24 h. Cytospin preparations were subjected to autoradiography by a standard emulsion dipping method and were examined by a pathologist to confirm the labeled cells as tumor cells.

7. It is essential to provide conditions that will allow the selective growth of tumor cells. The specially developed surface of culture dishes, while acting as

an adhesion surface to stimulate growth of many tumor cell lines, cannot be used for primary cultures because it also stimulates the growth of normal tissue fibroblasts, which are likely to be present in all surgical samples. Early methods extended clonogenic procedures and used agar as a substrate for tumor cell growth to prevent fibroblast growth *(41,42)*. Artificial extracellular matrices can also fulfill this function *(37–39)*. Our method of coating 96-well plates with a thin layer of agarose not only prevents fibroblast growth but also has the advantages that it is inexpensive and that it facilitates the harvesting of cultures.

8. Tumor tissue is normally exposed to an equivalent of a 5% oxygen atmosphere and can be damaged when exposed suddenly to 20% oxygen. Changes may be likened to those in reperfusion injury, which occurs in heart, brain, and other tissues following reversal of temporary ischemia *(43,44)*. The resulting generation of active oxygen species, either by stromal cells or by the tumor cells themselves, may lead to apoptosis *(45)*. In order to minimize the toxic effects of oxygen radicals, cultures should be grown in an atmosphere of 5% oxygen and 5% carbon dioxide.

9. Paclitaxel is used as an inhibitor of mitosis (and thus cell division) at the maximum drug concentration of 2 μM. Other mitotic inhibitors tested include vincristine (maximum concentration 30 nM) and docetaxel (maximum concentration 2 μM). The drugs cisplatin and carboplatin are used at maximal concentrations (15 μM and 40 μM), respectively, corresponding approximately to the maximal concentrations achieved in clinical trials. Since cyclophosphamide requires in vivo metabolic activation, it cannot be used directly, and 4-hydroperoxycyclophosphamide is used at a maximal concentration of 40 μM. This compound is converted spontaneously to 4-hydroxycyclophosphamide, which is thought to contribute to active alkylating species in vivo *(20)*. The topoisomerase poisons etoposide, doxorubicin, and camptothecin were used at maximal concentrations of 10 μM, 0.2 μM, and 0.5 μM, respectively.

10. There are a number of assumptions in the analysis reported in **Fig. 2** that must be addressed. The drug used to inhibit cell division, which is the basis of the stathmokinetic method, must not in itself induce apoptosis in G_1- or S-phase, and must also not cause G_1-phase arrest. Paclitaxel can induce apoptosis in its own right, but this is likely to occur after mitotic arrest *(49)*. If paclitaxel induced apoptosis, one would expect that higher concentrations would give rise to decreased thymidine incorporation, whereas a definite "plateau" effect is observed in most cases *(13)*. With occasional cultures, very high paclitaxel concentrations give reduced thymidine incorporation, perhaps suggesting an induced slight slowing of the cell cycle. However, this is not observed with paclitaxel concentrations around 200 nM, which generally provide a maximal effect.

11. The incorporation of ^{3}H-thymidine has been used in this technique because it provides an "S-phase window" on the cell cycle that allows a kinetic model (*see* **Fig. 2**) to be applied. Other methods of assessing cell proliferation, such as protein staining *(2,46)*, tetrazolium dyes *(3,47)*, and ATP bioluminescence *(48)*,

measure the total cell population and are difficult to apply to primary cultures because of the loss of stromal and other cells during the course of culture. Labeling with ^{3}H-thymidine provides a further advantage that appropriate cytological examination of cells labeled at the end of the incubation time can confirm whether the proliferating cells are tumor cells.

12. The culture time has been chosen as 7 d because it provides a reasonable time frame for data to be incorporated into potential clinical decisions on treatment. Additionally, the culture time should be sufficiently short to ensure that nutrients in the growth medium are not exhausted, but long enough to allow drug-induced cell loss. The cell density of the cultures when they are set up is critical because if it is too low there will be insufficient thymidine labeling for accurate results, and if it is too high, cell proliferation will cease before the cells are harvested. For this reason it is important to determine that the number of cells growing at the end of the culture time is linearly related to the number of cells inoculated.

13. As shown in **Fig. 4**, data for a cytotoxic agent was analyzed by comparing the effect of the agent on 3H-thymidine incorporation with that of an inhibitor of cell division (the mitotic poison paclitaxel). An example for cisplatin is shown in **Fig. 6**, each point on the graph representing one sample. The distance along the horizontal axis defines the maximal mitotic arrest induced by paclitaxel (*see* **Subheading 4.2.3.**). The relationship between the maximal logarithmic reduction by paclitaxel (P), culture incubation time (t) and measured culture doubling time (T) for a series of cell lines was previously found to be approximated by the equation $p = 0.54 \times t/T$ (correlation coefficient $= 0.90$) *(13)*. This equation can be used to estimate the doubling time of the primary cultures (t = 7 d) and is shown at the top of the graph.

14. At the maximal concentration used, cisplatin induces efficient G_2-phase arrest. Thus, in the absence of induced cell death, it would have a very similar effect to a mitotic inhibitor on the dynamics of the cell population (indicated by the diagonal line). However, if it induces apoptosis as well as G_2-phase arrest, it would have a greater effect. The distance of the points below the diagonal line provides an indication of cisplatin-induced cell loss. The graph shows that while many of the points cluster relatively closely to the diagonal line, a few are a considerable distance away, probably indicating drug-induced cell loss.

15. The technique can also be applied to new drug development, for instance the case of inhibitors of EGF receptor tyrosine kinase. Binding of EGF to its receptor activates its cytoplasmic tyrosine kinase, setting in motion a cascade of signals that are necessary for stimulation of cellular proliferation and suppression of apoptosis *(23,24)*. A variety of inhibitors of the tyrosine kinase domain have been identified, including some that possessing 50% inhibitory concentrations for the isolated receptor of less than 10 pM *(25)*. This raises the question of what effects such inhibitors have in primary cultures. We have previously shown that 6-amino-4-[(3-bromophenyl)amino]-7-(methylamino)quinazoline, a selective inhibitor of EGF receptor tyrosine kinase, is also an inhibitor (at nanomolar

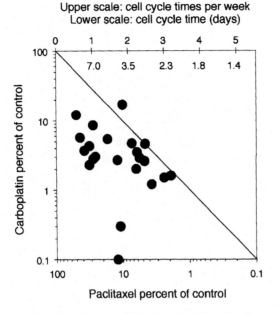

Fig. 6. Data from primary cultures of lung cancer samples from 21 patients. Each point compares the maximal effect of paclitaxel with that of cisplatin at an added concentration of 15 μM. The estimated cycle time can be derived from the upper axis. The concentration of cisplatin is sufficient to cause G_2-phase arrest, and if this is the only effect the point should lie close to the diagonal. It apoptosis is induced in addition to G_2-phase arrest, the points will lie below the diagonal.

concentrations) of ^{3}H-thymidine incorporation in primary cultures from lung cancer *(14)*. **Figure 7** shows results from 17 patients plotted against the corresponding results for paclitaxel, and the pattern contrasts with that for cisplatin (*see* **Fig. 6**). Although the drug inhibits ^{3}H-thymidine incorporation by more than 50% in most of the cultures, the maximal percentage reduction of ^{3}H-thymidine incorporation is less than that caused by paclitaxel. The results suggest that the drug's main effect may be cell-cycle arrest.

16. DNA damage induced by radiation or DNA damage-inducing drugs may also induce G_1-phase arrest, which is generally dependent on the function of the p53 protein *(50)*. Because this is at least partially reversible, it would give a false impression of induced cell loss in graphs of the type shown in **Fig. 6**. This has been investigated in detail, using both cell culture and flow cytometry, for a series of p53-wild type melanoma cell lines exposed to radiation *(51)*. G_1-phase arrest was observed initially but reversed by 2–3 d. Such an effect may thus not contribute substantially to the differential when measured after 7 d, but cannot be ruled out completely.

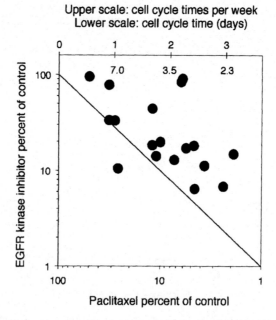

Fig. 7. Data from primary cultures of lung cancer samples from 17 patients. Each point compares the maximal effect of paclitaxel with that of a 4-anilinoquinazoline inhibitor of EGF receptor tyrosine kinase *(14)* at a concentration of 10 n*M*.

References

1. Hoffman, P. C., Mauer, A. M., and Vokes, E. E. (2000) Lung cancer. *Lancet* **355,** 479–485.
2. Finlay, G. J., Baguley, B. C., and Wilson, W. R. (1984) A semiautomated microculture method for investigating growth inhibitory effects of cytotoxic compounds on exponentially growing carcinoma cells. *Anal. Biochem.* **139,** 272–277.
3. Scudiero, D. A., Shoemaker, R. H., Paull, K. D., Monks, A., Tierney, S., Nofziger, T. H., et al. (1988) Evaluation of a soluble tetrazolium/formazan assay for cell growth and drug sensitivity in culture using human and other tumor cell lines. *Cancer Res.* **48,** 4827–4833.
4. Alley, M. C., Scudiero, D. A., Monks, A., Hursey, M. L., Czerwinski, M. J., Fine, D. L., et al. (1988) Feasibility of drug screening with panels of human tumor cell lines using a microculture tetrazolium assay. *Cancer Res.* **48,** 589–601.
5. Weinstein, J. N., Kohn, K. W., Grever, M. R., Viswanadhan, V. N., Rubinstein, L. V., et al. (1992) Neural computing in cancer drug development—predicting mechanism of action. *Science* **258,** 447–451.
6. Scherf, U., Ross, D. T., Waltham, M., Smith, L. H., Lee, J. K., Tanabe, L., et al. (2000) A gene expression database for the molecular pharmacology of cancer. *Nature Genet.* **24,** 236–244.

7. Ross, D. T., Scherf, U., Eisen, M. B., Perou, C. M., Rees, C., Spellman, P., et al. (2000) Systematic variation in gene expression patterns in human cancer cell lines. *Nature Genet.* **24,** 227–235.

8. O'Connor, P. M., Jackman, J., Bae, I., Myers, T. G., Fan, S. J., Mutoh, M., et al. (1997) Characterization of the p53 tumor suppressor pathway in cell lines of the National Cancer Institute anticancer drug screen and correlations with the growth-inhibitory potency of 123 anticancer agents. *Cancer Res.* **57,** 4285–4300.

9. Wilson, G. D. and McNally, N. J. (1991) Measurement of cell proliferation using bromodeoxyuridine, in *Cell Proliferation in Clinical Diagnosis* (Hall, P. A., Levison, D. A., and Wright, N. A., eds.), Springer-Verlag, London, pp. 113–139.

10. Steel, G. G. (1977) Basic theory of growing cell populations, in *Growth Kinetics of Tumours*, 1st ed. (Steel, G. G., ed.), Clarendon, Oxford pp. 56–85.

11. Komaki, R., Milas, L., Ro, J. Y., Fujii, T., Perkins, P., Allen, P., et al. (1998) Prognostic biomarker study in pathologically staged N1 non-small cell lung cancer. *Int. J. Rad. Oncol. Biol. Phys.* **40,** 787–796.

12. Sirzen, F., Zhivotovsky, B., Nilsson, A., Bergh, J., and Lewensohn, R. (1998) Higher spontaneous apoptotic index in small cell compared with non-small cell lung carcinoma cell lines; lack of correlation with Bcl-2/Bax. *Lung Cancer* **22,** 1–13.

13. Baguley, B. C., Marshall, E. S., Whittaker, J. R., Dotchin, M. C., Nixon, J., McCrystal, M. R., et al. (1995) Resistance mechanisms determining the *in vitro* sensitivity to paclitaxel of tumour cells cultured from patients with ovarian cancer. *Eur. J. Cancer* **31A,** 230–237.

14. Baguley, B. C., Marshall, E. S., Holdaway, K. M., Rewcastle, G. W., and Denny, W. A. (1998) Inhibition of growth of primary human tumour cell cultures by a 4-anilinoquinazoline inhibitor of the epidermal growth factor receptor family of tyrosine kinases. *Eur. J. Cancer* **34,** 1086–1090.

15. Baguley, B. C., Marshall, E. S., and Finlay, G. J. (1999) Short-term cultures of clinical tumor material: potential contributions to oncology research. *Oncol. Res.* **11,** 115–124.

16. Smith, J. A. and Martin, L. (1973) Do cells cycle? *Proc. Natl. Acad. Sci. USA* **70,** 1263–1267.

17. Cross, F., Roberts, J., and Weintraub, H. (1989) Simple and complex cell cycles. *Annu. Rev. Cell Biol.* **5,** 341–395.

18. Eastman, A. (1990) Activation of programmed cell death by anticancer agents: cisplatin as a model system. *Cancer Cells* **2,** 275–280.

19. Marshall, E. S., Finlay, G. J., Matthews, J. H. L., Shaw, J. H. F., Nixon, J., and Baguley, B. C. (1992) Microculture-based chemosensitivity testing: a feasibility study comparing freshly explanted human melanoma cells with human melanoma cell lines. *J. Natl. Cancer. Inst.* **84,** 340–345.

20. Ludeman, S. M. (1999) The chemistry of the metabolites of cyclophosphamide. *Curr. Pharmaceut. Design* **5,** 627–643.

21. Cross, P., Marshall, E. S., Baguley, B. C., Finlay, G. J., Matthews, J. H. L., and Wilson, W. R. (1994) Assessment of proliferative assays for radiosensitivity of

tumor cell lines using high throughput microcultures. *Rad. Oncol. Invest.* **1**, 249–260.

22. Marshall, E. S., Matthews, J. H. L., Shaw, J. H. F., Nixon, J., Tumewu, P., Finlay, G. J., et al. (1994) Radiosensitivity of new and established human melanoma cell lines: comparison of [³H]-thymidine incorporation and soft agar clonogenic assays. *Eur. J. Cancer* **30A**, 1370–1376.

23. Bridges, A. J. (1996) The epidermal growth factor receptor family of tyrosine kinases and cancer: can an atypical exemplar be a sound therapeutic target? *Curr. Med. Chem.* **3**, 211–226.

24. Mendelsohn, J. and Fan, Z. (1997) Epidermal growth factor receptor family and chemosensitization. *J. Natl. Cancer. Inst.* **89**, 341–343.

25. Bridges, A. J., Zhou, H., Cody, D. R., Rewcastle, G. W., McMichael, A., Showalter, H. D., et al. (1996) Tyrosine kinase inhibitors. 8. An unusually steep structure-activity relationship for analogues of 4-(3-bromoanilino)-6,7-dimethoxyquinazo-line (PD 153035), a potent inhibitor of the epidermal growth factor receptor. *J. Med. Chem.* **39**, 267–276.

26. Finlay, G. J. (1992) *In vitro* systems for anti-cancer drug screening, in *The Search for New Anti-Cancer Drugs*, 1st ed. (Waring, M. J. and Ponder, B. A., eds.), Kluwer, Dordrecht, pp. 55-85.

27. Hamburger, A. W. and Salmon, S. E. (1977) Primary bioassay of human tumor stem cells. *Science* **197**, 461–463.

28. Courtenay, V. D., Selby, P. J., Smith, I. E., Mills, J., and Peckham, M. J. (1978) Growth of human tumour cell colonies from biopsies using two soft-agar techniques. *Br. J. Cancer* **38**, 77–81.

29. Rubin, R. and Baserga, R. (1995) Insulin-like growth factor-I receptor. Its role in cell proliferation, apoptosis, and tumorigenicity. *Lab. Invest.* **73**, 311–331.

30. Kovar, J., Stunz, L. L., Stewart, B. C., Kriegerbeckova, K., Ashman, R. F., and Kemp, J. D. (1997) Direct evidence that iron deprivation induces apoptosis in murine lymphoma 38C13. *Pathobiology* **65**, 61–68.

31. Leist, M., Raab, B., Maurer, S., Rosick, U., and Brigelius-Flohe, R. (1996) Conventional cell culture media do not adequately supply cells with antioxidants and thus facilitate peroxide-induced genotoxicity. *Free Radic. Biol. Med.* **21**, 297–306.

32. Brower, M., Carney, D. N., Oie, H. K., Gazdar, A. F., and Minna, J. D. (1986) Growth of cell lines and clinical specimens of human non-small cell lung cancer in a serum-free defined medium. *Cancer Res.* **46**, 798–806.

33. Singletary, S. E., Baker, F. L., Spitzer, G., Tucker, S. L., Tomasovic, B., Brock, W. A., et al. (1987) Biological effect of epidermal growth factor on the in vitro growth of human tumors. *Cancer Res.* **47**, 403–406.

34. Meredith, J. E., Fazeli, B., and Schwartz, M. A. (1993) The extracellular matrix as a cell survival factor. *Mol. Biol. Cell.* **4**, 953–961.

35. Ruoslahti, E. and Reed, J. C. (1994) Anchorage dependence, integrins, and apoptosis. *Cell* **77**, 477–478.

36. Frisch, S. M., Vuori, K., Ruoslahti, E., and Chanhui, P. Y. (1996) Control of adhesion-dependent cell survival by focal adhesion kinase. *J. Cell. Biol.* **134,** 793–799.
37. Baker, F. L., Spitzer, G., Ajani, J. A., Brock, W. A., Lukeman, J., Pathak, S., et al. (1986) Drug and radiation sensitivity measurements of successful primary mono-layer culturing of human tumor cells using cell-adhesive matrix and supplemented medium. *Cancer Res.* **46,** 1263–1274.
38. Parkins, C. S. and Steel, G. G. (1990) Growth and radiosensitivity testing of human tumour cells using the adhesive tumour cell culture system. *Br. J. Cancer* **62,** 935–941.
39. Girinsky, T., Lubin, R., Pignon, J. P., Chavaudra, N., Gazeau, J., Dubray, B., et al. (1993) Predictive value of *in vitro* radiosensitivity parameters in head and neck cancers and cervical carcinomas: preliminary correlations with local control and overall survival. *Int. J. Rad. Oncol. Biol. Phys.* **25,** 3–7.
40. Tanigawa, N., Kitaoka, A., Yamakawa, M., Tanisaka, K., and Kobayashi, H. (1996) *In vitro* chemosensitivity testing of human tumours by collagen gel droplet culture and image analysis. *Anticancer Res.* **16,** 1925–1930.
41. Weisenthal, L. M., Dill, P. L., Kurnick, N. B., and Lippman, M. E. (1983) Comparison of dye exclusion assays with a clonogenic assay in the determination of drug-induced cytotoxicity. *Cancer Res.* **43,** 258–264.
42. Gazdar, A. F., Steinberg, S. M., Russell, E. K., Linnoila, R. I., Oie, H. K., Ghosh, B. C., et al. (1990) Correlation of *in vitro* drug-sensitivity testing results with response to chemotherapy and survival in extensive-stage small cell lung cancer: a prospective clinical trial. *J. Natl. Cancer. Inst.* **82,** 117–124.
43. Lefer, A. M. and Lefer, D. J. (1993) Pharmacology of the endothelium in ischemia-reperfusion and circulatory shock. *Annu. Rev. Pharmacol. Toxicol.* **33,** 71–90.
44. Levine, R. L. (1993) Ischemia—from acidosis to oxidation. *FASEB J.* **7,** 1242–1246.
45. Slater, A. F., Stefan, C., Nobel, I., van den Dobbelsteen, D. J., and Orrenius, S. (1995) Signalling mechanisms and oxidative stress in apoptosis. *Toxicol. Lett.* **82–83,** 149–153.
46. Skehan, P., Storeng, R., Scudiero, D., Monks, A., McMahon, J., Vistica, D., et al. (1990) New colorimetric cytotoxicity assay for anticancer-drug screening. *J. Natl. Cancer. Inst.* **82,** 1107–1112.
47. Finlay, G. J., Wilson, W. R., and Baguley, B. C. (1986) Comparison of *in vitro* activity of cytotoxic drugs toward human carcinoma and leukaemia cell lines. *Eur. J. Cancer Clin. Oncol.* **22,** 655–662.
48. Sevin, B. U., Peng, Z. L., Perras, J. P., Ganjei, P., Penalver, M., and Averette, H. E. (1988) Application of an ATP-bioluminescence assay in human tumor chemosensitivity testing. *Gynecol. Oncol.* **31,** 191–204.
49. Jordan, M. A., Wendell, K., Gardiner, S., Derry, W. B., Copp, H., and Wilson, L. (1996) Mitotic block induced in HeLa cells by low concentrations of paclitaxel (taxol) results in abnormal mitotic exit and apoptotic cell death. *Cancer Res.* **56,** 816–825.

50. Fan, S. J., Eldeiry, W. S., Bae, I., Freeman, J., Jondle, D., Bhatia, K., et al. (1994) p53 gene mutations are associated with decreased sensitivity of human lymphoma cells to DNA damaging agents. *Cancer Res.* **54,** 5824–5830.
51. Parmar, J., Marshall, E. S., Charters, G. A., Holdaway, K. M., Shelling, A. N., and Baguley, B. C. (2000) Radiation-induced cell cycle delays and p53 status of early passage melanoma lines. *Oncol. Res.* **12,** 149–155.

38

The Hollow Fiber Assay

Leslie-Ann M. Hall, Candice M. Krauthauser, Roseanne S. Wexler, Andrew M. Slee, and Janet S. Kerr

1. Introduction

The hollow fiber assay is a unique in vivo model that allows simultaneous evaluation of up to 6 different cell lines in 2 physiological separate compartments. It was developed by Hollingshead et al. *(1)* as a preliminary rapid screen for assessing novel putative chemotherapeutic compounds prior to their evaluation in the mouse xenograft model. The hollow fiber model has a shorter evaluation time and a reduced compound requirement compared to traditional xenograft models. The model allows for the effective pairing of a novel compound with the appropriate cell line by its capacity to utilize multiple cell lines.

The hollow fiber assay has been used for the identification of tumor lines, which are sensitive to cytotoxic agents and for selection of treatment regimens for experimental compounds *(1,2)*. It has also been further optimized for the evaluation of compounds with defined mechanisms of actions, specifically cell cycle inhibitors, by selection of an initial cell density that generated a greater window of cell growth *(3)*. NCI-H460, non-small cell lung carcinoma, optimized using this approach, was treated with cisplatin (Platinol-AQ), a DNA damaging agent. A 70% growth inhibition resulted, which was comparable to the performance of cisplatin in the traditional xenograft model *(3)*. Krauthauser et al. *(4)* have used this model to study the effect of tetracycline-regulated gene expression in cell lines that did not form tumors in the xenograft model.

The hollow fiber assay has also shown utility in mechanistic studies. The expression of selected proteins can be investigated from the cells grown in the hollow fibers and corresponding bone marrow from treated and nontreated

From: *Methods in Molecular Medicine, vol. 74: Lung Cancer, Vol. 1: Molecular Pathology Methods and Reviews*
Edited by: B. Driscoll © Humana Press Inc., Totowa, NJ

animals through the use of Western-blot analysis *(3)*. This approach allows for a comparison of the effect of compounds on the cells within the fiber and the bone marrow, a cellular compartment that is sensitive to many therapeutic agents. The cells can also be extracted from the fiber and analyzed for protein concentration using standard protein assays and for the presence of compound levels using high-performance liquid chromatography (HPLC) or mass spectrometry.

The hollow fiber assay is not a replacement for traditional xenograft studies where the host-cell interactions are more complex. It does, however, offer an effective screening tool that is fast and uses minimal quantities of compound. However, the model requires considerable hands-on time and consists of the following steps: preparing fibers, preparing cells, loading fibers, implanting fibers, removing fibers, assaying for cell viability by MTT (3-4,5-dimethyl-thiazol-2-yl-2,5-diphenyl-tetrazolium bromide) dye conversion assay, and calculating percent net growth.

The data generated from the assay are expressed in terms of percent net growth, because it is not possible to consistently remove every cell from the fiber. However, estimations on the actual cell counts removed from the fiber can be determined by constructing standard curves from in vitro viability studies. Subsequent cell counts can then be estimated utilizing these standard curves.

1.2. Study Design

The hollow fiber assay is composed of in vitro and in vivo studies conducted in parallel. The day 0 in vitro study is used for determining the percent net growth in the test and control fibers. Other in vitro time points are run in parallel with the in vivo study as controls for the assay and/or as reference points for the dosing schedule. Fibers are loaded with cells and allowed to equilibrate/stabilize overnight before dispensing into in vitro and in vivo studies. The fibers can be implanted into two different physiological compartments (subcutaneous [sc] and/or peritoneal [ip] sites). The cells are allowed to equilibrate and grow in vivo for 3 d before beginning a dosing regimen. On d 3, fibers are removed from a group of animals to establish the percent net growth at the beginning of the treatment. In vitro fibers are also tested at this point as a control for the assay. Animals are dosed from d 3 to d 7 with study termination on d 7. All endpoints described herein were arbitrarily assigned and can be adjusted to suit the study; therefore, it is important to assess the growth profile of each cell line in vivo prior to conducting any studies. The growth profiles are typically conducted by varying cell densities implanted into the sc and ip compartments over a 7–10 d period and determining cell viability by the MTT dye conversion assay at d 3, 7, and 10 (*see* **Fig. 1**). Based on the growth characteristics of each cell line the appropriate cell-loading concentration and study termination points can be determined (*see* **Note 1**).

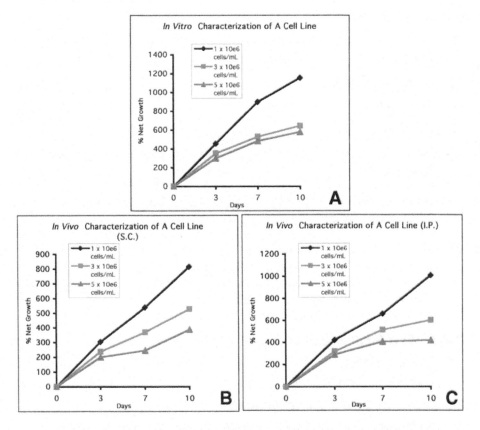

Fig. 1. Typical growth profiles of varying cell densities in vitro (**A**) and implanted in the subcutaneous (**B**) and intraperitoneal (**C**) compartments over 10 d.

2. Materials

2.1. Preparation of Fibers

1. Polyvinylidene fluoride (PVDF) hollow fibers: 500,000 dalton molecular weight exclusion, 1.0 mm ID (Spectrum Medical Industries, #S9320101-4 for white, blue, green and yellow).
2. 70% Ethanol (EtOH).
3. Nalgene Instrument/Pipet Sterilizing Pan, polypropylene (VWR #62662-751).
4. Autoclavable Polypropylene Bags, Scienceware (12″ × 24″) #H13185-1224 (Bel-Art Product, Pequannock, NJ).
5. Sterilization Pouches, 5″ × 10″ (Propper Manufacturing Co., Long Island, NY #024010).
6. BD Intramedic Luer Stub Adapter, Sterile (Clay Adams Brand #427564).
7. Diack Sterilization Monitors 256F/121C (Diack #H15912-30).
8. Syringes (50cc).

2.2. Cells

1. Appropriate complete medium.
2. Hemacytometer or cell counting device.

2.3. Loading Fibers

1. Prepared fibers,
2. Cell suspension.
3. Smooth-jawed needle holder with scissors.
4. Bacti-Cinerator III Heat Chamber (Oxford Labware, St. Louis, MO, #8889-001007).
5. Syringes (5 and 10 mL).
6. BD Intramedic Luer Stub Adapter, Sterile (Clay Adams Brand #427564).
7. 6-Well tissue culture plates.
8. Dressing forceps with serrated tips: 4.5″ (for handling fibers) and 6″ (for removing sterile fibers from the Nalgene sterilizing pan).
9. 500 cm^2 Square tissue-culture dish, sterile (VWR 25382-327).
10. Mixer (Clay Adams Brand Nutator Mixer, Becton Dickinson, Sparks, MD) (Innovative Medical Systems, Ivyland, PA).
11. Lab Marker, black (VWR Brand #52877-310).

2.4. In Vitro Fiber Study

1. Complete medium.
2. 6-Well tissue culture dishes.

2.5. Implanting Fibers into Animals

1. Nude mice, minimum of 5 wk old (Taconic Farms, Germantown, NY).
2. Loaded fibers.
3. Instruments.
   a. Iris Scissors, straight (4.5″).
   b. Cancer-implant needles (Trocar), 11-gauge by Popper & Sons (VWR #20068-792).
   c. ADSON tissue forceps, 4.75″ with 1 × 2 teeth (for holding skin and/or peritoneal lining); dressing forceps with serrated tips, 4.5″ (for handling fibers).
   d. Clip applier (Roboz, Rockville, MD #RS9260).
   e. Wound clips (Auto Clips) MikRon Precision Inc. (Biomedical Research Instruments, Rockville, MD #205016).
4. Hot bead sterilizer (Biomedical Res. Instruments, Rockville, MD #55-2000).
5. Metofane (Methoxyflurane) (Mallinckrodt Vet. #556850) (*see* **Note 13**).
6. Betadine or povidone-iodine topical solution, USP swabs (James Alexander Corp., Blairstown, NJ #773).
7. Alcohol pads.
5. Gauze pads.
6. Bell jar.

7. Isoflurane (AIRCO Rare & Specialty Gases).
8. FORANE (Isoflurane), Sensor Device Inc. (SDI). VAPORTEC Series 5 (Viking Medical Products, Medford Lakes, NJ).

2.6. Removal of Fibers

1. 6-Well tissue-culture plate.
2. Complete medium.
3. Instruments.
   a. Scissors, 5″, Sharp-Blunt Points.
   b. Dressing forceps with serrated tips, 4″ (for handling fibers) and ADSON tissue forceps, 4.75″ with 1 × 2 teeth (for holding skin and/or peritoneal lining).
4. CO_2 (to euthanize animals).

2.7. MTT Dye Conversion Assay

1. DMSO (dimethyl sulfoxide).
2. MTT #M2128 (Sigma #M-2003, St. Louis, MO).
3. Protamine sulfate (Sigma #P-4380).
4. 24- and 96-Well plates.
5. Microtiter plate reader.

3. Methods
3.1. Fiber Preparations

The hollow fibers are available in four colors: white, yellow, blue, and green. Additional distinctive groups can be prepared by marking the end of the fiber segments with a black lab marker during the loading process. The fibers are purchased in approx 36″ segments. The following procedure describes preparation of dry hollow fibers. Spectrum Medical Instruments now provides fibers already prepared and stored in 70% EtOH.

1. Cut fibers into 6″ sections. The fibers are closed at the end by the cutting process.
2. Open each end of the 6″ section by gently squeezing on the end.
3. Put approx 500 mL of 70% EtOH into the Nalgene Instrument/Pipet Sterilizing Pan. Adjust volume to completely cover the 6″ fiber sections.
4. Fill a 50cc syringe with 70% EtOH and place the BD intramedic luer stub adapter on the end of the syringe. (Any size syringe may be used.)
5. Insert the adapter into one end of the fiber section and flush 70% EtOH through the fiber.
6. Place the EtOH prepared fiber into the pan of 70% EtOH.
7. Repeat process for each fiber segment.
8. Check that the fibers are completely covered with 70% EtOH and cover the pan.
9. Label the pan (fiber color, 70% EtOH, and date) and store pan at room temperature.
10. Soak fibers in the 70% EtOH for a minimum of 3 d and up to 2 wk.

11. Place approx 500 mL of deionized (dI) water into a Nalgene Instrument/Pipet Sterilizing Pan.
12. Fill a 50cc syringe with dI water and place the BD intramedic luer stub adapter on the end of the syringe. (Any size syringe may be used.)
13. Insert the adapter into one end of the 70% EtOH soaked fiber and flush dI water through the fiber.
14. Place the dI water flushed fiber into the dI water pan.
15. Repeat process for each 70% EtOH soaked fiber section.
16. Adjust dI water volume to completely cover the fiber sections and add the Diack sterilization monitor to the pan. The Diack tube should be completely submerged in the water and the attached string should hang over the edge of the pan. Cover the pan with a lid.
17. Label the pan with the fiber color, dI water, and date.
18. Place the pan in an autoclave bag, seal bag (with autoclave tape) and sterilize.
19. Sterilize on a liquid setting with drying time (*see* **Note 2**). After the sterilization cycle allow the pan to cool.
20. Carefully remove the autoclave bag and place the pan in a biosafety cabinet.
21. Check the Diack sterilization monitor to determine that the pan contents have been sterilized. The fibers can now be loaded with cells or stored until needed (*see* **Note 3**).

3.2. Cells

1. The cells are grown under standard growth conditions.
2. Remove cells from the flask by standard method (i.e., trypsinization).
3. Determine cell count by using a hemacytometer or equivalent method.
4. Resuspend cells to the appropriate concentration in complete medium.
5. Place cells on ice until ready for use.
6. Fill 50-mL tubes with complete medium (medium with the required additives for growth of the cells) and place on ice.
7. Prepare 6-well culture dishes by adding 2–4 mL of complete medium to each well and storing dishes at 2–8°C. Prepare sufficient dishes or wells to hold 4–10 2 cm cell-loaded fiber sections. The more fibers placed in the well, the more medium needed/well. All the fiber sections need to be completely covered with medium.
8. Place the prepared 6-well plates into the refrigerator until needed in the fiber-loading process.

3.3. Fiber Loading

Sterile technique is required for loading cells into the prepared sterile fibers. The cells should be loaded into the fibers in a biosafety cabinet and sterile gloves (or apply 70% EtOH to nonsterile gloves before use) should be used for handling all materials (sterile fibers, sterile instruments and cells).

1. Sterilize 2 pair of dressing forceps and 1 pair of needle holders with scissors for each cell preparation.
2. Prepare the work area by thoroughly wiping out the biosafety cabinet with 70% EtOH.
3. Place the following items into the biosafety cabinet: the fiber pan, the Bacti-Cinerator III Heat Chamber and a sterile tray (500cm² Square tissue-culture dish) for the actual fiber loading. (Either the lid or the bottom half of the 500 cm² square tissue culture dish can be used for fiber loading.) A new dish should be used for each cell line. To maintain sterility, only open the culture dish in the biosafety cabinet.
4. Position a flat ruler under the fiber loading tray to use for measuring the fiber sections.
5. Prepare mixer to hold cell-suspension syringe. A suitable set-up would be as follows:
   a. Place a sterile, 15 mL conical tube on top of a small ice pack/freezer gel pack.
   b. Wrap a paper towel across the tube and around the ice pack.
   c. Attach tape to the paper towel to hold the tube in place on the ice pack and to secure the ice pack on the mixer.
   d. Place the mixer set-up into the biosafety cabinet and remove the top of the 15-mL conical tube (*see* **Note 4**).
6. Place the 50-mL tube of complete medium into the biosafety cabinet.
7. In the biosafety cabinet, attach a luer stub adapter to a 10-mL syringe and fill the syringe with complete medium from the 50-mL tube.
8. Pour the balance of the complete medium into the fiber-loading tray and place the 10-mL syringe on the edge of the fiber-loading tray with the luer stub adapter directed downward on the tray.
9. In the biosafety cabinet, attach another luer stub adapter to a 5-mL syringe.
10. Rock the tube containing the cell suspensions 2–3 times before filling the 5-mL syringe.
11. Place the 5-mL syringe into the 15-mL tube set-up on the mixer. Start the mixer so the cells are gently rotated.
12. Place the sterile instruments (2 pairs of dressing forceps and needle holder with scissors) on the edge of the fiber loading dish in the biosafety cabinet.
13. Turn on the Bacti-Cinerator Heat Chamber.
14. Remove approx 6 fiber sections from the pan using 1 pair of forceps and place them on the fiber-loading tray (*see* **Note 5**). Pick-up one fiber and hold it loosely between fingers. Flush cold, complete medium through the fiber using the 10-mL syringe to remove any residual water from the fiber.
15. Place the fiber in the medium on the fiber-loading dish (*see* **Note 6**). Repeat the process with all the fibers on the dish.
16. Remove the 5-mL syringe containing the cell suspension from the mixer and rock it back and forth 2–3 times to ensure the cells are mixed. Pick-up one

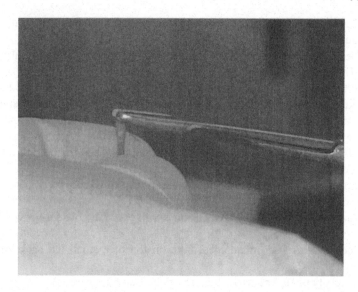

Fig. 2. Heat-sealing the end of cell-loaded fiber using needle holder.

medium-filled fiber and hold it loosely looped between fingers, such that both ends of the fiber are facing upward.

17. Flush the cell suspension through the fiber to fill it (*see* **Note 7**). Return the syringe containing the cell suspension to the 15-mL conical tube on the mixer.

18. Place the end of the needle holder into the Bacti-Cinerator Heat Chamber and hold it there for approx 4–8 s.

19. Use the hot needle holder to seal one end of the fiber by closing the needle holder around the end of the fiber and slightly pulling with the needle holder to stretch the fiber end shut (*see* **Note 8**). The needle holder should be hot enough to slightly melt the fiber end and allow the end of the fiber to stretch-out with a slight pull of the needle holder. The needle holder should not be hot enough to completely burn the end of the fiber (*see* **Fig. 2**).

20. Release the sealed end of the fiber from fingers and using the same procedure (*see* **Subheading 3.3., steps 18,19**) seal the other end of the fiber at or slightly below the fluid level in the fiber.

21. Place the sealed fiber back into the medium on the fiber-loading dish.

22. Repeat this process (*see* **Subheading 3.3., steps 16–21**) with all the fibers on the fiber-loading dish.

23. Using the second pair of forceps, position the cell-loaded fiber in the fiber-loading dish on top of the ruler (the ruler is located under the fiber-loading dish).

24. Hold one end of the fiber in place over the ruler with the forceps.

25. Use the ruler to measure 2-cm segments and mark the segments on the fiber by clamping the needle holder (cold) at each location. This process will make crimp

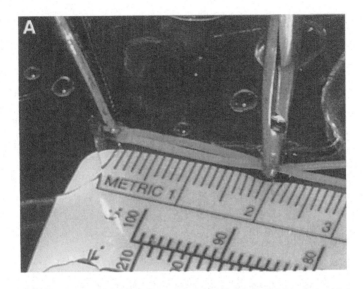

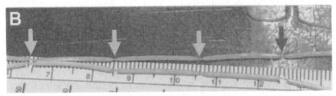

Fig. 3. (**A**) Marking 2 cm segments on the cell-loaded fiber by positioning the fiber near the ruler (located under the fiber-loading dish) and using the needle holder to crimp the location. (**B**) Cell-loaded fiber that has been marked every 2 cm using a needle holder. The arrows indicate the crimp marks. This process allows for equal-sized implant fibers.

marks on the fiber and will allow for preparing equal-sized implant fibers for the study (*see* **Fig. 3A** and **B**).

26. Repeat this process (*see* **Subheading 3.3., steps 23–25**) for each fiber on the fiber loading dish.

27. Pick-up one fiber and position it such that the thumb and fourth (ring) finger will be below the 2-cm crimp mark and the index and middle finger will be above the 2-cm crimp mark (*see* **Notes 9**).

28. Place the needle holder into the Bacti-Cinerator for 4–8 s. The needle holder should only be hot enough to slightly melt the fiber but not completely burn through the fiber. Clamp the needle holder over the 2-cm mark on the fiber while slightly pulling the fiber in opposite directions with each set of fingers. The fiber will have a stretched/transparent-look at this location (*see* **Note 8**) and will be sealed on both ends (*see* **Fig. 4**). Using the scissor portion of the needle

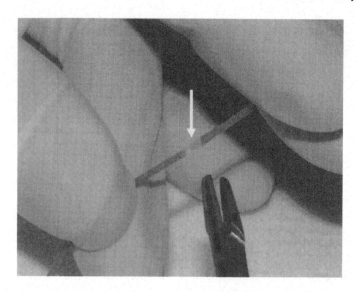

Fig. 4. Cell-loaded fiber that has been heat-sealed at the 2-cm crimp mark. The arrow indicated the heat-sealed area, which has a stretched/transparent appearance. The fiber is sealed at both ends of this area. Scissors are then used to separate the sections.

holder, cut off the 2 cm section in the middle of the stretched section or heat seal (*see* **Fig. 5**).

29. Place the 2-cm section in the medium on the fiber-loading dish.
30. Repeat process (*see* **Subheading 3.3., steps 28, 29**) at each 2-cm crimp mark on the fiber.
31. Repeat process (*see* **Subheading 3.3., steps 27–30**) with all the fibers on the fiber-loading dish.
32. Remove the 6-well plate from the refrigerator and place it in the biosafety cabinet. Put the 2-cm cell-loaded fiber sections into the wells and return the plate to 2–8°C.
33. Repeat entire process (*see* **Subheading 3.3., steps 14–32**) until all study fibers are prepared.
34. Place the 6-well culture dishes containing the 2-cm sections into the 37°C incubator with 5% CO_2 overnight.
35. Prepare a key of the fiber color, cell line, and/or condition for each study. Additional fiber colors can be prepared by applying a black lab marker to the end of any color of the hollow fibers (*see* **Note 10**).

3.4. In Vitro (Parallel) Assay

Before the implantation process, fiber sections are set aside for the parallel in vitro study. The in vitro time points tested for viability by the MTT dye conversion assay should also correspond with in vivo study actions.

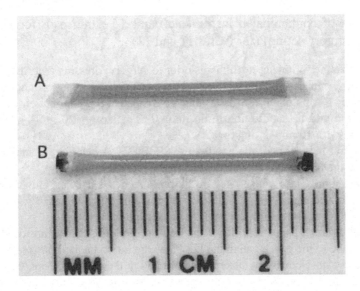

Fig. 5. Finished 2-cm cell-loaded implant fibers: **(A)** standard, unaltered color and **(B)** standard color distinguished by the application of a lab marker during the fiber-loading process.

Timepoints

In Vitro	In Vivo Study Actions
Day 0	Fibers are implanted into study animals (only in vitro fibers tested for viability).
Day 3	Dosing begins for study animals and in vivo fibers are also collected from a group of the study animals.
Day 7	Study terminated and in vivo fibers are collected from study animals.

1. Label separate 6-well plates for in vitro termination time points: d 0, d 3, and d 7. Four fibers of each cell line or condition being evaluated are needed at each in vitro time point.
2. In the biosafety cabinet, pipet 2 mL of complete pre-warmed medium/well.
3. Remove the plates containing the 2-cm cell-loaded fiber sections from the incubator. Place 4 cell-loaded fiber sections of each cell line or condition/well in each of the in vitro 6-well plates.
4. Perform the MTT dye conversion assay on d 0 in vitro fibers as described in **Subheading 3.7.**

3.5. Implantation of Fibers into Animals

Set-up for fiber implantation requires a hood for use of metofane, an animal recovery area with heating pad and a bell jar to anesthetize the animals. Additional items needed but not required are a hot bead sterilizer (for quick sterilization of contaminated instruments) and a heating pad (for placement under the surgery set-up) (*see* **Notes 11** and **12**).

1. Sterilize the following instruments prior to surgery: dressing and ADSON tissue forceps, cancer-implanting needles (trocars), iris scissors, wound clips, clip applier, Q-tips or cotton balls, and gauze pads (for application of betadine solution and to handle nonsterile items). Sterilize for 20 min on instrument setting with 10 min drying time.
2. Wipe out the inside of the hood with 70% EtOH. A heating pad may be placed inside the hood at the intended work area.
3. In the hood, place gauze pads in the bottom of the bell jar and add metofane to slightly dampen the pads. Place the separator over the gauze pads (the pads should not stick through the holes in the separator).
4. Place a gauze pad in the lid of the bell jar. Holding the lid upside down add metofane to the gauze pad in the lid. Place the lid on the bell jar (*see* **Note 13**).
5. Prepare "nose cones" by placing a gauze pad in the tip of a 50-mL conical tube. Carefully add metofane to only the gauze pad. Remove any metofane spilled on the inside of the tube.
6. Place sterile pads over the heating pad (optional) and/or intended work area being careful not to touch the intended surgery area on the pad.
7. Place sterile instruments, alcohol pads, and betadine sticks on the sterile pad. If available, turn on the hot bead sterilizer.
8. Position 6-well plates containing the cell-loaded fibers near intended surgery site for easy access during the implantation process.

3.5.1. SC Surgery (see **Note 14**)

1. Anesthetize the animal (mouse) in the bell jar containing the metofane.
2. Remove the animal from the bell jar and position on abdomen with the nose inside the "nose cone" but not touching the gauze pads. This will help to keep the mouse anesthetized through the entire implantation process.

   Apply betadine to the nape of the neck and then wipe the area with alcohol (pad).
3. Using ADSON tissue forceps, pick up the skin at the base of the neck. Cut a slit (0.5–1.0 cm) in the skin through the connective tissue.
4. Continue to hold the skin up (forming a tent) and insert dressing forceps into the incision. Open and close the forceps under the skin a couple of times to clear a pocket for implanting the fibers and then release the skin.
5. Using dressing forceps, load fibers into the trocar.
6. Again, pick-up the skin at the incision, place the trocar into the incision and push the base to place the fibers caudally under the skin (*see* **Fig. 6**).
7. Remove the trocar and use the ADSON tissue forceps to hold the skin on both sides of the incision closed.
8. Use a clip applier to close the incision with a wound clip. Typically 1 clip is all that is needed.

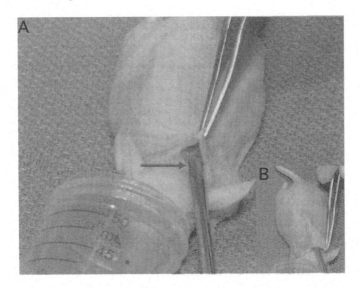

Fig. 6. sc Surgery (**A**) A smll incision is made through the skin. The arrow indicates fibers that have been loaded into the trocar. The trocar is inserted into the incision to place the fibers under the skin. (**B**) The fibers are then further positioned on the back of the animal with the trocar.

9. Put the animal in the recovery area or prepare for ip fiber implantation.
10. Recover the animal by placing it in a warm area and monitoring the breathing (*see* **Note 15**). The animal should be moving around within a few minutes and can be returned to the cage.

3.5.2. IP Surgery

1. The ip fiber implantation process requires the insertion of fibers into the peritoneal cavity; therefore, it is crucial to take necessary precautions to minimize contamination. Wear sterile gloves, minimize contaminating gloves by using the sterile gauze pads to touch anything that is not sterile including handling the mice, lids on the 6-well plates, alcohol pad packaging, and the holder on the betadine stick.
2. Position the animal on its side with the nose inserted in the "nose cone."
3. Thoroughly disinfect the abdomen with betadine and then wipe the area with a alcohol pad.
4. Use the ADSON tissue forceps to pick-up the skin on the side of the abdomen. With the scissors, make a small incision (0.5–1.0 cm) through the skin.
5. Move the ADSON tissue forceps into the incision and pick-up the intraperitoneal lining. Make an incision (0.5–1.0 cm) through the lining being careful not to nick/cut any organs beneath the lining.

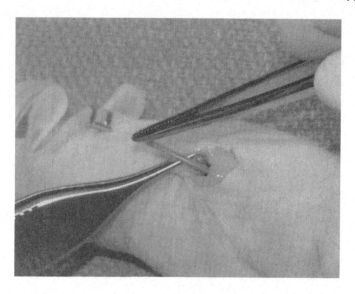

Fig. 7. ip Surgery: A small incision is made through the skin and the peritoneal lining. Fibers are implanted into the cavity using forceps.

6. Hold the intraperitoneal lining up (forming a tent) and carefully insert the fibers into the cavity using the dressing forceps. Lay the fibers flat under the intraperitoneal lining and do not disrupt the placement of the organs (*see* **Fig. 7**).
7. Use the forceps to hold the intraperitoneal lining incision closed and then take the ADSON tissue forceps to hold the skin incision closed as well as the ip lining.
8. Remove the forceps that were holding only the intraperitoneal lining and use this hand to close both incisions with the clip applier. Typically 1–2 clips are needed to close the incisions.
9. The animal may now be placed in recovery (*see* **Subheading 3.5.1., step 10**) or prepared for the sc fiber implantation (*see* **Subheading 3.5.1., step 2**).
10. Repeat implantation process for all study animals

3.6. Fiber Removal

1. Prepare 6-well culture dishes for collecting the fibers to be removed from the study animals by adding 2 mL of pre-warmed complete medium to each well (*see* **Note 16**).
2. Euthanize the animals with CO_2 (but no more than 5–10 animals at a time) and collect the fibers promptly.
3. Remove the fibers from the sc site by lifting the skin near the fibers with ADSON tissue forceps and making an incision through the skin parallel to the fibers with scissors (sharp-blunt point scissors).

4. Make another incision above the fibers and fold the skin back.
5. Use dressing forceps to remove the fibers from under the skin.
6. Gently wipe the fibers off with a kimwipe and place them in the medium of the appropriate collection well.
7. Position the animal on its side, lift the skin on the abdomen with ADSON tissue forceps, and cut crosswise through the skin.
8. Cut a large opening in the skin and fold the skin back.
9. Lift the peritoneal lining with forceps and make an incision through the lining being careful not to cut the fibers.
10. Cut a large opening in the lining and carefully remove the fibers using dressing forceps (*see* **Note 17**). Gently wipe the fibers with a kimwipe and place them in the appropriate collection well.
11. Dispose of animals according to in-house procedures.

3.7. MTT Dye Conversion Assay

3.7.1. Reagent Preparation

1. Protamine Sulfate. Prepare a 2.5% solution of protamine sulfate in saline and filter (0.2 micron). Store at 2–8°C (*see* **Note 18**).
2. MTT: Prepare a 5 mg/mL stock of MTT in saline and filter (0.2 micron). The solution should be yellow in color and is light-sensitive (cover container with foil). Store at 2–8°C.
3. MTT Working Solution: Prepare a 1 mg/mL solution of MTT from the 5 mg/mL stock in the appropriate complete medium. Warm the working solution in a 37°C waterbath before use.

3.7.2. Assay

1. Add 1 mL of MTT working solution (1 mg/mL) to well containing 2 mL of complete medium and fibers.
2. Incubate at 37°C in 5% CO_2 for 4 h.
3. Aspirate MTT-medium solution from well.
4. Wash fibers by adding 2 mL of 2.5% protamine sulfate solution to each well. Store at 4°C overnight.
5. Perform a second wash with 2.5% protamine sulfate solution the following day at 4°C for a minimum of 2 h (*see* **Note 19**). Remove the fibers from the protamine sulfate and gently wipe off with kimwipe.
6. Place one fiber into each well of a 24-well culture dish and then cut each fiber in half (*see* **Note 20**). Label wells/plates clearly to indicate termination date, fiber location, treatment and animal number.
7. Allow the fibers to dry by placing the culture dishes in a biosafety hood, near the vent/air flow (*see* **Note 21**). The formazan is light sensitive; therefore, the plates should be covered and/or stored in the dark.
8. Extract the formazan by adding 250 µL of dimethyl sulfoxide (DMSO) to each well (fiber). Cover the plate with aluminum foil.

9. Place plates on a shaker at a low to medium speed for 4 h at room temperature. (The shaker speed should be sufficient to shake the samples but not splash the DMSO out of the wells.)
10. Transfer 150 μL of the extracted material from each well to a 96-well plate.
11. Read the 96-well plate at 540 nm on a microplate reader.

3.7.3. Calculations

1. At study termination the viable cell mass contained within the hollow fibers is determined by using the "stable-end point" MTT dye conversion assay. The results are expressed in terms of percent net growth. The d 0 in vitro time point is the most critical measurement for interpreting the results. The percent net growth is calculated by normalizing the data in terms of the d 0 in vitro result. This time point establishes the state of the cells at the initiation of the study and all results are expressed relative to cell growth from this starting point.
2. The d 3 in vitro result is used as a control for the assay. This time point typically marks the beginning of the dosing regimen and shows that the cells are continuing to grow in the hollow fibers. The d 3 in vivo result indicates the starting cell growth for the implanted fibers. Both the in vitro and in vivo data for this time point are expressed in relationship to the d 0 in vitro result.
3. The d 7 in vitro result is also a control for the assay that marks the cell growth in the hollow fibers at the study termination point. The in vivo result indicates the cell growth for the implanted fibers at the end of the dosing regimen and end of study. These results are also expressed in relationship to d 0 in vitro result.
4. Net growth formula:
   (sample OD – d 0 in vitro mean OD/ d 0 in vitro mean OD) × 100

3.8. Cell Growth Profiles

Prior to conducting any studies it is important to establish the growth characteristics of each cell line in hollow fibers in vivo and in vitro.

1. For each cell line prepare several different concentrations of cells (0.5×10^6 – 1×10^7 cells/mL) as described in **Subheading 3.2.**
2. Load prepared fibers with the varying cell concentrations as described in **Subheading 3.3.**
3. Set-aside fibers for the parallel in vitro study described in **Subheading 3.4.** and add fibers for a d 10 termination point.
4. Implant fibers into both physiological compartments (sc and ip) as described in **Subheading 3.5.**
5. Perform MTT assay (*see* **Subheading 3.7.**) on d 0 in vitro fibers the day of implantation.
6. Collect in vitro and in vivo fibers at d 3, 7, and 10 (*see* **Subheading 3.6.**) and assess for viability using the MTT assay.

Construct growth curves and determine optimum cell concentration and study termination points (*see* **Fig. 1**) with percent net growth vs time (*see* **Note 22**).

3.9. Cell Count Estimations

Because it is not possible to reproducibly flush all the cells from the fiber at study termination, in vitro standard curves can be constructed to define cell number with OD readings. Utilizing the MTT dye conversion assay an estimate of the cell count within the fibers can be determined.

1. For each cell line prepare different concentrations of cells from 1×10^4 to 1×10^7 cells/mL (or cover the concentration range expected for your studies).
2. Load each concentration of cells into at least 4 fiber sections, as described in **Subheading 3.3.**).
3. Place the loaded fibers into 6-well plates (4 fiber sections/well) containing 2 mL of appropriate complete medium.
4. Store 6-well plates (with and without loaded fiber sections) at 2–8°C until all cell concentrations have been loaded into fibers.
5. After all cell concentrations have been loaded into fibers, add 1 mL of the MTT working solution to each well and incubate at 37°C with 5% CO_2 for 4 h. Follow MTT assay procedure as described in **Subheading 3.7.**
6. Determine the mean OD for each cell concentration. The intra-assay variability can be determined for each concentration by calculating standard deviation and percent coefficient of variation (%CV).
7. Construct a standard curve with the cell concentrations and the mean OD values.
8. Repeat process (*see* **Subheading 3.9.**, steps 1–7) twice to allow for interassay variability in cell count estimations.
9. Construct a final standard curve for each cell line with mean values from the multiple curves (*see* **Fig. 8**).
10. Approximate cell numbers can be determined in subsequent hollow fiber studies using the OD values with the corresponding in vitro standard curve.

3.10. Total Protein/Western-Blot Analysis

1. Cut the ends of the fibers off. Use a syringe (with the BD intramedic luer stub adapter attached) containing the appropriate buffer to flush the cells out of the fiber.
2. For total protein the fibers can be flushed with 0.2 mL of a sample buffer containing aprotinin, leupeptin, and 4-(2-aminoethyl)-benzenesulfonyl fluoride (aebsf) into eppendorf tubes. The samples are then vortexed, heated at 97°C for 3 min, and stored at –70°C until evaluated by standard protein assay.
3. For Western-blot analysis the fibers can be flushed with a Tris-HCl sample buffer containing sodium dodecyl sulfate (SDS), glycerol, and β-mercaptoethanol into

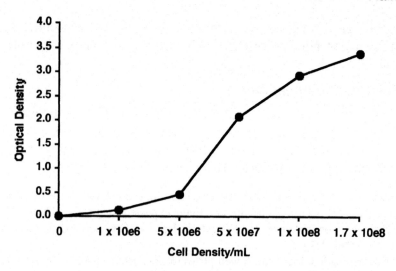

Fig. 8. Example of standard curve used for cell-count estimations in the fibers.

eppendorf tubes. The sample buffer used for the protein assay can also be used for Western-blot samples with the addition of dithiothreitol.

4. The samples are then heated for 5 min at 95°C and stored at –70°C until evaluated.

5. The cellular proteins can be separated by SDS-polyacrylamide gel electrophoresis (PAGE), transferred to nitrocellulose, probed with the specific primary antibody and visualized with a substrate system using standard techniques.

4. Notes

1. A typical set-up for a (dosing) study with 1 cell line, 25 animals, implantation at 2 sites and 7-d study termination:

   A. Animals:
      1. 5 animals for d 3 in vivo termination point.
      2. 10 animals for controls (dosed from d 3–7 with vehicle control).
      3. 10 animals for treatment (dosed from d 3–7 with compound/drug).

   B. Total fiber count would be 62. (Prepare additional fibers, [approx 15%] for unexpected incidents to give a total of 71 fibers.)
      1. 12 fibers for in vitro parallel study (4 fibers/termination point); termination points would be d 0, d 3, and d 7.
      2. 25 fibers for sc implantation (1 fiber implanted sc/animal).
      3. 25 fibers for ip implantation (1 fiber implanted ip/animal).

   C. Schedule
      1. Fibers would be implanted in animals on d 0. In vitro fibers designated for d 0 would be tested by the MTT dye conversion assay.
      2. On d 3, 5 animals would be euthanized and fibers removed from the sc and ip compartments to determine cell viability at the beginning of the

dosing regimen. Day 3 in vitro fibers would also be tested by the MTT dye conversion assay at this time.

3. On d 3, dosing would begin for the 10 treated and untreated animals.
4. Animals would be dosed from d 3 to d 7.
5. On d 7 the study would terminate with the collection of all the in vivo fibers from the treated and untreated animals. The MTT dye conversion assay would be performed on the in vivo fibers and d 7 designated in vitro fibers as described in **Subheading 3.7.**

2. The sterilization time is dependent on the container, liquid volume and container contents. Prior to sterilization of fibers, optimize the sterilization time for the specific materials and equipment being used. Optimize by placing a measured volume of water into the appropriate container with a Diack sterilization monitor and varying the sterilization time until the monitor indicates sterilization was obtained. A typical sterilization cycle for a Beta Star autoclave using a $45.6'' \times 15.2'' \times 6.7''$ container with approx 150 fiber sections in 500 mL of dI water was 70 min on the liquid setting with 20 min drying time.

3. The fibers will remain sterile if handled properly (only open container in a biosafety cabinet). For extended storage monitor the water level in the container and add sterile water as needed.

4. The tube is used to hold the cell suspension syringe, the ice pack is used to keep the cell suspension cold and the mixer is used to keep the cells suspended through out the fiber-loading process. (This set-up allows for an even distribution of viable cells loaded into the fibers.)

5. The number of fiber sections removed at a time is dependent on the amount of time needed to load the fibers. Process fibers in numbers that can be completed in 10–15 min to minimize the amount of time the cells are at room temperature on the fiber-loading tray. Designate this pair of forceps for removal of fibers from the fiber pan only and position them such that they are not contaminated by any other items used in the process.

6. Fibers must remain wet during processing. Dry fibers have a white appearance. Fibers that dry during processing must be discarded.

7. The cell suspension will feel cool to the touch as it passes through the fiber near the fingers. Depending on the cell density, a change in appearance may also be observed.

8. If the fiber is white in color (vs transparent) at the heat seal then the ends are not sealed.

9. This is suggested fingering for sealing off the 2-cm fiber sections. The objective is to hold the fiber around the 2-cm crimp mark in a manner to ultimately allow pulling in opposite directions with fingers.

10. Additional fiber colors can be prepared by applying a black lab marker to the end of any color of the hollow fibers. The hollow fibers are prepared as previously described (*see* **Subheadings 3.1.** and **3.3.**). The lab marker is applied during the cell loading process and the separation of the 2-cm sections. After the cell suspension is flushed through the fiber (*see* **Subheading 3.3., steps 16, 17**),

the needle holder is warmed in the Bacti-Cinerator for 2–4 s and then clamped over the tip of the lab marker for 2–3 s. The needle holder is placed back in the Bacti-Cinerator and the fiber end is sealed as described in **Subheading 4.3., steps 19, 20**. The process is repeated with the lab marker before sealing the other end of the cell-loaded fiber (*see* **Subheading 3.3., step 20**). Seal all the cell-loaded fibers on the dish with the application of the lab marker and the process continues as described in **Subheading 3.3., steps 23–26**. After the 2-cm sections have been marked with the needle holder, the needle holder is again warmed in the Bacti-Cinerator for 2–4 s and then clamped over the tip of the lab marker for 2–3 s. The needle holder is placed back into the Bacti-Cinerator and the process of separating the 2 cm sections continues as described in **Subheading 3.3., steps 27–29**. The 2-cm fiber section will have black marks on the sealed ends that distinguish the fiber as a different color (*see* **Fig. 4B**). The process is repeated with the application of the lab marker before the separation of the next 2-cm section.

11. A hot bead sterilizer, if available, allows for quick sterilization of instruments that become contaminated during the implantation process.

12. A heating pad can also be used under the surgery set-up to keep the anesthetized animal warm during the ip surgery.

13. Metofane was typically used (in a hood) to anesthetize animals in our hollow fiber studies. Metofane is no longer available but isoflurane is a suitable substitute with the appropriate equipment. **Figure 9** is one example of an isoflurane set-up (A FORANE (Isoflurane), Sensor Device Inc. (SDI). VAPORTEC Series 5).

14. The implantation process works best with two people. One person handles the mice (animals) and performs sc surgeries. The second person can then remain sterile to perform the more invasive ip surgeries.

15. If the animal's breathing is shallow, try gentle pats on the chest or a gentle breath toward the nose.

16. Prepare sufficient culture dishes to collect separate wells for the surgery sites (2) and for each animal.

17. The fibers implanted into the ip cavity tend to shift and may be found underneath or between organs. A careful search is sometimes required.

18. Protamine sulfate is slow to go into solution so gradually add the protamine sulfate to the saline with continuous mixing.

19. The second protamine sulfate wash should be a minimum of 2 h and a maximum of 2 wk. The plates are maintained at 2–8°C during this time.

20. If lab marker was applied to the end of fiber during the loading process then the crimped, marked ends of the fiber must also be removed.

21. Drying usually takes at least 12 h. Fibers should be completely dry before continuing the process.

22. A typical set-up for the growth profile of 1 cell line:
    A. Fibers
       1. 1 fiber color/cell density (3 different densities) = 3 colors of hollow fibers.
       2. 5 mice/termination point (d 3, d 7, and d 10 termination\points) = 15 mice.

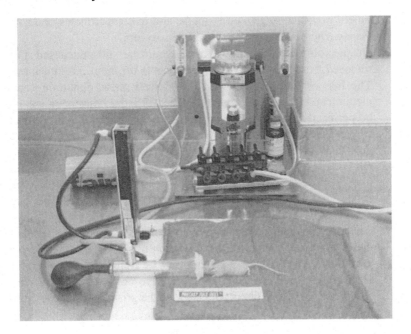

Fig. 9. An isoflurane set-up.

3. sc and ip implantations = 2 sites.
4. Four fibers/cell density/termination point for the in vitro parallel study (day 0, day 3, day 7, and day 10 termination points).
5. Total fiber count/cell density = 46 fibers. (Prepare additional fibers, [approx 15%] as back-up [unexpected incidents] for a total of 53 fibers. Also, 2 test fibers/cell density/site could be evaluated since each site can hold up to 6 fibers. This would increase the fiber count/cell density to 76, excluding additional fibers.)
   in vitro study (4 fibers × 4 termination points) = 16 fibers.
   in vivo, sc = (1 fiber × 15 mice) = 15 fibers.
   in vivo, ip = (1 fiber × 15 mice) = 15 fibers.

B. Schedule
1. Fibers would be loaded with varying cell densities on a Thursday. The fibers would be incubated overnight in an incubator at 37°C with 5% CO_2.
2. Fibers would be set-aside in 6 well plates for in vitro parallel study on Friday. Four plates would be prepared for each termination point (d 0, d 3, d 7, and d 10) with 4 fibers/cell density/well and labeled appropriately. The MTT dye conversion assay would be performed on the d 0 in vitro fibers. The plate would be stored at 2–8°C (second wash) until all the growth profile fibers were collected.

3. Fibers would be implanted in the sc and ip compartments of 15 mice on Friday. There would be 1 fiber/cell density/site.

4. On the following Monday, 5 mice would be euthanized and the fibers removed from the sc and ip compartments for the d 3 termination point. The fibers would be collected into 6-well plates containing complete medium and labeled appropriately. The MTT dye conversion assay would be performed on these in vivo fibers as well as the d 3 in vitro parallel study. The plates would be stored at 2–8°C (second wash) until all the growth profile fibers were collected.

5. On Friday (1 week after implantation), 5 mice would be euthanized and the fibers removed for the d 7 termination point (same procedure as described for d 3 in **step 4**). Again the MTT dye conversion assay would be conducted on the in vivo and in vitro fibers and the plates stored.

6. On the following Monday the growth profile study would be terminated at the day 10 time point with the collection of the last set of in vivo and in vitro fibers. The final set of plates would be stored at 2–8°C overnight.

7. On Tuesday or Wednesday the MTT dye conversion assay would be completed for all the fibers collected for the growth profile (*see* **Subheading 3.7.2., steps 6–11**).

Acknowledgments

A special thanks to Eric Wexler of Bristol-Myers Squibb Company for his photographic expertise.

References

1. Hollingshead, M. G., Alley, M. C., Camalier, R. F., Abbott, B. J., Mayo, J. G., Malspeis, L., and Grever, M. R. (1995) In vivo cultivation of tumor cells in hollow fibers. *Life Sci.* **57,** 131–141.

2. Hollingshead, M., Plowman, J., Alley, M., May, J., and Sausville, E. (1999) The hollow fiber assay, in *Relevance of Tumor Models for Anticancer Drug Development* (Fiebig, H. H. and Burger, A. M., eds.), Karger, Basel, Switzerland, pp. 109–120.

3. Hall, L. M., Krauthauser, C. M., Wexler, R. S., Hollingshead, M. G., Slee, A. M., and Kerr, J. S. (2000) The hollow fiber assay: continued characterization with novel approaches. *AntiCancer Res.* **20,** 903–912.

4. Krauthauser, C. M., Hall, L. M., Wexler, R. S., Slee, A. M., Mitra, J., Enders, G. H., and Kerr, J. S. (2001) Regulation of gene expression and cell growth *in vivo* by tetracycline using the hollow fiber assay. *AntiCancer Res.* **21,** 869–872.

Index